Understanding Medical Education

Evidence, Theory and Practice

Understanding Medical Education

Evidence, Theory and Practice

EDITED BY

Tim Swanwick

London Deanery
London, UK

WILEY-BLACKWELL

A John Wiley & Sons, Ltd., Publication

This edition first published 2010, © 2010 by The Association for the Study of Medical Education

Blackwell Publishing was acquired by John Wiley & Sons in February 2007. Blackwell's publishing program has been merged with Wiley's global Scientific, Technical and Medical business to form Wiley-Blackwell.

Registered office: John Wiley & Sons Ltd, The Atrium, Southern Gate, Chichester, West Sussex, PO19 8SQ, UK

Editorial offices: 9600 Garsington Road, Oxford, OX4 2DQ, UK
                        The Atrium, Southern Gate, Chichester, West Sussex, PO19 8SQ, UK
                        111 River Street, Hoboken, NJ 07030-5774, USA

For details of our global editorial offices, for customer services and for information about how to apply for permission to reuse the copyright material in this book please see our website at www.wiley.com/wiley-blackwell

Library of Congress Cataloging-in-Publication Data

Understanding medical education : evidence, theory, and practice / edited by Tim Swanwick. – 1st ed.
        p. ; cm.
    Includes bibliographical references and index.
    ISBN 978-1-4051-9680-2 (pbk.)
    1. Medicine–Study and teaching.   I. Swanwick, Tim.   II. Association for the Study of Medical Education.
    [DNLM: 1. Education, Medical–methods–Collected Works.   2. Education, Medical–organization & administration–Collected Works.   W 18 U55 2010]
    R845.U53 2010
    610.76–dc22

                                    2010013901

A catalogue record for this book is available from the British Library.

Set in 9 on 11 pt Palatino by Toppan Best-set Premedia Limited
Printed and bound in Spain by GraphyCems

6   2012

Contents

List of contributors

Mark A. Albanese
Director of Research
National Conference of Bar Examiners;
Professor Emeritus
Departments of Population Health Sciences and Educational
    Leadership and Policy Analysis
School of Medicine and Public Health
University of Wisconsin-Madison
Madison, Wisconsin, USA

Antony Americano
Director of Corporate Services
London Deanery
University of London
London, UK

Janet Askham
Research Director
Picker Institute Europe
Oxford, UK

Dinesh Bhugra
Professor of Mental Health and Cultural Diversity
Institute of Psychiatry, King's College London;
Honorary Consultant at the Maudsley Hospital
London, UK

David Blaney
Chief Executive of ASME;
Undergraduate Dean, Hull York Medical School
York, UK

Alan Bleakley
Professor of Medical Education
Peninsula Medical School
Plymouth, UK

Katharine A.M. Boursicot
Reader in Medical Education
Barts and the London;
Reader in Medical Education and Head of Assessment
Queen Mary's School of Medicine
London, UK

Paul Bradley
Director of Clinical Skills
Peninsula Medical School
Plymouth, UK

Julie Brice
Academic Support Manager
Peninsula College of Medicine and Dentistry
Plymouth, UK

Graham Buckley
Chairman, ASME
Edinburgh, UK

Bill P. Burdick
Associate Vice President for Education
Foundation for Advancement of International Medical Education
    and Research;
Co-Director
FAIMER Institute;
Clinical Professor of Emergency Medicine
Drexel University College of Medicine;
Philadelphia, Pennsylvania, USA

Deborah Cohen
Senior Clinical Medical Research Fellow
Individual Support Programme, School of Medicine
Cardiff University
Wales, UK

Ian Cooper
Language and Communications Specialist
Individual Support Programme
School of Medicine
Cardiff University
Wales, UK

Oonagh Corrigan
Senior Lecturer in Clinical Education Research
Peninsula Medical School
Plymouth, UK

Kate Ellis
Academic Standards and Policy Officer
Peninsula College of Medicine and Dentistry
Plymouth, UK

Kevin Eva
Associate Professor and Associate Chair
Department of Clinical Epidemiology and Biostatistics
McMaster University
Hamilton, Ontario, Canada
Editor of the Wiley-Blackwell journal, *Medical Education*

Martyn Evans
Professor of Humanities and Principle
John Snow College, Durham University
Durham, UK

Eamonn Ferguson
Professor of Health Psychology
University of Nottingham
Nottingham, UK

Della Freeth
Professor of Professional Education
Queen Mary University London
London, UK

Jill Gordon
Professor of Medical Education
Medical Humanities Unit
Centre for Values, Ethics and Law in Medicine
University of Sydney
Sydney, Australia

Janet Grant
Professor of Education Medicine and Director
Open University Centre for Education in Medicine
Milton Keynes, UK

Larry D. Gruppen
Chair
Department of Medical Education
University of Michigan Medical School
Ann Arbor, Michigan, USA

Jan Illing
Head of Medical Education Research Group
Durham University
Durham, UK

Brian Jolly
Director
Centre for Medical and Health Sciences Education
Monash University
Melbourne, Australia

David M. Kaufman
Professor, Faculty of Education
Director, Learning and Instructional Development Centre
Simon Fraser University
Burnaby, British Columbia, Canada

Tara J. Kennedy
Assistant Professor
Department of Pediatrics
University of Toronto
Toronto, Ontario, Canada

Jean Ker
Director
Clinical Skills Centre;
Senior Lecturer in Medical Education
University of Dundee
Dundee, Scotland, UK

John Launer
Associate Director
London Deanery
London, UK

Lorelei Lingard
Professor, Department of Medicine
Director, Centre for Education Research and Innovation
Schulich School of Medicine and Dentistry
The University of Western Ontario
London, Ontario, Canada

Bridget Lock
Director of Medical Education
Princess Royal University Hospital
Farnborough, UK

Andrew Long
Associate Dean
London Deanery;
Officer for Assessment
Royal College of Paediatrics and Child Health
London, UK

Karen V. Mann
Professor
Division of Medical Education
University of Manchester
Manchester, UK

Clare Morris
Associate Dean
Bedfordshire and Hertfordshire Postgraduate Medical School
University of Bedfordshire
Luton, UK

Peter McCrorie
Professor and Head
Centre for Medical and Healthcare Education
St George's, University of London
London, UK

Jean McKendree
Senior Lecturer in Medical Education
Hull York Medical School
Hull, UK

Judy McKimm
Associate Professor and Pro Dean (Health and Social Practice)
Unitec, New Zealand

John J. Norcini
President and CEO
Foundation for Advancement of International Medical Education
and Research
Philadelphia, Pennsylvania, USA

Geoff Norman
Professor of Clinical Epidemiology and Biostatistics
McMaster University
Hamilton, Ontario, Canada

Fiona Patterson
Director
Organisational Psychology Research Team
City University
London, UK

John Pitts
Retired, formerly
Associate Director in Educational Research
NHS (Severn and Wessex Deanery);
Honorary Research Fellow
University of Winchester
Winchester, UK

Trudie E. Roberts
Head of the School of Medicine and
Director of the Medical Education Unit
University of Leeds
Leeds, UK

Melody Rhydderch
Occupational Psychologist
Individual Support Programme
School of Medicine
University of Cardiff
Wales, UK

Lambert W.T. Schuwirth
Associate Professor for Assessment of Medical Competence and
    Performance
University of Maastricht
Maastricht, The Netherlands

John Spencer
Professor in Medical Education in Primary Health Care and
    Education Development
University of Newcastle
Newcastle, UK

Yvonne Steinert
Associate Dean for Faculty Development
Director of the Centre for Medical Education;
Professor of Family Medicine
McGill University
Montreal, Quebec, Canada

Cees P.M. van der Vleuten
Scientific Director
School of Health Professions Education
University of Maastricht
Maastricht, The Netherlands

David Wall
Deputy Regional Postgraduate Dean
West Midlands Deanery;
Professor of Medical Education
Staffordshire University
Stoke-on-Trent, UK

Casey B. White
Assistant Dean for Medical Education
Assistant Professor of Medical Education
University of Michigan Medical School
Ann Arbor, Michigan, USA

Diana F. Wood
Director of Medical Education and Clinical Dean
School of Clinical Medicine
University of Cambridge
Cambridge, UK

Foreword

Education and learning have always been important parts of medicine- how we learn, how we assist learning and how we can best continue to learn, are all components of the process. Over the centuries these processes have changed radically; from essentially book learning and observation, to the introduction of anatomy and the formal study of the human body, through the development of the process of clinical examination, backed up by pathology to the beginning of laboratory work.

The complexity of modern medicine has added a much greater dimension to the learning. As the determinants of disease become clearer so the range of topics to cover and understand grows. Thus in addition to understanding the molecular basis of illness there is a need to consider social and economic issues in determining health, lifestyle choices, and the environment, and the wider public health.

How do we put all of this together? How do we develop a curriculum? How much needs to be learned at each stage of the process? And how do we assess the progress of the student and doctor? How do we ensure that we keep practice up to date and that continuing learning becomes an in built part of medical practice? How do we build it into our genes? How can we use the new learning technologies such as e-learning and simulation to best effect?

In addition to all of this we have seen a resurgence of interest in education itself and real wish to under-stand more fully the principles and practices involved. This requires the development of research tools and methods of assessment if we are to take learning to an even higher plane.

Patients, and the public, are central to this, in two ways. First and foremost, the purpose of all of this is to help patients and their families deal with illness, the consequences of the diagnosis and the effects of treatment. Communication skills are key to this. The role of the doctor is to act as a healer and this requires a wide range of skills which are regularly updated and reviewed. Patients also point the way for us in the aspects of clinical practice.

The second role of the patient is to help the student or the doctor in the learning process. Increasingly patients give their time and skills to help us do better and we should recognise how much they contribute the education of the profession.

This splendid book covers these topics and many more. It makes the process of learning and assessment readily accessible and should stimulate new ideas and better ways of improving the care we give to patients and the public.

Sir Kenneth C. Calman
Chancellor
The University of Glasgow

Preface

Understanding Medical Education

Understanding Medical Education was launched as a series of monographs in September 2006, and was the brainchild of Association of Medical Education's then Chief Executive, Frank Smith. It has provided an outstanding success, selling over 40 000 copies worldwide. The series was designed to meet the needs of all newcomers to medical education including those studying at certificate, diploma or masters level and contributors have included experts from all walks of medical education from across the world. These popular monographs have now been collected into a single core textbook, providing a comprehensive guide to the theoretical and academic bases to modern medical education practice.

This accessible and timely reference will support all those working in medical education across the spectrum of undergraduate education, through postgraduate training to continuing professional development. As well as providing practical guidance for clinicians, teachers and researchers, *Understanding Medical Education* should be a first 'port-of-call' for anyone engaged in medical education as an academic discipline. The book is a unique resource which should prove invaluable for anyone involved in the development of healthcare professionals, in whatever discipline, wherever they are in the world.

An on-line edition of the complete book together with individual chapter downloads are available at www.wileymedicaleducation.com.

Editor: Professor Tim Swanwick

Tim Swanwick MA FRCGP MA(Ed) FAcadMed has a broad range of experience in medical education and is based at the London Deanery where he is currently the Director of Professional Development. Tim is a Visiting Professor at the University of Bedfordshire, a Visiting Fellow at the Institute of Education and an Honorary Senior Lecturer of Imperial College. He has researched and published widely on many aspects of medical education and sits on the Executive and Council of ASME and the Academy of Medical Educators.

Association for the Study of Medical Education

The Association for the Study of Medical Education seeks to improve the quality of medical education by bringing together individuals and organisations with interests and responsibilities in medical and healthcare education. The association is unique in that it draws its members from all areas of medical education and from all specialties. It provides a forum for debate and the exchange of information, and an international network for the promotion of knowledge and expertise in medical education.

Acknowledgements

Such a major undertaking is a team effort and thanks must go to Graham Buckley and the *Understanding Medical Education* advisory board for their support and guidance, Jill Cropper for her expert copy editing, Brian Cairns at the publishing house, *Blue Square* and to Nicky Pender and the ASME team for their unfailing administrative support. Thanks also to Martin Davies and Carla Hodge at Wiley-Blackwell for helping to convert the *Understanding Medical Education* series into such an impressive and attractive volume.

Introduction: Understanding Medical Education

Tim Swanwick and Graham Buckley

It was the nuclear physicist and father of the hydrogen bomb, Edmund Teller, who once wrote (perhaps rather worryingly) 'confusion is no bad thing; it is the first step towards understanding'.(1, p. 79) Newcomers to the field of medical education could be forgiven for being confused. Medical education is a busy, clamorous place where a host of pedagogical practices, educational philosophies and conceptual frameworks collide. It is a place where academic journals vie for attention, institutions and professional bodies compete for political leverage, and the wheel of reform and 'improvement' revolves faster than, and often independently of, the cycle of evaluation and research. And it is a place of increasing accountability and regulation because of its proximity to one of the prime sociopolitical concerns of government, that of the health of its people.

It was the desire to develop evidence-based policy and practice in this complex arena that led to the establishment of the Association for the Study of Medical Education (ASME) in 1957. The past 50 years have seen a burgeoning of literature in the field. This is both a help and a challenge to the clinician taking on responsibilities for teaching, assessment and educational supervision. The range and diversity of relevant theory and research is now almost overwhelming, and in 2006 ASME recognised the need for a succinct yet comprehensive guide to the rich literature now underpinning best practice in medical education. *Understanding Medical Education* aims to be that guide.

What is Medical Education?

Medical education as we know it today spans three sectors: undergraduate, postgraduate and the continuing professional development of established clinicians. But it has not always been that way and Abraham Flexner – whose seminal report on the transformation of the American medical school system we celebrate the centenary of this year(2) – would not have recognised the attention currently given to the design, management and quality assurance of structured training in the postgraduate years, still less the need to instigate regulatory systems to ensure the ongoing personal and professional development of practising clinicians.

Medical education's ultimate aim is to supply society with a knowledgeable, skilled and up-to-date cadre of professionals who put patient care above self-interest, and undertake to maintain and develop their expertise over the course of a lifelong career. Medicine has a privileged position in society and, as a result, medical education is itself set apart from the humdrum of higher education. In many countries it luxuriates in separate funding streams and higher rates of remuneration for its clinical teachers; is the beneficiary of status and patronage through its colleges, academies and professional institutions; and is a formidably powerful, and predominantly conservative, political lobby, more than occasionally a source of frustration for those who seek to modernise health services.

Within the confines of this academic and political preserve lies the discipline of medical education; although one could question whether medical education is a discipline in its own right or an idiosyncratic collection of concepts appropriated from other educational fields, perfused with a technical rationality borne out of the dominance of bioscience within medicine. There are certainly a number of predominant educational assumptions, such as experiential learning and reflective practice, and favoured curricular approaches borrowed from other fields – witness the transplantation of competency-based education from vocational training. But medical education is not just a magpie and has made, and continues to make, its own significant advances and contributions to the wider educational literature. Many of these unique and major developments are expounded within this book: problem-based learning, simulation, structured assessments of clinical competence, supervision and the use of e-learning to name but a few.

Challenges and Preoccupations

Another characteristic of medical education is that it is, as Cooke and her colleagues note, 'in a perpetual state of unrest'.(3, p. 1339) A constant stream of reports issues from regulators, commissions, enquiries and task forces urging reform. This may just reflect the sluggish response to change and innate conservatism of our profession and educational institutions. This is not, as it happens, a new phenomenon. In the UK, George Pickering, writing as far back as 1956, offers us the wry observation that 'no country has produced so many excellent analyses of the present defects of medical education as has Britain, and no country has done less to implement them'.(4, p. 113) We suspect that Britain is not alone in this regard. But the frequency of such reports increases and the clarion calls for change are ever louder. So what are the current preoccupations of medical education and society's expectations of it?

To begin at the beginning, getting the right students and later on the right trainees training in the right specialty is crucial. In a competitive and litigious environment, the importance of having demonstrably fair selection processes is unarguable. Good person–job fit is essential to productivity, quality and job satisfaction. In Chapter 24, Fiona Patterson and Eamon Ferguson identify just how difficult getting all this right can be. Predicting who will make a good doctor is critically dependent on what the role of the doctor will be 10–15 years into the future, something that is increasingly uncertain. So are there generic attributes that we can select for? What selection methods should we use? And to encourage the recruitment of well-rounded practitioners, should entry to medical school be graduate only?

Having selected the right students and, with luck, matched the right trainees to the most suitable postgraduate training programme, what about the *quality* of the education and training? In Chapter 26, Oonagh Corrigan and colleagues discuss the different discourses around this thorny concept, but a key and very current concern for most developed countries is reduced patient contact time. It was Flexner's mentor, William Osler, who brought students and patients closer together through his educational philosophy that medicine was 'learned by the bedside and not in the classroom' (5, p. 188) and the practical introduction of residency programmes. Both are now threatened by the concerns over patient safety, expansion of medical student numbers, regulatory requirements on working hours and a staggeringly accelerated patient throughput. Patients undergoing gall bladder operations in Osler's day were in hospital for several weeks. The procedure now is carried out on a day-patient basis. At almost every stage of training, learners see fewer patients, do less to them and as a consequence find themselves increasingly unprepared for practice.(6)

A related concern is patient safety. Medicine is not only faster-paced, it is also more hazardous. As Cyril Chantler has succinctly put it:

> *Medicine used to be simple, ineffective and relatively safe. Now it is complex, effective and potentially dangerous.*(7, p. 1178)

One of the responses to reduced opportunities for contact with patients and more hazardous interventions has been the widespread adoption of simulation across all fields and stages of medical education. The availability of sophisticated technologies now enables high-fidelity reproduction of complex patient scenarios. Students and doctors in training no longer need to carry out procedures for the first time on real patients – the skills of ophthalmoscopy, venepuncture and catheterisation can all be learned in the skills laboratory. Full-immersion scenarios also offer the opportunity to work on non-technical areas such as team working, leadership and situational awareness. But questions remain about transfer to the authentic setting, an issue that is explored in depth by Jean Ker and Paul Bradley in Chapter 12.

Growing concerns over patient safety have influenced not only the way medicine is practised – with the widespread introduction of protocols, checks and audit – but also the degree to which doctors are now publicly accountable. In the UK, high-profile cases such as Bristol,(8) Alder Hey(9) and Shipman(10) have ushered in a new era of accountability and this year sees the introduction of relicensing for all medical practitioners in Britain. Patient safety issues also permeate undergraduate medicine. Protecting patients within a teaching and learning environment while producing competent doctors who will maintain their knowledge, attitudes and skills is a major challenge for those who design undergraduate curricula.

Increasing accountability is just one facet of a new social compact with patients; a compact, no longer based on blind and unquestioning trust, but on true partnership. As John Spencer, writing with Judy McKimm, highlights in Chapter 13, we see increased patient involvement across the board in both teaching and learning, and also in decision making about how medical education is organised, governed and its resources allocated. Patients are now also intimately involved in the selection and assessment of both undergraduate students and postgraduate trainees, and feedback from patients is a routine feature of continuing professional development and reaccreditation processes.

One of the corollaries of the above is that there is a growing recognition of the need to professionalise clinical teaching.(11) The pressures for this are channelled through professional bodies, but also arise from an increase in the expectations of students and doctors in training about the quality of the learning opportunities they are afforded. Clinical teachers and others with responsibilities for medical education increasingly look for academic support and accreditation of their expertise, and one of the target groups of *Understanding Medical Education* are newcomers to medical education, whether undergraduate or postgraduate, including those studying at certificate, diploma and masters levels. Such professional credentialling of medical educators is a burgeoning industry in Europe and North America and reflects a more general trend of the 'professionalisation' of medical education. Professionalisation has produced a new breed of scholarly educators and, coming as they do from a bioscientific background, a desire for evidence-informed medical education practice.

This raises questions about the nature of medical education research and again we see worlds colliding. In a recent exchange in ASME's academic journal,

Medical Education, a series of articles considered whether it is helpful to construe medical education as a medical or a social science.(12,13) Monrouxe and Rees capture captures the essence of the debate.

> *Medical education research has benefited from its association with 'hard' medical science in that this has encouraged the engagement of clinicians in research activities. However, this gain is offset by a particular loss represented by the failure (of some) to understand that medical education is about people, and the way we think, act and interact in the world. Medical education research is not a poor relation of medical research; it belongs to a different family altogether.* (13, p. 198)

Curriculum design continues to evolve, with problem-based learning now influencing the majority of medical school courses. Postgraduate medical education is also in the throes of curricular change, with many specialties formerly taught to implicit and informal curricula now articulating explicit and public curriculum statements for the first time. The tensions these developments produced are closely examined in the chapters by Janet Grant, Mark Albanese, and Clare Morris and David Blaney. Curriculum delivery is also challenged by the emerging possibilities of information technology (many of which are addressed by Jean McKendree in Chapter 11), and we are at the foot of a steep learning curve when it comes to embedding e-learning in all levels of education and training.

There are macro-political concerns too, around the commissioning of medical education and its responsiveness to service needs. The demographics are changing: at the beginning of the 21st century the developed world is already experiencing the demands of an increasingly elderly population with complex healthcare needs, and across the world we see a health inequalities gap that shows no signs of narrowing. Rising patient expectations and an ease of access to information present challenges not only in how care is delivered, but where and by whom. Managers within all healthcare systems are waking up to the fact that the majority of their future employees already work in their health services and that significant investment may need to be diverted from training new and inexperienced practitioners into developing and supporting their existing workforce.

Finally there is the vexed question of 'what is a doctor?' (or any other healthcare professional for that matter). With significant overlaps in knowledge and skills developing, what unique features does a doctor bring to the bedside or office, and what do we mean by a professional in the 21st century? Friedson argues that the professions, societal groups based on expertise, altruism and self-scrutiny, will never disappear, but will merely shrink in size as much of their work is taken on by a deprofessionalised operating core of medical technicians.(14) Others, such as Donald Berwick, disagree and see:

> *the reinvention of professionalism in a world on new terms of engagement; complexity, interdependence, pervasive hazard,*
> *a changing distribution of power and control and borne on the back of technology, distributed, democratised capacities…* (15, p. 130)

What is certain is that at no point in the past has the medical profession had to engage so actively with these debates, and the question 'what are we educating for?' has never been so important.

Scholarship and the Pursuit of Excellence

Understanding Medical Education began life as a series of free-standing monographs commissioned by the Association for the Study of Medical Education. The aim of the series was to provide an authoritative, up-to-date and comprehensive resource summarising the theoretical and academic bases to modern medical education practice, with contributions from experts in all walks of medical education. Although its authors come from Europe, Australasia and North America, we believe that it offers a worldwide perspective on contemporary practice. Most importantly, *Understanding Medical Education* aims to be both accessible and useful to the reader. The intention is that after reading one of the chapters that follow the reader will not only be better informed about their field of interest, but able to assimilate their new knowledge into their clinical teaching or academic activities.

Boyer's expanded definition of 'scholarship' takes us beyond the narrow confines of research to consider the need to recognise and reward not only the scholarship of 'discovery' but also that of integration of new knowledge, its application to social practice and teaching.(16) The aim then is to develop both scholarly educators and educational scholars. This is hugely important for medical education as the vast majority of medical educators are not researchers, nor indeed do they have the opportunity to work across disciplinary boundaries to integrate new knowledge. What they can be, and often are, are excellent teachers and scholarly agents of change and improvement within medical education. This highlights a perennial problem in medical education, namely that funding for academic institutions, either through grants or vehicles such as the Research Assessment Exercise,(17) is linked strongly to research output. Similarly, teaching in clinical settings usually plays second fiddle to clinical productivity. This has led to a situation where both academic and service institutions continue to emphasise staff involvement in activities other than teaching, an activity that remains largely unrewarded and unrecognised, and a challenge that new professional bodies such as the Academy of Medical Educators have set out to address.(11)

Medical education is complicated, contested and highly political. In a complex and uncertain world, we need to make the best decisions for the future that we can. For that, we need both scholarly medical educators and educational scholars. We hope that this book may contribute to their development.

References

1 Teller E, Teller W and Talley W (1991) Hypotheses non fingo. Chapter 5 in: *Conversations on the Dark Secrets of Physics*. Perseus Publishing, Cambridge, MA.

2 Lexner A (1910) *Medical Education in the United States and Canada: a report to the Carnegie Foundation for the Advancement of Teaching*. Carnegie Foundation for the Advancement of Teaching, New York.

3 Cooke M, Irby DM, Sullivan W and Ludmerer KM (2006) American medical education 100 years after the Flexner Report. *New England Journal of Medicine*. 355: 1339–44.

4 Pickering GW (1956) The purpose of medical education. *British Medical Journal*. 2(4968): 113–16.

5 Osler W (2003) Quoted in: Silverman ME, Murray TJ and Bryan CS (eds) *The Quotable Osler*. American College of Physicians – American Society for Internal Medicine, Philadelphia, PA.

6 Illing J, Davies C and Bauldauf B (2008) *How Prepared are Medical Graduates to Begin Practice. A comparison of three diverse medical schools*. Report to Education Committee of the General Medical Council. General Medical Council, London.

7 Chantler C (1999) The role and education of doctors in the delivery of healthcare. *Lancet*. 353: 1178–81.

8 Bristol Royal Infirmary Enquiry (2001) *Learning from Bristol: the report of the public inquiry into children's heart surgery at the Bristol Royal Infirmary 1984–1995* (www.bristol-inquiry.org.uk; accessed June 2009).

9 Redfern M (2001) *The Royal Liverpool Children's Inquiry Report* (The Alder Hey report) (www.rlcinquiry.org.uk; accessed June 2009).

10 Smith J (2005) *Shipman Fifth Report. Safeguarding Patients: lessons from the past – proposals for the future* (www.the-shipman-inquiry.org.uk; accessed June 2009). ·

11 Swanwick T (2009) Teaching the teachers – no longer an optional extra. *British Journal of Hospital Medicine*. 70: 176–7.

12 Bligh J and Brice J (2007) The Academy of Medical Educators: a professional home for medical educators in the UK. *Medical Education*. 41: 625–7.

13 Monrouxe LV and Rees CE (2009) Picking up the gauntlet: constructing medical education as a social science. *Medical Education*. 43: 196–8.

14 Friedson E (1988) *Profession of Medicine: a study of the sociology of applied knowledge*. University of Chicago Press, Chicago.

15 Berwick D (2009) The epitaph of profession. *British Journal of General Practice*. 59: 128–31.

16 Boyer EL (1997) *Scholarship Reconsidered: priorities of the professoriate*. Jossey-Bass, San Francisco, CA.

17 Higher Education Funding Council for England, Scottish Funding Council, Higher Education Funding Council for Wales, Department for Employment and Learning NI. Research Assessment Exercise (www.rae.ac.uk; accessed June 2009).

Principles of curriculum design

Janet Grant

KEY MESSAGES

- The curriculum is made up of all the experiences learners have that enable them to reach their intended achievements from the course.

- A curriculum statement should enable learners, teachers and managers to know and fulfil their obligations in relation to the course. It should describe intended learner achievements, content to be covered (the syllabus), teaching, learning, supervision, feedback and assessment processes, entry requirements and course structure.

- A syllabus is simply a list of the main topics of a course of study. This is only part of the curriculum.

- The way in which a curriculum for medical education is designed depends on the designers' views about how students learn, how medicine is practised, social responsibility and accountability, the role of the knowledge base, professional values and health service development.

- The curriculum design process should ask what is the purpose of the educational programme, how will the programme be organised, what experiences will further these purposes and how can we determine whether the purposes are being attained?

- There is no body of evidence that shows that there is one best choice for framing a curriculum as a whole or any of it parts. A curriculum should simply be fit for the purpose and context of its day.

Introduction

My bookshelves are a history of medical education. I chose some books at random to determine whether the years had produced different ideas about curriculum design. Partially they had, and partially they had not. In 1961,(1) the debate was around instructional skill based on ideas about how students learn. The curriculum was to be made up of objectives and experiences with relatively traditional divisions of content, but all based on the health needs of society, the philosophy of scientific thinking and the professional characteristics of physicians. In 1972,(2) the advice was to define aims and objectives in behavioural terms (not so different from today's preoccupation with competences, perhaps), and also that curricula should offer what the student and community require – not what is convenient for medical school staff to offer. Teachers were advised to try to integrate their teaching more effectively and give students some choice over what they learn. By 1982(3) and 1983,(4) a systems approach to educational design was advocated, with an emphasis on teaching methods aimed at delivering the learning objectives in the knowledge that active student involvement in learning was a likely effective strategy. By 1989,(5) it seemed reasonable to devote entire books to the question of how the curriculum might be structured to facilitate learning appropriate to clinical practice.

We can see from this snapshot that ideas develop and have roots in previous thinking. Ideas of integration, a focus on students learning rather than teachers teaching, a need for teachers to learn how to do their job well, a focus on outcomes, albeit expressed as objectives, and a recognition of the responsibility of the school to respond to societal need and to prepare the student for professional practice have been current for many years. But the same ideas can give rise to different curriculum designs and to different processes of reaching that design. The design principles that we have now are based on the professional choices that curriculum designers make. Those choices are informed by the theories and social conditions of the day, and by the values and experiences of the medical profession doing its best to produce the next generation of doctors fit for its changing purpose.

Jolly and Rees(6) admit that there is a need for rational, open and accountable curriculum design processes. They eloquently describe the accompanying lack of evidential basis for how best to do this, but conclude that:

> Although curriculum design is an imprecise and arbitrary rubric, such a code is needed: systematic and arbitrary is somewhat better than capricious.

Curriculum design in medical education is an arena in which many battles are fought. There are many different views and values about, for example, what medical

Understanding Medical Education: Evidence, Theory and Practice. Edited by T Swanwick. © 2010 Association for the Study of Medical Education.

students should learn, how they should learn it, what qualities we want them to develop, where the science base stands, where skills of communication and examination should be acquired, how long it should all take and whether we want to frame their task in terms of outcomes or competences.

There are equally as many views about how a curriculum should be developed and structured. And given that in education it is often difficult to find incontrovertible research findings on which to base decisions, there are no evidence-based approaches to curriculum design that we could meaningfully quote. This means that vogues in curriculum design ebb and flow in response to the dominant concerns of society and the professions, just as they ebb and flow in relation to teaching and learning methods, curriculum evaluation and even assessment of learning.

All these factors make a heady cocktail, which ensures that the business of curriculum design, development and review will never close. Eisner(7) talks of 'curriculum ideologies', which are 'the value premises from which decisions about practical educational matters are made'. These can be very strong, so that, as Toohey(8) says, 'Alternative views are literally "unthinkable"'. And so zealousness for a particular curriculum model develops, as she says, on beliefs that are 'so commonly held in the discipline, that they are accepted without question'. And because curriculum theory is based largely in ideology rather than evidence, this continuing spiral of changing views will never cease.

To muddy this pool even further, the issues around curriculum design at the basic (medical school), postgraduate and continuing education levels are very different. In medical school, we have students who have everything to learn and a school that has the responsibility and opportunity to ensure that they do and the right to call on the student's time and fill it with activities that reflect the school's view of curriculum.

At the postgraduate level, learning occurs in the context of clinical practice. Our student now is a young doctor who still has much to learn and examinations to pass, but also has clinical duties to fulfil. Much of the learning is dependent on the clinical work that is experienced, and teachers and curriculum planners only have limited power to organise the days of a postgraduate trainee.

At the stage of continuing professional development, every doctor has become an autonomous professional, each with a unique history of experience and many with unique learning needs arising out of their professional practice. For most, there is little protected time and minimal finance for learning. At this point, the idea of a set curriculum might seem to be an unworkable irrelevance. Instead, we might simply guide senior doctors to identify their own learning needs, design their own learning and reinforce that in their own practice.(9)

Here, therefore, the principles of curriculum design are discussed only as they apply to medical school and postgraduate training. Enduring principles are presented that will stand the tests of time, changes of fashion and the many different contexts across the world in which medical curricula are applied. The principles outlined should be flexible enough to yield different types of curricula in different hands. A question not discussed here concerns whose hands they might be. We assume that a curriculum is best designed by teams that include subject specialists, clinical and non-clinical teachers, learners and teachers, educationalists, managers and, of course, patients.

What Is Curriculum? Definition and Standards

Educators and philosophers have addressed the question of what to teach and how to teach it at least since Plato wrote *The Republic* in about 360 BCE. It might seem surprising, then, that it is only relatively recently, perhaps in the last 40 to 50 years, that curriculum design has become a topic of debate in its own right, although the initial concerns about the nature of curricula arose with the advent of mass schooling in the late 19th century.(10) Until that point, curricula were defined by elite and specialist groups, and a curriculum statement (whether explicit or implicit) might contain only the content to be studied, and perhaps the time to be taken and the teaching method to be used.

Nowadays, however, this will not do. For reasons discussed in the next section, a curriculum statement now would be regarded as satisfactory only if it addresses the wider experience of the learner and the context of learning as well as the content and quality control of the enterprise. The curriculum should guide the learner, the teacher and educational managers. At the same time, it should leave room in its implementation for the creative and individual professionalism of the teacher, and for the individual preferences of the learner, given that both are clear about what is to be achieved.

The specification of intended curriculum outcomes (expressed in whatever terms) is, in almost all cases, non-negotiable, not least because the curriculum is the basis for planning and developing the assessment system. If there is no agreed curriculum, how can we develop an objective, representative, valid and reliable assessment system? Simply, we cannot.

Every country has some kind of guidance in relation to curricula at all stages. But few set actual standards for how a curriculum should be stated, what its component parts should be, and how it should be developed, implemented and used. In the UK such standards are set by the General Medical Council (GMC) now incorporating the Postgraduate Medical Education and Training Board (PMETB). There are no national curricula for continuing professional development, because at this stage practitioners need to identify their own learning needs from their practice.(9)

In many countries, curricula are set by the state; in others they are set by regulatory or professional bodies. In the US, the Liaison Committee on Medical Education sets accreditation standards that contain guidance on many key aspects of curriculum, but not on how to frame the curriculum statement itself. The UK offers a similar statement at the undergraduate level and specific standards for curriculum design at the postgraduate level, which allow the development of different curriculum statements that meet those set standards. Increasingly, medical educators at all levels are comparing their own curricula and medical education and training processes with the standards set by the World Federation for Medical Education (WFME).

Definition

Although much is written about curriculum, definitions are few and far between. Accordingly, the curriculum subcommittee of PMETB reviewed curriculum theories, the context of medical education, and the needs of teachers, trainers and regulators. As a result, a definition of curriculum was developed and adopted (*see* Box 1.1). Curricula that comply with this definition will offer all stakeholders a clear description of requirements and expectations. The definition, although developed for postgraduate training, is appropriate to all levels.

Standards for curriculum design

Curriculum standards address much more than the syllabus content of the course. For example, the guidance in the GMC's *Tomorrow's Doctors*(12) – which formed the basis of quality inspections of medical schools until 2010 – addresses a wide range of issues from the core knowledge, skills and attitudes expected of students on graduation to systems of assessment and arrangements to ensure the health and safety of patients.

In the US, the Liaison Committee on Medical Education sets accreditation standards for American Medical Schools as a condition for licensure of their graduates. Not surprisingly, among the accreditation standards are some fundamental curriculum issues (*see* Box 1.2).

In the postgraduate arena, the UK's regulator, the PMETB developed specific standards against which all postgraduate curricula are formally judged and approved before implementation. These standards themselves reflect the factors and theories that best describe the vision and values of the Board,(13) the view taken of the learning process, and the key contexts and factors that influence medical education. These are discussed further in the next section. Although the standards shown in Box 1.3 were developed for curricula in postgraduate medical education, there is no reason why they should not equally be applied to any level of medical education and training in any location.

Such standards try to decrease the distance between the three coexisting types of curriculum identified by Coles:(14)

BOX 1.1 What is a curriculum?(11)

A statement of the intended aims and objectives, content, experiences, outcomes and processes of an educational programme, including:

- a description of the training structure (entry requirements, length and organisation of the programme, including its flexibilities, and assessment system)
- a description of expected methods of learning, teaching, feedback and supervision.

The curriculum should cover both generic professional and speciality-specific areas.

The syllabus content of the curriculum should be stated in terms of what knowledge, skills, attitudes and expertise the learner will achieve.

BOX 1.2 Areas addressed by the Liaison Committee on Medical Education Accreditation standards

- Institutional setting
  - governance administration
  - academic environment
- Educational programme for the MD degree
  - educational objectives
  - structure
  - teaching and assessment
  - curriculum management
  - evaluation of programme effectiveness
- Medical students
  - admissions
  - student services
  - the learning environment
- Faculty
  - number
  - qualifications and functions
  - personnel politics
  - governance
- Educational resources
  - finances
  - general facilities
  - clinical teaching facilities
  - information resources and library services

BOX 1.3 Postgraduate Medical Education and Training Board curriculum standards

Standard 1: Rationale

(a) The purpose of the curriculum must be stated, including its overall role in the relevant postgraduate training.

(b) The curriculum must state:
   - how it was developed and consensus reached
   - how content and teaching/learning methods were chosen
   - how the curriculum was agreed and by whom
   - the role of teachers and trainees in curriculum development

(c) The appropriateness of the stated curriculum to the stage of learning and to the speciality in question must be described.

(d) Linkages of the curriculum to previous and subsequent stages of the trainee's training and education should be clarified.

(e) The curriculum must be presented in relation to programmes and posts within those programmes.

Standard 2: Content of learning

(a) The curriculum must set out the general professional and speciality-specific content to be mastered.
   - Knowledge, skills, attitudes and expertise must be addressed.
   - Recommendations on the sequencing of learning and experience should be provided, if appropriate.
   - The general professional content should include a statement about how *Good Medical Practice* is to be addressed.

(b) Content areas should be presented in terms of the intended outcomes of learning matched to identifiable stages of training, where appropriate:
   - what the trainee will know, understand, describe, recognise, be aware of and be able to do at the end of the course.

(c) Content areas should be linked to guidance on recommended learning experiences.

Standard 3: Model of learning

The curriculum must describe the model of learning appropriate to the speciality and stage of training.

- General balance of work-based experiential learning, independent self-directed learning and appropriate off-the-job education.
- How learning for knowledge, skills, attitudes, and expertise will be achieved.

Standard 4: Learning experiences

(a) Recommended learning experiences must be described that allow a diversity of methods covering, at a minimum:
   - learning from practice
   - opportunities for concentrated practice in skills and procedures
   - learning with peers
   - learning in formal situations inside and outside the department
   - personal study
   - specific teacher inputs

(b) Educational strategies that are suited to work-based experiential learning and appropriate off-the-job education should be described.

Standard 5: Supervision and feedback

(a) Mechanisms for ensuring feedback on learning must be recommended and required.

(b) Mechanisms for ensuring supervision of practice and safety of doctor and patient must be defined.

Standard 6: Managing curriculum implementation

Indication should be given of how curriculum implementation will be managed and assured locally and within programmes. This should include:

- intended use of the curriculum document by trainers and trainees
- means of ensuring curriculum coverage
- suggested roles of local faculty in curriculum implementation
- responsibilities of trainees for curriculum implementation
- curriculum management in posts and attachments within programmes
- curriculum management across programmes as a whole.

Standard 7: Curriculum review and updating

(a) Plans for curriculum review, including curriculum evaluation and monitoring, must be set out.

(b) The schedule for curriculum updating, with rationale, must be provided.

(c) Mechanisms for involving trainees and lay persons in (a) and (b) must be set out.

Standard 8: Equality and diversity

This curriculum should describe its compliance with anti-discriminatory practice.

The Postgraduate Medical Education and Training Board was subsumed into the General Medical Council in April 2010. Despite the merger, these curriculum standards remain current and in use at the time of publication of this book.

- the curriculum on paper
- the curriculum in action
- the curriculum the learner experiences.

Further afield, the World Federation for Medical Education (WFME) has set, piloted and evaluated quality improvement standards for all aspects of medical education at all stages to 'promote the highest scientific and ethical standards in medical education, initiating new learning methods, new instructional tools and innovative management of medical education. These are all aspects of curriculum.

The WFME standards(15) address:
- mission and outcomes
- the educational programme
- the learning and training process
- assessment of learning
- students and trainee characteristics and needs
- staffing and faculty
- educational resources and training settings
- evaluation of the educational programme and process
- governance and administration
- curriculum renewal.

These standards are already widely used for self-studies within medical schools and for accreditation purposes. They support the emerging consensus recognition that curriculum design must encompass much more than a statement of the content to be covered in the course.

A note of caution

The standards cited all require the curriculum designer to think about the intended product and character of the course, its rationale, values or mission. Without these elements, standard setting for curricula becomes a dangerous and instrumental undertaking, apt to serve only political or economic purposes. 'Aims-talk', as Noddings(16) calls it, is the first and most important element of curriculum design and its most important standard.

Factors that Influence Curriculum Design

It can be seen from the PMETB curriculum definition and standards that a comprehensive curriculum statement is much more than a syllabus statement, which simply sets out the topic headings or content of a course or a programme. Writing a curriculum is a process that demands consideration of values, beliefs and choices. It deserves a review of evidence and a development process, which sends out messages about quality assurance and recognition of all the stakeholders.

The days when subject experts or workforce managers alone wrote down what was to be learnt are now past. These days, curriculum design encompasses

---

BOX 1.4 Influences and effects on medical curricula

Influence	Example of effect
Theories of learning	Learner-centred design, for example, problem-based
Theories of professional practice	Integrated curricula Teamwork Ethics
Social values	Socially responsible medical schools Widening participation curricula
Knowledge base expansion	Core and options curriculum
Professional	Communication skills training Professionalism
Health service development	Community-oriented curricula Multiprofessional elements
Political	Shorter curricula for faster production of medical workforce
Accountability and transparency	Outcomes-based curricula Objectives-based curricula

---

many other factors that derive from the democratisation of social processes, the development of educational theory, political imperatives and economic concerns. Box 1.4 highlights some influences on modern medical curricula and their areas of effect.

Each of the influences cited here has had its effect, and the residue of each of those effects remains to become incorporated in the new generation of curriculum, making each new reformulation richer than the previous models.

The evolution of curriculum models and learning theories is addressed below. But the other factors, which are not part of the academic discourse, are equally as important in shaping ideas about curriculum. Some of these factors affect the content of the curriculum, and some affect its design. For example, theories of professional practice have arisen around the sorts of ideas that are embodied in the UK General Medical Council's statement on *Good Medical Practice*, which defines a set of common content for professional behaviour and values.(17) This document covers such issues as professional standards for clinical care, maintaining good medical practice, educational activity, and relationships with patients, colleagues and teams. It is a professional statement and the PMETB standards (*see* Box 1.3) recognise this.

Another highly influential statement is that of the Royal College of Physicians and Surgeons of Canada(18) on the essential roles and key competencies of specialist physicians. This statement addresses

the qualities of a doctor that every educational programme should facilitate:
• medical expert
• communicator
• collaborator
• manager
• health advocate
• scholar
• professional.

Such statements not only contribute to the vision that an organisation has of its intended product, but will also affect directly the content and style of the curriculum. On the other hand, social drivers for accountability and transparency have determined the use of clear outcomes, amenable to peer or lay input and review. Political imperatives have often pushed curricula to be more aware of issues of the cost and speed of workforce production. From this, we should be aware that choice of curriculum design or model is not an objective entity but is socially, professionally, academically and politically constructed.

At any one point, curriculum design is a child of its time.

Curriculum models

Curriculum models have been the subject of academic and management theory since the mid-20th century when Tyler first put forward the idea that:

> ...it is very necessary to have some conception of the goals that are being aimed at. These educational objectives become the criteria by which materials are selected, content is outlined, instructional procedures are developed and tests and examinations are prepared.(19)

Although Tyler adopted a relaxed view of how objectives should be framed, this approach still allowed a 'transmission model'(20) of learning, which focuses on the teacher's rather than the learner's activity. Despite Mager coining the subsequent term 'instructional objectives', and taking a harder line on expressing objectives in measurable terms, his simultaneous intention was to change that focus and emphasise the importance of student achievement rather than teacher activity.(21) At the same time, he was much more prescriptive about exactly how those achievements should be specified: in behavioural, observable terms that were amenable to assessment. And so the use of the curriculum as the foundation of assessment became a central tenet.

There followed a raft of curriculum theorists who found that the Mager and Tyler models did not encompass all types of valued learning. So, for example, Eisner(7) introduced the idea of problem solving and expressive objectives or expressive outcomes, leading us on to a current dominant view of curriculum formulation. Some theorists tried to break free from curriculum models that specified outcomes in whatever form. So Stenhouse,(22) for example, proposed a process model that focused on the processes of acquiring, using and evaluating the knowledge of the discipline.

In more recent times, the idea of a competence-based curriculum, which was originally introduced in practical vocational subjects, has held sway. Its suitability as a basis for assessments, its commonsense appeal, its analytical basis and its implicit message that if we could define competences, we can ensure that learners acquire them and be assured by relevant testing that this is so, all make a competence model attractive. I have myself argued that competences alone cannot describe the skills of a profession.(23) Some prominent writers, such as Hyland,(24) have suggested that the competence movement in curriculum design is little more than an economically driven derivative of the behavioural school.

> This attempt to specify exactly what is to be achieved and measured is, of course, nothing more than reconstituted behaviourism...Constructed out of a 'fusion of behavioural objectives and accountability'..., the movement provided irresistible appeal to those seeking accountability and input–output efficiency in the new economic realism of the 1980s.

Perhaps this does ring some bells today.

The twin factors of accountability and efficiency of education or training appeal to medicine, which has become increasingly concerned about demonstrating transparency and public accountability in times of increasing litigation. The contextual climate of a hard-pressed health service, limited resources, and managerial and political imperatives has made the appeal of the model very alluring.

We can see from these examples of curriculum models that their use is a function of instrumental pragmatism, values and ideologies, political, social and managerial imperatives, and of the ideas that are current about how people learn. This means that selection of a curriculum model is a process that requires careful thought and open justification. That justification is unlikely to be in terms of research evidence; it will be in terms of ideology.

Theories of learning

An important factor in the development of new curriculum models has been the burgeoning field of learning research and theory. Not unexpectedly, there is a symbiotic relationship between learning theory and curriculum models. While objectives-based curriculum models were predominant, so was behavioural theory. While behavioural theory has declined, however, assessment theory and managerial imperatives have taken over to ensure that the behavioural aspects of curriculum definition still remain, albeit in new guises.

Learning theory has entirely changed its stance on effective pedagogy during the past half century. As with every other aspect of education, learning theory and consequent pedagogical practice is a never-ending work in progress. Ideas change. So, we have seen that at the time of the objectives-based curriculum models, behavioural theory was also in its prime, and the role of the teacher in shaping behaviour was a main focus. High on the best-seller list were books that explained how to teach, not how students learn. But even those books, and some were excellent, strayed into recognising the students' responsibility for learning.(25)

But things have changed, and in the past 20 to 30 years, the focus has moved away from teaching and towards learning. Jacques quotes Nicol,(26) who explains that nowadays, the teacher:

> …encourages participation, dialogue and interaction by students with course materials and with each other. The teacher should function as a facilitator of learning, intellectually critical, stimulating and challenging, but within a learning context that emphasises support and mutual respect.

Surely in this we can see the roots of curriculum models such as problem-based learning. And just as educational theory develops and is applied across the whole range of education, we have seen problem-based learning applied in such diverse arenas as design, chemical engineering and the arts. So learning theories are powerful in their practical effects on educational practice.

Around this current view of effective learning requiring activity on the part of the learner has developed a panoply of ideas about the components of this approach. So in medical education, as in every other form of education, we have seen a considerable body of published work on approaches to learning, on learning styles, group work and the social context, on the trainer–learner relationships and the value system in which learning occurs. Such ideas have a direct effect on curricula and the models of curriculum that are adopted.

Specific theories of learning are too many and varied to report, although there are some key ideas that have persisted and have influenced curriculum design. Adult learning theory,(27) which promotes active self-directed learning towards personally relevant goals, despite its lack of evidence base, seems to have an intuitive appeal and has been widely cited as the basis for curriculum and course design. For example, the University of New Mexico School of Medicine is recognised for its approach to '…adapting adult learning theory to medical education'.(28)

Other key theoretical frameworks that medical education has chosen to use include the dichotomy between deep and surface-level process approaches to learning.(29) The former is characterised by an active concern in the student to seek the underlying meaning, the wider picture, the relationship between different information and experiences, the logic of the argument, and the need to question and understand. Surface-level processors, on the other hand, take a passive approach and seek to learn the content, acquire the knowledge and get the right answers.

Our knowledge of learning styles and approaches has clear implications for curriculum design in terms of teaching skills and methods, learning opportunities and assessment.(30) Curricula that dissuade students from simple rote learning and encourage deep processing have now become the dominant form. And curricula can affect a learner's approach to learning. So McManus *et al.* point out(31) that:

> Formal education, particularly effective formal education, can also alter study habits and learning styles… Intercalated degrees increase deep and strategic learning and decrease surface learning at medical school…Deep and strategic learning also relate to the clinical experience gained by medical students, making it possible that greater patient involvement during undergraduate clinical training, rather than mere reliance on textbook learning to pass exams, a characteristic of surface learners, will also reduce surface-disorganised approaches to work.

The learning theories that inform today's curriculum design seem to be very far from the ideas of behavioural theories of learning, and from the idea that the knowledge base of the discipline must first be learnt before its application can be attempted. Today's trajectory of learning is flatter, with integration being the hallmark throughout the course, and deep learning in the context of practice its aim.

Yet at the same time as these developments, we also have seen the rise of competence-based curriculum frameworks, which seem strangely to hark back to the days when curricula were based on the attainment of set objectives and the underlying theory was distinctly behavioural. This contradiction remains unresolved in the competence-based curricula of today, which simultaneously rely on student-centred learning methods.

Theory and practice of the discipline

Of course it is not only theories of how students learn that affect the design of curricula. Theories about the discipline of medicine itself have also been paramount in changing the face of curricula. It has been more than 50 years since the first appearance of an integrated curriculum in practice in Case Western Reserve Medical School in Cleveland, Ohio. As they describe their own history:

> Already a leading educational institution for more than a century, the School of Medicine in 1952 initiated the most advanced medical curriculum in the country, integrating the basic and clinical sciences, focusing on organ systems and featuring an introduction to patients and clinical work in the first year. Many other medical schools followed suit.(32)

But now it is almost universally accepted that the practice of medicine requires this integration of its component parts: of science and clinical experience, knowledge, skills and attitudes, judgement and problem solving, even of continuing to learn through reflection on practice. So whereas in former times a curriculum for medicine might have offered its component constituents of science, clinical skills and experience to facilitate clinical judgement, leaving the integration of these to the learner, this learning trajectory has been superseded and the integrated context of practice now is reflected in the integrated nature of curricula. The curriculum is increasingly for practice(33) rather than simply to acquire the elements of professional knowledge, skills and attitudes for later application.

A further aspect of professional practice that has influenced curriculum design is the advent of teamworking in medicine. As healthcare has become more complex, working practices have changed and healthcare managers seek more cost-effective ways of delivering high-quality care. So, many medical schools have developed their curricula to offer:

> ...exciting opportunities for inter-professional learning which will prove invaluable as you prepare to join the healthcare teams of the future.(34)

Very recently, the whole question of professionalism and how it is acquired has gripped the profession and its educational institutions worldwide. Such issues have arisen from a series of trigger crises that the profession itself experienced in standards of practice and in changing practices, as well as in the changing role of doctors in society, market forces and accountability within the healthcare system, and society's changing relationship with the professions in the light of greater universal education and wider access to previously protected knowledge. Each of these ideas has its direct effect on the design of curricula. It has already been suggested by one key working group(35) that medical schools should 'consider introducing professional values early into the undergraduate medical course...' and that '...each student's professional values should be assessed throughout their training to ensure their fitness to practise'.

> Another major influence on curriculum design has been the move of health service provision into the community, along with the realisation that medical schools themselves have a social responsibility.

Curriculum design then, is subject to a wide variety of influences in relation to the profession of medicine, the healthcare service and society as a whole. Each curriculum design team must decide for themselves which of these they will choose to characterise their own work (*see* Box 1.5).

The Purpose and Components of Curriculum Design

Curriculum design has two components: the structure of the curriculum, and its content. Battles are fought and choices made in both arenas.

BOX 1.5 Where's the evidence?

Although there is much research published about different curriculum models, and teaching and learning strategies, there is no evidence to suggest that there is a 'best' template for curriculum design. This is partly because a curriculum is made up of many components and there is little evidence to suggest that even for any one of these there is a 'best choice' for all circumstances. Curricula have many different specific purposes and therefore many different designs. Their effectiveness can only be judged against their intended purposes. And few share exactly the same purpose, beyond intending to produce safe and responsible doctors.

This makes comparative or controlled research almost impossible.

So each curriculum designer must decide on the purpose of the curriculum and then search the literature for the relevant evidence about the likely effect of each curriculum component in serving that purpose. Convincing evidence may sometimes be difficult to find. So curriculum designers will often rely on their professional judgement and values and should always seek to gather their own evidence about the effects of their own curriculum.

Prior to the 1960s, curriculum change was best described as unplanned 'drift'.(36) But from that point, Kelly(37) records that educationalists recognised the need for planned innovation to keep pace with societal changes, while maintaining standards and values, and taking advantage of new theoretical underpinnings. At the same time, the idea of the curriculum as a total description of the intentions, mechanisms, context and outcomes of education took hold. The curriculum must explain and justify itself, describe the intended learning experiences and their rationale and explore the likely effects of the students' exposure to them.

A curriculum is therefore a document that must:

- tell the learner exactly what to expect including the methods of student support
- advise the teacher what to do to deliver the content and support the learners in their task of personal and professional development
- help the institution to set appropriate assessments of student learning and implement relevant evaluations of the educational provision
- tell society how the school is executing its social responsibilities.

The curriculum should present a reasoned picture of the subject to be studied and define the teaching and learning processes, and the intended outcomes of that study.

It can be seen that the curriculum is a powerful tool and for that reason is often the focus of battles for power and control. The major theorists of our time have seen that curriculum is the instrument for a more humane and socially accountable society. In medicine, the current trend for greater involvement of the community and its healthcare needs, and of patients and their families in curriculum development is a reflection of this tenet.

Steps in Curriculum Design

Despite the differences of view that have existed over the years and between different practitioners and theorists, all are generally agreed that the process of curriculum design must answer the following central questions, originally set out by Tyler in 1949.(19)

- What is the purpose of the educational programme?
- How will the programme be organised?
- What experiences will further these purposes?
- How can we determine whether the purposes are being attained?

The curriculum designer must make choices about how to answer each of these questions. We have seen that those choices are influenced by a number of contextual factors, but what are the options that are available at each stage? The next sections set out some of those options.

It must be said, however, that although these steps and their subsections are discussed below serially, in real life, many such decisions occur in parallel, or in a different order, because they are so tightly interdependent and are a function of local conditions. Figure 1.1 summarises the steps that most curriculum writers agree should be undertaken in the process of curriculum design and lists the sorts of options that the curriculum designer must choose between at each stage.

How do we express the overall purpose of an educational programme?

The purpose of a programme is often based on a set of aims, or a mission statement, such as the WFME standards require, or a statement of professional values such as that of the CanMeds project mentioned above, or a 'vision statement' such as that developed by the University of Sheffield Medical School, which encompasses the general intentions, values and characteristics of the curriculum. For example, the Sheffield vision statement deals with:

- the qualities of the intended graduates
- the method of expressing the intentions of the curriculum (outcomes-based)
- the curriculum structure (integrated, patient contact, community experience, facilitating student learning and student choice)
- curriculum organisation (based on body systems, progressively presenting undifferentiated patient problems)

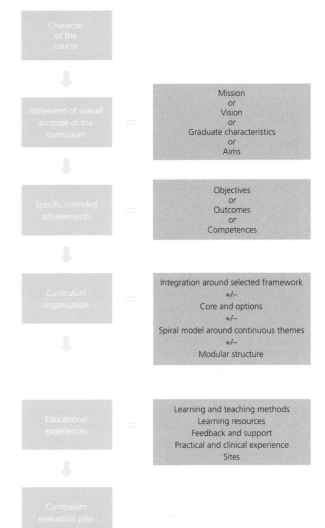

Figure 1.1 Steps and options in curriculum design.

- the instructional approach (a spine of problem, case- and patient-based integrated learning activities complemented by a range of other teaching and learning activities, with an increase in systematic teaching of some components to ensure competence in key areas)
- student learning approach (progressively more self-directed, supported by information technology resources, distance learning and activities)
- the assessment system (formative and summative based on the defined outcomes)
- the curriculum management system and team
- the curriculum monitoring and improvement system.

Thus a vision statement addresses all the central curriculum design issues and must be the result of extensive discussion and consultation with all the relevant stakeholders and experts. Such consultation is fundamental to a properly managed change process,(38) and in Sheffield, it took nearly a year to complete.(39)

On another level, Brown University School of Medicine(40) chose to think about the intended achievements of its curriculum in terms of the abilities of successful doctors. It derived, through consultation, nine such abilities:

1 effective communication
2 basic clinical skills
3 using basic sciences in the practice of medicine
4 diagnosis, management and prevention
5 lifelong learning
6 self-awareness, self-care and personal growth
7 the social and community contexts of healthcare
8 moral reasoning and clinical ethics
9 problem solving.

In the end, a comparison of the statements of different types shows that they express very similar ideas. What is important is that the statement of purpose of the programme is made. How it is made is for local choice.

Underpinning the overall purposes of the curriculum will be a set of values that pervade the thinking or the aspirations of the school. Many years ago, these value choices were set out in the SPICES(41) model (Figure 1.2) as a series of dimensions between two extremes. It is still helpful to consult this model at the first stage of curriculum planning. But we should be clear that no automatic value judgements should be attached to either dimension; for example, apprenticeship learning is still regarded as fundamental to medical training, and the potential narrow instrumentality of a planned systematic approach is recognised as having its dangers in professional training.

How can we describe specific intended achievements?

There are many ways to express what it is that a curriculum is intended to achieve. We have seen that the choice of how to express this is often as much a function of social context and educational fashion or belief as it is of any objective evidence of effect. The importance of this stage of planning is twofold; it will:
- define the content of the course
- be the basis of the assessment blueprint.(42)

Not surprisingly, this is another contentious area: every department and teacher will want to have their own subject properly represented in the curriculum, and a team-based approach that matches the organisation of the curriculum is advisable, with iterative consultations following a properly managed change process.(38)

Essentially, what the curriculum intends to achieve is most commonly expressed in one of the following ways:
- As *objectives*, expressed as the specific knowledge, skills and attitudes that the student will display at the end of the course. As we have seen, the objectives model became predominant after the Second World War, when reconstruction was most efficiently tackled in a managerial way, leading to observable and measurable changes, after the chaos of the preceding period.
- As *intended outcomes,* stated in clear and precise terms, which will allow the designer to specify the learning experiences that will facilitate achievement of the stated outcomes. For many, this is a return to Tyler's original idea of objectives.(43)
- As *competences* to be achieved and assessed, again expressed in terms that bear similarity to objectives but are often thought of in relation to the ultimate intended performance that the competences underpin.

There has been a furious debate around the use of these terms, and what they mean, how they differ, what they imply and how they are used. It has been argued that a simple statement of competences alone cannot reflect the complex nature of a profession or the central skill of professional judgement.(23) It was Stenhouse's belief that a statement of behavioural objectives cannot address socialisation and problem solving,(44) which are processes fundamental to a profession.

It has also been argued that such 'product-orientated curricula' are disempowering for the learners and take control of learning away from the learner,(45) and possibly disempower teachers similarly. In this, an outcomes-based curriculum would be incompatible with a learner-centred approach to learning, yet the two, in many curricula, attempt to coexist.

	Innovative approaches	Traditional strategies
1	Student-centred	Teacher-centred
2	Problem-based	Information gathering
3	Integrated	Discipline-based
4	Community-based	Hospital-based
5	Electives	Standard programme
6	Systematic	Apprenticeship-based

Figure 1.2 Educational strategies in curriculum development: the SPICES model.(41).

Specific guidance on the specification of outcomes has been offered and makes its similarity to the objectives-based model clear. In outcome-based education:

> Decisions about the curriculum are driven by the outcomes the students should display at the end of the course. In outcome-based education, product defines process. [It]…can be summed up as 'results-orientated thinking' and is the opposite of 'input-based education' where the emphasis is on the educational process and where we are happy to accept whatever is the result. In outcome-based education, the outcomes agreed for the curriculum guide what is taught and what is assessed.(46)

It is not surprising that the instrumental nature of this approach has given rise to some controversy. Key writers have sometimes opted to use these terms interchangeably,(40) equating outcome-based and competency-based as the same thing in practical terms.(47) We could equally say that objectives are not very different. An outcome might be:

> Obtains history in relation to possible underlying causes including cardiovascular and non-organic causes.(39)

It would be difficult to say in what way this is different from a competence or an objective. And it really does not matter, because statements such as this are fit for purpose. It is a debate with no conclusion, and perhaps the answer really does not matter. What is important is fitness for purpose, and the main purposes of stating the intended achievements of the curriculum are:

- to inform learners of what they should achieve
- to inform teachers of what they should help the learners to achieve
- to be the basis of the assessment system, so that everyone knows what will be assessed
- to reflect accurately the nature of the profession into which the learner is being inducted and the professional characteristics that must be acquired.

Regardless of the rhetoric surrounding these different ways of describing what a curriculum should achieve, the important point is that this is done in terms specific enough to guide planning, assessment and review, and to give students and teachers appropriate expectations. Perhaps it is high time that medicine found a new and more appropriate way of describing its qualities (*see* Box 1.6).

How will the programme be organised?

Once the overall intentions of the curriculum and its more specific intended achievements are defined and agreed, the curriculum must be written to reflect the intended organisation of the course. The main current organisation models are:

- integration
- core and options
- spiral model
- modular.

These options are not mutually exclusive and many curricula display elements of them all. So an integrated curriculum with a modular core of mandatory content

---

BOX 1.6 Focus on: Competence and competency

The terms 'competence' and 'competency' seem to be the focus of concern and debate. But in education, preoccupation with definition of terms is, perhaps, to miss the point. In dictionary terms, these are alternative words with the same meaning. Both simply mean 'the ability to do something; the ability to perform a given task'. So there is no contest between competence and competency – it is simply a matter of which word you care to use. But this definitional fact does not stop a semantic debate raging.

It seems that in common curriculum parlance, a competence is a specific, measurable entity (knowledge, skill, behaviour) that the learner should display by the end of the programme. But this does not mean that the possessor of the competences will translate into performance. And so, in education, the term 'competency' sometimes seems to be used to suggest the underlying propensity to turn competence into performance.

The underlying pedagogical theory seems to be that if we can define the competences that make up professional performance, then we can aim the teaching programme at them and make it more efficient and effective. This theory is flawed.

If the acquisition of competences in turn leads to competency to perform, this will be because the separate competences have been used repeatedly in concert in the context of complex professional practice to gather information, to process it, to make judgements and decisions, to solve problems, to make interventions, to deal with and interact with peers, colleagues and patients, and to think in multidimensional terms about personal, interpersonal, ethical, financial, managerial, multiprofessional and evidence-based factors.

So a curriculum that bases self on the specification of competences is only recognising the first step on a path that leads to the competency that is the precursor of the ultimate complex professional performance. And if we spend too long in debating definition, perhaps we are no more than sublimating our energies and closing our eyes to more difficult questions.

---

and student-selected options, which contain topics that are revisited in increasing depth at successive stages of the curriculum, is quite possible and possibly the most common approach among new curricula.

Integration

A curriculum based on separate disciplines is not integrated. The knowledge and skills are presented in silos and the integration has to occur entirely in the student's head through use in practice. An integrated curriculum, however, organises the material to be learnt around an entity that is more related to practice.

Curriculum integration can be managed as either horizontal integration between different subject areas or vertical integration between the clinical and basic sciences. Integrated curricula in medical schools across the globe are now too numerous to mention and it seems likely that, in time, curricula worldwide will adopt both vertical and horizontal integration. This can be a threatening development for some departments, especially in basic sciences, which often feel that they are likely to lose their identity. But if integration is properly managed, and the curriculum content properly defined, every department should be able to track its own contribution to the curriculum as a whole.

There can be little doubt(48) that the early clinical experience vertical integration offers students is beneficial to their motivation and satisfaction, their acclimatisation and professional induction, and their confidence and ability to reflect on and appraise their own skills. It can strengthen and broaden learning and intensify the relevance of the course to ultimate clinical practice.

The adoption of integration implies a complete reorganisation of the curriculum and so decisions must be made about the basis for that integration. In other words, what will be the framework around which the content of the curriculum will be arranged? There are many choices.

- In Sheffield, the curriculum was designed around an agreed list of presenting clinical problems derived from published sources and other curricula, added to locally and then rated by clinical teachers for their importance. A blueprint for each problem was then constructed, which defined the curriculum content and outcomes.(39)
- In Manchester,(49) the core problem-based curriculum was organised around index clinical situations (ICSs) for which new graduates must have a required level of competence. These ICSs were derived in consultation with primary and secondary care clinicians, who then defined the knowledge and skills base for each one in a variety of specific domains, including technical, contextual, intellectual and interpersonal.

Equally, the basis for integration could be bodily systems, age, patient cases or any other grouping. Each approach has its advantages and disadvantages. Within the chosen framework, however, the specific content to be covered can be specified in terms of repeated and consistent curriculum themes that run vertically through the whole course. This is described further below in relation to module design.

Core and options

This specification of mandatory and optional sections of the curriculum was a response to the perceived problem of content overload in medical education. It has been widely used in medical schools and is cur-

rently under consideration in postgraduate training. Given that this is the central, mandatory content of the curriculum, 'core' can mean different things. But if a core and options model is chosen, then the basis on which the core is selected must be known and agreed. To date, there is no adequate evidence base to suggest that one way of identifying the core is better than any other.(50) Harden and Davis(51) set out the possibilities:

- the essential aspects of each subject or discipline
- the essential competencies for practice
- areas of study relevant to many disciplines.

A fourth possibility is a study of only those disciplines deemed essential, but this approach 'has caused great alarm among some teachers, and justifiably so'.(51) At medical school, it is generally thought that students must gain knowledge and experience of all major disciplines.

There are many ways of determining the content of the core curriculum, ranging from modified Delphi processes(52,53) and other formal consultations, to statistical and epidemiological methods, critical incident techniques and more informal consultative and team-based work. Whatever method is chosen, it should be well understood and publicised, and properly managed according to a timescale. It should involve all interested parties and stakeholders and bear in mind the vision of the school.

Options can then be built around the core and given timetabled slots or blocks to offer students choices in their learning and career development, and the opportunity for more self-directed study. Some guidance can be provided: for example, options can be provided in different categories such as basic sciences, core extension studies, laboratory specialties, social and community sciences, education and management. Students may then be required to undertake options in a variety of these areas.

Some medical schools have an 'options bank', which departments and teachers add to and students then select from. These would normally be well-defined elements with a defined assessment plan, each of which would be able to accommodate a limited number of students. It is also possible to allow students to design their own options, either within certain headings or freely but according to set criteria about planning, process and outcomes against which the option can be marked and assessed.

Spiral model

The principle of the spiral curriculum, first elaborated by the titan educationalist Jerome Bruner,(54) is that students should revisit material at increasing levels of complexity as they progress through the course. Thus, for example, the themes of clinical methods, ethics and health promotion, and their accompanying attitudes, knowledge and skills, were designed into the Dundee curriculum(55) to be revisited in more complex ways during the four main stages of the course, which dealt with normal structure, function and behaviour, then abnormal structure, function and behaviour, then clinical practice and, finally, on-the-job-learning.

Thus the features of the spiral curriculum are that:(56)

- topics, themes or subjects are revisited on a number of occasions throughout the course
- there are increasing levels of difficulty
- new learning is related to previous learning
- the competence of the learner increases.

Module-based

A module is a self-contained unit of study. It should have its own outcomes (however expressed), activities and assessments. Students tend to take more than one module of study at a time. Modules are planned according to the curriculum framework selected. In an integrated course, modules will tend to have similar structures, with the vertical themes of the course that spiral through the curriculum being addressed in each module. So, for example, a module on cardiovascular disease might have its content decided in relation to curriculum themes of:

- clinical sciences
- basic sciences
- behavioural sciences
- population sciences
- clinical skills
- interpersonal skills and professional behaviours.

The module might then be taught around a number of index cases, which illustrate these themes and the necessary content. It is in the nature of modules that there is some flexibility in the order in which they are taught.

How do we determine the experiences that will further those purposes?

The experiences that students have will be selected on the basis of the planning and design work that has been carried out in the previous steps. The choices that must be made are in relation to:

- learning and teaching methods, including learning resources, feedback and support
- practical and clinical experience, including sites.

Learning and teaching methods, including learning resources, feedback and support

Decisions about learning and teaching methods will flow from the planning of previous stages. For example, if a self-directed, independent learner is an intended product of the course, then learning methods that encourage that will be used. But there is no one-to-one relationship between course intentions and teaching and learning methods. Every curriculum designer has a range of choices that could lead to the same outcomes. And although it might be true, for example, that problem-based learning fosters active learning

and encourages deep learning and integration, it is not the only way of achieving those aims.

Likewise, although problem-based learning can be an entire curriculum approach, more frequently it is used for just part of a curriculum – either in the first couple of years or as just one type of teaching and learning method as part of a curriculum that also includes other approaches. Problem-based learning does itself contain a variety of learning methods, and although there is now no commonly agreed definition of problem-based learning,(57) all definitions do tend to emphasise small group learning, authentic problems that stimulate the self-directed learning process (often carefully defined), and acquisition of knowledge and problem-solving skills.

The curriculum designer can choose from the following, at a minimum, each of which has a positive role to play:

- clinical skills laboratories, including communication skills training
- clinical experience, inpatient, ambulatory and community
- study guides describing what is to be learnt and relating this to available learning opportunities(58)
- lectures
- seminars and tutorials
- independent or guided group work
- simulations
- practicals
- resource-based learning, including e-learning and library work
- formative assessment, appraisal and feedback on learning.

The curriculum designer should state what balance of these methods might be desirable and expected. But the method selected alone will not determine effect on learning unless it is used in an appropriate manner. Thus problem-based learning has variable effects on the acquisition of knowledge,(59) and any teaching or learning method, whether apparently learner-centred or not, which has a heavy workload, high contact hours, excessive material or an emphasis on coverage, is likely to push students towards a surface approach to learning.(60) Likewise, any educational method that displays an appropriate motivational context, a high degree of learner activity, interaction with peers and teachers, and a well-structured knowledge base (which might be where problem-based learning sometimes falls down) will encourage a deep approach.(61)

The role of assessment as an instrument of learning, especially if used formatively for that purpose only, should not be overlooked and should be considered with other interventions such as appraisal and regular structured and supportive feedback sessions.

Practical and clinical experience, including sites

In basic medical education, and perhaps even beyond, a wide range of knowledge, skills and attitudes can be acquired as effectively in the community as in hospital settings.(62) So if the curriculum has the intention of producing graduates with an interest in practice in the community,(63,64) then primary care might be developed as a major provider of teaching, learning and experience, offering effective integrated teaching.(65) Four types of community-based teaching have been identified.(66)

- Community-orientated teaching: teaching in and about the community
- Agency-based teaching: teaching involving community healthcare providers other than primary care physicians
- General practice-based teaching: either specific clinical teaching or an attachment
- Specialist teaching in the community: specialist subjects taught by hospital practitioners in a community setting.

Equally, such knowledge and skills can also often be achieved in hospital settings. The choice of location is to be decided by the curriculum designers in light of the previous steps. Finally, the role of skills laboratories in helping students to acquire basic and more advanced clinical and communication skills in a safe, structured environment before using these with patients should also be considered as part of the curriculum design process.

How can we determine whether the purposes are being attained?

Whether the purposes of the curriculum are attained should be measured in two ways. First, a robust assessment system that is properly blueprinted on to the curriculum will measure students' attainment of the intended learning outcomes of the programme. Second, a curriculum evaluation strategy that addresses the views and experiences of all stakeholders will offer information about how the curriculum in practice fulfils or does not fulfil its purposes. On the basis of assessment and evaluation findings, the curriculum can be reviewed and renewed to ensure that it remains fit for purpose. But the assessment of student learning, evaluation of the curriculum in practice and curriculum renewal are topics for another occasion.

References

1 Miller G (ed.) (1961) *Teaching and Learning in Medical School.* Harvard University Press, Cambridge, MA.
2 Simpson MA (1972) *Medical Education. A Critical Approach.* Butterworths, London.
3 Cox KR and Ewan CE (eds) (1982) *The Medical Teacher.* Churchill Livingstone, Edinburgh.
4 Newble D and Cannon R (1983) *A Handbook for Clinical Teachers.* MTP Press, Boston, MA.
5 Balla JI, Gibson M and Chang AM (1989) *Learning in Medical School. A Model for the Clinical Professions.* Hong Kong University Press, Hong Kong.
6 Jolly B and Rees L (eds) (1998) *Medical Education in the Millennium.* Oxford University Press, Oxford.
7 Eisner EW (1994) *The Educational Imagination: on the design and evaluation of school programs (3e).* Macmillan, New York.
8 Toohey S (1999) *Designing Courses for Higher Education.* Society for Research into Higher Education and Open University Press, Buckingham.
9 Grant J, Chambers E and Jackson G (1999) *The Good CPD Guide.* Reed Business Information, Sutton, Surrey.
10 Flinders DJ and Thornton SJ (2004) *The Curriculum Studies Reader (2e).* RoutledgeFalmer, New York.
11 Grant J, Fox S, Kumar N and Sim E (2005) *Standards for Curricula.* Postgraduate Medical Education and Training Board, London. (http://www.pmetb.org.uk/index.aspx?articleid=662).
12 General Medical Council (2003) *Tomorrow's Doctors. Recommendations on Undergraduate Medical Education.* GMC, London.
13 For a statement of the PMETB Vision and Values see http://www.pmetb.org.uk/index.aspx?articleid=377
14 Coles CR and Gale Grant J (1985) ASME medical education research booklet no 1. Curriculum evaluation in medical and health-care education. *Medical Education.* **19**(5):405–22.
15 World Federation for Medical Education (2003) *WFME Global Standards for Quality Improvement. Trilogy.* WFME Office: University of Copenhagen, Denmark (www.sund.ku.dk/wfme/).
16 Noddings N (2003) *Happiness and Education.* Cambridge University Press, Cambridge.
17 General Medical Council (2001) *Good Medical Practice (3e).* GMC, London.
18 The Royal College of Physicians and Surgeons of Canada (1996) *Essential Roles and Key Competencies of Specialist Physicians. CanMeds2000 – skills for the new millennium.* Report of the Societal Needs Working Group. Canadian Medical Education Directions for Specialists 2000 Project (http://rcpsc.medical.org/publications/index.php).
19 Tyler RW (1949) *Basic Principles of Curriculum and Instruction.* University of Chicago Press, Chicago.
20 Jacques D (2000) *Learning in Groups. A Handbook for Improving Group Work (3e).* RoutledgeFalmer, London.
21 Mager R (1975) *Preparing Instructional Objectives (2e).* Fearon-Pitman Publishers, Belmont, CA.
22 Stenhouse L (1975) *An Introduction to Curriculum Research and Development.* Heinemann, Oxford.
23 Grant J (2000) The incapacitating effects of competence. A critique. *Journal of Health Sciences Education.* **4**(3): 271–7.
24 Hyland T (1993) Competence, knowledge and education. *Journal of Philosophy of Education.* **27**(1): 57–68.
25 McKeachie WJ (1951–69) *Teaching Tips. A Guidebook for the Beginning College Teacher (1–6e).* DC Heath and Company, Lexington, MA.
26 Nicol D (1997) *Research on Learning and Higher Education Teaching.* UCoSDA briefing paper 45. Universities and Colleges Staff Development Agency, Sheffield.
27 Knowles M (1979) *The Adult Learner: a neglected species?* Gulf, Houston, TX.
28 http://hsc.unm.edu/som/admissions/curriculum.shtml
29 Marton F and Säljo R (1976) On qualitative differences in learning I and II. *British Journal of Educational Psychology.* **46**(1/2): 4–11, 128–48.
30 Newble DI and Entwistle NJ (1980) Learning styles and approaches: implications for medical education. *Medical Education.* **20**(3): 162–75.

31 McManus IC, Keeling A and Paice E (2004) Stress, burnout and doctors' attitudes to work are determined by personality and learning style: a twelve-year longitudinal study of UK medical graduates. *BioMed Central Medicine.* 2(29).

32 http://casemed.case.edu/admissions/medicine_f.htm

33 Fish D and Coles C (2005) *Medical Education: developing a curriculum for practice.* Open University Press, Maidenhead.

34 http://www.som.soton.ac.uk/prospectus

35 Royal College of Physicians (2005) *Doctors in Society. Medical Professionalism in a Changing World.* Royal College of Physicians of London, London.

36 Hoyle E (1971) How does the curriculum change? In: Hooper R (ed.) *The Curriculum: context, design and development.* Oliver and Boyd in association with The Open University Press, Edinburgh.

37 Kelly AV (1999) *The Curriculum. Theory and practice.* Paul Chapman Publishing, London.

38 Gale R and Grant J (1997) Managing change in a medical context: guidelines for action. AMEE guide no. 10. *Medical Teacher.* 19: 239–49.

39 Newble D, Stark P, Bax N and Lawson M (2005) Developing an outcome-focused core curriculum. *Medical Education.* 39: 680–7.

40 Smith SR and Dollase R (1999) AMEE guide no. 14. Outcome-based education. Part 2 – planning, implementing and evaluating a competency-based curriculum. *Medical Teacher.* 21(1): 15–22.

41 Harden RM, Sowden S and Dunn WR (1984) Educational strategies in curriculum development: the SPICES model. *Medical Education.* 18: 284–97.

42 Newble D, Jolly B and Wakeford R (eds) (1994) *The Certification and Recertification of Doctors.* Cambridge University Press, Cambridge.

43 Prideaux D (2000) Emperor's new clothes: from objectives to outcomes. *Medical Education.* 34: 168–9.

44 Stenhouse L (1975) *An Introduction to Curriculum Research and Development.* Heinemann, London.

45 Rees C (2004) The problem with outcomes-based curricula in medical education: insights from educational theory. *Medical Education.* 38: 593–8.

46 Harden RM, Crosby JR and Davis MH (1999) AMEE guide no. 14. Outcome-based education. Part 1 – an introduction to outcome-based education. *Medical Teacher.* 21(1): 7–14.

47 Harden RM, Crosby JR, Davis MH and Friedman M (1999) AMEE guide no. 14. Outcome-based education. Part 5 – from competency to meta-competency: a model for the specification of learning outcomes. *Medical Teacher.* 21(6): 546–52.

48 Dornan T, Litttlewood S, Margolis SA, Spencer J and Ypinazar V (2006) BEME guide. How can experience in clinical and community settings contribute to early medical education? A BEME systematic review. *Medical Teacher.* 28(1): 3–18.

49 O'Neill PA, Metcalfe D and David TJ (1999) The core content of the undergraduate curriculum in Manchester. *Medical Education.* 33(2): 114–20.

50 D'Eon M and Crawford R (2005) The elusive content of the medical school curriculum: a method to the madness. *Medical Teacher.* 27(8): 699–703.

51 Harden RM and Davis MH (1995) AMEE guide no. 5. The core curriculum with options or special study modules. *Medical Teacher.* 17(2): 125–48.

52 Alahlafi A and Burge S (2005) What should undergraduate medical students know about psoriasis? Involving patients in curriculum development: modified Delphi technique. *British Medical Journal.* 330: 633–6.

53 Syme-Grant J, Stewart C and Ker J (2005) How we developed a core curriculum in clinical skills. *Medical Teacher.* 27(2): 103–6.

54 Bruner J (1977) *The Process of Education (2e).* Harvard University Press, Cambridge, MA.

55 Harden RM, Davis MH and Crosby J (1997) The new Dundee medical curriculum: a whole that is greater than the sum of the parts. *Medical Education.* 31: 264–71.

56 Harden RM and Stamper N (1999) What is a spiral curriculum? *Medical Teacher.* 21(2): 141–3.

57 Gijbels D, Docht F, Van den Bossche P and Segers M (2005) Effects of problem-based learning: a meta-analysis from the angle of assessment. *Review of Educational Research.* 75(1): 27–61.

58 Harden RM, Laidlaw JM and Hesketh EA. AMEE guide no. 16. Study guides – their use and preparation. *Medical Teacher.* 21(3): 248–65.

59 Albanese MA and Mitchell S (1993) Problem-based learning: a review of the literature on its outcomes and implementation issues. *Academic Medicine.* 68: 52–81.

60 Gibbs G (1992) Improving the quality of student learning through course design. In: Barnett R (ed.) *Learning to Effect.* SRHE and Open University Press, Buckingham.

61 Biggs JB (1989) Approaches to the enhancement of tertiary teaching. *Higher Education Research and Development.* 8(1): 7–25.

62 Murray E, Jolly B and Modell MA (1999) A comparison of the educational opportunities on junior medical attachments in general practice and in teaching hospital: a questionnaire study. *Medical Education.* 317: 170–6.

63 Bligh J (1999) Is it time for a community-based medical school? *Medical Education.* 33(5): 315.

64 Nazareth I and Kaya M (1999) Medical education in the community – the UNITRA experience. *Medical Education.* 33: 722–4.

65 Worley P, Silagy C, Prideaux D, Newble D and Jones A (2000) The Parallel Rural Community Curriculum: an integrated clinical curriculum based in rural general practice. *Medical Education.* 34: 558–65.

66 McCrorie P, Lefford F and Perrin F (1994) *Medical Undergraduate Community-based Teaching: a survey for ASME on current and proposed teaching in the community and in general practice in UK universities.* ASME occasional publication no. 3. ASME, Dundee.

Teaching and learning in medical education: how theory can inform practice

David M Kaufman and Karen V Mann

> **KEY MESSAGES**
> - Understanding theory can enhance the use of effective teaching and learning strategies.
> - The learner is an active contributor in the learning process.
> - Learners interact actively with the curriculum, patients and teachers in a complex, changing environment.
> - The entire context of learning is important, rather than any single variable, and includes interactions of all the variables.
> - Values, attitudes and the culture of the profession are often learned implicitly and without explicit teaching or awareness of learning.
>
> - Learning is enhanced when it is relevant, particularly to the solution and understanding of real-life problems and practice.
> - Individuals' past experience and knowledge are critical to how they learn.
> - Learning has an emotional aspect to it that is often under-recognised and can influence the learning significantly.
> - Individual learners are capable of self-regulation, that is, setting goals, planning strategies and monitoring their progress.
> - The ability to reflect on one's practice (performance) is critical to lifelong, self-directed learning.

Introduction

How can educational theory inform our practice? Several writers have described a gap between theory and practice. Indeed, this perception has led practitioners in many professions to conclude that theory is in an ivory tower, not useful or relevant to those in practice. Educators are no exception.(1) However, as professional practice is better understood, it is clear that theory has the potential both to inform practice and to be informed by it.

Our purpose in this chapter is to describe eight selected approaches to education theory and explore their implications for the practice of medical education. We use the term 'theory' in a general sense, that is, as a set of assumptions and ideas that help to explain some phenomenon. Knowles(2) put this succinctly more than 25 years ago, defining a theory as: 'a comprehensive, coherent, and internally consistent system of ideas about a set of phenomena'.

Each of the theoretical approaches we describe is consistent with Knowles' definition. The eight theoretical approaches discussed are:

Understanding Medical Education: Evidence, Theory and Practice.
Edited by T Swanwick. © 2010 Association for the Study of Medical Education.

- adult learning principles(3)
- social cognitive theory(4)
- reflective practice(5)
- transformative learning(6)
- self-directed learning(7)
- experiential learning(8)
- situated learning(9)
- learning in communities of practice.(10)

We selected these because we believe them to be particularly useful in the context of the issues facing medical education today. We will describe each theoretical formulation, highlighting its major constructs, and present implications of the theory for educational practice, followed by a specific example drawn from medical education. We will conclude with a consideration of the connections and commonalities among the eight theories, so that readers may make these connections within their own practice.

Adult Learning Principles

The purpose of adult education has been the subject of a number of typologies.(11–15) Generally, these accord with a list proposed by Darkenwald and Merriam,(15) namely:
- cultivation of the intellect
- individual self-actualisation

- personal and social improvement
- social transformation
- organisational effectiveness.

A number of theoretical frameworks have developed around these functions, which Merriam(16) has grouped into three categories. The first category is based on *adult learning characteristics*, in which the best-known framework is 'andragogy'.(3) Also in this group is Cross'(17) 'Characteristics of Adults as Learners' model, based on differences between adults and children across personal and situational characteristics.

The second category emphasises the *adult's life situation*. Two theories have been proposed in this category, Knox's Proficiency Theory(18) and McClusky's Theory of Margin.(19) The third category focuses on *changes in consciousness*. Several models in this category emphasise reflection upon experience and environment. Mezirow's Perspective Transformation(20) (discussed later) and Freire's Theory of Conscientization(21) are the best-developed models in this category.

Merriam and Caffarella(22) have provided an excellent summary of the various theory-building efforts in adult learning. They conclude that no single theory fares well when judged by the criteria of comprehensiveness (i.e. includes all types of learning), practicality and universality of its application. They also assert that a phenomenon as complex as adult learning will probably never be adequately explained by a single theory. Although these theoretical frameworks provide implications for practice, few have actually been applied widely in adult education practice. Knowles'(3) andragogy is the exception. The remainder of this section focuses on and andragogy, its implications for practice and an example of its use in undergraduate medical education.

Andragogy

Malcolm Knowles(3) first introduced the term 'andragogy' to North America, defining it as 'the art and science of helping adults learn'. Knowles did not present andragogy as an empirically based theory, but simply as a set of four assumptions,(3) to which a fifth was later added (*see* Box 2.1).(23)

Andragogy has its roots in humanistic psychology through the work of Maslow(24) and Rogers.(25) The core basis of andragogy is that the attainment of adulthood is marked by adults coming to view themselves as self-directed individuals. Knowles' 'model of assumptions' has given adult education a 'badge of identity' that distinguishes the field from other areas of education, for example, childhood schooling.(26) Bard(27) has asserted that andragogy 'probably more than any other force, has changed the role of the learner in adult education and in human resource development' (p. xi). However, it has also caused enormous controversy, debate and criticism. The early

---

> **BOX 2.1 Andragogical assumptions(3,23)**
>
> 1 As a person matures, their self-concept moves from that of a dependent personality towards one of a self-directing human being. Adults are capable of determining their own learning needs, and of finding the means to meet them.
>
> 2 An adult accumulates a growing reservoir of experience, which is a rich resource for learning. This experience can be brought to bear on new learning, and enhance the new learning significantly. It can also provide an effective context for the acquisition of new knowledge and skills.
>
> 3 The readiness of an adult to lean is closely related to the developmental tasks of their social role. Adults value learning that integrates with the demands placed on them in their everyday life.
>
> 4 There is a change in time perspective as people mature, from future application of knowledge to immediacy of application. Thus an adult is more problem centred than subject centred in learning. Generally, adults value learning that can be applied to authentic problems that they encounter in everyday life.
>
> 5 Adults are more motivated to learn by internal factors rather than external ones. The internal desire to succeed, the satisfaction of learning and the presence of personal goals have a greater effect on *maintaining* [italics added] motivation than external incentives and rewards.

---

criticism led Knowles to later modify his model by describing andragogy and pedagogy as a continuum, and suggesting that the use of both teaching methods is appropriate at different times in different situations, regardless of the learner's age.(23)

It is widely accepted that andragogy is not really a theory of *how* adults learn, the assumptions being merely descriptions of the adult learner.(28) Furthermore, even the assumptions have been questioned as prescriptions for practice.

Others argue that andragogy may in time become a theory, but through empirical studies of the assumptions. At least, andragogy captures general characteristics of adult learners and offers guidelines for planning instruction with learners who tend to be at least somewhat independent and self-directed (29).

Implications for educational practice

There are several implications for practice that can be derived from the theories of adult learning which have at their heart the fact that an adult's life situation is quite different from that of a child. Merriam and Caffarella(22) discuss these differences in three areas: context, learner and learning process.

Context

Children are dependent on others for their well-being, while adults have assumed responsibility for managing their own lives. Typically, being a learner is only one of several roles played concurrently by adults. Additionally, the principles that have guided approaches to teaching children, and which have been applied to learners of all ages, have focused on generalised learning in the school setting.(30) In contrast, adults generally learn and function in settings where situation-specific skills are required to resolve relevant problems.

Learner

As Knowles has described,(3) there are significant differences between adults and children that must be addressed in the learning process. These include the need of adults to be self-directing, their large reservoir of experience, the relationship of their readiness to learn to their social role, their desire for knowledge that can be immediately applied to current relevant problems and their internal motivation to learn.

Learning process

Three non-cognitive factors have been shown to affect adult learning:

- pacing (e.g. through deadlines for assignments or adhering to a schedule)
- meaningfulness
- motivation.(22)

Pacing of learning through deadlines or other pressures may adversely affect learning, since adults have many competing demands. Also, adults tend to perform poorly on learning tasks that are not meaningful, or which do not fall within their domain of interest.

The ideas presented thus far can be formulated as a set of principles to guide adult learning activities. Several writers have proposed principles or 'tips' for practitioners.(23,31) Knowles(23) himself drew seven principles from the assumptions of andragogy, which are presented here (*see* Box 2.2).

Social Cognitive Theory

Social cognitive theory(4), formerly social learning theory(32), acknowledges the social (interactive) aspect of learning and unites two approaches to understanding learning. These are the behaviourist approach, which emphasises the influence of the environment on our actions, and the cognitive approach, which emphasises the importance of cognition in mediating our learning and functioning.

These two approaches are united in a basic tenet of social cognitive theory, which posits that our actions, learning and functioning are the result of a continuous,

---

BOX 2.2 Principles of adult learning(23)

1 An effective learning climate should be established. Learners should be comfortable, both physically and emotionally. They should feel safe and free to express themselves without judgement or ridicule.

2 Learners should be involved in mutual planning of methods and curricular directions. Involvement will help assure that collaboration occurs in the content and learning process. It will also increase the relevance to the learners' needs.

3 Learners should be involved in diagnosing their own learning needs. Once again, this will help to ensure meaningfulness and will trigger learners' internal (intrinsic) motivation. It will also promote self-assessment and reflection, and effective integration of learning.

4 Learners should be encouraged to formulate their own learning objectives. The rationale for this is the same as for 3, above. Learners are thus encouraged to take control of their learning.

5 Learners should be encouraged to identify resources and to devise strategies for using them to accomplish their objectives. This principle connects adult learning needs to practical resources for meeting their objectives, and also provides motivation for using such resources for a specific and focused purpose.

6 Learners should be helped to carry out their learning plans. One of the key elements of motivation is expectancy of success. Learners will become discouraged and lose their motivation if a learning task is too difficult. Also, too much pressure without support can lead to a decrement in learning.

7 Learners should be involved in evaluating their own learning. This is an essential step in a self-directed learning process that requires critical reflection on experience, a specific example of which(5) is discussed later in this paper.

---

dynamic, reciprocal interaction among three sets of determinants: personal, environmental (situational) and behavioural. Personal factors include the individual's attitudes, perceptions, values, goals, knowledge and all previous experience. Environmental factors encompass all those influences that may reward or hinder actions and the achievement of goals. Bandura notes explicitly that 'personal and environmental factors do not function as independent determinants; rather, they determine each other. People create, alter and destroy environments. The changes they produce in environmental conditions, in turn, affect their behaviour and the nature of future life' (p. 23).(4) Bandura further states that behaviour, rather than being a 'detached by-product' of persons and situations, is itself an interacting determinant in the process.

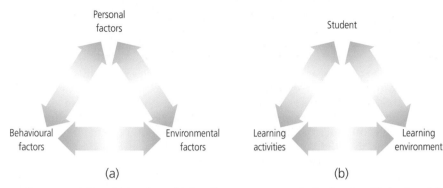

Figure 2.1 Diagrammatic representation of (a) reciprocal interaction among personal, situational and behavioural factors; (b) the same factors using a medical education example.

Figure 2.1 shows the interactions schematically and how these might apply to medical education.

Bandura asserts that the relative influences exerted by each of the three sets of factors will vary for different activities, different individuals and different circumstances. For example, when environmental conditions exert a powerful influence they will prevail. In a medical education example, when trainees are thrust into the busy environment of a clinical ward they will do what is required to get the job done and to meet expectations. In other cases, the behaviour and its feedback will be a major influence. For instance, when students are learning and practising a new skill, the feedback from this will have a strong influence. Finally, in those instances where situational influences are relatively weak, personal factors will exert the strongest regulatory influence. To complete our example, when not pressed by powerful environmental forces students may choose to learn a new skill or to learn more about talking with patients. These choices will be affected by the student's own values, perceived needs and individual goals. There may also be interaction within each factor as they exert an influence on each other. The simple example provided here is not intended to convey lack of complexity; rather, it is to emphasise the ongoing, dynamic nature of our interaction with our environment.

Environmental influences can affect people in ways other than their behaviour, as when thoughts and feelings are modified through observing others' behaviour (modelling), teaching or social persuasion. Thoughts do not arise in a vacuum. Individual perceptions and understandings are developed and verified through both direct and vicarious experience, judgements of others and by inference from what is already known.(4) (p. 27).

Basic human capabilities

Bandura views humans as possessing five basic capabilities that underpin our learning and functioning in all situations.

Symbolising capability

Almost every aspect of our lives is touched by our remarkable ability to use symbols to transform our experience into a form that can be internalised and serve as a guide to future actions. This ability enables us, when confronted with a new problem, to test possible solutions symbolically, rather than laboriously trying out each alternative.

Forethought capability

Most of our behaviour is regulated by thought. We anticipate the likely outcomes of our actions and plan goals for ourselves and courses of action to maximise the likelihood of obtaining them. Also, as noted, images of desirable future events can become motivators of our current behaviour.

Vicarious capability

If learning occurred only through performing actions and experiencing their effects, learning and development would be slow, tedious and enormously inefficient. Fortunately, much learning that can be acquired through direct experience can also be acquired or facilitated vicariously through observation of other people's actions and their consequences. This applies to social development, especially where, in some situations, new behaviours can only be conveyed effectively by modelling. Even if learning can occur in other ways, the ability to learn vicariously distinctly shortens the process.

Self-regulatory capability

In social cognitive theory, the capability for self-regulation is central. Much of our behaviour is regulated primarily by our internal standards and our evaluative reactions to our own actions. Any discrepancies between our actions and those standards activate a self-evaluation, which will influence our subsequent behaviour. Self-evaluation is our personal guidance system for action. We exercise self-regulation or self-directedness by arranging facilitative environmental conditions using our images of future events as guides and creating incentives for our efforts.

Self-reflective capability

Perhaps the most distinctive is the capability for self-reflection, whereby we can analyse our experiences and think about our thought processes. Cognitive theorists refer to this as metacognitive capability. Through self-reflection we gain understanding about ourselves, our behaviour and the world around us.

A central concept in social cognitive theory is *self-efficacy*; the individual's judgement about his or her ability to carry out a specific task or activity (*see* Box 2.3).

BOX 2.3 Focus on: Self-efficacy(33)

According to Bandura, a central type of thought that affects action is people's judgements of their capabilities to deal with different realities, or their *self-efficacy*. This judgement influences what people choose to do, how much effort they invest in activities, how long they persist in the face of disappointment and whether tasks are approached anxiously or assuredly. Judgements about our personal efficacy, whether accurate of faulty, arise from four main information sources.

- Performance attainments – our own performance is the most influential source of efficacy because it is based on authentic experience of mastery. Successes raise our efficacy appraisals; failures generally have a lowering effect, especially if they occur early in the learning and they do not reflect lack of effort or difficult situations. Once strong positive efficacy perceptions are developed, occasional failures do not have a marked effect. Feelings of capability are generally task-specific, though they can generalise to other, similar tasks.

- Vicarious experience – observing other similar people perform successfully can raise our own beliefs that we can perform similar tasks. This source of information is particularly effective when people are encountering new tasks and have little experience on which to base their perceptions.

- Verbal persuasion – we have all had the experience of trying to convince people that they possess capabilities that will enable them to achieve what they seek. If the heightened efficacy that the persuasion is attempting to achieve is realistic, it can be influential, particularly in affecting the amount of effort individuals put into a task.

- Physiological state – people often judge their capability based on the messages received about their physiological states. We frequently interpret arousal in taxing situations as an ominous sign of vulnerability, and tend to expect more success when we are not tense and aroused.

Implications for educational practice

Understanding the concepts of ongoing dynamic interactions, basic human capabilities and how people form their conceptions of their abilities allows us to plan a learning environment that is most conducive to maximising each individual's development. We will consider some implications of this theory for effective teaching and learning; in particular, five learning processes (that build on the basic capabilities) that can be brought to bear in medical education:

- modelling or demonstration
- a clear objective, goal or desired outcome
- provision of task-relevant knowledge
- guided practice and feedback
- opportunities for learners to reflect on their learning.

Modelling or demonstration of the desired process or skill facilitates vicarious learning through observation. This opportunity not only shortens the learning process, it is often essential when new skills are being acquired. Demonstration can help students to form an image of the desired skill/behaviour, which can be used as a guide for action and as a standard of performance against which to monitor their personal progress. Finally, learner perceptions of efficacy are increased by observing someone else perform successfully.

A *clear objective*, goal or image of the desired outcome enhances learning. It builds on our capability for forethought, providing a guidepost for monitoring and directing our progress appropriately. Awareness of the goal also increases expenditure of energy and effort and stimulates the development of strategies to reach the goal.

Learners require *task-relevant knowledge*. They must have the basic building blocks to use as a foundation for newly acquired knowledge and skills. It maybe knowledge related to content or process, but it must be relevant to the individual's prior knowledge and skills, and to the current goal. Further, learners may need stimulation and assistance to activate prior knowledge, to relate it to the new learning. This knowledge promotes students' views of themselves as capable of the task. Otherwise, their perceptions of their efficacy are likely to be low, which will affect both developing efficacy perceptions and their future performance.

Guided practice of a new skill with feedback allows learners to develop positive efficacy perceptions about the task, and to experience successes rather than failures in that crucial early learning period. Practice promotes the internalisation of personal standards, which can then be used in self-regulation and self-evaluation. Corrective feedback is integral to effective learning. Without feedback, the level of performance achieved is lower. Similarly, feedback is less effective in improving performance when it is not related to a goal or desired level of achievement.(33)

Finally, and arguably most critically, learners require *opportunities to reflect* on their learning, to consider their strategies, to determine whether new approaches are required to achieve their goal and to draw lessons for future learning. Reflection also allows the integration of new experiences into existing experience and knowledge. Finally, it allows the learner to build accurate and positive perceptions of efficacy, based on their experience.

In summary, social cognitive theory provides us with several important constructs that may inform our educational practice. They include the concept that learners are constantly interacting with their environment and their actions and consequences. Many of the characteristics that we seek are present as basic capabilities common to all. Rather than creating these characteristics, learning opportunities can be created to develop and build on them. Finally, we can have some confidence that people are inherently self-directed. Given the appropriate conditions and support, they will set goals, develop strategies to attain them and monitor their progress regularly.

Reflection and Reflective Practice

The concepts of *reflection* and the *reflective practitioner* are at the centre of the epistemology of professional practice. They borrow from and link three previously well-established epistemologies: positivism, interpretive theory and critical theory.(5,34) The positivistic view of science assumes that theory is a scholarly pursuit that may be unrelated to practice. It is only the predictive value of theory that is of practical value. Reflection in professional practice extends this view by proposing that theory and practice inform each other.

As knowledge is embedded in practice, practitioners are positioned to test and revise theories through practice. They do so by reflection and action. The reflective process, as such, serves as a bridge in the theory–practice relationship.

It ties the reflection to the interpretive model. The interpretive epistemology proposes that theory is interpreted in light of personal current and past experiences. Theory guides or enlightens action and understanding. Lastly, the concept of reflective practice shares with critical theory the observation that theory is intimately linked to practice through a process of critical thinking and examination. This process permits professionals to break free from established paradigms and reformulate the ways in which practice, problems and problem solving are viewed. This reframing is part of learning and change. It is how practice helps organise theory.(5,35) Reflective practice then becomes a vehicle for learning effectively.

Al-Shehri *et al.*(35) and Moon(36) reviewed definitions and approaches to reflection and reflective practice found in the educational literature. Clift *et al.*(37)

analysed issues and programmes that encourage reflective practice in education. But it is Schön who has perhaps been most influential in our understanding of reflective practice. Schön(5,38) summarises the need for a new scholarship that recognises knowing-in-action, on-the-spot experimentation (reflection-in-action) and action research.

Principles of reflective practice

Schön's works(5,38,39) are based on the study of a range of practice professions. Schön argues that formal theoretical knowledge, such as that acquired in the course of professional preparation, is often not useful to the solution of the messy, indeterminate problems of real-life practice. Central to his premise is the need for professional scholarship and the recognition of an epistemology of professional practice. The reflective practitioner incorporates these principles by relating professional knowledge to practical competence and professional activity. By linking theory to practice, both can inform each other.

Professionals develop zones of mastery around areas of competence. They practise within these areas as if automatic. Schön terms this a professional's 'knowing-in-action'. Indeed, practising one's profession has been likened to riding a bicycle. Occasionally the bicycle skids.(40) This occurs in response to a surprise or the unexpected. Two types of reflection are triggered at this time: 'reflection-in-action' and 'reflection-on-action'.(5)

Reflection-in-action involves the three activities of
- reframing and reworking the problem from different perspectives
- establishing where the problem fits into learned schema (i.e. already existing knowledge and expertise)
- understanding the elements and implications present in the problem, its solution and consequences.

Reflection-on-action, which occurs later, is a process of thinking back on what has happened in the situation to determine what may have contributed to the unexpected, and how this situation may affect future practice.

Both are iterative processes whereby insights and learning from one experience may be incorporated into future 'knowing-in-action'.(5,38)

Other approaches to reflection and learning from experience have also been influential.(40–42) Boud *et al.*(43) also outline an iterative process comprising three main phases, beginning with the *experience*. The second phase involves returning to the experience and, through reflective processes, dealing with both negative and positive feelings about it, and re-evaluating it. The last aspect of the process Boud *et al.* labelled 'outcomes', in which new perspectives on experience can lead to a change in behaviour and a readiness for application and commitment to action. These authors view reflection as the key to learning effectively. They also emphasise the importance of recognising the emotional aspects of experience that accompany effective learning from experience.

Moon(36) views reflection as the catalyst that moves surface learning to deep learning. Deep learning can be integrated with current experience and knowledge, resulting in rich cognitive networks that the individual can draw on in practice.

Similar characteristics are found across a number of reflective models.

- They describe reflection as a series of iterative steps or levels.
- They generally define levels of reflection, from superficial, descriptive levels to deeper levels.
- Generally, the deeper reflective levels are regarded as more difficult to achieve, although they hold greater potential for learning and growth.

There also appears to be a dynamic relationship between reflective practice and self-assessment, both explicitly and implicitly. The ability to self-assess depends on the ability to reflect accurately on one's practice, and the ability to reflect effectively relies heavily on accurate self-assessment.(44)

In the workplace, true professionals are known for their ability for on-the-spot experimentation and improvisation, their commitment to ongoing practice-based learning and their self-directed reflective learning skills. It is these collective skills that permit professionals to continually and subtly learn from practice, adapt to change and maintain their competence. The core capabilities of professionals are tied to a number of essential skills. Professionals recognise and value the traditional form of knowledge, that is, that gained in school or in study, as well as experiential knowledge, that is, that gained through experience and practice. In the context of their practice, they use both these forms of knowledge to continually reshape their approach to problems, solutions, actions and outcomes. This creative process, sometimes called wisdom or artistry, occurs in response to new meanings, insights and perspectives gained through reflection on current and past experiences. It leads to continued learning and ongoing competence within a profession.(5)

Reflection has frequently been viewed as an individual professional activity. In some cases, reflecting inadequately or inaccurately on one's performance can lead to circular, 'single-loop' learning, which can often lead to confirmation of current behaviours rather than to questioning and identifying areas for learning.(45) For this reason, reflection is increasingly suggested as a collective activity whereby individuals can share individual insights and reflections, and increase their collective and individual learning.(46) The evidence surrounding reflective practice is summarised in Box 2.4.

BOX 2.4 Where's the evidence: Reflective practice

Despite the observation that reflection has been described in several different fields, and much has been written about it in the respective literatures, the research literature in the field is relatively early in its development. A review(41) of the research across medicine, nursing and other health professions suggests the following.

- Reflective thinking is seen in practising professionals and in students across a variety of heath professions, including nursing, dentistry, medicine and health sciences.
- Reflection appears to serve a number of purposes. In medicine, it appears to occur most naturally in response to complex and new problems.(42) However, it is also demonstrated in anticipation of challenging situations.(47)
- The phenomenon of reflection is not unitary. Several elements and aspects of reflection have been demonstrated. The tendency to reflect and reflective ability vary across individuals and across situations.
- Attempts to measure and classify reflective thinking have resulted in validated instruments which demonstrate the differences exist and are measurable. Generally, it seems that deeper levels of reflection are achieved less often and are more difficult to achieve.
- It appears that reflective ability can be developed. Strategies associated with reported changes in reflective ability used small group resources and activities such as portfolio and journal keeping.
- Several factors appear to constantly influence reflection both negatively and positively. These include environment, time, maturity, effective guidance and supervision, and the organisational culture.
- Reflective practice appears to be linked to learning, particularly to deep learning, the development of self-regulated learning and the development of professional identity.(36)

Implications for educational practice

Reflective practitioners are able to assess a situation from the perspectives of both theoretical background and practical experience. They must be able to bridge successfully the theory–practice gap and apply both aspects of learning while examining the situation from all perspectives. Reflectivity in practice is a learned skill of critical thinking and situation analysis.

As reflection, practice-based learning and action based on these are all skills to be learned and applied, opportunities to acquire them must be available.

The mentor or teacher models, shares and fosters this creative process in the presence of future and current practitioners. The skills required for reflection must be developed in professional courses within our undergraduate, graduate, clinical and continuing medical education areas. Initially, the mentor or teacher models, shares and demonstrates the skills. He or she facilitates the learners' abilities to perceive options and alternatives, to frame and reframe problems. He or she also assists the learners to reflect on the actions and options they chose, and on what knowledge and values may have influenced their choice. Finally, teachers assist students to consider critically what they have learned and integrate it into their existing knowledge.

Once the learner has gained sufficient experience and insight into the profession, the teacher's role becomes one of facilitating systematic experiential learning, on-the-spot experimentation, and reflection on process, action and outcomes. Teachers observe and comment positively on situations in which the learner's reframing has occurred.(40) This helps the learner to become consciously aware of the process of reflection.

A dilemma in incorporating reflective practices into our educational programmes is to select those strategies that will facilitate its active development, and to select activities that are relevant to practice. Some literature has addressed this issue when considering the merits of journals and portfolios. However, there has been a move to incorporate more critically reflective activities across the continuum.

Several authors(35,48–53) have linked reflective practice to adult learning theory, self-directed learning, curriculum development, and effective professional education and knowledge translation.

Slotnick(41) linked Schön's work to how physicians learn in practice. He emphasised the importance of thinking while solving problems (reflection-in-action) and thinking after problem solving (reflection-on-action). These two activities are required for clinicians to gain new insights and perspectives around practice-based problems, problem solving and practice itself. Ongoing learning, maintenance of competence and improved practice will result.

Slotnick(41) outlined related principles and implications for learners and teachers in practice. Parboosingh(54) adopted the Schön model to assist in understanding how practitioners change and develop professionally. According to Parboosingh, to remain current, physicians require both an understanding of their areas of competence (mastery) and the ability to think reflectively. These two concepts are embedded in the epistemology of professional practice.

Shapiro and Talbot,(40), like Slotnick(41) and Parboosingh(52,54), reinforced the importance of practice context. They proposed that an understanding of artistry within the process of practice is required, and adopted Schön's model(38) to aid in this understanding. Specifically, Shapiro and Talbot(40) applied the reflective practice model to family medicine. The

authors described how to teach professional artistry. They proposed that open learning environments encourage a continual reshaping of practice-based learning, along with the development of continuous competence.

Lockyer *et al.*(46) explored how reflection could be used in both classrooms and practice, to enhance the integration of knowledge and its translation into professional practice.

Palmer *et al.*(47) addressed curriculum design issues specific to professional education and reflection. Using the nursing profession as the context, they described roles for lecture-practitioners, mentors (coaches) and mentees. To define the content or skill-set for a reflective curriculum, they borrowed from Atkins and Murphy.(44) They identified five skills as essential to partake in reflection:
- self-awareness
- description
- critical analysis
- synthesis
- evaluation.

Palmer *et al.*(47) also provided guidance specific to assessing reflective learning.

Crandall(42) notes the value of using Schön's model for all levels of the medical education continuum. She outlines how clinical teachers can use it to assist learners, and provides evidence through clinical teacher interviews that stages of Schön's model occur during effective clinical learning events. Specific evidence is provided for all five stages that Schön recommends:
1 knowing-in-action
2 surprise
3 reflection-in-action
4 experimentation
5 reflection-on-action.

Crandall offers strategies for implementing the reflective practice across the medical education continuum, and provides possible advantages for this.

Al-Shehri *et al.*(35) described two roles for providers of continuing medical education in fostering self-directed experiential learning, in which reflection is core; to sustain motivation for such an approach in established practitioners and to 'devise ways of sharing individual experience which both interpret and enhance learning' (p. 251). The authors make a number of suggestions as to how these tasks may be accomplished. Westberg and Jason(55) also offer practical approaches for fostering reflection in medical education, before, during and following experience. They emphasise the importance of the learning environment in effectively fostering reflection.

Lastly, Moon(56) proposes a process of reflection to promote transfer of new learning to practice. She describes this four-phase framework in the context of continuing education workshops and short courses, wherein participants are helped to address four questions.

Transformative Learning

Mezirow's concept of transformative learning has developed over 20 years into a comprehensive and complex theory.(6,48,51) Transformative learning theory defines learning as the social process of constructing and internalising a new or revised interpretation of the meaning of one's experience as a guide to action. In other words, transformative learning involves helping adults to elaborate, create and transform their meaning schemes (beliefs, feelings, interpretations, decisions) through reflection on their content, the process by which they were learned and their premises (social context, history and consequences).(51) Transformative learning can be contrasted with conventional learning that simply elaborates the learner's existing paradigm, systems of thinking, feeling or doing, relative to the topic. Although learning is increased, the learner's fundamental structure is maintained. Transformative learning changes the learner's paradigm so radically that, although it may retain the old perspective, it is actually a new creation. Critical reflection and rational discourse are the primary processes used in learning. The core of transformative learning in Mezirow's(51) view is the uncovering of distorted assumptions or errors in learning.

Empowerment of learners is both a goal and a condition for transformative learning. An empowered learner is able to participate fully and freely in critical discourse and the resulting action. This requires freedom and equality, as well as the ability to assess evidence and engage in critical reflection.(48) Reflection is a key concept in transformative learning theory. Mezirow(51) defines it as the process of critically assessing the content, process or premises of our efforts to interpret and give meaning to an experience. He distinguishes among three types of reflection:

- *content reflection* – an examination of the content or description of a problem
- *process reflection* – examination of the problem-solving strategies being used
- *premise reflection* – questioning the problem itself, which may lead to a transformation of belief systems.

Perspective transformation may be the result of a major event in one's life, or the cumulative result of related transformations in concepts, beliefs, judgements or feelings. The most significant learning involves critical reflection around premises about oneself. This kind of learning is triggered by a disorienting dilemma that invokes self-examination and a critical assessment of assumptions. Through a process of exploring options for new roles, relationships and actions, new knowledge and skills are acquired. This leads to planning and implementing a new course of action, provisionally trying new roles, renegotiating relationships and forming new ones, and building competence and self-confidence.

Mezirow(6) explains that discourse is a crucial process, and refers to a special kind of dialogue in which the focus is on content and attempting to justify beliefs by giving and defending reasons, and by examining the evidence for and against competing viewpoints.

Transformative learning is a complicated, emotional process requiring significant knowledge and skill to implement effectively.(53) A new paradigm emerges only after the old one becomes dysfunctional, and it is the task of the transformative educator to challenge the learner's current perspective. A paradigm shift will occur only if the learner perceives the existing paradigm to be significantly inadequate in explaining his or her experience. However, the new paradigm appears only after a period of disorientation during which no clear paradigm remains. It is typical for the learner to resist letting go of the old paradigm and beginning the transition to the new one. During this process, the teacher–learner relationship may intensify enormously because the learner may begin to resent the teacher or feel anger towards him or her. Often learners feel a complex love–hate for the teacher who intentionally assisted in the collapse of their existing paradigm.

Successful transformative learning questions assumptions (this is a key to the process), provides support from others in a safe environment, provides challenge, examines alternative perspectives and provides feedback. New assumptions are tested in the authentic settings or in discussion with others.

Implications for educational practice

How can educators promote and support transformative learning? First, educators need to take a reformist perspective, rather than a subject-centred or consumer-oriented perspective.(57) In a subject-centred perspective, the educator is the expert authority figure and designer of instruction. In a consumer-oriented perspective, the educator is a facilitator and resource person. In a reformist perspective, essential to transformative learning, the educator is a co-learner and provocateur; they challenge, stimulate and provoke critical thinking.(53) Box 2.5 illustrates Cranton's(53) stages before, during and following transformative learning.

Cranton(53) provides the following guidelines for transformative educators.

- Promote rational discourse. Remember that rational discourse is a fundamental component of transformative learning and part of the process of empowering learners.
- Promote equal participation in discourse. This can be done by stimulating discussion through a provocative incident or controversial statement.
- Develop discourse procedures (e.g. stay on topic, summarise) and avoid using own position to make dismissive statements.

BOX 2.5 Stages of change in transformative learning(53)

Stage of change	Through
Initial learner development	Freedom to participate Comfort Learner decision making
Learner critical self-reflection	Questioning assumptions Consciousness raising Challenging assumptions
Transformative learning	Revision of assumptions Educator support Learner networks Action
Increased empowerment	Critical self-reflection Transformative learning Autonomy

- Develop group facilitation skills (e.g. dominant participant, silent participant).
- Encourage decision making by learners. This can be done by making the process open and explicit.
- Encourage critical self-reflection. This can be accomplished by challenging learners, asking critical questions and proposing discrepancies between learners' experiences and new or conflicting information. To be successful here, a climate of openness and supportiveness needs to be established.
- Consider individual differences among learners. Learners should be assisted in becoming more aware of their own learning styles and preferences. The educator needs to develop a strong awareness of how learners vary in the way they think, act, feel and see possibilities.
- Employ various teaching/learning strategies. Many strategies are effective, for example: role playing (with skilful debriefing), simulations and games, life histories or biographies, exposure to new knowledge, journal writing (with self or others' feedback) and critical incidents arising in the practice setting.

Self-directed Learning

Self-directed, lifelong learning (SDL) is increasingly essential in the development and maintenance of professional competence and is a hallmark of best practice.

Those responsible for professional education, including that of physicians, are challenged to create curricula that ensure the development of these skills and the evaluation methods needed to ascertain their achievement.

The literature on SDL has developed along two overlapping pathways. The first has framed self-direction as a goal towards which individuals strive, reflecting a humanistic orientation such as that described by Maslow(58) and Brockett and Hiemstra.(59) These models imply achievement of a level of self-actualisation, along with the acceptance of personal responsibility for learning, personal autonomy and individual choice.

The second line of development has framed SDL as a method of organising learning and instruction, with the tasks of learning left primarily in the learners' control. Early development included linear models, where learners moved through a series of steps to reach their learning goals (e.g. Knowles(60)). Later models have described the self-directed learning process as more interactive, involving opportunities in the environment, the personal characteristics of learners, cognitive processes, the context of learning and opportunities to validate and confirm self-directed learning collaboratively. Examples of this are seen in several models clearly described by Merriam and Caffarella.(61) This line of development also includes models of instruction such as those of Grow(62) and Hammond and Collins,(63) which present frameworks for integrating self-directed learning into formal educational settings.

Candy(7) has clarified the field of SDL significantly, bringing educators closer to understanding the specific characteristics to identify, develop and evaluate in the self-directed learner. Candy(7) identified approximately 100 traits associated with self-direction, clustered around four dimensions:
- self-directedness, including personal autonomy
- self-management in learning
- learner control of instruction
- the independent pursuit of learning.

Self-directed learning is an integral aspect of several theoretical approaches, including the cognitive, social learning, humanist and constructivist. As noted earlier, the social learning approach views individuals as inherently self-regulating, with self-direction as a natural activity. The humanist approach views self-direction as evidence of higher levels of individual development.

The cognitive perspective recognises the need to build rich, interconnecting knowledge structures, based on existing knowledge, which allow continuing incorporation of new learning. The constructivist perspective recognises the unique personal and social construction of knowledge that occurs in different learners. Self-directed learning elements can also be seen in the ability to learn from experience through critical reflection, which allows learners to identify their personal learning needs and to be aware of, monitor and direct the growth of their knowledge, skills and expertise.

Generally, self-direction is a natural human process that can occur inside or outside of formal settings. SDL does not exclude formal activities such as lectures or courses. It is the learner's choice of activities to meet and manage a particular learning goal that denotes self-direction. A number of factors in the learner and in the environment will affect the learner's ability to be self-directing.

- The learners' view of themselves as learners is also an influencing factor. Learners who view themselves as competent, with the skills to learn in a variety of situations, are more likely to be self-directed and independent.
- Sometimes the demands of the learning situation influence the capacity for self-direction. Where the situation demands that certain (particular) knowledge and skills are non-negotiable, or where the situation requires the learner to reproduce exactly what has been taught, the capacity for self-direction may be obscured.
- Self-direction is, to some degree, a function of subject matter mastery. As the learner builds a base of relevant knowledge and skills, the capacity to be self-directed is enhanced. This basic knowledge is held by some to be essential for effective SDL. For others who promote learning based on activation of prior knowledge, there are few learning situations where the learner is completely lacking relevant knowledge to engage a learning task.
- Much of professional learning is situated learning; that is, the learning is inseparable from the situation in which the knowledge is used. Similarly, professional knowledge and acumen become embedded in practice, and part of the professional's 'knowing-in-action'.(38) Learners may require a cognitive guide and opportunities to participate in their community of practice and the knowledge embedded in it.(60,61)
- Knowledge is also socially constructed, in that it is built from mutually understood perceptions and assumptions. Learners' participation in the social construction of knowledge through discussion and participation provides a cultural basis for their self-direction.
- Knowledge is dependent on context for its meaning, its structure in memory and its availability. Understanding and experience of a broad range of discipline-relevant contexts encourage self-direction in transferring knowledge to other appropriate contexts.

Comprehensive measures of self-directedness are few. Two scales have been used sufficiently to have achieved validation.(64,65) The Self-Directed Learning Readiness Scale (SDLRS) was developed by Gugliemino(64) as a tool to assess the degree to which people perceive themselves as possessing the skills and attitudes conventionally associated with SDL. The Oddi(65) Continuing Learning Inventory is a 26-item scale that purports to identify clusters of personality characteristics that relate to initiative and persistence

in learning over time, through a variety of learning modes.

The ability to self-assess is critical to effective self-directed learning. To properly direct one's ongoing learning, and to assess where and what learning is required, the individual must be able to assess his or her current practice with reasonable accuracy. A recent review of the self-assessment literature suggests that our current understanding of self-assessment is insufficient and that our ability to assess our own performance is limited. Eva and Regehr(66) suggest that accurate self-assessment requires a knowledge of appropriate performance, and of the criteria by which to judge it. They further suggest that several sources of information may be necessary for accurate self-assessment, including feedback from others about one's performance. It is also important to better understand the cognitive, affective and psychomotor bases of self-assessment to effectively promote the development of self-assessment capacity.

A more detailed look at self-assessment and self-regulated learning is provided elsewhere in this book.

Implications for educational practice

There are a number of important implications for curricula, teaching and learning in medical education, all of which are facilitated by the creation of a supportive learning environment where learners feel safe to ask questions and to admit to not understanding. Learners must have the opportunity to develop and practise skills that directly enhance effective SDL. These include competency at asking questions and a critical appraisal of new information.

Learners also need to acquire multiple approaches to learning, along with the ability to decide when each is appropriate. For ongoing SDL, however, *deep learning* skills,(67) which involve understanding principles and concepts, and elaborating the relationships among them, are most likely to support self-direction. Making use of learners' existing knowledge structures, and assisting them to add to and enrich those structures and understand similarities and dissimilarities, encourages the individual to understand his or her knowledge base and to identify gaps. A fundamental skill in self-direction is that of critical reflection on one's own learning and experience. Learners must practise and develop skills at reflecting on all aspects of their learning to determine additional learning needs and to set goals accordingly. Miflin *et al.*(68) describe an attempt to introduce SDL into graduate medical education in a university in Australia. Lack of clarity of what constitutes self-direction forced a reconsideration of the curriculum.

Critical to the achievement of both explicit and implicit curriculum goals is congruence between the goals and the assessment methods.(19) Assessment will invariably drive learning and give the strongest messages to learners about the real goals of the curriculum. Although there are genuine attempts to do otherwise, too frequently assessment methods reward teacher-directed, fact-oriented learning, and do not reward or evaluate the learners' achievement of self-directed learning.

Experiential Learning

Kolb's experiential learning theory(8) is derived from the work of Kurt Lewin,(69) John Dewey(70) and Jean Piaget.(71) Lewin's(69) work in social psychology, group dynamics and action research concluded that learning is best achieved in an environment that considers both concrete experiences and conceptual models.

Dewey(70) constructed guidelines for programmes of experiential learning in higher education. He noted the necessity of integrating the processes of actual experience and education in learning. Piaget's(71) research regarding cognitive development processes constituted the theory of how experience is used to model intelligence. Abstract thinking, including the use of symbols, is closely linked to learners' adaptation to their environment. Thus, Kolb's experiential learning theory is a model of learning based on research in social, educational and cognitive psychology and education.

Kolb's theory can be used as a framework in interpreting and diagnosing individual learners, as well as designing learning environments.(72) Kolb's four learning environments are

- affectively oriented (feeling)
- symbolically oriented (thinking)
- perceptually oriented (watching)
- behaviourally oriented (doing).(73)

Within these environments, grasping and transforming experiences are the two constituent activities of learning tasks.(74) There are two components of the grasping phenomena: concrete experience, which filters directly through the senses, and abstract conceptualisation, which is indirect and symbolic. The transforming experience also consists of two processes: reflection and action. One, or a combination of the four activities (concrete experience, abstract conceptualisation, reflection and action) may be used in learning.(8) Learning is enhanced if students are encouraged to use all four components (*see* Figure 2.2).

This section explores Kolb's learning environments in more depth by presenting practical implications for planners of educational programmes, teachers and learners. Educational formats for delivering experiential learning activities are also included.

Implications for educational practice
Programme planners

There are three major guideposts for directing experiential instructional activities.(75) First, experiential

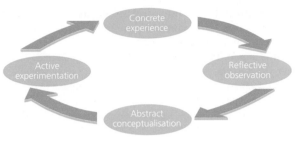

Figure 2.2 Kolb learning cycle.

learning methods and procedures are bridges connecting a learner's existing level of understanding, philosophies, affective characteristics and experiences with a new set of knowledge, abilities, beliefs and values. Second, in experiential learning the learner adopts a more assertive role in assuming responsibility for his or her own learning. This leads to a shift in the power structure from the traditional relationship between teacher and learner. Last, experiential learning involves the transfer of learning from an academic mode to one that involves more practical content.

More specifically, in the affectively oriented environment, learners experience activities as though they were professional practitioners.(8,74) The learner's present values and experience generate information. In the symbolically oriented environment, the learner uses experiences to develop skills or concepts that can provide the right answer or the best solution to a problem.(8,74) The source of information is primarily conceptual. In the perceptually oriented environment, the learner views concepts and relationships from different perspectives.(8,9)

Behaviourally oriented activities focus on specific problems or practices to which learners apply their competencies.(8,76)

Teachers

The roles and actions of teachers depend on the particular learning context.(8,76) In the affectively oriented environment they act as role models and relate to the learner as friendly advisors. They deliver information quickly and tailor it to the needs and objectives of individual learners. Teachers monitor progress by encouraging ongoing discussion and critique without constricting guidelines to inhibit students.

In the symbolically oriented environment: 'The teacher is accepted as a body of knowledge, as well as a timekeeper, taskmaster, and enforcer of events',(8) in order for the learner to reach a solution or a goal.(8,76) Success is compared against the correct or best solution by objective criteria. The teacher provides guidelines regarding terminology and rules.

In the perceptually oriented environment, teachers act as process facilitators, emphasising process rather than solution. They also direct and outline connections between discussions. Learners evaluate answers and define concepts individually. Performance is not measured against rigid criteria but by how well learners use predetermined professional criteria.

In the behaviourally oriented environment, teachers act as mentors and reflect on their background when giving counsel. There are a few guidelines. Learners manage their own time and focus on 'doing'.(8,76) It is essential that the learner complete the task using professional standards.

Learners

In the affectively oriented environment the learner must work with people, be perceptive to encompassing values and feelings, and become engaged in a learning group in a concrete experience.

In the symbolically oriented environment learners study quantitative data to test their theories and postulations.(74,76) Using unique ideas and action plans, learners develop and conceptualise their experiences and models. This relates to the experience of abstract conceptualisation.

The perceptually oriented environment encourages the learner to analyse and manage data with an open mind.(74,76) The learner must learn to see things with a broad point of view, compose complete plans of action and conjecture about the implications of ambiguous circumstances. The learner undergoes the transformative experience of reflective observation by openly approaching the learning activity.

In the behaviourally oriented environment learners must make their own choices in order to locate and exploit potential opportunities, committing themselves to meet predetermined goals and objectives. They are encouraged to adapt to uncertainty and shifting circumstances, and to guide others. This relates to the transforming experience of active experimentation.

Caffarella(75) describes a number of formats for experiential learning activities in medical education in a variety of settings, from practical clinical environments to strictly academic arenas. Depending on the format, the teacher may form a strict regimental relationship with the learner or may foster a caring bond.

Learners along the medical educational continuum use various experiential learning methods. These may include apprenticeship, internship or practicum, mentoring, clinical supervision, on-the-job training, clinics and case study research.

Situated Learning

Situated learning belongs to those theories of learning that have a socio-cultural basis, which view learning and development as occurring via transformation through participation in community activities. Learners transform their understanding, roles and responsibilities as they participate.(9,76,77)

In contrast to some of the theoretical models already discussed, where learning is a one-sided process in which either the teacher or the learner is responsible, situated learning is about *participation*. Learning occurs through collaboration with other learners and more senior community members in carrying out activities with purposes connected explicitly with the history and current practices of the community.(78) New learners enter the community of practice and learn through a process of legitimate peripheral participation in which they perform the less vital tasks of the community. As they take on more responsibility learners move towards the centre. As they participate increasingly in the community's practice they come to understand the particular knowledge that distinguishes that community from others.

A central tenet of situated learning is then that learning occurs through social interaction. Learners acquire knowledge from talk of the community. They also learn to talk to and participate in the community. The community offers a variety of relationships and exemplars from whom to learn, including masters, more advanced apprentices and finished products. Learners learn how masters walk, talk and conduct their lives; observe what other learners are doing and what is needed to become part of the community. Through this participation they learn about the values and shared knowledge and practices of the community. They learn how people in the community 'collaborate, collude and collide, and what they enjoy, dislike, respect and admire'.(78)

For Lave and Wenger, the opportunity to learn around relationships with other apprentices and to observe the masters' (senior practitioners) practice creates the curriculum in the broadest sense. Learners can develop a view of what the whole enterprise is about, and what there is to learn. 'Engaging in practice, rather than its object, may be a condition for the effectiveness of learning'.(78)

What is the *relationship of situated learning to other learning theories*? Situated learning allows a broad view of learning that relates to several other conceptions of learning, both long-standing and more recent.

Situated learning shares with social cognitive theory(4) the view that learning occurs in a dynamic interaction between the learner and the environment. Situated learning suggests that learning is not separate from social influences. The context in which teaching and learning occur is critical to learning itself, and learning is culturally and contextually specific.(79) Learning occurs within social relations and the practices that occur there.

Situated learning also holds that some knowledge related to a task is only present in the context or location of the task. Brown *et al*.(80) described situated cognition and emphasised the idea of cognitive apprenticeship. Cognitive apprenticeship supports learning in a domain by enabling students to acquire, develop and use cognitive tools in authentic domain activity. This happens in practice as teachers guide learners through processes of framing problems and applying disciplinary knowledge to their solution. In the process, teachers provide a scaffold for the learner's development, which can be withdrawn gradually as the learner gains more knowledge and experience.

Situated learning as described by Lave and Wenger(9) extends beyond the acquisition of concepts and structures by the individual and includes all of the learning in the learning environment. It views the community and learning opportunities as a way of structuring learning resources, with pedagogical activity (teaching) as only one resource among many.

Situated learning theory was originally a means for studying the learning that occurs through apprenticeship.(9) Traditionally, apprenticeship has been viewed as a relationship between the master or senior practitioner and the novice or learner. Through apprenticeship, the learner comes to understand the content and process of professional practice. Situated learning provides a way of understanding the process whereby apprentices acquire knowledge and skills through following and attempting to be like the master. In the situated learning model, the apprenticeship is actually to the whole community, and much of the learning occurs in the relationships between people, rather than inside the individual learner's head.

Situated learning also relates closely to notions of informal learning. According to Eraut,(81) informal learning is a significant dimension of the learning that occurs in the course of our work. He suggests that it is implicit, unintended, opportunistic and unstructured, and often occurs in the absence of a teacher. Learning about how things are done, exposure to a variety of different approaches and practical approaches to problems occur daily. There is still much to understand about it; however, the evidence that informal learning and learning from others in the workplace occurs is convincing. This is in contrast to the image of independent learners that is embedded in much of formal medical education.

Informal learning with its corollaries of implicit learning – 'the acquisition of knowledge independent of conscious attempts to learn and in the absence of explicit knowledge about what was learned'(82) – and tacit knowledge – 'that which we know but cannot tell'(83) – will be covered in more detail in the context of the medical apprentice elsewhere in this book.

Situated learning also relates to experiential learning, or learning by doing. Experiential learning has as its goal the integration of conceptual models and concrete experience,(8) and of actual experience and education. Again, situated learning extends the concept to include the experiential learning as occurring within a context. It also extends the notion of experiential learn-

ing beyond the individual learner, as it views the learner as contributing to, and participating in, the shared experience of the community.

In addition to all the above theoretical relationships, situated learning is entirely in keeping with constructivism. Constructivism views learning as a process of active participation in problem solving and critical thinking. Through these processes, learners construct their own knowledge and understanding of the world based on their previous knowledge and experience. Knowledge is integrated into previously existing concepts and schemata, which gradually become richer and more connected.

Postmodern constructivist approaches do not view the locus of knowledge as in the individual. Rather they view learning as a social constructivist process. Learning and understanding are social; cultural activities and tools are essential to conceptual development that will allow learners to develop the skills and standards that are valued by the community.(79) In the context of situated learning, knowledge may be constructed not only individually, but jointly by communities and the individuals who are members.

Implications for educational practice

Situated learning is relevant to medical education in many ways and at all levels of the continuum of education. Apprenticeship remains a pervasive teaching and learning method in physician learning. Learners in undergraduate and postgraduate medical education programmes are assigned to various clinical and community sites where they are immersed, to a greater or lesser degree, in the work of the community, performing minor tasks and striving to learn from the more advanced learners and mentors in the community.

Increasingly, medical and health professional educations are recognised as a process of professional socialisation. Hafferty and Franks (84) articulated the notion of three levels of curriculum as including formal, informal and hidden. The *formal curriculum* represents that which is stated. The *informal curriculum* may include both explicit and serendipitous goals, and is found in the interaction between teachers and learners, and clinical environments, other students, personal interests and goals. Part of the informal curriculum may also be what Hafferty termed the *hidden curriculum*, which may be seen in the practices and routines of the community, particularly in relation to coping and thriving. The hidden curriculum often teaches values and moral judgements, and may be found especially in the institutional policies, language, assessment strategies and allocation of resources of an institution. Clearly, these curricula all exist and are enacted in the context of situated learning in medicine. Not all messages of the hidden curriculum are negative. Both negative and positive aspects have been described. Often these are unintentionally imparted through actions, discussions and relationships among members of the community. This relates the notion of situated learning closely to role modelling, as the senior members of the community enact through their behaviours, both tacitly and explicitly, how problems of the discipline are approached, how colleagues are regarded and how knowledge is built.

When learners are involved in clinical placements, participation in the actual daily round of activities is important in enhancing the effectiveness of their learning. Clearly, the longer the engagement in a community, the greater the opportunity to participate meaningfully. Where attachments are short, learners may remain at the periphery and feel little participation in the community. Special attention may be needed to identify how their participation can been sured and enhanced.

Faculty (teachers) enact several roles concurrently. As in the perspective of social learning theory, they are modelling skills, knowledge, values and attitudes that learners observe, along with how those actions are received in the community.

Beyond role modelling, faculty are also demonstrating how knowledge is built, understood and how practices evolve. This aspect of talk offers both challenges and advantages.

Learners who participate in and listen to the talk of the community are able to learn in a contextualised way. However, the nature and content of the talk become important considerations. As teachers, we need to be mindful of our talk, and open to reflecting on it with learners. Learning through observation is also vulnerable to misunderstanding, as learners will interpret what they observe in light of their current experience and understanding.(85) It is important to find opportunities and demonstrate willingness to discuss and reflect on experience with learners.

Participation in the work of the clinical site or community is a key to this understanding of learning. Situated learning suggests that all members of the community are involved. In the case of medical education this means that more senior learners and other health professionals can all enhance the learners' participation.

Different fields of medicine have distinct knowledge and skill bases. However, there will still be some aspects that are common to all, including communication with patients, ethical approaches and grounding of actions, basic clinical skills, etc., in which learners can participate across their fields of experience As faculty, we need to think carefully about how we can promote participation among learners.

Building on the advantage of situated learning, we have the opportunity to rethink our students' experience and consider all the ways we have available to promote their learning. However, this involves thinking of learners as part of our learning environment, rather than as temporary adjuncts to it.

Communities of Practice

Lave and Wenger(9) first proposed the term *community of practice* (CoP) to capture the importance of activity in integrating individuals within a community, and of a community in legitimising individual practices. Within this context, they described a trajectory in which learners move from legitimate peripheral participant to full participation in the CoP. The concept of legitimate peripheral participation means that access to a CoP, its resources and activities provides a means for newcomers to learn through observation and gradually deepen their relationship to the CoP. Barab *et al.*(86) defined a CoP as 'a persistent, sustaining social network of individuals who share and develop an overlapping knowledge base, set of beliefs, values, history and experiences focused on a common practice and/or mutual enterprise'.

Wenger(10) proposed three constituent parts of a CoP: *mutual engagement, joint enterprise* and a *shared repertoire*. Mutual engagement involves both work-related and socio-cultural activities, achieved by interaction, shared tasks and opportunities for peripheral participation. Joint enterprise refers to the need for the group to respond to a mandate for itself, and not simply an external mandate. Finally, a shared repertoire involves the 'routines, words, tools, ways of doing things, stories, gestures, symbols, genres, actions or concepts that the community has adopted in the course of its existence'.(10) Wenger(10) summarised his conceptual framework for a social theory of learning comprising four components that are 'deeply interconnected and mutually defining'. All of these should be present in a true CoP. The components include the following:

- *Meaning* – learning as experience. Members talk about their experience and create shared meaning.
- *Practice* – learning as doing. Members talk about the shared ideas and resources that can sustain action.
- *Community* – learning as belonging. Members talk about the community process and how they are learning and developing competence.
- *Identity* – learning as becoming. Members talk about how learning changes who they are.

Therefore, we can see that the concept of a CoP is complex and multidimensional, serving multiple purposes both for individuals and the subcommunities that participate in the full community.

The primary purpose of CoPs is knowledge translation. Knowledge translation has been defined as 'the exchange, synthesis and ethically sound application of knowledge – within a complex system of interactions among researchers and users – to accelerate the capture of the benefits of research … through improved health, more effective services and products, and a strengthened health care system'(87) .

More recently, other terms have been proposed for essentially the same broad concept. These terms include knowledge mobilisation,(88) knowledge utilisation,(89) knowledge exchange,(90) knowledge management(91) and knowledge brokering,(92) all of which involve an active exchange of information among various stakeholders, such as researchers, healthcare providers, policy makers, administrators, private sector organisations, patient groups and the general public. Partnerships are at the heart of all knowledge translation activity,(87) and effective knowledge translation is dependent on meaningful exchanges among network members for the purpose of using the most timely and relevant evidence-based, or experience-based, information for practice or decision making.

In the field of continuing medical education, the limitations of traditional workshop/presentation models are becoming apparent.(93) It is now recognised that there is a need for continuous learning to occur in the context of the workplace, and for reflection-in-practice and reflection-on-practice to be supported.(5) Knowledge translation is essential to shortening the path from evidence to application of that evidence in practice, and CoPs provide an opportunity to embed learning within a clinical context. A highly effective way to learn about complex issues is through experience, application and discussion with mentors and peers in the same or similar contexts. Relevant learning occurs when the participants in the CoP raise questions or perceive a need for new knowledge. Using Internet technology enables these discussions to occur in a timely manner, and records of these can be archived for later review or by those who missed the discussion.

There are a number of key factors that influence the development, functioning and maintenance of CoPs.(94) The legitimacy of the initial membership is important. Commitment to the desired goals of the CoP, relevance to members and enthusiasm about the potential of the CoP to have an impact on practice are also key. On the practical side, a strong infrastructure and resources, such as good information technology, useful library resources, databases and human support, are essential attributes.

Skill in accessing and appraising the knowledge sources is important, as is the skill in bridging this knowledge to practice. Providing the above-mentioned key factors requires strong, committed and flexible leaders who can help guide the natural evolution of the CoP. If professional learning is to flourish, it is critical that a blame-free culture is established in which community members can learn from positive and negative experiences.(95)

Some writers have outlined some key questions to address in establishing a CoP.(96)
- How will the community be formed and evolve?
- nd when will members join?
- do members do and how will they interact?
- .... will the CoP be supported by the members' organisation(s)?

- What value will members and their organisations receive?

Others have suggested principles for cultivating CoPs.(97) CoPs are dynamic entities and need to be designed for adaptability and large growth. They should combine the perspectives of both insider members and outsider participants, and all members should be valued regardless of their level of participation. Both public and private spaces are necessary and need to be related. A critical principle is that the CoP must provide value to its members, otherwise participation will be minimal or absent. Although familiarity is important, challenge and excitement need to be provided to keep the energy high. Finally, CoPs have a rhythm they need to settle into, one that works for its members (*see* Box 2.6).

Virtual communities of practice

Virtual (online) communities play a socialisation role to the same extent as real communities do.(98) The theoretical foundation of virtual communities is based on social cognitive theory and situated learning. Henri and Pudelko(98) have proposed three components of the social context of activity in virtual communities – the goal of the community, the methods of initial group creation, and the temporal evolution of both the goals and the methods of the group – leading to the development of four different types of community. Figure 2.3 illustrates that a CoP requires a highly cohesive group with a clear goal.

Box 2.7 dissects the characteristics of these four types of community further. It demonstrates that although many types of virtual community can exist, they may not be true CoPs. The virtual CoP generally arises from an existing, face-to-face CoP in which professional practice is developed through sharing

---

BOX 2.6 Factors for success of a community of practice

Lave and Wenger(9) suggest that the success of community of practice depends on five factors:

- the existence and sharing by the community of a common goal
- the existence and use of knowledge to achieve that goal
- the nature and importance of relationships formed among community members
- the relationships between the community and those outside it
- the relationship between the work of the community and the value of the activity

Wenger(10) later added the idea that achieving the shared goals of the community requires a shared repertoire of common resources, e.g, language, stories and practices.

knowledge among members. Through this interaction, new practices may be developed and identification with the community can occur.

Some writers have distinguished 'soft' from 'hard' knowledge.(99) Soft knowledge can be gathered in a domain through sharing solutions to a particularly difficult problem, describing idiosyncrasies of particular tools, equipment or processes, and recounting and reflecting on challenging events (i.e. recounting war stories). This refers to the implicit or tacit knowledge in a domain. CoPs are central to the creation and maintenance of soft knowledge. Hard knowledge, in contrast, is stored in databases and documents. It is highly explicit and codified. A key question is whether a virtual CoP can effectively share soft knowledge, which tends to be situated in specific contexts. This is a question that requires further research.

Virtual CoPs are a recent phenomenon, and studies on their effectiveness to enhance learning have not yet

been carried out. Parboosingh(100) advocates conducting evaluation studies that focus on how the CoP takes advantage of the technology, rather than how the technology affects the CoP.

Implications for educational practice

This chapter integrates the concepts of knowledge translation and CoPs. These ideas have many obvious applications in the medical education arena, and a number of these CoPs are emerging in various specialties. The application outlined in this section is a CoP for palliative care practitioners and students. This is an excellent application because palliative care is a truly interdisciplinary field that involves subcommunities of various specialties, including oncologists, family physicians, nurses and social workers. These subcommunities need to interact in CoPs, but the various professional groups also need to interact with each other around specific topics and cases. This provides an excellent model for continuing medical education, and also provides an environment for training residents, interns and medical students. Since many participants are acquiring and applying new knowledge in this field, scaffolding learners through an evolving continuum from simulation to participation to codetermined interactions is an effective instructional approach.(101) For example, family physicians, residents and nurses who have trained with oncology specialists may begin with simulated cases. They then learn to participate in real cases supported by learning materials and/or clinicians until they are able to operate as full participants. The scaffolding process proposed here uses a staged approach for bridging from a learner (knowledge) identity to a participant (practitioner) identity. This approach is consistent with the constructivist(102) view of learning that espouses the learner as central in the educational process. The advantages of the situated learning

Figure 2.3 Different forms of virtual communities of practice according to their context of emergence. Adapted from Henri and Pudelko(98) (p. 476).

BOX 2.7 Principal descriptors of the four types of virtual communities (adapted from Henri and Pudelko)(98, p. 485)

	Community of interest	Goal-oriented community	Learning community	Community of practice
Purpose	Gathering around a common topic of interest	Created to carry out a specific task	Pedagogical activity proposed by the instructor	Stems from an existing, real community
Activity	Information exchange	Sharing of diverse perspectives and production of objects commissioned by the mandate	Participation in discussions of collective topics	Professional practice development through sharing knowledge among members
Learning	Knowledge construction for individual use	Knowledge construction from diverse knowledge systems towards collective use	Knowledge construction by carrying out social situated activities	Appropriation of new practices and development of involvement

approach over the traditional didactic approach are discussed above in the section on situated learning.

A CoP implemented in a community-based learning environment could include specialist and non-specialist practitioners in palliative care, as well as residents and medical students (clerks). It would aspire to achieve a number of different aims, based on the challenges by Richardson and Cooper.(103)

- Engage all trainees in a research culture (i.e. encourage evidence-based practice).
- Provide an opportunity for participants to identify with their peers and supervisors.
- Encourage cross-site discussion to explore shared theory, methodological and practical issues.
- Provide a forum for discussion and a recognised channel for communication and collaboration.
- Facilitate high-quality supervision to ensure adequate access to teaching and learning for all practitioners.
- Foster scholarly interaction and good supervisory practice to stimulate dialogue among students and supervisors across sites.

We are asserting that linking medical students, their community preceptors and medical school specialists in an online CoP can greatly enhance the learning and practice experience of all participants. A recent study(104) demonstrated that students assigned to community practices for their paediatric clerkship perform as well as, or better than, students assigned to academic medical centres in written examinations. An online CoP approach can build on this positive finding and perhaps provide an even more effective community experience for medical students. A side benefit could be the improvement in teaching and supervisory methods used by their preceptors.

Connections

In this paper, we have presented eight theoretical approaches to learning, each of which has the potential to inform our practice as educators. Fo reach theoretical approach we have set out the underlying framework and principles and provided examples of its application. The application of educational theory to practice has always been somewhat eclectic. This is not unusual in applied sciences such as education. To make this exposition of theory as useful as possible to our educational practice, it is helpful to consider the relationships among the theoretical frameworks, and the consistency of messages and themes that can be drawn from all of them to inform teaching and learning. Some of these common themes are presented here.

All theoretical frameworks view the learner as an active contributor in the learning process. In each of the theoretical approaches discussed here the learner actively interacts with a changing, complex environment. The curriculum can no longer be viewed as something that is transmitted to, or acts upon, the students, be they undergraduate, postgraduate or practising physicians. There is an important element of human agency. Moreover, in practice, the physician-learner is stimulated to learn through interactions in the practice environment.

The entire context of learning is more important than any one variable alone. The learning environment is complex. It includes learners, faculty, patients, colleagues, resources and other workers. It is both the interacting and the independent effect of all these variables that result in the learning environment, whatever the level of learner. Learning is accomplished both through direct experience and vicariously, and from many interactions in this complex system. Consequently, we must analyse as many factors in the environment as possible when planning, implementing and evaluating our educational programmes. In learning from practice, physicians solve complex problems that occur in the environment of the patient, family, physician and community. All of these influence the effectiveness, nature and outcomes of learning.

Learning is integrally related to the solution and understanding of real-life problems. For adult learners, learning is most effective and motivating when it is relevant to the solution of real-life needs or problems. This is obvious in the learning that occurs in reflective practice, where the new learning is triggered by the surprise encountered in a problem in practice. Experiential learning in real-life problems leads to ongoing mastery and competence. Similarly, learning around clinical problems, both in the clinic and in the classroom, represents learning to solve the authentic tasks of the profession and of future professional practice.

Individuals' past experience and knowledge are critical in learning, in actions and in acquiring new knowledge. At all levels, learning must be connected to relevant experience, or compatible with the learner's existing knowledge. Past experience and knowledge will affect perceptions of self-efficacy, which will, in turn, affect the choice of new experiences and goals. Learners' past experience is important in providing a framework for acquisition of new knowledge. In practice, the new learning opportunities identified will depend substantially on the individual's existing experience and knowledge.

Learners' values, attitudes and beliefs influence their learning and actions, and building learners' self-awareness in this area is important for their development. These values, attitudes and beliefs are central to learners' willingness to attempt new actions. They affect virtually everything that learners think, as well as their interactions with mentors, peers and patients. Various processes exist to modify these, such as reflective observation, perspective transformation, role modelling and feedback on action.

Individuals as learners are capable of self-regulation, that is, of setting goals, planning strategies and evaluating their progress. Adult learners are viewed as self-motivated and directed, pursuing those learning objectives relevant to personal goals. They are inherently self-regulating, and the process of reflection implies a learning that arises directly out of experience. In planning learning experiences we must regard these not as skills we have to teach students, but as skills and abilities that need to be developed and enhanced.

The ability to reflect on one's practice (performance) is critical to lifelong, self-directed learning. At the heart of all these theoretical approaches is the belief that we can learn from our experience, incorporating it into our existing knowledge and skills. This opportunity for reflection requires an early introduction to a systematic approach to facilitate reflection. Reflection is not merely description of experience, but analysis of it. It is not a natural and intuitive ability, and it must be developed through practice. It is critical to becoming an effective lifelong learner, as it also enables learners to develop and apply standards to their performance, decide what further learning needs to occur, and continue their learning over a professional lifetime.

Applying these theories to medical education requires practice. Medical educators need to acquire and study relevant literature to better understand these theories, and to participate in a community of peers who have a common interest in this area. Through the process of practising the application of each theory, receiving feedback from learners and peer observers, and reflecting-on-practice, medical educators will continue to improve in their teaching role.

Acknowledgement

We would like to acknowledge Dr Penny Jennett in the Faculty of Medicine of the University of Calgary for her co-authorship of a previous ASME monograph on which this chapter is based.

References

1 Tripp D (1993) *Critical Incidents in Teaching. Developing Professional Judgement.* Routledge, London.

2 Knowles M (1973) *The Adult Learner: a neglected species.* Gulf Publishing, Houston, TX.

3 Knowles MS (1980) *The Modern Practice of Adult Education.: from pedagogy to andragogy (2e).* Cambridge Books, New York.

4 Bandura A (1986) *Social Foundations of Thought and Action. A Social Cognitive Theory.* Prentice-Hall, Englewood Cliffs, NJ.

5 Schön DA (1983) *The Reflective Practitioner: how professionals think in action,* pp. 57–60. Basic Books, New York.

6 Mezirow J (1994) Understanding transformation theory. *Adult Education Quarterly.* **44**(4): 222–44.

7 Candy PC (1991) *Self-direction in Lifelong Learning.* Jossey-Bass, San Francisco, CA.

8 Kolb DA (1984) *Experiential Learning: experience as the source of learning and development.* Prentice Hall, Englewood Cliffs, NJ.

9 Lave J and Wenger E (1991) *Situated Learning: legitimate peripheral participation.* Cambridge University Press, New York.

10 Wenger E (1998) *Communities of Practice: learning, meaning, and identity.* Cambridge University Press, New York.

11 Selman G and Dampier P (1990) *The Foundations of Adult Education in Canada.* Thompson Educational Publishing, Toronto.

12 Hallenbeck W (1960) The function and place of adult education in American society. In: Knowledges MS (ed.) *Handbook of Adult Education in the United States,* pp. 29–38. Adult Education Association of the USA, Chicago.

13 Verner C and Booth A (1964) *Adult Education.* Centre for Applied Research in Education, New York.

14 Jarvis P (1985) *The Sociology of Adult and Continuing Education.* Croom Helm, London.

15 Darkenwald G and Merriam SB (1982). *Adult Education: foundations o f practice.* Harper & Row, New York, pp. 43–64.

16 Merriam SB (1987) Adult learning and theory building: a review. *Adult Education Quarterly.* **37**(4): 187–98.

17 Cross KP (1981) *Adults as Learners.* Jossey-Bass, San Francisco, CA.

18 Knox AB (1980) Proficiency theory of adult learning. *Contemporary Educational Psychology.* **5**: 378–404.

19 McClusky HY (1970) *An approach to a differential psychology of the adult potential.* In: Grabowski SM (ed.) *Adult Learning and Instruction,* pp. 80–95. ERIC Clearinghouse on Adult Education, Syracuse, NY.

20 Mezirow J (1981) A critical theory of adult learning and education. *Adult Education.* **32**: 3–27.

21 Freire P (1970) *Pedagogy of the Oppressed.* Herder and Herder, New York.

22 Merriam SB and Caffarella RS (1991) *Learning in Adulthood: a comprehensive guide.* Jossey-Bass, San Francisco, CA.

23 Knowles MS *et al.* (1984) *Andragogy in Action: applying modern principles of adult learning.* Jossey-Bass, San Francisco, CA.

24 Maslow AH (1970) *Motivation and Personality (2e).* Harper & Row, New York.

25 Rogers C (1968) *Freedom to Learn.* Charles E Merrill, Columbus, OH.

26 Brookfield S (1986) *Understanding and Facilitating Adult Learning.* Jossey- Bass, San Francisco, CA.

27 Bard R (1984) Foreword. In: Knowles MS and Associates (eds) *Andragogy in Action,* p. xi. Jossey-Bass, San Francisco, CA.

28 Hartree A (1981) Malcolm Knowles' theory of andragogy: a critique. *International Journal of Lifelong Education.* **3**(3): 203–10.

29 Merriam SB (1996) Updating our knowledge of adult learning. *Journal of Continuing Education in the Health Professions.* **16**(3): 136–43.

30 Resnick LB (1987) Learning in school and out. *Educational Researcher.* **16**: 13–20.

31 Zemke R and Zemke S (1981) 30 things we know for sure about adult learning. *Training.* **18**: 45–9.

32 Bandura A (1977) *Social Learning Theory.* Prentice-Hall, Englewood Cliffs, NJ.

33 Bandura A (1982) Self-efficacy mechanism in human agency. *American Psychologist.* **37**: 112–47.

34 Carr W and Kemmis S (1983) *Becoming Critical: knowing through action research.* Deakin University Press, Geelong, Victoria.

35 Al-Shehri A, Stanley I and Thomas P (1993) Continuing education for general practice. Systematic learning from experience. *British Journal of General Practice.* **43**: 249–53.

36 Moon J (1999) *Reflection in Learning and Professional Development.* Kogan Page, London.

37 Clift R, Houst WR and Pugach M (eds) (1990) *Encouraging Reflective Practice in Education: an analysis of issues and programs.* Teachers College Press, New York.

38 Schön DA (1987) *Educating the Reflective Practitioner: toward a new design for teaching and learning in the professions.* Jossey-Bass, San Francisco, CA.

39 Schön DA (1995) The new scholarship requires a new epistemology. *Change.* **27**(6): 26–34.

40 Shapiro J and Talbot Y (1991) Applying the concept of the reflective practitioner to understanding and teaching family medicine. *Family Medicine.* **23**(6): 450–6.

41 Slotnick HB (1996) How doctors learn: the role of clinical problems across the medical school-to-practice continuum. *Academic Medicine.* **71**(1): 28–34.

42 Crandall S (1993) How expert clinical educators teach what they know. *Journal of Continuing Education in the Health Professions.* **13**: 85–98.

43 Boud D, Keogh R and Walker D (eds) (1985) *Reflection: turning experience into learning.* Kogan Page, London.

44 Atkins S and Murphy K (1993) Reflection: a review of the literature. *Journal of Advanced Nursing.* **18**(8): 1188.

45 Jennett PA, Lockyer JM, Maes W, Parboosingh IJ and Lawson D (1990) Providing relevant information on rural practitioners: a study of a medical information system. *Teaching and Learning in Medicine.* **2**(4): 200–4.

46 Lockyer J, Gondocz ST and Thivierge RL (2004) Knowledge translation: the role and place of practice reflection. *Journal of Continuing Education in the Health Professions.* **24**: 50–6.

47 Palmer A, Burns S and Bulman C (eds) (1994) *Reflective Practice in Nursing: the growth of the professional practitioner.* Blackwell Scientific Publications, Oxford.

48 Mezirow J (1991) *Transformative Dimensions of Adult Learning.* Jossey-Bass, San Francisco, CA. and academia. *Journal of Continuing Education in the Health Professions* **10**(3): 237–43.

49 Lockyer J, Woloschuk W, Hayden A, McCombs B and Toews J (1994) Faculty perceptions of their role as consultants to practising physicians. *Academic Medicine.* **69**(10): S13–15.

50 Beecher A, Lindemann J, Morzinski J and Simpson D (1997) Use of the educator's portfolio to stimulate reflective practice among medical educators. *Teaching and Learning in Medicine.* **9**(1): 56–9.

51 Mezirow J *et al.* (1990) *Fostering Critical Reflection in Adulthood.* Jossey-Bass, San Francisco, CA.

52 Jennett PA, Parboosingh IJ, Maes WR, Lockyer JM and Lawson D (1990) A medical information networking system between practitioners

53 Cranton P (1994) *Understanding and Promoting Transformative Learning: a guide for educators of adults.* Jossey-Bass, San Francisco, CA.

54 Parboosingh J (1996) Learning portfolios: potential to assist health professionals with self-directed learning. *Journal of Continuing Education in the Health Professions.* **16**(2): 75–81.

55 Westberg J and Jason H (2001) *Fostering Reflection and Providing Feedback. Helping Others Learn from Experience.* Springer Series on Medical Education. Springer, New York.

56 Moon J (2004) Using reflective learning to improve the impact of short courses and workshops. *Journal of Continuing Education in the Health Professions.* **24**: 4–11.

57 Brookfield SD (1990) *The Skillful Teacher: on technique, trust and responsiveness in the classroom.* Jossey-Bass, San Francisco, CA.

58 Maslow AH (1968) *Toward a Psychology of Being (2e).* Van Nostrand Reinhold, New York.

59 Brockett RG and Hiemstra R (1991) *Self-direction in Adult Learning: perspectives on theory, research and practice.* Routledge, New York.

60 Knowles MS (1975) *Self-directed Learning: a guide for learners and teachers.* Association Press, New York.

61 Merriam SB and Caffarella RS (1999) *Learning in Adulthood (2e).* Jossey-Bass, San Francisco, CA.

62 Grow G (1991) Teaching learners to be self-directed: a stage approach. *Adult Education Quarterly.* **41**(3): 125–49.

63 Hammond M and Collins R (1991) *Self-directed Learning: critical practice.* Nichols/GP Publishing, New York.

64 Gugliemino LM (1977) Development of the self-directed learning readiness scale. Unpublished doctoral dissertation. University of Georgia, Athens, GA.

65 Oddi LF (1986) Development and validation of an instrument to identify self-directed continuing learners. *Adult Education Quarterly.* **36**(2): 97–107.

66 Eva KW and Regehr G (2005) Self-assessment in the health professions: are formulation and research agenda. *Academic Medicine.* **80**: 547–54.

67 Entwistle N and Ramsden R (1983) *Understanding Student Learning.* Croom Helm, London.

68 Miflin B, Campbell CB and Price DA (1999) A lesson from the introduction of a problem-based graduate entry course: the effects and different views of self-direction. *Medical Education.* **33**: 801–7.

69 Lewin K (1951) *Field Theory in Social Sciences.* Harper & Row, New York.

70 Dewey J (1938) *Experience and Education.* Kappa Delta Phi. Touchstone, New York.

71 Piaget J (1971) *Psychology and Epistemology.* Penguin Books, Harmondsworth.

72 Holzer SM and Andruet RH (1998) A multimedia workshop learning environment for statics. Virginia Polytechnic Institute and State University, Blacksburg, VA. Workshop presented at ASEE Conference and Exposition, Seattle, WA.

73 Lee P and Caffarella (1994) Methods and techniques for engaging learners in experiential learning activities. In: Jackson L and Cala RS (eds) *New Directions for Adult and Continuing Education 62,* pp. 43–54. Jossey-Bass, San Francisco, CA.

74 Fry R and Kolb B (1979) Experiential learning theory and learning experiences in liberal arts education. *New Directions for Experiential Learning.* **6**: 79–92.

75 Caffarella RS (1992) *Psychological Development of Women: linkages to the practice of teaching and learning in adult education.* ERIC Clearinghouse on Adult, Career and Vocational Education, Columbus, OH.

76 Rogoff B, Matusov E and White C (1996) Models of teaching and learning: participation in a community of learners. In: Olsen DR and Torrance N (eds) *The Handbook of Education and Human Development: New Models of Learning, Teaching, and Schooling,* pp. 388–415. Blackwell, Oxford.

77 Rogoff B (2003) *The Cultural Nature of Human Development.* Oxford University Press, New York.

78 Lave J and Wenger E (2002) Legitimate peripheral participation in communities of practice. In: Harrison R, Reeve F, Hanson A and Clarke J (eds) *Supporting Lifelong Learning. Perspectives on Learning,* pp. 1111–26. RoutledgeFarmer, London.

79 Palinscar AS (1998) Social constructivist perspectives on teaching and learning. *Annual Review of Psychology.* **49**: 345–75.

80 Brown JS, Collins A and Duguid P (1989) Situated cognition and the culture of learning. *Educational Researcher.* **18**: 32–42.

81 Eraut M (2000) Non-formal learning and tacit knowledge in professional work. *British Journal of Educational Psychology.* **70**: 113–36.

82 Reber A (1995) *Implicit Learning and Tacit Knowledge: an essay on the cognitive unconscious.* Oxford University Press, New York.

83 Polyani M (1958) *Personal Knowledge: towards a post-critical philosophy.* Routledge and Kegan Paul, London.

84 Hafferty F and Franks R (1994) The hidden curriculum, ethics teaching and the structure of medical education. *Academic Medicine.* **69**: 861–71.

85 Coulehan J and Williams PC (2001) Vanquishing virtue: the impact of medical education. *Academic Medicine.* **76**: 598–605.

86 Barab SA, Barnett M and Squire K (2002) Developing an empirical account of a community of practice: characterizing the essential tensions. *The Journal of the Learning Sciences.* **11**(4): 489–542.

87 Canadian Institutes of Health Research (CIHR) (2004) *Knowledge Translation Strategy: 2004–2009: innovation in action.* CIHR, Ottawa.

88 Social Sciences and Humanities Research Council (SSHRC) (2006) Knowledge mobilization – the transfer, dissemination, and use of human sciences knowledge. In: *SSHRC Department Performance Report 2004–05.* SSHRC, Ottawa (http://www.tbs-sct.gc.ca/rma/dpr1/04-05/SSHRC-CRSHC/SSHRC-CRSHCd4504_e.asp; accessed 29 October 2006).

89 Caplan N (1978) The two communities theory and knowledge utilization. *American Behavioral Scientist.* **22**: 459–70.

90 Oftek E and Sarvary M (2002) Knowledge exchange and knowledge creation: should the emphasis shift in a competitive environment. INSEAD working paper.

91 WHO (2006) Bridging the 'know–do' gap in global health (http://www.who.int/kms/en/; accessed 6 October 2006).

92 Canadian Health Services Research Foundation (CHSRF) (2003) *The Theory and Practice of Knowledge Brokering in Canada's Health System.* A report based on a CHSRF consultation and a literature review. CHSRF, Ottawa.

93 Davis DA, Thomson MA, Oxman AD and Haynes RB (1992) Evidence for the effectiveness of CME. A review of 50 randomized controlled trials. *Journal of the American Medical Association.* **268**: 1111–17.

94 Lathlean J and LeMay A (2002) Communities of practice: an opportunity for interagency working. *Journal of Clinical Nursing.* **11**: 394–8.

95 Triggs P and John P (2004) From transaction to transformation: information and communication technology, professional development and the formation of communities of practice. *Journal of Computer Assisted Learning.* **20**: 426–39.

96 Millen DR, Fontaine MA and Muller MJ (2002) Understanding the benefits and costs of communities of practice. *Communications of the ACM.* **45**(4): 69–73.

97 Wenger E, McDermott R and Snyder W (2002) *Cultivating Communities of Practice: a guide to managing knowledge.* Harvard Business School Press, Boston, MA.

98 Henri F and Pudelko B (2003) Understanding and analyzing activity and learning in virtual communities. *Journal of Computer-Assisted Learning.* **19**: 474–87.

99 Kimble C, Hildreth P and Wright P (2001) Communities of practice: going virtual. In: Malhotra Y (ed.) *Knowledge Management and Business Model Innovation*, pp. 220–34. Idea Group Publishing, Hershey, PA, London.

100 Parboosingh JT (2002) Physician communities of practice: where learning and practice are inseparable. *Journal of Continuing Education in the Health Professions.* **22**: 230–6.

101 Hung D and Tan SC (2004) Bridging between practice fields and real communities through instructional technology. *International Journal of Instructional Media.* **31**(2): 1–8.

102 Vygotsky LS (1978) *Mind in Society: the development of higher psychological processes.* Harvard University Press, Cambridge, MA.

103 Richardson B and Cooper N (2003) Developing a virtual interdisciplinary research community in higher education. *Journal of Interprofessional Care.* **17**(2): 173–82.

104 White CB and Thomas AM (2004) Students assigned to community practices for their pediatric clerkship perform as well or better on written examinations as students assigned to academic medical centers. *Teaching and Learning in Medicine.* **16**(3): 250–4.

Problem-based learning

Mark A Albanese

KEY MESSAGES

- Problem-based learning (PBL) has become one of the dominant forms of medical education in the world.
- Universal features of PBL:
  - a patient problem serving as the stimulus for learning
  - small group instruction, usually between six and eight students per group
  - instructors serving as facilitators/tutors.
- PBL problems are critical to the process and need to meet specific criteria.
- PBL facilitators/tutors need to be instructed in how to fulfil their role.
- PBL requires planning for physical and instructional resources to be available.
- Recent implementations of PBL curricula show a trend towards hybridisation, with lectures providing cognitive scaffolding for basic sciences in support of PBL.

- Implementation of PBL in the clinical years can homogenise the experience to meet competencies, but care should be exercised that it does not supplant patient contact.
- Assessments of PBL have been fraught with methodological problems; however, PBL has generally shown high student satisfaction, high faculty satisfaction, and a trend towards improved clinical knowledge and functioning.
- Recent assessments of PBL have suggested that hybrid curricula produce increases in performance in both the basic science and clinical years in the order of a small to medium effect size. There is also evidence that there may be a differential effect in which some students who have performed relatively poorly in previous schooling do well, and those who have done well in the past do relatively poorly, indicating that there may be a need to tailor instruction to students' needs.

What Is Problem-based Learning?

Problem-based learning (PBL) began at McMaster University, when it opened in 1969. In designing the curriculum for the newly opened university, the originators borrowed heavily from different disciplines, including case studies from business.(1) Howard Barrows and Victor Neufeld both came to McMaster in 1970, an event that would lead to the two being largely responsible for PBL being exported throughout the world. In an effort to clarify what exactly PBL is, Barrows published a taxonomy of PBL in 1986.(2) This taxonomy was anchored at one end by what has been called case-based learning, in which a completely digested patient case is presented by an instructor, and at the other end by what Barrows refers to as reiterative PBL.

PBL can be characterised as an instructional method that uses patient problems as a context for students to acquire knowledge about the basic and clinical sciences. 'The basic outline of the PBL process is: encountering the problem first, problem-solving with clinical

reasoning skills and identifying learning needs in an interactive process, self-study, applying newly gained knowledge to the problem, and summarizing what has been learned'(3) (p. 15.) In Barrows' original reiterative form, the PBL process concludes with students evaluating the information resources they used and then analysing how they might have better managed the patient problem. In recent years, other methods of PBL have been developed, and the Maastricht 7-Step method,(4) a 'how to do it' list of instructions to the tutor and student, has become increasingly popular (*see* Box 3.1).

In reiterative PBL:

- The process begins with a patient problem. Resources accompanying the problem included detailed objectives, print materials (originally primarily book chapters), audiovisual resources (originally slide-tape shows), multiple-choice self-assessment exercises and resource faculty.
- Students work in small groups, sometimes called tutorial groups. Six to eight students per group are often recommended.
- The small groups are moderated by one or more faculty facilitators (sometimes called tutors).
- Students determine their own learning needs to address the problem, make assignments to each other to obtain necessary information, and then

Understanding Medical Education: Evidence, Theory and Practice. Edited by T Swanwick. © 2010 Association for the Study of Medical Education.

BOX 3.1 How to: Organise a PBL tutorial using the Maastricht 7-step method(4)

Step 1: Identify and clarify unfamiliar terms presented in the scenario; scribe lists those that remain unexplained after discussion.

Step 2: Define the problem or problems to be discussed; students may have different views on the issues, but all should be considered; scribe records a list of agreed problems.

Step 3: 'Brainstorming' session to discuss the problem(s), suggesting possible explanations on the basis of prior knowledge; students draw on each other's knowledge and identify area of incomplete knowledge; scribe records all discussion.

Step 4: Review Steps 2 and 3 and arrange explanations into tentative solutions; scribe organises the explanations and restructures if necessary.

Step 5: Formulate learning objectives; group reaches consensus on the learning objectives; tutor ensures learning objectives are focused, achievable, comprehensive and appropriate.

Step 6: Private study (all students gather information related to each learning objective).

Step 7: Group shares results of private study (students identify their learning resources and share their results); tutor checks learning and may assess the group.

return to report what they have learnt and continue with the problem. This happens repeatedly as students secure more information and keep probing deeper into the problem.

- Students return for a final debriefing and analyse the approach they took after receiving feedback on their case report.
- Student evaluation occurs in a small group session and is derived from input from self, peers and facilitators.

There are many derivatives of these approaches that have been used and called PBL. Dolmans *et al.*(5) indicate, 'Although PBL differs in various schools, three characteristics can be considered as essential: problems as a stimulus for learning, tutors as facilitators and group work as stimulus for interaction' (p. 735). While, the 'McMaster Philosophy' had three key features,

- self-directed learning
- PBL
- small group tutorial learning,

the only characteristic that cuts across all of what has passed as PBL is that learning is based on a patient problem. While purists probably consider such variations on PBL to be corruptions of the basic PBL process, I think it is important to explore how the various elements of PBL continue to make the learning experience

valuable. Who knows, we may ultimately find that the only thing that is really important is for learning to be structured around patient cases and that the small-group elements and facilitating tutors are incidental. However, it will take time and creative research to determine how these differing elements of PBL interact to achieve the goals of PBL.

Problems

Characteristics of problems

There are seven qualities required of an appropriate PBL problem. It should:

- present a common problem that graduates would be expected to be able to handle, and be prototypical of that problem
- be serious or potentially serious – where appropriate management might affect the outcome
- have implications for prevention
- provide interdisciplinary input and cover a broad content area
- lead to an encounter of faculty members' objectives
- present an actual (concrete) task
- have a degree of complexity appropriate for the students' prior knowledge.(6)

The structure or format of the problem, sometimes called a case, provides room for a lot of variability. It can range from brief paragraphs describing a symptom or set of symptoms (e.g. chest pain), to elaborate paper or computer simulations or even the use of simulated patients. It can be relatively unorganised, unsynthesised and open-ended, a form that Barrows(2) suggests promotes the application of clinical reasoning skills, structuring of knowledge in useful contexts and the development of self-directed learning, and will also be more motivating. One example of this type of format is the Problem-based Learning Modules (PBLMs), a specialised written simulation that provides flexibility for students to pursue almost unlimited types of enquiry. There are other forms that provide more structure. The Focal Problem, developed at Michigan State, for example, starts with a written narrative of a clinical problem as it unfolds in a real-life setting. In this design, after descriptions of significant developments occur, 'stop and think' questions are inserted for students to ponder. This approach helps students to focus on the steps in the decision-making process used in solving problems that may have more than one viable solution.(7–9) These varied problem designs and computer-based variants may all have a role at some point in a PBL curriculum. More structured formats might be better placed early in the curriculum when students will be challenged by even the simplest clinical scenarios, while the less structured formats may be more effective after students gain clinical experience and comfort with the PBL method. However, this recommendation is based more on theory and intuition than on any specific research.

Sources of problems

There are a number of resources from which PBL cases can be obtained. MedEdPORTAL is a resource developed by the Association of American Medical Colleges (www.aamc.org/mededportal) as a repository of peer-reviewed materials for medical education, facilitating the dissemination of educational scholarship. Cases submitted for review are evaluated by peers for their quality, and contact information is made available in a searchable database. Anyone interested in using a case can then contact the authors to work out an arrangement for using the case.

The PBLMs described earlier are available from Southern Illinois University (http://www.pbli.org/shopping/pblms.htm). PBLMs are actual patient cases in a book format that permits free enquiry. The learner can ask the patient any question in any sequence and get the patient's response, and perform any item of the physical examination in any sequence and learn the result as in the real clinical situation. Any laboratory and diagnostic test can be ordered in any sequence as well. Whatever can be done with the real-life patient in terms of history taking, physical examination and the ordering of laboratory tests can be done with the PBLM. A separate 'User's Guide' provided with each PBLM can be used with any of the PBLMs in the series and provides the key for free enquiry. There is also a section in the PBLM that allows learners to follow the course of the patient under the care of the physicians responsible for the actual case. PBLMs are copyrighted and cannot be reproduced. The Tutorial Process Videotape set demonstrates the proper use of a PBLM in a tutorial group.

There is also the Health Education Assets Library (HEAL; http://www.healcentral.org), which is a repository of peer-reviewed materials for medical education, facilitating the dissemination of educational scholarship. HEAL is a collaborative university-based project started in 2000 by three universities. It is committed to open access to high-quality resources in perpetuity worldwide and to sharing developed tools in an open source environment.

Problem selection issues

In a PBL curriculum, the problems are the central feature of the curriculum. It is essential that the problems provide a developmentally appropriate sequence that addresses key skills and abilities that lead students to developing competence. Any given case can address a multitude of objectives besides the medical content, such as population health, epidemiology, communication skills, health literacy, spousal abuse and prevention. The challenge is to ensure that the cases meet their stated objectives and that the pathway that students take through the case invariably leads to

their achieving the case objectives. This is more difficult to achieve than one might think. Hays[10] warns of biases in PBL problems towards more acute problems in the younger age groups, urban healthcare and dominant culture issues. He further elaborates that many problems that have objectives pertaining to rural health describe poor healthcare in rural settings and patients having to be rescued by clinicians in large teaching hospitals. In addition, objectives addressing the healthcare of indigenous peoples often illustrate dominant culture stereotypes. These biases can work at cross-purposes to the desired objectives from which they were drawn.

In addition to the biases that can creep into the cases themselves, it is difficult to ensure that all student groups achieve the objectives of the cases, particularly for cases that are relatively unstructured. The gain in student independence and development of self-directed learning skills with progressively less-structured cases must be balanced by the potential for students to miss dealing with some of the anticipated objectives of a case. Research on whether students achieve case objectives shows variable results. Dolmans *et al.*[11] found that 62% of faculty-generated objectives were definitely identified by the 12 tutorial groups they studied. Coulson and Osborne[12] analysed learning issues identified by students in PBL groups and compared them with learning objectives that faculty deemed essential. Groups identified an average of 61% of the essential learning objectives.

One additional issue related to problems is their use in the clinical years. One would expect that a patient would be the best possible PBL problem. However, there has been an increasing trend towards introducing formal PBL tutorial groups into the clinical years. The merits of having such formal PBL tutorial groups in the clinical years are not altogether clear. Dornan *et al.*[13] conducted interviews with 14 general physicians after the University of Manchester extended PBL tutorial groups into the clinical years. The physician comments are poignant as they describe the loss of student excitement in clinical discovery that has accompanied the students' preoccupation with their PBL cases. From a non-physician perspective, it would seem a tragedy if PBL were to supplant readily available clinical mentoring by seasoned physicians. However, this type of instruction is becoming increasingly difficult to provide. Clinicians' comments about the wards included: 'falling numbers of beds, shorter lengths of stay, changing work patterns, pressure on staff and a narrower range of "material" were seen as constraints' (p. 167). The outpatient realm fared little better, with comments that dealt with space constraints, work pressure, productivity targets, patient expectations and the time-cost of teaching. As the clinical environment appears to be increasingly hostile to teaching, PBL may need to be the fallback to maintain clinical education at a reasonable level of quality. This may be especially true if medical education continues to progress towards competency-based education and students will need to demonstrate core skills that may not be reliably obtained during the general course of clinical education.

Facilitators/Tutors

Selection and training of facilitators
Selection
In the original McMaster PBL curriculum, Neville and Norman state that tutors were not required to have any particular content expertise other than that contained in the tutorial guides. This was a conscious choice because it was believed that content experts would be unable to resist the temptation to lecture to the students, thereby short-circuiting the student's opportunity to apply the knowledge that they might have to address the biomedical problems contained in the tutorial. Miflin(14) argues that given the norms of the time when PBL originated, tutors were expected to be physicians and general medical expertise was an unstated assumption underlying the qualifications of tutors. In subsequent research, several studies found better learning outcomes if the facilitator/tutor had content expertise.(15,16) Zeitz and Paul(17) argue that these two studies were experiments in PBL in a larger, traditional curriculum and that the learners were novices regarding PBL. In their experience, when novices 'first attempt problem-based learning, the outcomes are better if the faculty facilitators are content "experts"'. However, after one to two months, students enrolled in a PBL curriculum are so acculturated and so highly skilled in student-centred, self-directed learning that they are no longer so dependent on the facilitator. Zeitz and Paul further argue that in practice it is not feasible for facilitators to be content experts for all problems that they will facilitate. What they have found is that facilitators need to develop 'case expertness' by facilitating the case between three and five times. I would argue that what we need to determine is not whether tutors need to be content experts, but what is the minimum content expertise and group facilitation expertise needed for tutors to be effective.(18) As far as what is needed regarding tutor expertise is concerned, I think the title of Miflin's article summarises our current understanding: 'Problem-based learning: the confusion continues'.

Training
Facilitators need to be given specific guidelines about how they are to interact with students. Moving from content expert to facilitator is not necessarily natural for many faculty members, so practising the role during training will be helpful. The use of 'standardised' students, a group of people who are trained to act like students, can make the practice closer to the real thing than it might otherwise be. However, it can be expensive and the fidelity of the simulation to real life may be difficult to maintain.

Facilitators should also be given all information about the case and any associated reading or materials that students will be given, as well as materials that will allow them to guide students in their search for knowledge. This includes the 'next steps' that students are expected to take. Anything that can help facilitators reach the case expertness described by Zeitz and Paul (17) more quickly is useful.

Facilitators also need to be prepared for students' reaction to the experience. If students are used to having faculty members serving as content deliverers, rather than facilitators, the transition to this type of relationship can be rocky. Initially, facilitators need to be prepared for students responding to their answering questions with questions by giving them a look that says, 'I pay X zillion dollars for this education, the least you can do is answer my question.' Over time, students learn that the facilitator is not there simply to answer their questions, but early on it can be a difficult adjustment for both students and facilitators.

Bowman and Hughes(19) use a clinical psychology framework and the similarity between PBL and small groups in clinical psychology to argue that PBL may be susceptible to the regressive and task-avoiding behaviours seen in clinical psychology groups. They cite four shared characteristics that can promote these problems: extended contact time (often more than six hours per week), non-directive role of tutor that facilitates uncertainty, the unpredictable nature of group process and the potential intimacy of PBL. While these characteristics may induce undesirable behaviour in students, Bowman and Hughes argue that the facilitator is also susceptible. To avoid tutor problems (wanting to be 'one of the gang', liked by students, in control, subverting the primary task with a new agenda, having a relationship with a student), training and follow-up should provide the following, according to Bowman and Hughes:
- clear statements of the primary task of PBL tutors
- clear boundaries on the staff role and availability
- ongoing review and monitoring of tutor work
- social activities that are friendly but not intimate.

They argue for establishing monthly supervision, peer observation and mentoring for all PBL tutors.

How many facilitators per group?
The number of facilitators needed per group has not really been studied in a controlled manner, but there are practical considerations that lead to the conclusion that more than one will stretch facilitator resources pretty thin. There have been studies that examined the impact of having fewer than one facilitator per group. Farrell *et al.*(20) explored the use of a single facilitator who circulated among four groups, each of which had

from three to four students in an ophthalmology section for second-year medical students. The authors found improvements in learning that were comparable to those made by students who had a more traditional ophthalmology experience, and high student satisfaction as well. Khaliq(21) reported substantial increases in student satisfaction ratings after introducing problem-solving exercises into lectures. In the problem-based course on public health for first-year medical students at the University of Wisconsin, we used two facilitators rotating among five groups (this was replicated with five different sets of facilitators and student groups). Each facilitator pair was composed of a methodologist and a clinical epidemiologist. The ability of the facilitators to discuss issues relative to their own experience base seemed to be synergistic, but there was substantial variability among the five different replications.

Small Groups

Optimal size
Recommendations for optimal group size tend to be anecdotal. Dr David Matheson, a member of the PBL Best Practices Consortium (see Acknowledgements for details), offers the suggestion that 'groups should contain no more than seven members and no fewer than five. More than seven results in too many opportunities for reluctant members to hide. Fewer than five puts the spotlight on members permanently and removes much of the opportunity for "think" time.' Another member of the Consortium, Dr Gail Swarm, states, 'We have groups here that range from six to eight students. Having groups of seven students really seems to be a "magical" number.'

A search of Pubmed using the terms 'PBL' and 'small-group size' yielded no hits, so I can offer no more than the additional recommendation that group sizes over 10 are no longer small.(6) Also, an even number of group members will make it more difficult to obtain a majority vote than will an odd number. Depending on whether or not one thinks that negotiating one's way out of tied votes is a skill worth promoting, this may or may not be desirable. There may be literature from business, counselling or psychiatry that could provide more insight into optimal small-group sizes for problem-solving exercises, but I will leave that to others.

Composition
The groups should be composed of students, of course, but what varieties? They come in many different shapes and sizes. Generally, I would recommend randomisation, but stratified according to gender and academic ability. Also, students who are 'couples', especially if married, should be assigned to different groups because having them in the same group has a high likelihood of disrupting the desired group dynamics.

Randomisation can do some unusual things, which is why statisticians acknowledge that error (usually 5%) is a possibility in any given statistical test. So, for things that may impact on group functioning, I would recommend 'improving on chance' by ensuring their representation is consistent with that of the larger group. If there are 50% females in the class, I would suggest identifying those groups that do not have equal numbers of males and females and evening them out.

I recommend stratifying by academic ability because it has been shown to have a very lasting impact on physician careers. Gonnella *et al.*(22) followed graduates of Jefferson Medical College who were in deciles based on first-year medical school grades into residency. They found a linear trend indicating that academically low performers were much less likely to thrive by various criteria. I would suggest stratifying so the groups are balanced in their representation by three levels of ability: bottom 25%, middle 50% and top 25%. There are a number of challenges to stratifying by academic ability in a PBL curriculum. First, it may not be possible to determine who is in the bottom 25%, let alone at other levels of performance, by the grading methods that are used in a PBL curriculum. For example, if a pass/fail grading system is used, it is almost impossible to determine who is in the bottom 25%. Barring direct academic measures in medical school, I would recommend using admissions test performance. In the US, the Medical College Admissions Test (MCAT) can be used, as it has been shown to correlate relatively strongly with performance in medical school ($r \approx 0.60$).(23) Scores that average below 8 (the national mean of all who take the test and a point about one standard deviation below the mean for all those who are actually admitted to medical school) on the primary subtests (biological and physical sciences and verbal reasoning) can serve as a reasonable substitute. For non-North American schools, admissions test performance that puts the students one or more standard deviations below the mean of admits can be used.

Structure (role assignments)
It has become increasingly clear that just throwing a group of students together with a problem is not necessarily going to yield something useful. Guidelines and role assignments are often recommended to help students make a start on how to organise themselves to do productive work. Barrows(3) (pp. 60, 61) recommends that students assume three separate administrative roles to make the process work smoothly:
• PBL module reader
• action master list handler
• recorder.
In the context Barrows was describing, students were working through what they called PBL modules. They

were also instructed to formulate action lists. So, Barrows recommends having one student in the role of module reader, another handling the list of actions that need to be taken and a third who is a general recorder of activities.

David Matheson states, 'While it may be true that the world is run by those who turn up [Woody Allen], attendance at PBL sessions has to be mandatory to avoid group erosion and to underline the seriousness of the enterprise. Groups need rules and standards of acceptable behaviour. I have tried groups without rules, groups with minimal rules [such as be considerate of others] and all sorts of variations in between. In the end, each such group has decided to set out basic norms of acceptable behaviour comprising of, for example, when interruption is permitted, the attitudes towards latecomers, whether eating was allowed during a session, what to do if the tasks for the day were completed before time was out and so on. Importantly, these rules work best when generated by the group.'

Technology is also becoming a problem for small-group management and may interfere with problem solving. Dr Stephen Davis, another member of the PBL Best Practices Consortium, provides a number of recommendations regarding ground rules for technology use, which are summarised in Box 3.2.

Time management

Dr Dennis Baker, another member of the consortium, notes, 'It has been my experience that when students identify learning issues the learning issues are stated in very general terms which can lead to learning inefficiencies and additionally when the students come back together to discuss the learning issues the discussion of them can be lengthy and unfocused.' PBL adherents may not consider this type of situation to be necessarily bad, but simply the stage that students need to go through to become effective problem solvers. It may also be that the facilitator should play a role in helping the students to see that their learning issues may not be sufficiently well delineated to yield productive searches. However, if it persists and students do not seem to be making progress in delineating clearer and more specific learning issues, the facilitator should take a more assertive role in pointing out the elements of the learning issues that are unclear before allowing students to go off on their independent assignments.

The facilitator should assist the groups by noting the time and pointing out how much progress needs to be made before they finish. This role should actually be taken over by the students themselves as they become more skilled in working in small groups. However, there may be some value in having a formally appointed timekeeper role if it becomes apparent that discussion gets out of control and the group continually runs over the allotted time.

Resources

Space requirement

David Matheson recommends that rooms be dedicated to PBL and used only by an individual group. 'This helps create a sense of group cohesion and gives the group a place to call "home".' However, dedicated space in today's crowded health sciences learning centres can be hard to come by. As schools respond to the anticipated shortage of physicians by increasing class sizes, they will be even more hard-pressed to supply dedicated space for PBL groups. While it is not hard to see how dedicated space would be a desirable feature, it is not necessarily clear that the lack of dedicated space will have detrimental effects on student learning.

Computing resources

Matheson suggests that rooms need at least two networked computers to allow groups to access internet resources. He further recommends that the room should be Wi-Fi enabled so that anyone who wishes to can use the network via a laptop. However, the use of technology can have its drawbacks. Kerfoot *et al.*(24) noted that a large plasma screen monitor with internet access distracted students from engaging in problem solving as they searched the Internet for answers to questions. Thus, care needs to be exercised so problem-solving exercises do not devolve into

---

> ### BOX 3.2 How to: Deal with information technology
>
> - Discussion is still supreme (as opposed to reading off a screen).
> - Laptop work must be related to the group's tasks (no personal email, chat or other surfing/playing).
> - System should be used for sharing information.
> - Scribe should control the technology for the session.
> - Wrap-up should include evaluation of how the technology is being used.
> - Group agrees on what they believe is appropriate use.
> - Give immediate feedback if technology is being used inappropriately.
> - Agree that it is not appropriate to look up work that should have been prepared.
> - Purpose of technology is to enhance group effectiveness.
> - Quick look-ups allowed ≤60 seconds.
> - Single, group-only computer – no individual users.
> - Add a spot for this in the facilitator evaluation of students (appropriate use of technology).
> *http://oucom.ohiou.edu/fd/group_ground_rules.htm*

students using small-group time to look for answers on the Web.

Instructional resources

A well-stocked library is an important need for students in a PBL curriculum. Nolte(25) found that library use of reserve books increased 20-fold after introducing a PBL course on neurobiology into the curriculum. With the more recent advent of the Internet and online references, having internet access is essential. Literature search software such as Pubmed is critical. Having general web-searching capability with software such as Google and Ask Jeeves will be useful for looking for non-library references including policy statements and current events. However, as Kerfoot *et al.* noted, there need to be guidelines for internet usage to avoid having the problem-solving process subverted by web searches.

Whiteboards and blackboards are also beneficial. Some schools have adopted electronic blackboards that enable electronic capturing of the material students write on the board.

Lectures can be an instructional resource, but Barrows recommends limiting them to 1–1.5 hours per day(3) (p. 46). Barrows also recommends that basic science research staff should be a resource available to meet with students for 4–6 hours per week(3) (p. 50).

With new learners, there is a danger of having too many resource options. Students can get bogged down looking for information and give too little attention to problem solving, a problem similar to the one that Kerfoot *et al.* noted with plasma screen computer access to the Web.

Creature comforts

The instructional environment in the small group should be informal and as low-stress as possible. Lighting should be sufficient to see all types of educational resources that will be shared. The environment (chairs) should be comfortable, but not so comfortable as to make it difficult for students to stay awake. Students should be able to bring food and drink into the meeting room. Ready access to a refrigerator and even microwave helps make the room comfortable. David Matheson recommends having access to such things as a kettle, cups and teaspoons. If possible, it is desirable for each PBL group to have its own dedicated room where they can leave things out knowing that they will not be disturbed before the next time they meet.

Standardised patients

As early as 1973, Barrows and Tamblyn reported using standardised patients for both teaching and assessing students in PBL groups.(26) When learning communication skills and physical examination skills, it can be especially useful to have standardised patients who

can meet with PBL groups. Depending on the goals of the session, patients may need to be coached in the art of teaching and in the components of the examination that are being learnt. In cases where the goal is simply to give students an opportunity to work through the history and physical examination with a 'real' person, there may not be the need for such extensive training. However, it should be clear what the purpose of the session is in the determination of the training/skill needs of the standardised patients when the session is being scheduled. Generally, standardised patients are expensive to deploy and their use should be carefully considered in relation to the benefits derived. Patient involvement in medical education is discussed in detail in Chapter 13.

Organisation and Grading

Administration and governance

According to Barrows,(3) PBL is most compatible with what has been called an organ-based curriculum, in which courses are aligned with different organs of the body. Thus, a course on the cardiovascular system would have the anatomy, physiology, biochemistry and so on, of the system all integrated. Because patient problems are often localised to a single organ system, it seems logical that PBL would be consistent with an organ-based curriculum.

However, organising staff for organ-system teaching and PBL can be difficult because most medical schools are organised around discipline-based departments (e.g. pathology, anatomy, surgery). Interdisciplinary collaboration can be difficult to sustain in a disciplinary-based medical school because it cuts across the organisational structure of the medical school, thereby requiring extra resources to sustain (effort to contact people who are at greater distances, travel to meetings outside the department, more people to share academic credit with, less return on effort, etc.). Thus, while there is the excitement and energy of developing new organ-based curricula and PBL when a new dean arrives and marshals resources for the new curriculum, maintenance when the 'newness' wears off and resources are needed for other pressing matters is a challenge (this has been recognised as a problem for interdisciplinary research efforts).

Some newer medical schools in the US are organising themselves differently from what has traditionally been the case. For example, Florida State University, a recently opened medical school with a PBL curriculum, has organised itself around five departments that can be considered interdisciplinary: biomedical sciences; medical humanities and social sciences; clinical sciences; geriatrics; and family medicine and rural health. The University of New Mexico School of Medicine, another school with a PBL curriculum, has grouped its biological sciences into five departments: biochemistry and molecular biology; cell biology and physiology; molecular genetics/microbiology; neurosciences; and pathology. Organ-based curricula and PBL require interdisciplinary collaboration to be most effective. The interdisciplinary structure of these departments is more likely to sustain an organ system and PBL curriculum in the face of administrative changes and budget reductions because they require fewer resources to maintain than is the case in a medical school with discipline-based departments.

Programme evaluation

It is desirable to have both formative and summative evaluation processes in place. Formative evaluation is timed to identify and resolve small problems before they become big problems. Summative evaluations are designed to assess how effective the total learning experience has been.

For formative evaluation purposes, Barrows(3) recommends that the course coordinator meets weekly with groups. One of the advantages of modern technology is the ability of students to report issues as they occur through either email or posting to a web site. Students should be encouraged to report issues that are detracting from their learning experience as early as possible. Confidentiality should be assured because the PBL process is such a personal one that any criticisms can be misinterpreted or taken very personally. This becomes especially problematic with formative evaluation because it occurs while the PBL process is still in progress.

Summative evaluation relies on information that is generally collected after the completion of the learning experience. The goal is to determine the effectiveness of the experience. Student ratings are the most commonly used summative evaluation data. Students' success in achieving programme goals and objectives can also be a source of information. For PBL curricula in the preclinical years, ratings of preceptors in the clinical years have been useful. For entire curricula, the ratings of graduates and the residency supervisors of the graduates have also been useful. Performance on objective examinations, especially external ones such as the United States Medical Licensing Examination (USMLE) Step exams in the US, can also serve as summative evidence. However, they have been criticised as being not very sensitive to the types of skills that PBL is attempting to develop. Generally, one is better off using a range of different types of data to evaluate a programme and PBL is no different. Each type of data that one collects generally has its own weaknesses, but in aggregate the weaknesses can be mitigated. Over the past 15 years, the effectiveness of PBL has been the subject of at least eight separate literature reviews with somewhat controversial results. I will return to this in the final section when I deal with the impact of PBL.

Grading systems

Grading students in PBL offers challenges because there is the desire for collaborative learning among students. If the grading system is not properly designed, it can work at cross-purposes to this goal. In particular, if grading is competitive, with a fixed quota for the highest grades (e.g. reserve honours grades for the highest 16%), students may be unwilling to help other students for fear that they would disadvantage themselves. There is also the component of PBL that has students working in groups and producing reports that are group work. Distinguishing individual performance in this type of activity is difficult and generally imprecise. A pass/fail grading system is most compatible with these elements of PBL. However, many staff and students believe that a pass/fail grading system does not provide the motivation for, or recognition of, achieving excellence. To recognise excellence, an honours grade beyond pass is sometimes added. The other concern is that staff appear to be loathe to award failing grades. To distinguish poorer performance in a way that staff appear to be more likely to use, a marginal or low pass grade is sometimes used as a buffer between fail and pass. Which system to use depends on the goals and aspirations of the school and the proclivities of its staff. The good thing is that if the grading system does not work, it can always be changed.

Student Evaluation

Evaluating student performance in PBL is challenging; it would take an entire separate publication to treat it adequately. Here, I give a brief overview of selected methods that have been used. For each, I describe the method and briefly note its major strengths and weaknesses. For readers who are interested in more detailed descriptions of methods used to evaluate students in PBL, I refer you to Nendaz and Tekian,(27) and for an excellent reference on how to write test items and an analysis of the strengths and weaknesses of various approaches to student assessment, I recommend a free online manual.(28)

Multiple-choice exams

The use of multiple-choice examinations, including true/false and the extended matching variety, is common because of the ease of scoring. Writing multiple-choice questions that are appropriate for PBL, however, presents a formidable challenge and one that some would argue is not possible. Generally, there is no better way of covering a breadth of content more efficiently. Whether multiple-choice tests can assess the content at the level of problem solving that PBL is designed to promote is an open question. There are those who believe that well-written multiple-choice questions are capable of assessing these problem-solving skills, and there are those who believe otherwise. At the very least, writing such sophisticated questions is a very complex skill, one that is unlikely to be particularly prevalent among the staff who are generally tasked to do this at the typical medical school.

That said, there is a form of multiple-choice examination that has been relatively widely used to assess PBL. The Progress Test has been used at the University of Maastricht since the early 1980s.(29) A version was adopted at McMaster University in 1992. A Progress Test reflects the end objectives of the curriculum and samples knowledge across all disciplines and content areas relevant for the medical degree. The Maastricht exam was composed of 250 true/false questions, while the McMaster exam contained 180 multiple-choice questions. At Maastricht the Progress Test is administered four times per year to all students in the medical school, while McMaster administers its test three times per year to all students. The Maastricht Progress Test has been found to have a strong correlation with a test on clinical reasoning (r = 0.93).(30) The McMaster version of the Progress Test was submitted to an extensive psychometric analysis and showed test–retest reliabilities over successive administrations ranging from 0.53 to 0.64, and predictive validity of the cumulative score was approximately 0.60.(31)

The main problem with a Progress Test is that it is inefficient. What I mean by inefficient is that neophyte examinees spend a lot of time answering questions the answers to which they can only hope to guess at (advanced clinical questions), and advanced examinees spend a lot of time answering questions that are too primitive for them (they answer them correctly with little thought needed). Measurement specialists prefer to administer relatively short tests that are appropriate for the learner's level and then scale the results to place the learner on an ability continuum. This, however, requires relatively advanced measurement methods (e.g. Item–Response Theory), lots of data and fairly sophisticated technical support. If the Progress Test is the only major knowledge evaluation taking up students' time in the curriculum, some inefficiency is probably acceptable.

Short-answer questions

Using a PBL scenario and then having students write their response at various stages of what would be the PBL process has the potential for being effective in assessing aspects of PBL, probably with less challenge than with the multiple-choice type question. Getting students to give answers to how they would respond in the first stage of the PBL process should be relatively easy to do in this format. After the first stage, however, it becomes more complicated. Should students' responses to the first stage be used in subsequent stages? If so, the answers will be idiosyncratic for each student and grading them objectively becomes exceedingly challenging. Also, if a student does poorly in an

earlier stage, their later responses may be wrong, but correct given what they did earlier. Should they be given full credit, partial credit or no credit for these later answers? Generally, it is not good practice to have items that are linked in this manner. The answers to the questions are not independent and weighting them properly becomes problematic. A way around the linkage would be to provide a standard set of student choices for earlier stages, and ask the student to indicate what they would do now. This avoids the lack-of-independence problem but introduces an element of artificiality into the process. Some students would not have taken the earlier route through the case, and that makes it difficult for them to take the case from that point forward. Clearly, there are challenges in using short-answer questions to mirror the PBL process. Using short-answer as opposed to supplying the alternatives in a multiple-choice question solves the potential for students to get the answer correct by guessing, but does so with substantial added costs for grading.

Essay and modified essay questions

Essay questions provide the least structure and have the potential to offer insight into the thought processes underlying students' choices when confronted with a patient problem. However, a student who is not very skilled at writing essays could appear to be less accomplished than they are simply because they do not write well. Saunders *et al.*(32) describe what they call modified essay questions. Each modified essay question covered nine areas of primarily internal medicine content. Each area was scored as fail, pass or good answer/above average. The advantage of the essay-type questions is in their relative ease of construction. The disadvantage is in their complexity and time necessary for scoring. Achieving reliable scores among graders is a major challenge, not to mention getting the essays graded in a timely manner.

Simulations

Simulations in medical education were first described by McGuire and Babbott in 1967.(33) At that time, technology involved the use of latent image pens that uncovered answers printed on paper that were only able to be disclosed by the use of the fluid contained in the pens. Unfortunately, such technology ended relatively abruptly in the late 1970s; urban rumour has it that the fluid was found to be a carcinogen. However, computers picked up where the 'carcinogen' left off, and today computer simulations are quite sophisticated. The USMLE Step 3 exam uses computer simulations as part of its assessment. In a PBL simulation, a student is presented with a case and after giving it consideration, they indicate the next steps to be taken. The computer then shows the results of these actions. This proceeds until the designated end point of the simulation is reached. Some simulations end with the diagnosis, others end with management of the patient until the problem resolves itself or the virtual patient dies.

Computer simulations, the most likely ones to be encountered today, are complex and expensive to create. Grading student choices can also be complex if it must take into account every choice a student makes in working through what may be a complex process. Some simulations get around this problem by grading according to whether the desired end point is reached and not whether the desired route is taken to reach the end point. Other simulations are interested in the process that is taken as well as whether the end point is reached. These are the most complex simulations to grade.

Triple jump exercise

The primary goal of a triple jump exercise is to assess clinical problem-solving and self-directed learning skills. In a triple jump exercise, students discuss a written clinical scenario and identify the related learning goals, review the learning materials individually, and return to present their conclusions and judge their own performances. Students sometimes have 3 hours to complete their exercise, sometimes a week. This type of assessment is often used for formative evaluation purposes. It is less used for grading purposes because it is time-consuming, limiting the number of scenarios that can be evaluated, and as a result scores tend to be contextually bound to the specific problem assessed. I personally think the name choice is unfortunate because it is too close to the negative term 'jumping through hoops' – thrice.

Objective Structured Clinical Exams

Objective Structured Clinical Examinations (OSCE)s are performance-based examinations in which students rotate from station to station.(34) Stations often use standardised patients, computer simulations, literature search facilities, manikins and other types of 'hands-on' experience. The strengths of the OSCE are its face validity and standardised clinical experience for all examinees. There are relatively few other ways of assessing complex skills and abilities such as communication skills with the same degree of standardisation and reliability. The primary limitation of the OSCE pertains to its cost. It requires substantial infrastructure to administer: personnel to recruit, train and manage standardised patients and facilities. For a more detailed discussion of the OSCE, see Chapter 17.

Peer evaluations

Peer evaluation has a certain appeal because it is what clinicians do on a daily basis in practice. For students, however, they are still learning the profession and what it means to be a professional. They may be competing with one another for grades, accolades and residency positions. Peer evaluation can have a markedly disruptive effect on group dynamics. Care should be taken if peer evaluation is to be used for grading students, particularly if the group is to reconvene after an assessment episode.

Facilitator evaluations

Facilitator ratings of students are often used in PBL. Because the facilitator is present for the small-group meetings and can observe the interactions that occur, they can provide a unique perspective on each of the students' contributions. With time, the facilitator tends to adopt an increasingly less prominent role as students become more skilled in managing their own activities. This provides the facilitator with even more opportunity to observe and evaluate the contributions of different students to the group work. However, making the facilitator evaluation a major factor in grading can be disruptive to the dynamics of the PBL groups as students posture for the facilitator.

Self-evaluations

One of the goals of PBL is to develop self-directed learning skills in students. A key component of achieving this goal is the ability to accurately assess one's strengths and weaknesses and identify ways to address one's weaknesses. Self-assessment is then a key to achieving self-directed learning skills. However, it is not clear if anyone is really good at doing this. Studies of self-assessment have demonstrated that poor performers tend to overestimate their performance and high performers tend to underestimate their performance.(35,36) Such tendencies are fairly pervasive across skills. As a consequence, using self-assessments in grading may penalise the high performers and give undeserved increases in grades to the poorest performers (lowest 25%). While self-assessment is a good activity for students to experience, it should be used with great care in assigning grades.

The Theoretical Basis for Problem-based Learning

The concept of contextual learning is often used to support PBL. The basic premise is that when we learn material in the context of how it will be used, it promotes learning and the ability to use the information. In PBL, the problem is usually portrayed in the real-life context of a patient coming to visit a doctor or some variation. Colliver(37) criticises the contextual learning argument on the grounds that it was drawn from a weak research finding and that almost all clinical education occurs in the contextually relevant process of patient care. However, other theories provide more compelling support.

Information-processing theory

Information-processing theory has been argued to underlie PBL.(38) This theory involves: prior-knowledge activation, encoding specificity and elaboration of knowledge. Prior-knowledge activation refers to students using knowledge they already possess to understand and structure new information. Encoding specificity refers to transfer of learning being more likely to occur when the situation in which something is learnt more closely resembles the situation in which it will be applied. Elaboration of knowledge refers to information being better understood and remembered if there is opportunity for elaboration (discussion, answering questions, etc.). These three elements are commonly a part of PBL. They also have relatively strong documentation from the larger education and psychology literature. That encoding specificity incorporates most of the salient features of contextual learning theory suggests that information processing theory provides a more comprehensive and parsimonious basis of theoretical support for PBL than does contextual learning theory alone.

Cooperative learning

Cooperative learning is another concept that supports PBL. Cooperative learning situations are those where individuals perceive that they can reach their goals if and only if the other group members also do so. The small group format used in PBL often fits this definition. Qin *et al.*(39) conducted a meta-analysis of studies assessing the effect of cooperative versus competitive learning on problem solving. Cooperation was operationally defined by the presence of joint goals, mutual rewards, shared resources and complementary roles among members of a group. Competitive learning situations were those where individuals perceived that they can reach their goals if and only if the other participants cannot attain their goals. Competition was operationally defined by the presence of a goal or reward that only one or a few group members could achieve by outperforming the others. Problem solving was defined by situations that required participants to form a cognitive representation of a task, plan a procedure for solving it, execute the procedure and check the results. Their study spanned the 20th century. The authors concluded that overall, 'co-operation resulted in higher-quality problem solving than did competition'. One possible reason for the success of cooperative learning is that it enables material to better mesh with students' level of cognitive development. In cooperative efforts, learners exchanged ideas and corrected each other's errors more frequently and effectively than did individuals competing with each other. It is possible that students who are struggling to understand the material are more likely to be able to identify the sources of other students' misunderstandings than is the expert instructor.

Self-determination theory

Self-determination theory distinguishes between two types of motivating conditions: controlled and autonomous.(40) Controlled motivators are termed maladaptive and include external demands and contingencies as well as 'introjected regulation', which are internalised contingencies about what they 'should' do. These are all accompanied by either explicit or implicit rewards or punishments, or in the case of the introjected regulation, what they term 'intrapsychic' or internal representations of rewards and punishments (self-aggrandisement and self-derogation). Under controlled forms of motivation, people act with a sense of pressure and anxiety. In educational situations, this takes the form of learning that is rote, short-lived, and poorly integrated into students' long-term values and skills. It does not take much of a leap to infer that many traditional curricula are steeped in controlled forms of motivation. Autonomous motivators are those personally endorsed by the learner and reflect what the individual finds interesting and important. They include learners engaging in an activity simply because it is interesting and enjoyable, as well as situations in which the learner has identified with its value for functioning as a physician. In contrast to the external element of the rewards and punishments administered in controlled motivating conditions, autonomous motivation involves behaving with a sense of volition, agency and choice. Williams *et al.*(40) cite research which has demonstrated that, relative to controlled motivation, autonomous motivation for learning promotes greater conceptual understanding, better academic performance, higher academic achievement, stronger feelings of competence, enhanced creativity, a preference for optimal challenge over easy success, more positive feelings while learning, a tendency to cope more positively with failures and setbacks, greater persistence and better psychological adjustment.

A learning climate that promotes autonomous motivators includes one in which educators take the perspectives of students into account, provide relevant information and opportunities for choice, and encourage students to accept more responsibility for their own learning and behaviour. It also includes teachers being meaningfully involved in students' learning through dialogue, listening, asking students what they want, providing satisfying rather than superficial replies to student-generated questions, providing information and advice, and suspending judgement when soliciting the opinions and reactions of students. Such an environment minimises pressure and control while encouraging a high level of performance. Clearly, autonomous motivators can be employed in either a PBL or a traditional curriculum. However, autonomous motivators would seem to be especially compatible with collaborative learning environments. Furthermore, PBL would seem to be an easier fit with autonomous motivators than would be the traditional curriculum.

Control theory(41)

Control theory posits that all behaviours are based on satisfying one or more of five basic needs. It further posits that one cannot make someone do something, especially learn, unless to do so satisfies some need of the person doing it. Control theory argues that people keep mental images in their head and attach them to whichever needs they satisfy. People feel pleasure when a need is satisfied and pain when a need is frustrated. The five basic needs proposed by control theory are:

- survive and reproduce
- belong and love
- gain power
- be free
- have fun.

Control theory argues that everything we do is initiated by a satisfying picture of that activity that we store in our heads as a pleasant memory. We choose our behaviours, including emotions. For instance, rather than saying one is depressed, one should say I am choosing to be depressed. Behaviours are a person's best attempt to gain control of their lives, 'to reduce the difference between what we want at the time and what we see is available in the real world'. Control theory argues that one must meet one or more needs in order to influence another person. The reason instruction fails is that it fails to meet the needs of the learner. It would seem that small group PBL satisfies the following needs:

- freedom – less structured time, students can choose when to meet and what they are to do next
- power – students have the power to determine their learning needs
- love and belonging – small groups and facilitators become much more personally involved with one another than in the lecture
- fun – the most dominant finding is that both students and faculty enjoy PBL
- survive and reproduce – students helping students promotes survival.

These four theories/concepts are potential explanations for why PBL works. There are likely to be others that apply as well. In my experience, they all have elements that appear to predict well the behaviour of students. Perhaps the best advice is to hedge your bets and incorporate all elements of the four theories into the PBL you use.

Effectiveness of PBL

The question that has dogged PBL since its inception has been to what degree does it produce the types of change in learners that it was designed to produce?

This includes self-directed learners who have a deeper knowledge of their discipline and who are better prepared to apply the science of medicine to patient care. Demonstrating these changes, however, has been a daunting challenge. Over the past 40 years, there have been hundreds of studies designed to test these differences, and at least eight major reviews since 1990 (5–7,29,42–45).

The attempts to do systematic reviews have either resorted to a very small set of controlled studies [see Vernon and Blake(46); Newman(47); Colliver(37)] or adopted a thematic approach [see Berkson(42)] or what might be called a 'best evidence approach' that used effect sizes when possible and a thematic approach when not [see Albanese and Mitchell(6)]. For those who are certain that PBL is the best thing since sliced bread, these reviews have been disappointing. Newman summarised the earlier reviews as:

> Vernon and Blake (1993) concluded 'results generally support the superiority of the PBL approach over more traditional academic methods.' Albanese and Mitchell (1993) whilst acknowledging the weaknesses of the research literature concluded that PBL was more nurturing and enjoyable and that PBL graduates performed as well and sometimes better on clinical examinations and faculty evaluations. However, they also concluded that PBL graduates showed potentially important gaps in their cognitive knowledge base, did not demonstrate expert reasoning patterns, and that PBL was very costly. Berkson (1993) was unequivocal in her conclusion that 'the graduate of PBL is not distinguishable from his or her traditional counterpart'. She further argued that the experience of PBL can be stressful for the student and faculty and implementation may be unrealistically costly. The two more recent reviews also came to differing conclusions. Van den Bossche and colleagues (2000) concluded that PBL had a positive robust effect on the skills of students but a negative non-robust effect on knowledge. The review by Smits and colleagues (2002a) concluded that there was no consistent evidence that PBL is superior to other educational strategies in improving doctors knowledge and performance. (p. 13) Newman's review was no more encouraging. Only for the outcome 'accumulation of knowledge' were there more than three studies that met the inclusion criteria. For this outcome, of 39 effect sizes computed, 16 favoured the PBL group and 23 the control. Generally, the state of the literature was not sufficient to make much out of it in his pilot review.

However, I think the analysis of PBL must make a distinction between those studies conducted before and from 1993. The three reviews that came out that year apparently moved curricula towards what might be called hybrids, a combination of structured activities directed at giving students the disciplinary conceptual frameworks (usually via lecture) combined with substantial time devoted to PBL. At the risk of 'cherry picking' only the studies that have shown posi-

BOX 3.3 Effect sizes for MCAT, Step 1 and Step 2 for pre-PBL, transition and post-PBL classes

	1996	1997	1998–2005/6
Variable	Pre-PBL	Transition year	PBL years (range)
MCAT	−0.23	−0.18	−0.06 (−0.17 to 0.07)
Step 1	−0.25	−0.10	0.30 (0.10 to 0.60)
Step 2	−0.50	0.00	0.38 (0.25 to 0.50)

tive results, I will highlight what I think have been some of the findings of interest in that period. One of the more compelling studies comes from 10 years of experience with PBL at the University of Missouri-Columbia. Hoffman *et al.*(48) present results for the USMLE Steps 1 and 2, and residency director perceptions of their graduate versus all other graduates for the period one year before implementation of PBL (1996 graduating year) and post implementation (1997–2006 graduating years). The performances of the classes on the MCAT were also presented to demonstrate to what extent USMLE performance diverged from the pattern of MCAT scores. Hoffman presented their results as effect sizes, with national means and standard deviations serving as comparison values for those from Missouri. Hoffman's results were presented in graph form; I estimated their values from the graphs to arrive at effect sizes for the year before PBL was implemented, the transition year (first year of PBL) and the mean effect size over the eight to nine years during which PBL was operating. The results are shown in Box 3.3.

Using MCAT effect sizes as an index for student entering academic ability, one would expect the Step 1 and Step 2 effect sizes to be comparable unless the curriculum somehow affected the students' ability in a disproportionate way. In the pre-PBL year, the Step 1 effect size was almost identical to the MCAT effect size, which was approximately one-quarter of a standard deviation below the national mean. The Step 2 effect size was even more negative, approximately one-half standard deviation below the national mean. There was a relatively dramatic improvement in the transitional year that continued for the eight to nine years since PBL was introduced into the curriculum. In that period, the MCAT effect sizes have risen from −0.23 to −0.06, but the changes in Step 1 and Step 2 have been stunning, rising to 0.30 and 0.38, respectively. Thus, during the PBL period, Step 1 and Step 2 performance exceeded, by over one-third of a standard deviation, that which would have been predicted from MCAT scores. Even more impressive is that the improvement in scores has been sustained over such a long period. The type of PBL used in the curriculum

at Missouri would probably be termed hybrid. They have about 10 hours of lecture concurrent with an equal amount of time spent in PBL. This exceeds the limit on lectures that Barrows(3) recommended (1.5 hours per day; 7.5 hours per week). One other point is that concurrent with implementing PBL, they reduced the class size from 112 to 96 students. While the smaller class size may have had some impact on the findings, it is hard to believe that this alone could have made such a large difference.

Examples of other recent findings include the survey responses Schmidt *et al.*(49) obtained from 820 of 2,081 (39%) graduates of a PBL school and 621 of 3,268 (19%) graduates of a traditional school in the Netherlands regarding self-ratings of professional competence. For interpersonal competencies such as working in a team, interpersonal skills and skills required for running meetings, the PBL graduates rated themselves more skilled by an effect size of a whopping 1.30. For PBL-related competencies such as self-directed learning, problem solving and information gathering, the PBL graduates rated themselves as more highly skilled by an effect size of 0.78. For general academic competencies and task-supporting competencies, the differences were 0.14 and 031, respectively, which are small yet more positive for PBL graduates.

Schafer *et al.*(50) recently reported a randomised trial of PBL versus traditional curricula regarding basic science and clinical knowledge. Students who had applied for the PBL track but due to limits on numbers were randomly assigned to the PBL track ($N = 122$) or to the traditional track ($N = 129$), and the remaining students in the traditional track ($N = 617$) were compared at three time points (beginning of first, third and fifth semester) using a 200-item progress test (1/3 basic science, 2/3 clinical). The results showed comparable gains by all groups on the basic science portion of the exam; however, by the third administration performance on the clinical section by the PBL students exceeded that of the other two groups by effect sizes greater than 1.17.

My colleagues and I have(51) examined the relationship of undergraduate science grade point averages (SGPA) to Step 1 failure rate for students in a PBL track and traditional track at one medical school and those at three other traditional medical schools. The relationship between the total MCAT score and Step 1 failure is shown in Figure 3.1.

The SGPA cutpoints represented in Figure 3.1 were obtained by 'cutting off' the group of examinees who fell below the cutpoint, and computing the percentage of them who failed Step 1. Thus, for 3.0, the examinees who had an SGPA below 3.0 were separated off and the percentage of them who failed Step 1 was determined and plotted on the graph. Although the overall failure rates for the three different groups were not different by a large margin (2%), the pattern by which the three different groups reached the overall failure

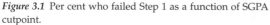

Figure 3.1 Per cent who failed Step 1 as a function of SGPA cutpoint.

rate was strikingly different for the PBL track. While the traditional track and the three traditional medical schools had a relatively linear relationship between SGPA and Step 1 failure rate, the PBL school had almost no failures among those with SGPA values below 3.0. However, for SGPA values between 3.0 and 3.4, the PBL students had a much higher failure rate. Beyond an SGPA of 3.4, the failure rates of the different schools merged together.

These results raise the spectre that PBL may be better for some students, particularly those who have had relatively poor grades in prior course work (SGPA < 3.0), and worse for students who did relatively well, but not stellar, in prior course work (SGPA = 3.0–3.4). These results need to be confirmed with other schools but may explain why the results from studies of PBL have been so variable. If some students do better and others do worse, effects will be difficult to find as they will cancel each other out (*see* Box 3.4).

Summary

Beginning a PBL curriculum is not for the faint-hearted. There is much infrastructure that needs to be put into place, and there may be increased costs. While the effectiveness of PBL appears to be gaining better documentation, and we are gaining a better understanding of how to do PBL, there is still much we need to learn. In the meantime, it is important for anyone involved in implementing PBL to keep in mind what it is that one is trying to accomplish. Dolmans *et al.*(5) identified four important processes underlying PBL based on recent learning principles that provide a good synopsis of what one is trying to accomplish with PBL. These four processes are that learning should be a:
- constructive process
- self-directed process
- collaborative process
- contextual process.

By a constructive process, we mean that learning is an active process by which students 'construct or recon-

BOX 3.4 Where's the evidence: For the effectiveness of PBL?

A summary

Reviews of PBL have generally been disappointing, showing at best that PBL is no worse than the traditional curriculum, but not consistently better. In recent years, more schools have moved to hybrid curricula, and there have been some notable successes and intriguing complexities identified.

Hoffman *et al.* present results for the United States Medical Licensing Examination (USMLE) Steps 1 and 2, and residency director perceptions of their graduate versus all other graduates that showed effect sizes over one-third of a standard deviation beyond what would be expected based on the student's entering academic performance.

Schmidt *et al.*'s survey of graduates of a PBL school and traditional school in the Netherlands regarding self-ratings of professional competence found effect sizes from 0.78 to 1.3 for PBL-related competencies.

Schafer *et al.* reported a randomised trial of PBL versus traditional curricula regarding basic and clinical knowledge and found PBL students' performance on the clinical knowledge section exceeded that of the other groups by effect sizes greater than 1.17.

My colleagues and I examined the relationship of Medical College Admission Test (MCAT) and undergraduate science grade point averages (SGPA) to Step 1 failure rate for students in a PBL track and traditional track at one medical school and those at three other traditional medical schools. The relationship between the total MCAT score and SGPAs and Step 1 failure indicated that some students who do less well academically have lower-than-expected Step 1 failure rates and others who do better academically have higher-than-expected Step 1 failure rates in a PBL curriculum. This suggests that the problem demonstrating PBL effects may be due to differential effect for differing students.

struct their knowledge networks'. A self-directed process is one where learners are involved in planning, monitoring and evaluating the learning process. A collaborative learning process is one in which the social structure involves two or more students interacting, with a common goal, shared responsibilities, mutual dependency and a need to reach agreement through open interaction. A contextual process recognises that learning is context bound and that transfer to different contexts requires confronting cases or problems from multiple perspectives. No matter how someone decides to implement PBL ultimately, it is important that as they design their experience they keep clearly in mind what they are trying to accomplish and do not become distracted from their goal.

BOX 3.5 Focus on: The PBL Best Practices Consortium

PBL has been in existence for over 30 years. While there has been much research on it, there are elements that can best be described as relying on superstition and tradition. In establishing the PBL Best Practices Consortium, my goal was to develop a collection of individuals who were actively involved in conducting PBL, and tap their collective wisdom. I have defined a best practice as something that you wish someone had or did tell you before you started. Dues for enrolling in the group are the submission of one or more best practices that one wishes to share (although I have included some members who wanted to be involved in the e-conversations who were not actively involved in PBL). These enrolment dues were some of the sources of the recommendations in this paper (all attributed). I also plan to send monthly questions to the group, to collect a compendium of best practices. Through this means, I hope to dispel myths, or at least provide justification for their existence.

Acknowledgements

In addition to the literature cited I draw upon comments from selected members of the PBL Best Practices Consortium; Dennis Baker, Stephen Davis, David Matheson and Gail Swarm. Members of the consortium offer best practices, things they wish someone had told them (or did tell them) about how to implement PBL, in response to monthly questions that I post to the group. Participation in the consortium is free and anyone can become a member by emailing me at maalbane@wisc.edu. (Box 3.5) (details correct at the time of writing).

References

1 Neville AJ and Norman GR (2007) PBL in the undergraduate MD program at McMaster University: three iterations in three decades. *Academic Medicine.* **82**(4): 370–4.

2 Barrows HS (1986) A taxonomy of problem-based learning methods. *Medical Education.* **20**: 481–6.

3 Barrows HS (1985) *How to Design a Problem-based Curriculum for the Preclinical Years.* Springer, New York.

4 Wood DF (2003) ABC of learning and teaching in medicine: problem based learning. *British Medical Journal.* **326**: 328–30.

5 Dolmans DHJM, De Grave W, Wolfhagen IHAP and van der Vleuten CPM (2005) Problem-based learning: future challenges for educational practice and research. *Medical Education.* **39**: 732–41.

6 Albanese MA and Mitchell S (1993) Problem-based learning: a review of literature on its outcomes and implementation issues. *Academic Medicine.* **68**: 52–81.

7 Jones JW, Bieber LL, Echt R *et al.* (1984). A problem-based curriculum – ten years of experience. In: Schmidt HG and de Volder ML (eds) *Tutorials in Problem-based Learning*, pp. 181–98. Van Gorcum, Assen, Maastricht.

8 Wales CE and Stager R (1972) Design of an educational system. *Engineering Education* **62**: 456–9.

9 Pawlak SM, Popovich NG, Blank JW and Russell JD (1989) Development and validation of guided design scenarios for problem-solving instruction. *American Journal of Pharmaceutical Education.* **53**: 7–16.

10 Hays R (2002) Problems with problems in problem-based curricula. *Medical Education.* **36**: 790.

11 Dolmans DHJM, Gijselaers WH and Schmidt HG (1992) Do students learn what their teachers intend they learn? Guiding processes in problem-based learning. Paper presented at the Annual Meeting of the American Educational Research Association, San Francisco, CA, April.

12 Coulson RL and Osborne CE (1984) Insuring curricular content in a student-directed problem-based learning program. In: Schmidt HG and de Volder ML (eds) *Tutorials in Problem-based Learning*, pp. 225–9. Van Gorcum, Assen, Maastricht.

13 Dornan T, Scherpbier A, King N and Boshuizen H (2005) Clinical teachers and problem-based learning: a phenomenological study. *Medical Education.* **39**: 163–70.

14 Miflin B (2004) Problem-based learning: the confusion continues. *Medical Education.* **38**: 921–6.

15 Eagle CJ, Harasym PH and Mandin H (1992) Effects of tutors with case expertise on problem-based learning issues. *Academic Medicine.* **67**: 465–9.

16 Davis WK, Nairn R, Paine ME *et al.* (1992) Effects of expert and non-expert facilitators on the small-group process and on student performance. *Academic Medicine.* **67**: 470–4.

17 Zeitz HJ and Paul H (1993) Facilitator expertise and problem-based learning in PBL and traditional curricula. *Academic Medicine.* **68**(3): 203–4.

18 Albanese M (2004) Treading tactfully on tutor turf: does PBL tutor content expertise make a difference? *Medical Education.* **38**: 916–20.

19 Bowman D and Hughes P (2005) Emotional responses of tutors and students in problem-based learning: lessons for staff development. *Medical Education.* **39**(2): 145–53.

20 Farrell T, Albanese MA and Pomrehn P (1999) Problem-based learning in ophthalmology: a pilot program for curricular renewal. *Archives of Ophthalmology.* **117**: 1223–6.

21 Khaliq F (2005) Introduction of problem-solving activities during conventional lectures. *Medical Education.* **39**: 1146–7.

22 Gonnella J, Erdmann J and Hojat M (2004) An empirical study of the predictive validity of number grades in medical school using three decades of longitudinal data: implications for a grading system. *Medical Education.* **38**: 425–34.

23 Julian ER (2005) Validity of the Medical College Admission Test for predicting medical school performance. *Academic Medicine.* **80**(10): 910–17.

24 Kerfoot BP, Masser BA and Hafler JP (2005) Influence of new educational technology on problem-based learning at Harvard Medical School. *Medical Education.* **39**(4): 380–7.

25 Nolte J, Eller P and Ringel SP (1988) Shifting toward problem-based learning in a medical school neurobiology course. In: *Research in Medical Education, 1988: Proceedings of the Twenty-Seventh Annual Conference*, pp. 66–71. Association of American Medical Colleges, Washington, DC.

26 Barrows HS and Tamblyn RM (1976) An evaluation of problem-based learning in small groups utilizing a simulated patient. *Journal of Medical Education.* **51**: 52–4.

27 Nendaz MR and Tekian A (1999) Assessment in problem-based learning medical schools: a literature review. *Teaching and Learning in Medicine.* **11**(4): 232–43.

28 Case S and Swanson D (2001) *Constructing Written Test Questions for the Basic and Clinical Sciences* (3e). National Board of Medical Examiners, Philadelphia (http://www.nbme.org/PDF/2001iwg.pdf; accessed 24 October 2006).

29 Van der Vleuten CPM, Verwijnen GM and Wijnen WHFW (1996) Fifteen years of experience with Progress Testing in a problem-based learning curriculum. *Medical Teacher.* **18**: 103–9.

30 Boshuizen HP, van der Vleuten CP, Schmidt HG and Machiels-Bongaerts M (1997) Measuring knowledge and clinical reasoning skills in a problem-based curriculum. *Medical Education.* **31**: 115–21.

31 Blake JM, Norman GR, Keane DR *et al.* (1996) Introducing progress testing in McMaster University's problem-based medical curriculum: psychometric properties and effect on learning. *Academic Medicine.* **71**: 1002–7.

32 Saunders NA, McIntosh J, McPherson J and Engel CE (1990) A comparison between University of Newcastle and University of Sydney final-year students: knowledge and competence. In: Nooman ZM, Schmidt HG and Ezzat ES (eds) *Innovation in Medical Education: an evaluation of its present status*, pp. 50–63. Springer, New York.

33 McGuire CH and Babbott D (1967) Simulation technique in the measurement of problem-solving skills. *Journal of Educational Measurement.* **4**(1): 1–10.

34 Harden RM, Stevenson M, Downie WW and Wilson GM (1975) Assessment of clinical competence using objective structured examination. *British Medical Journal.* **1**: 447–51.

35 Kruger J and Dunning D (1999) Unskilled and unaware of it: how difficulties in recognizing one's own incompetence lead to inflated self-assessments. *Journal of Personality and Social Psychology.* **77**(6): 1121–34.

36 Ward M, Gruppen L and Regehr G (2002) Measuring self-assessment: current state of the art. *Advances in Health Sciences Education.* **7**: 63–80.

37 Colliver J (2000) Effectiveness of problem based learning curricula. *Academic Medicine.* **75**: 259–66.

38 Schmidt HG (1983) Problem-based learning: rationale and description. *Medical Education.* **17**: 11–16.

39 Qin Z, Johnson DW and Johnson RT (1995) Cooperative versus competitive efforts and problem solving. *Review of Educational Research.* **65**(2): 129–43.

40 Williams GC, Saizow RB and Ryan RM (1999) The importance of self-determination theory for medical education. *Academic Medicine.* **74**(9): 992–5.

41 Glasser W (1986) *Control Theory in the Classroom.* Harper & Row, New York.

42 Berkson L (1993) Problem-based learning: have the expectations been met? *Academic Medicine.* **68**(10): S79–88.

43 Norman GR and Schmidt HG (1992) The psychological basis of PBL. A review of the evidence. *Academic Medicine.* **67**(9): 557–65.

44 Smits P, Verbeek J and De Buisonje C (2002) Problem based learning in continuing medical education: a review of controlled evaluation studies. *British Medical Journal.* **324**: 153–6.

45 Van den Bossche P, Gijbels D and Dochy F (2000) Does problem based learning educate problem solvers? A meta-analysis on the effects of problem based learning. Paper presented at the VII EDINEB Conference, Newport Beach, CA, June 21–3, 2000.

46 Vernon DTA and Blake RL (1993) Does problem-based learning work? A meta-analysis of evaluative research. *Academic Medicine.* **68**: 550–63.

47 Newman M (2003) *A Pilot Systematic Review and Meta-Analysis on the Effectiveness of Problem Based Learning.* On behalf of the Campbell Collaboration Systematic Review Group on the effectiveness of problem based learning. University of Newcastle, Learning and Teaching Support Network, Newcastle.

48 Hoffman K, Hosokawa M, Blake R *et al.* (2006) Problem-based learning outcomes: ten years of experience at the University of Missouri-Columbia School of Medicine. *Academic Medicine.* **81**(7): 617–25.

49 Schmidt HG, Vermeulen L and van der Molen HT (2006) Long-term effects of problem-based learning on the attitudes of undergraduate health care students. *Medical Education.* **40**(6): 562–7.

50 Schafer T, Huenges B, Burger A and Rusche H (2006) A randomized controlled study on the progress in knowledge in a traditional versus problem-based curriculum. *Proceedings of the 2006 Annual Meeting of the Association for Medical Education in Europe*, Cotone Congressi, Genoa, Italy, 14–18 September. Abstract 10H2, p. 208.

51 Albanese MA, Colliver J and Dottl SL (2006) Disrupting the tyranny of prior academic performance. Does PBL help or hinder. *Proceedings of the 2006 Annual Meeting of the Association for Medical Education in Europe*, Cotone Congressi, Genoa, Italy, 14–18 September. Abstract 10H1, p. 208.

Further Reading

Albanese M (2000) Problem based learning: why curricula are likely to show little effect on knowledge and clinical skills. *Medical Education.* **34**: 729–38.

Albanese MA and Mitchell S (1993) Problem-based learning: a review of literature on its outcomes and implementation issues. *Academic Medicine.* **68**: 52–81.

Barrows HS (1985) *How to Design a Problem-based Curriculum for the Preclinical Years.* Springer, New York.

Davis MH and Harden RM (1999) AMEE medical education guide number 15: problem-based learning: a practical guide. *Medical Teacher.* **21**: 130–40.

Norman GR and Schmidt HG (2000) Effectiveness of problem-based learning curricula: theory, practice and paper darts. *Medical Education.* **34**: 721–8.

Interprofessional education

Della Freeth

KEY MESSAGES

- Interprofessional education (IPE) is just a special case of professional education, so knowledge about good practice for learning and teaching in a wide range of contexts can be applied directly to IPE.

- The uniqueness of IPE lies in deliberately creating heterogeneous groups. By bringing together participants from different professions around a particular task, it is anticipated that the increased diversity of knowledge and perspectives will enhance the learning of all.

- Healthcare is delivered by multidisciplinary teams so interprofessional practice is inevitable. IPE may help to develop insights, shared knowledge and teamwork skills that promote effective collaboration to deliver high-quality care efficiently.

- IPE is not limited to formally planned and overtly labelled blocks of content. Whenever practitioners meet in multiprofessional groups to address complex needs or service evaluations and improvements there is potential for learning. Serendipitous IPE can be a feature of daily practice.

- The *raison d'être* for IPE is to enhance professional practice: uniprofessional as well as interprofessional.

- Poorly planned and delivered IPE may be damaging if it generates a reluctance to engage in subsequent interprofessional collaboration or reinforces negative stereotypes.

Introduction

My starting position is that interprofessional education (IPE) is simply a special case of professional education, so all that we know about good practice in professional education applies to IPE too. What is different about IPE is a conscious decision to amplify the heterogeneity of learning groups.

Second, I view professional education as the range of formally planned and serendipitous experiences, which, aided by reflection and a process of trying things out, form and continually modify our professional knowledge and practical wisdom.

I stress this broad view of education, a vibrant patchwork of experiences informing a lifelong project of development, because too much that is said about education portrays it narrowly as formal units of planned content. This view is often further restricted by the expectation of delivery by especially designated people in especially designated places using currently approved means of transmission and assessment. This is not to argue against formally planned and overtly labelled IPE delivered by university faculty and experienced healthcare professionals in a range of learning environments. Rather, it is a plea that in addition to valuing the important contributions of formal IPE, we should notice and value the contributions of informal interprofessional learning. Both are inextricably linked to professional practice – hopefully high-quality interprofessional collaboration founded on complementary professional contributions to care.

Naturally, more will be said about formal IPE; after all serendipitous IPE happens spontaneously. But it is not quite that simple; geography, shared interests or problems, and organisational structures and cultures can promote or inhibit informal and serendipitous interprofessional learning. Some of these factors are amenable to re-engineering.

Defining Interprofessional Education

The most widely recognised and robustly debated definition of IPE is supplied by the UK Centre for the Advancement of Interprofessional Education (CAIPE):

> Interprofessional education occurs when two or more professions learn with, from and about each other to improve collaboration and the quality of care.(1)

CAIPE qualifies its definition further, stating that IPE includes:

> ... all such learning in academic and work-based settings before and after qualification, adopting an inclusive view of 'professional'.

A number of key points can be drawn from this definition. Namely, that:

Understanding Medical Education: Evidence, Theory and Practice.
Edited by T Swanwick. © 2010 Association for the Study of Medical Education.

- education is defined by the occurrence of learning
- 'with, from and about' necessitates *active* learning and implies learning based on some type of exchange
- the main aims are to improve collaboration and to improve care.

IPE then is, not just about a mixed group of people acquiring the *same* knowledge or developing the *same* clinical skill. This can be made clearer by oversimplifying for a moment. During the exchanges of active IPE, representatives of profession X will learn about the expertise and perspectives of representatives of profession Y; meanwhile representatives of profession Y learn about the expertise and perspectives of representatives of profession X. Hopefully, all participants learn something about themselves and their own professional practice. In this way, everyone learns something different and can subsequently use that learning to enhance working as a particular type of professional within a multidisciplinary team.

CAIPE also developed seven principles(1) to guide provision, commissioning, development and evaluation. Their vision of effective IPE is that it:

- works to improve the quality of care
- focuses on the needs of service users and carers
- involves service uses and carers
- encourages professions to learn with, from and about each other
- respects the integrity and contribution of each profession
- enhances practice within professions
- increases professional satisfaction.

Thus the concept is to learn to practise in ways that are better for the people we serve, and better for ourselves and our colleagues because we focus on making a useful contribution to a collaborative effort. It is about trying to create a climate within which the different contributions of any pertinent people and organisations are valued, and, as far as is possible, well understood and well coordinated (Box 4.1). IPE is not an instrument for creating generic health workers, smashing the power of professions or reducing funding. Box 4.2 reviews concepts related to IPE.

BOX 4.1 Seven principles of interprofessional education(1)

- Works to improve the quality of care
- Focuses on the needs of service users and carers
- Involves service user and carers
- Encourages professions to learn with, from and about each other
- Respects the integrity and contribution of each profession
- Enhances practice within professions
- Increases personal satisfaction

BOX 4.2 Focus on: Terms and activities

Interprofessional education (IPE) is inextricably linked to multiprofessional education (MPE) and uniprofessional education. MPE is normally taken to be occasions when members or students of two or more professions learn side by side for whatever reason. Often this is because they have a common need to address particular content. Shared lectures and shared clinical skills sessions are example of MPE. These only become IPE if active, exchange-based learning can be woven into the educational experience. MPE may provide some opportunities for informal or interprofessional learning during relatively undirected time, for example, breaks or small group work. This is not meant to suggest that MPE is a good first step towards IPE: several studies have found that MPE can lead to resentment.(2) If the benefits of an interprofessional gathering are not realised each group of participants can feel that their education is being 'diluted'.

Uniprofessional education will form the bulk of any pre-registration professional curriculum and may remain the mainstay of post-registration continuing education and workplace learning. Uniprofessional learning is, therefore, an extremely important venue for the development of knowledge, skills and attitudes that underpin interprofessional collaboration.

Unfortunately, from place to place, and author to author, there is inconsistency in the use of the terms IPE and MPE, and there is an unhelpful proliferation of terms used to describe IPE and MPE. For example, shared learning, common learning, interdisciplinary education and interagency training. There seems little point wading deeply into this 'semantic quagmire'.(3) It should be sufficient to remain mindful that when people use these competing and overlapping terms they *may* do so inconsistently, with a vision that differs from your vision and without a clear conception of the defining features of this type of education. It will always be necessary to ascertain 'what exactly is being spoken of here?'

Some writers regard IPE as old-fashioned and inappropriately focused, preferring interprofessional *learning* (IPL). While the shift to focusing on learning is an important educational movement, the most widely adopted view of IPE defines education by the occurrence of learning (*see* Box 4.1), rendering the IPE/IPL debate redundant.

The recognition of competing terms and fashions is important because an unthinking rejection of differently labelled work could dislocate us from a rich heritage of valuable insights catalogued under terms that are not familiar or not currently in vogue. On the other hand, unthinking acceptance may have us working at cross-purposes with others.

The Rationale for Interprofessional Education

The drivers for IPE have been well elaborated by a range of authors.(4–7) I do not intend to summarise their arguments here. Instead, I will sketch out some key points that underpin the perspective taken in this paper.

- Healthcare is delivered by multidisciplinary teams so interprofessional practice is inevitable. IPE may help to develop insights, shared knowledge and teamwork skills that promote effective collaboration to deliver high-quality care efficiently.
- The pace of change in the 21st century is very high and there seems to be no end to increasing workloads. Perhaps these pressures and an attendant perception of fragmentation increase the felt need for formally identified IPE, while in gentler times less formal interprofessional learning opportunities might have been spotted and developed with little need for overt labelling and resource allocation.
- Concerns to monitor and promote equality of opportunity may also increase pressure to overtly label IPE, particularly at the pre-registration level. Informality, while a great boon to creativity, can be too easily susceptible to unintended and unexamined bias. This is an area where it can be difficult to keep the balance right.
- In modern healthcare, traditional hierarchies, roles and boundaries are increasingly challenged because they are thought to inhibit the efficient delivery of sound care. IPE can make a range of contributions to the ongoing challenge and renegotiation of traditional ways of thinking and being. For example, it can help participants to appreciate the contributions of different members of the team; it can promote shared examination of multifaceted problems and the formation of team plans rather than a tangle of criss-crossing separate responses; it may promote healing and collaboration when external pressures have damaged collaborative practice in a particular setting.
- When things go wrong in healthcare, subsequent investigations all too frequently identify failures in teamwork and failures in communication, often interprofessional or interagency teamwork and communication. IPE is commonly suggested as a contribution towards curing or immunising against poor collaboration. This has intuitive appeal and provides hints as to the nature of the required IPE.
- Learning theories highlight the motivational importance of the gap between what people think they know and what they think they need to know. Jarvis,(8) in particular, highlighted this gap and used the term 'disjuncture'. Disjuncture (providing it is not overwhelmingly large) stimulates learning, and skilful educators down the ages have found ways to create or reveal constructive disjuncture. Slightly unfamiliar contexts, such as IPE, create disjuncture, revealing learning needs and motivating learners to close the gap. Furthermore, 'constructive friction' between a learning environment and learners' habitual approaches to learning can promote change and personal development.(9) IPE can be an excellent context for creating and harnessing appropriate levels of disjuncture and constructive friction.

By definition, IPE means bringing people from different groups together (physically or electronically). It is inevitable that this increases the complexity of agreeing mutually convenient times, finding a suitable venue and suitably skilled facilitators, and identifying or creating learning resources that suit all participants; then negotiating responsibility for the associated costs and, where relevant, navigating the restrictions of multiple assessment schemes.

If the ideas and skills you wish to develop in a particular learning experience are not focused on improving collaboration and improving the quality of care, there may be little gain in struggling to deliver that part of the overall curriculum on an interprofessional basis. This applies most strongly at the pre-registration level, where the number of potential participants can be huge and the assessment requirements of different professional curricula are least likely to match. Thus it is appropriate for most of each profession's curriculum to be delivered uniprofessionally. Nevertheless it would be alarming if no part of the pre-registration curriculum addressed the nature of high-quality interprofessional collaboration for the effective delivery of high-quality care. Thus there will be appropriate opportunities to add value to the curriculum through interprofessional learning.

At the postgraduate level, numbers are often smaller, assessment requirements may be more flexible and a higher proportion of educational activities will be concerned with improving the quality of collaboration and care for particular groups of patients or clients. Then the question 'why do IPE?' becomes 'why not do IPE?' Perhaps we should expect the majority of postgraduate education to be interprofessional.

Activities that do not allow each participating group to contribute and gain to more or less the same extent are unlikely to be a good foundation for sound IPE. The aim is for everyone to learn something productive through balanced exchanges, not for one group to plunder the expertise of another.

Some aspects of improving interprofessional collaboration and improving care can be addressed quite well on a uniprofessional basis, reducing the need for IPE. For example, uniprofessional team-based activity, such as problem-based learning groups or action learning sets,(10) may be a successful environment for facilitators to draw out learning about how teams function, the importance of diversity within team membership, the effects of people joining and leaving, and strategies for improving team functioning and individual contributions.

These uniprofessional learning experiences may be sufficient in some circumstances; or they may be seen as having an important role in laying firm foundations for subsequent IPE that stretches learners a little further. In addition to this theoretical and pragmatic rationale for IPE, the evidence base is summarised in Box 4.3.

The Diversity of Interprofessional Education

Elsewhere(11) I have described a spectrum of IPE with two dimensions: first, variation in emphasis, and second, variation in the degree of planning and formalisation. The emphasis dimension runs from a primary focus on interprofessional collaboration as the subject matter for the IPE(12–14) to a secondary focus on interprofessional collaboration and a primary focus elsewhere [e.g. particular client group,(15–19) particular professional skills,(20–23) policy innovation,(24,25) improving systems,(26,27) and responding to audit(28,29)]. Many IPE initiatives seek to pay balanced attention to interprofessional collaboration and some other substantive content.(30–32)

The planning and formalisation dimension recognises that unplanned interprofessional learning is very influential and should be acknowledged. This often happens in daily practice when members of different professions review their work together, or encounter something slightly out of the ordinary, causing them to pause, observe some aspect of overlapping concern more closely or seek out information from one another.

It is axiomatic that we cannot plan serendipitous learning so we may think that it does not concern us in our roles as curriculum developers, tutors, facilitators or mentors, but we can pay more attention to creating the right conditions for positive unplanned learning. I stress conditions for *positive* learning because negative unplanned learning happens rather easily. Either way, these conditions form the 'hidden curriculum'.(33,34) I shall return to this later.

Beyond serendipitous interprofessional learning there is *informal* interprofessional learning that occurs more predictably because of work systems or the structure of educational programmes and events. Multidisciplinary team reviews of specific cases or processes can be good examples of informal IPE. These may be labelled as team meetings, action learning, audit, quality circles, external inspection and so on, each with a different emphasis and potential for informal and formally recognised interprofessional learning. Many educational programmes and events

provide opportunities for informal IPE simply by bringing people together; conferences and safety-related updates are common examples. The training and debate associated with introducing new equipment, processes or clinical guidelines provide further opportunities for informal interprofessional learning. Some of the examples cited at the beginning of this section to emphasise the diversity of IPE might be regarded as largely informal IPE.(15,21,22,26–28)

Students from different professions are often in the same clinical areas at the same time, providing opportunities for informal IPE even if the logistics of making this a formal part of the relevant professional curricula are too difficult to contemplate. This may be because of constant changes in the clinical area, the unpredictable availability of contributing practitioners, a lack of funding for the formalisation process and to address sustainability, long time lags in curriculum change processes and so on. Nevertheless, if students and the clinicians who supervise them look out for opportunities for productive interprofessional exchange, valuable interprofessional learning can occur. Developing a habit of informal interprofessional learning can help students to mature into competent, collaborative professionals, confident with their own expertise and area of responsibility, willing to learn from and educate other professions.

The main dangers of promoting informal IPE and not paying attention to formal IPE include:
- the impossibility of monitoring equality of opportunity
- scope for duplication (although this should be limited if learners actively negotiate their learning with supervisors or colleagues)
- scope for individuals to avoid engaging with this important aspect of professional practice
- less motivation for engagement if the formal curriculum does not value interprofessional collaboration sufficiently to include appropriate interprofessional learning objectives, experiences and assessments.

It can be important for programme planners and course participants to be clear about where their IPE lies within the two-dimensional spectrum of IPE I have described. This clarity will help everyone to set realistic learning goals and to make sound decisions about inclusion and exclusion.

Designing Effective Interprofessional Education

There is growing understanding of the effectiveness of IPE (*see* Box 4.3). Effective IPE is simply good education with the added 'twist' of purposefully harnessing the knowledge, learning needs and dynamics of an interprofessional group. A wide range of learning

BOX 4.3 Where's the evidence: Interprofessional education

There are hundreds of peer-reviewed studies of interprofessional education (IPE), but their quality is variable and it is wise to pay most attention to the stronger studies.(35–37) Methodological approaches for studying IPE should be aligned with the aims, principles and processes of the particular IPE under evaluation also paying heed to the needs to improve practice, increase understanding and inform policy.(38) Since IPE varies widely in its intentions, style and contexts, and studies vary in their purposes and intended audiences, wide variation should be expected in approaches to studying IPE.

Nevertheless, for post-registration learners there is evidence that IPE (mostly embedded in quality improvement inititatives) can improve the quality of care and the quality of working lives. To name just a few examples:

- progress with reducing infections and need for supplemental oxygen in neonatal intensive care(15) and reducing costs(39)
- improved preventative care, including increased screening and immunisation rates(29,40,41)
- improved teamwork and fewer errors observed in emergency departments(24)
- reduced use of physical restraint in nursing homes(42)
- increased interprofessional participation in planning and reviewing care(43,44)
- smoother work systems.(18,26,28)

There are also good studies of interprofessional teamwork that can inform thinking about informal and serendipitous IPE, or identify needs for post-registration IPE.(45,46)

Pre-registration education is always an investment in the future based on a professional consensus about desired content, policy driver and economic realities. Viewed in isolation, most parts of any profession's curriculum will have a limited evidence base, and two questions serve to illustrate this: Do we know that the pharmacology content of medical education is effectively integrated in subsequent professional practice? What do we know about the effectiveness of studying ethics at the pre-qualification level? So if we view IPE as content, we should not expect there to be an extensive evidence base.

On the other hand, if we view IPE as an educational method the evidence base we might expect would relate to its acceptability to learners and faculty; IPE's success in increasing knowledge of the topics addressed, changing attitudes and changed behaviour; studies of development and delivery; and models of integration with the wider curriculum, including assessment matters. In many ways the structure of the IPE evidence base would be similar to the structure of the evidence bases relating to, say, problem-based learning,(47,48) simulation,(49,50) or supervision and mentoring,(51–53) while recognising these fields are all at different stages of development.

In fact, studies of pre-registration IPE have provided a wide range of insights. The list below is illustrative not exhaustive, and the examples referenced are just a small selection from an ever increasing pool.

- Sustainable models of delivery that, over time, can accommodate large numbers of students.(30,32,54)
- Variable responses from students from different professions.(2,30,32)
- The pace and level of IPE needs to be closely matched to participants' prior experience.(30)
- IPE can develop more positive perceptions of members and of other professions and constructive 'mutual inter-group differentiation' (*see* Box 4.4), and a more sophistication understanding or roles within teams.(20,55,56)
- IPE can usefully extend (but is not a substitute for) uniprofessional learning and students sometimes feel tension between profession-specific and interprofessional learning objectives.(20,54,57)
- Rehearsing interprofessional teamwork is valued.(20,54)
- An interprofessional clerkship in primary care increased the comprehensiveness of care and the number of patients seen by medical students.(54)
- IPE can increase interest in working in places or specialities where there are recruitment shortfalls.(58)
- Patients are pleased with care provided by interprofessional student teams.(54,59)
- Medical students sometimes feel less supported by clinical supervisors than other professions' students.(30,59)

theorists and adult educators(60–75) have developed overlapping theories of adults' and professional learning. Key principles include:
- the perceived relevance of the learning opportunity
- the perceived demands of the learning context
- the relationship of current learning to prior learning
- the learners' self-concepts.

In addition, from psychology we learn about the key features of practice and feedback.(76,77)

Poorly planned and delivered education of any type can waste resources and create ill will. Poor-quality IPE may be particularly damaging if it creates increased reluctance to engage in subsequent interprofessional collaboration or reinforces negative stereotypes. We should try particularly hard to avoid delivering bruising or otherwise demotivating IPE.

The perceived relevance of the learning opportunity

Adult learners are life-centred and problem-centred, motivated to develop their knowledge and skills when they encounter an idea, a task or a problem that matters to them in their current context.(60,70,73,78) This may be something that is not going well at the moment or simply something new that they wish to explore. It is difficult to engage with things that do not interest us and seem to have little relevance. Furthermore, IPE participants are likely to want to develop their knowledge and practice from multiple perspectives (as individuals, as members of a particular profession and as members of diverse teams) and their primary focus will vary over time and in response to external demands.

IPE normally addresses this personal, professional and team development by appealing to shared interest in delivering good care to *patients* [the 'object' of 'activity'(78)]. This is most obvious within post-registration IPE: commonly labelled as *quality improvement* (some examples are provided in Box 4.3). People may not even notice they are engaged in IPE: learning with, from and about each other to improve collaboration and the quality of care. Participants from diverse backgrounds are focused on and motivated by their shared practice-based problem.

Normally, establishing relevance and authenticity requires active attention from curriculum developers and facilitators. They will try to ensure that learning opportunities (in clinical practice, university and staff development settings) are well aligned with the anticipated participants' concerns, interests and levels of expertise. This can be particularly challenging for IPE because the diversity of concerns, interests and expertise may well be greater within an interprofessional group. While this diversity can stimulate learning and enjoyment, it can also overstretch the skills of the facilitators or the ingenuity of the curriculum developers who provide trigger material and structure to guide learners. It is wise to work with a manageable level of diversity and select a theme that is fairly easily recognised as relevant to all participants.

The perceived demands of the learning context

Learners' *perceptions* of the learning environment and what is expected from them (more than any objective reality) affect what and how they learn,(79–82) for example, whether they mainly seek to absorb and reproduce knowledge or behaviours from facilitators or learning materials; focus on understanding and generating new knowledge; hope to transform their professional lives; or to please important gatekeepers. Overloading learners is known to encourage a reproducing (surface) approach to learning, faulty learning, disengagement or, at best, a strategic approach.(68,83) Thus, for example, it is not helpful to place an optional, experiential interprofessional learning opportunity

shortly before a high-stakes summative assessment (usually examinations for individuals or external inspections, audits or reviews for service delivery teams). While this may seem too obvious to mention, it is surprisingly easy to overlook important conflicting demands faced by one or more of the groups from whom participation is desired. This will constrain their participation and alter the overall dynamics of the interprofessional learning. Such oversights are more easily avoided when care is taken to include a member of each participating group in the planning process.

Learners' perceptions are shaped by explicit and implicit messages. Explicit messages include:

* the course description (as published and as spoken by facilitators)
* perhaps a handbook containing aims or intended learning outcomes
* the learning materials and assessment requirements.

These all convey the 'target understanding'(84) curriculum developers, tutors and examiners have in mind.

Implicit messages, the 'hidden curriculum', include:

* perceptions of the importance of a particular learning opportunity based on, for example, who chooses to attend or otherwise contribute and the attitudes they display
* any attendance or assessment requirements
* whether the event is allocated a bright and airy room with access to adequate technology and refreshments
* whether the event is pushed to the fringes of the timetable such as late on Friday afternoon
* many other subtle ways of reinforcing or undermining the official explicit messages.

IPE can be enhanced or undermined by the explicit and implicit messages delivered and (more importantly) *perceived* about its relationship to the (properly) dominant activities of uniprofessional education and practising as a member of a particular profession.

The self-concept of the learner

Professional and interprofessional education address learners who wish mainly to see themselves as competent, self-directed, appropriately self-evaluative and exercising choice(60,65,67), in short, skilfully self-regulating.(85) Any education that attacks these aspects of self-concept will produce resistance and possibly rejection. Of course, it is perfectly reasonable to dislike coercion and to try to avoid embarrassment or failure. Successful education will challenge learners (cognitively and affectively) but will monitor and adjust the degree of challenge to maintain productive learning. IPE participants bring along their constantly evolving professional persona and expertise. Skilful curriculum planning and facilitation are needed to ensure that their expertise and values are acknowledged and that challenge is supportive. This is most easily achieved when levels of expertise are appropriate for the task at hand. A practical response in post-registration inter-professional practice development is to ensure that participants are drawn from the correct levels within their particular profession or specialisation: those who really know about the processes under scrutiny and those who have the ability to effect change in the relevant environments. For pre-registration IPE we may sometimes match participants to learning activities, but more often we will match learning activities to available participants. This means that IPE curriculum developers must take time to examine the anticipated participants' prior learning and competing learning needs.

Adults' need for self-direction coexists with a need for structure, particularly in unfamiliar learning milieu.(86,87) IPE will be less familiar than uniprofessional education, so at the beginning, participants may feel quite strongly that the programme details and facilitators' actions should structure the learning experience for them. As confidence grows, the participants will have less need for this 'scaffolding',(88,89) so it is sensible to focus on supporting learners in the early stages of a learning encounter and then shift in the direction of measured challenge.

Links to prior learning

Prior learning influences subsequent learning and this has many dimensions. Learning proceeds more quickly and is better retained if it relates to earlier experience and learning.(90) The accuracy or otherwise of earlier learning, particularly the understanding of key concepts, lays firm or shaky foundations for later learning. This has been shown to be especially important in scientific fields.(87,91) Learning from prior experiences may support or inhibit new learning by providing relevant or distracting procedural and technical knowledge, and supportive or undermining emotional associations.(60,61,92) Prior learning will also influence the approaches to learning with which IPE participants feel comfortable and habitually select. Facilitators and curriculum developers should try to maintain an up-to-date understanding of the probable prior learning (curricula and extent of practice experience) for the learners to whom each IPE initiative is addressed.

Some learners develop unhelpful approaches to learning,(93,94) and it may be very difficult for them to change these.(95) Skilful facilitators will not underestimate the degree of personal challenge that IPE might present to some learners as a result of their prior learning, and will work more closely with these learners to provide additional scaffolding.

Practice and feedback

Practice is important for the development and maintenance of skills and good habits. The type of practice that yields improvement and change is deliberate,(76) that is, conscious and effortful, attentive to the quality of current performance and actively seeking strategies to improve performance. The effortful nature of deliberate practice necessitates limited duration with adequate recovery periods. Formal education typically includes short periods of practice (e.g. performing clinical skills in a clinical area or skills laboratory, role playing, problem solving and guided reflection) and encourages subsequent practice by setting assignments or targets, or by revisiting earlier practice in subsequent sessions. Reflection(96,97) is rarely included as an example of deliberate practice, but effective reflection is effortful and self-evaluative, constantly seeking improvement and actively evaluating alternative strategies. Productive reflection is hard work and sometimes contains little intrinsic enjoyment; the rewards of reflection are deferred rewards of subsequently improved performance. The level of challenge and deferred gratification mean that it is not surprising that learners can be less than enthusiastic about engagement in the reflective elements of curricula.

Good education increases the likelihood of effortful, self-evaluative practice by motivating learners to desire improvement, providing guidance that aids self-evaluation and developing skills of reflection. IPE is often problem-focused, providing motivation for improvement. Self-evaluation and reflection on current performance are supported by skilful facilitation, the structure of the learning experience and well-chosen learning materials.

Feedback is an important element of promoting learning.(98,99) It can come from many sources; for example, it is sometimes inherent in the success or otherwise of the activity undertaken, and instructional technology such as simulators or e-learning materials can be programmed to provide regular feedback. Reactions from others (if noticed and interpreted) are important sources of feedback, and key sources include:

- patients and families
- peers and mentors
- people from different professions and organisations.

People with educational responsibilities (senior clinicians, mentors and supervisors, university faculty, staff development facilitators and all kinds of assessors) should move beyond reaction and provide structured feedback that identifies specific strengths and weaknesses and directs attention to ways of improving. Nevertheless, we cannot tell that feedback has been received and incorporated into learning unless things change, for example, performance improves or new strategies are tried and evaluated. Usually, feedback during IPE comes from peers or facilitators.

Interprofessional Education and the Curriculum

As highlighted in Chapter 1, curriculum design is not about identifying *the right way* to do things, but a matter of making value-laden choices that are fit for purpose within a particular context. This chapter argues that there is no ideal or essential location for IPE within a curriculum, rather that there are many opportunities for enhancing learning through IPE. Those selected will depend on the preferences of the curriculum developers and local opportunities. The choices made also reflect developers' conceptions of the purposes of IPE.

Some people think that IPE must occur as early as possible in pre-registration education to avoid the development of negative stereotypes and a preference for uniprofessional working over collaborative practice. But our students are not blank pages on which we write or empty vessels that we fill, they arrive with life-based and media-based stereotypes and a strong commitment to their chosen profession. Nevertheless, early IPE can work well, provided it is appropriate to learners' current knowledge, experience and learning needs.(100–103) It is worth remembering that junior students may be more biddable than their seniors, so absenteeism is less likely to be a problem at this stage. Well-received early IPE might encourage later engagement within a spiral curriculum(100,104) that revisits interprofessional collaboration with increasing levels of sophistication and challenge. It is important that each return to IPE builds on rather than repeats earlier interprofessional and uniprofessional learning; otherwise, disengagement and resistance are highly likely.

If local constraints make early IPE difficult, it may be more efficient to ensure that pre-registration curricula across the professions have elements that *systematically* and *explicitly* work towards developing skills and insights that will aid later engagement with IPE and collaborative practice. Later engagement might occur during the middle years when students have begun to build a reasonably secure technical knowledge base relating to their own profession; they have some experience of professional practice and they have begun to examine communication skills, teamworking, decision making, working in partnership with patients and carers, ethical practice, patient safety, the nature of professionalism, and the limits of knowledge and resources. At this stage students have some useful profession-specific knowledge and experiences that they can share and they tend to be hungry for new experiences.(58,105)

If engagement with formal IPE is delayed until the final years of pre-qualification curricula it will be particularly important to recognise the competing priorities of high-stakes examinations and securing a job for the following year. It is also important to remember that students will by now have experienced informal and serendipitous IPE while engaging with other things, particularly while gaining experience in various clinical areas. They would not want to feel that a new block in the curriculum, formally labelled as IPE, is repeating ground they have already covered. It must

be clear that any revisiting is raising the level of thinking and skills; this is what a spiral curriculum demands.(104) But interprofessional learning can be a logical pinnacle within a spiral curriculum and there are studies of IPE used this way.(20,106) In the closing months of pre-qualification curricula, students are naturally preoccupied with the impending responsibilities and realities of professional practice. IPE that speaks to these strongly felt learning needs is likely to be well received.

As mentioned earlier, interprofessional continuing professional development is often more natural than uniprofessional development in improving certain clinical practices and developing services. IPE at this level can help ensure that resources are used wisely, that effective and patient-centred care are the main priorities and, importantly, that attention is given to the quality of working lives.

Overtly labelling particular learning experiences as interprofessional offers the advantage of visibility for an important aspect of professional practice, but creating isolated interprofessional elements within the curriculum can make IPE vulnerable to attack and easy to cut when times are hard. My (probably controversial) suggestion is that sustainability may be more easily achieved if interprofessional learning is embedded as a taken-for-granted part of certain other strands of activity. There are many possibilities, but obvious choices include:
- clinical and service-based quality improvement initiatives where the embedded model is already well developed at the post-qualification level
- multiprofessional student teams shadowing real teams or providing supervised care (see next section for further discussion)
- curriculum strands that address patient groups whose needs can only be met through interprofessional or interagency collaboration
- patient-safety initiatives.

It has to be recognised that IPE will always present logistical challenges that are not so strongly felt in uniprofessional education. It may also present political and financial challenges.

Delivering Effective Interprofessional Education

Most modes of educational delivery could potentially have some application in IPE, but some are more naturally suited to the task. I shall consider four here.

Case-based and problem-based triggers
Many IPE experiences use real cases and incidents, or authored scenarios drawn from a synthesis of past experience to trigger learning. This is a natural format, because all the participating professions are likely to

be familiar with learning in this way and because relevance to the concerns of participants should be achievable. Well-selected or well-crafted triggers ensure that each profession can make a valued contribution.

I have avoided using the term problem-based learning (PBL) and should explain why. Often in IPE it is the problem focus that matters; it may not be necessary or appropriate to conduct the IPE as a PBL experience. A second reason is that different groups of participants may have different conceptions of PBL that have grown up within their uniprofessional experiences to suit their profession-specific needs. It is the same as with the earlier warning to be alert to whether everyone in the group you are working with means the same thing when they talk about IPE (*see* Box 4.2). It can be an unnecessary distraction for IPE participants to be told that they will engage in PBL and then find things do not proceed according to the formula that they associate with the term.

Simulation

The term simulation covers everything from table-top exercises and simple role play (e.g. a telephone call) to medium-fidelity simulation in clinical skills centres on to high-fidelity clinical simulations supported by sophisticated technology or highly skilled simulated patients (*see* Chapter 12). The purposes of simulation include:

- providing a safe learning environment that protects patients and learners, where mistakes can be allowed to occur as learning opportunities
- providing learning opportunities that do not disrupt the normal delivery of care
- speeding up or slowing the passage of time to enhance learning
- allowing repeated practice, preferably after feedback or self-assessment
- providing managed formative exposure to things not yet experienced or only rarely experienced
- creating appropriate levels of disjuncture to stimulate learning.

It is worth remembering that the fidelity of any simulation only needs to be as high as is necessary to achieve the intended learning. Costs can be contained by examining which aspects of a situation need to be simulated and looking for the simplest way to do this. Naturally, people fear failure and embarrassment. Some types of simulation offer scope for public humiliation and thus require particularly careful planning and skilful facilitation to avoid creating 'miseducative experiences'.(107)

Since professional practice is interprofessional, it makes sense for some simulation-based education to be interprofessional. Examples include extending earlier uniprofessional learning through the development of interprofessional scenarios for rehearsing aspects of communication with simulated patients(20,107) and rehearsing case and workload management.(102,108)

Shadowing

Reciprocated shadowing, with associated discussion and reflection, can make an excellent contribution to interprofessional understanding of roles, responsibilities, constraints, expertise and models of practice. Passive observation tends not to be integrated with earlier learning and is soon forgotten. Thus a shadowing experience needs structure and follow-up activities that promote active learning. This increases the chance that learning will become integrated in subsequent professional practice. Some wider IPE initiatives include shadowing elements.(32,109–111)

Clinical work in interprofessional student teams

A variety of initiatives has involved interprofessional student teams providing care under the supervision of qualified practitioners.(30,54,59,109,112,113) These models show how a rolling programme of IPE in a particular service delivery setting can, over time, allow large numbers of students to rehearse and reflect on interprofessional teamwork. Patients tend to be highly satisfied with care provided by interprofessional student teams,(54,59) and follow-up studies show that students retain strong and largely positive memories of this type of IPE.(114,115) However, these models can be vulnerable to sudden changes in the clinical area, resulting in loss of staff to provide the level of supervision students require or a change in the caseload rendering a clinical area too demanding for student teams. Studies have also noted that supervising student teams and facilitating effortful reflection can be a draining role for clinicians and faculty.(112,114)

A model that stops short of providing care involves interprofessional student team members assessing patients with complex needs and conducting an interdisciplinary case conference to integrate their findings and develop a care plan.(32) The students' care plan is then presented to members of the client's actual care team for discussion and (formative) assessment; *see* The assessment of interprofessional education section, below.

The Role of Facilitation

To enable *active* learning *with*, *from* and *about* members of other professions, IPE normally adopts some form of small group learning. Advice on facilitating small group learning has been ably addressed by a wide range of authors.(116–121) Their insights are directly applicable to IPE. The added dimensions of facilitating interprofessional small group work are, first, that IPE groups are deliberately heterogeneous; and second, that the aim of IPE is to harness the different perspectives, skills and insights of participants from different professions.

Uniprofessional groups contain learners from different cultures, of different ages, with different abilities, varying prior experiences and different levels of interest in the topic under consideration. Consequently, faculty and practice-based supervisors are already skilled in playing to the strengths of different learners and supporting everyone to make a valued contribution; providing tailored feedback and sufficient (but not too much) challenge; and managing group dynamics, including conflict. Thus, experienced teachers already have most of the skills they will need to facilitate IPE. Nevertheless, the greater diversity within an interprofessional learning group may stretch these skills. More effort is involved in finding out about the expertise and prior experience of participants, necessitating greater advance preparation to ensure that learning materials and activities are pitched at the correct level and allow all groups to contribute. It can be harder to draw out a valued contribution from a quiet learner if you are unsure of the relevant profession's contribution yourself, again pointing to the need for advance preparation. On the other hand, the diversity of the group can make for a rich variety of contributions that enthuses everyone; then the facilitator's main roles may be to keep an eye on the time and to help summarise learning and plans before everyone disperses.

For a comfortable learning experience, the content and pace of the IPE need to feel appropriate to all participants (this links to the importance of perceived relevance and perceived demands, discussed earlier). Indicative content, and by implication pace, will be set when the IPE is planned. But any exchange-based learning relies on participants' contributions and, therefore, the facilitator must continually evaluate contributions and learners' engagement to judge when to expand themes or deepen thinking, and when to move the group on to something new. The diversity of interprofessional groups might make this task more challenging.

Tutors grow accustomed to working with learners from particular professions (often the tutor's own profession) and profession-based norms for learning and teaching encounters. Translating their consequent style and expectations directly into IPE can cause alarm and discomfort to some participants. IPE facilitators try to remain vigilant for signs of discomfort or resistance. These might indicate that certain participants need extra support to begin to feel at ease with the IPE activities (see earlier discussion of learners' self-concepts and links to prior learning). For example, some IPE participants may find reflective practice a natural state, while others are rather uncomfortable with such self-examination. Succinct displays of certainty may be the carefully developed cultural norm for one group, but this could be seen as arrogant and narrow-minded by another group. In addition, similar terms may be used by different professions to mean rather different things. It is best not to assume that everyone means the same thing when they say problem-based learning, self-directed learning, OSCE, clinical skills and many other terms.

Discomfort generated by lack of familiarity with IPE or with particular approaches to teaching and learning may cause some participants to try to change the nature of the learning experience so that it becomes more familiar. The conflicting expectations of different groups mean it is possible facilitators will have to contend with participants trying to tug the learning experience in different directions. It may become necessary to reflect this process back to the group and ask them to suspend resistance for a while, or to negotiate an acceptable compromise with respect to the learning activities.

Gender balance and the balance of professional membership can affect group dynamics.(106) There may be opportunities for facilitators to allocate group membership in ways that increase the likelihood of productive interprofessional discussion. Interprofessional co-tutoring is one way to mitigate tutors' inadequate knowledge of all participating professions and their usual approaches to learning and teaching, but there are costs to be balanced. The extra cost of additional facilitators would need to be offset by larger groups or reduced contact time. In addition, co-facilitators can feel that their own professional expertise is under the spotlight to a greater extent than in their routine work; this can be experienced as enjoyable or nerve-wracking. It is also important that co-tutors role-model high-quality interprofessional collaboration, otherwise the credibility of the learning experience may be damaged.

Conflict may be more likely in a group where firmly held professional positions are being exposed to scrutiny. Facilitators need to develop skills to productively harness the energy of conflict and set clear limits on acceptable behaviour. The Contact Hypothesis,(122,123) which suggests how prejudice and its associated conflict might be reduced, highlights the importance of facilitators drawing out both similarities and differences between participating groups (*see* Box 4.4). Most IPE facilitators find that conflict remains productive and manageable if there is a central focus on patient-centredness and improving the quality of services. Improving the quality of working lives by improving team communication and local processes is also an effective central focus at the post-qualification level.

Is e-moderation for interprofessional e-learning the same as uniprofessional e-moderation? In most respects the answer should be yes, so general e-moderation advice will be sound.(117,124,125) Predictable differences for e-IPE might include an unbalanced dynamic if members of each profession already know

BOX 4.4 Focus on: The Contact Hypothesis

The Contact Hypothesis(122,123,126) was developed from studies of religious and racial tension. It suggests that hostility between social groups would be reduced if members experienced greater contact, provided a set of 'conditions' is met:(127)

- each group should have equal status
- interaction should be conducted in a cooperative atmosphere
- participants should be working towards common goal and experience successful joint working
- 'the authorities' should support the initiative – for IPE this would mean professional bodies, healthcare providers, universities, faculty and clinicians.
- participants should be made aware of group similarities and group differences – members of one group compare their group's characteristics (in-group) with the characteristics of other groups (out-group) in an effort to establish positively valued distinctiveness.(128) IPE can usefully encourage mutual inter-group differentiation so that there can be shared acknowledgement of valued aspects of each group's identity(129)
- participants should have positive expectations
- participants from different groups should perceive one another as typical members of their group.

Listed thus, it sounds like a tall order for any educational initiative. Nevertheless, people have found the Contact Hypothesis a useful framework for developing or evaluating IPE that seeks to address unhelpful stereotypes and expectations.(2,55,129–131) The list of conditions provides useful guidance for curriculum developers and facilitators and it is in harmony with key features of theories of adult learning examined above, particularly the section on learning opportunities and learners' self-concepts.

fellow e-learners from their own profession but are just 'meeting' the other professions' learners in their e-IPE set. This is most likely to happen at the pre-qualification level when learners from different disciplines, possibly attending courses at different campuses, 'meet' to undertake e-IPE. Blending this with initial face-to-face IPE can help even out the degree to which learners feel they know one another.

Continuing with the case of pre-registration e-IPE, the ebb and flow of different professions' courses mean that any e-IPE group designed to run over an extended period will encounter times when one or other group leaves campus to gain experience in clinical settings. Even if faculty have planned continuing e-IPE, learners' access to the relevant network platform may be curtailed and, furthermore, students' attention may be almost completely diverted to their clinical experiences. This can lead to a profession unofficially dropping out for a while, changing the experience for those who remain (particularly in the extreme case of only two participating professions when the e-IPE comes to an unscheduled halt).

On their return, the temporarily absent learners will find themselves behind with the wider group's learning and need to catch up. Learners from other professions may have become irritated by the disengagement, so e-moderators may have to help the group to reintegrate … and then another profession goes out for a month's clinical experience. Happily, the downside of disengagement and re-entry is counterbalanced: re-entering learners often invigorate the e-IPE with insights and questions drawn from their recent clinical experience. E-moderators can help to initiate this process by welcoming people back and asking questions that help learners to link their recent experience with the e-IPE themes. Similar fluctuations in engagement with e-IPE can be seen when each participating profession approaches important summative assessments.

The Assessment of Interprofessional Education

Should we assess IPE at all? It might be argued that immersion in the process of IPE is more important than assessment. However, most people perceive value in including some formative or summative assessment. But how should we approach this? I would argue that the key concept is 'constructive alignment',(132) that is, assessment that by its nature reinforces the intended outcomes of the IPE. Since IPE is extremely varied, we should expect assessment associated with IPE to be equally varied.

Beginning with the most straightforward form of IPE, interprofessional quality improvement initiatives, the most appropriate form of assessment will be indicators drawn from the process of service delivery, and there are several good examples in Box 4.3. Within these team-based initiatives it is not usually felt to be necessary to assess the outcomes of IPE at the level of individual practitioners.

Individual practitioners will be assessed while they are undertaking specialist training or an award-bearing course. Formative assessment may well take the form of feedback from colleagues and supervisors. Some of this will be informal, as needs and opportunities arise, but increasingly this is complemented by more structured feedback – perhaps from a range of colleagues from different professions. Structured feedback is based on expected competences and can span formative and summative assessment. Summative assessments must have clearly defined criteria, and this is quite a complex undertaking for competences associated with interprofessional collaboration, but surely no more complex than trying to assess many other aspects of professionalism.

Pre-registration IPE and award-bearing post-registration IPE have to contend with the assessment requirements of all the participating professions and university departments, and practicalities too. This can feel like a problem without a solution and it is common for no summative assessment to be attached to IPE. The risk is that curriculum strands without assessment are interpreted as less valued, making disengagement and absenteeism more likely. Consequently, the most basic form of assessment for pre-registration IPE can be meeting an attendance or participation requirement, not unreasonable if interprofessional collaboration is viewed as a core facet of professionalism.

Many initiatives prefer to offer opt-in IPE to avoid the necessity of managing recalcitrant learners. Some IPE is assessed formatively or summatively through knowledge tests, essays, reflective journals and group presentations in various media (e.g. posters, patchwork texts, film, drama or through the ubiquitous presentation of software slide shows). Presentations may be delivered to peers, tutors, relevant practitioners or service users, providing different emphases within any resultant feedback or discussion. Whatever the format, learners gain most from active engagement with the activities that are assessed; this may need to be pointed out to group members who appear to be aiming for minimal participation. Encouraging self-assessment and including peer-assessment can be helpful here.

Faculty need to decide whether to assess teams or individuals, but current assessment regulations may limit options. This may signal a need for longer term work to align assessments with the principles of IPE, perhaps beginning with securing permission to pilot innovative assessments.

Tidal Flows in Interprofessional Education

Whichever beach you are sitting on it is likely to feel as if interest in IPE comes and goes like the tide. This applies to areas of practice as well as geographical locations, and beaches differ with respect to the amount of variation between high and low tide.

IPE matching the description we started with has been recorded since the 1960s. While there is national variation, early foci often included interprofessional teamwork in mental health and learning disabilities services, community and primary care. The 1970s saw increased attention to child protection and palliative care, while the 1980s brought IPE relating to HIV/AIDS. By the end of the century interest had broadened considerably and IPE had developed for maternity care, rehabilitation, chronic illnesses, ethics and management, and, to address the needs of

an ageing population and increasingly dispersed families, cost containment and workforce shortages. Most IPE occurred between qualified practitioners. Postmillennium foci have included patient safety, particularly in hospitals; disaster planning spurred on by heightened fears of terrorism; and boosting levels of pre-registration IPE. Most of these foci have endured, although relatively little is now written about some of the early foci. Hopefully, interprofessional collaboration and learning are too well embedded to be remarkable.

For several years colleagues in the US felt that, having arrived early, the tide had gone out rather a long way for interest and resources relating to IPE. Concerns about patient and public safety seem to have turned that tide for a while. At the time of writing, interest in IPE in the UK seems to be on the ebb. Financial concerns caused by fairly rapid social and demographic changes are driving political, health services, organisational and educational changes. IPE is less central to the political agenda and difficult to maintain through organisational upheaval.

Meanwhile, IPE in Canada has recently been enjoying a golden age of widespread interest and investment. Other countries too witness rising and falling tides of interest in IPE, although the Nordic countries have been relatively successful in maintaining steady progress with embedding IPE at the pre- and post-registration levels. Within Australasia and North America a significant strand of IPE development is concerned with meeting the needs of underserved populations, particularly rural communities and indigenous peoples. If you sit on any beach long enough the tide will ebb and flow.

Acknowledgements

I should like to acknowledge helpful comments and advice from four colleagues – Hugh Barr, Jon Fuller, Ivan Koppel and Scott Reeves – on the ideas explored in this chapter.

References

1 CAIPE (2006) CAIPE re-issues its statement on the definition and principles of interprofessional education. *CAIPE Bulletin.* **26**: 3. (http://www.caipe.org.uk/index.php?&page=define&nav=1; accessed March 2007).

2 Carpenter J and Hewstone M (1996) Shared learning for doctors and social workers: evaluation of a programme. *British Journal of Social Work.* **26**: 239–57.

3 Leathard A (1994) Interprofessional developments in Britain: an overview. In: Leathard A (ed.) *Going Inter-professional: working together for health and welfare*, pp. 3–37 Routledge, London.

4 Barr H (2005) *Interprofessional Education: today, yesterday and tomorrow* (revised edition). Occasional Paper 1. Higher

Education Academy Learning & Teaching Support Network for Health Sciences and Practice, London. (http://www.health.heacademy.ac.uk/publications/occasionalpaper/occp1revised. pdf; accessed February 2007).

5 Leathard A (2003) *Interprofessional Collaboration: from policy to practice in health and social care.* Bruner-Routledge, Hove.

6 Irvine R, Kerridge I, McPhee J and Freeman S (2002) Interprofessionalism and ethics: consensus or clash of cultures? *Journal of Interprofessional Care.* **16**: 199–210.

7 Øvretveit J, Mattias P and Thompson T (eds) (1997) *Interprofessional Working in Health and Social Care.* Palgrave Macmillan, London.

8 Jarvis P (1983) *Adult Learning in the Social Context.* Croom Helm, Beckenham.

9 Vermunt J and Verloop N (1999) Congruence and friction between learning and teaching. *Learning and Instruction.* **9**: 257–80.

10 Brockbank A and McGill I (2003) *The Action Learning Handbook: powerful techniques for education, professional development and training.* RoutledgeFalmer, London.

11 Freeth D, Hammick M, Reeves S *et al.* (2005) *Effective Interprofessional Education: development, delivery and evaluation.* Blackwell, Oxford, pp. 14–21, 25.

12 Gilbert J, Camp R, Cole C *et al.* (2003) Preparing students for interprofessional teamwork in health care. *Journal of Interprofessional Care.* **14**: 223–35.

13 Cooper H, Spencer-Dawe E and Mclean E (2005) Beginning the process of teamwork: design, implementation and evaluation of an inter-professional education intervention for first year undergraduate students. *Journal of Interprofessional Care.* **19**: 492–508.

14 Van Staa AL, Visser A and van der Zouwe N (2000) Caring for caregivers: experiences and evaluation of initiatives for a palliative care team. *Patient Education and Counselling.* **4**: 93–105.

15 Horbar J, Rogowski J, Plesk P *et al.* (2001) Collaborative quality improvement for neonatal intensive care. *Pediatrics.* **107**: 14–22.

16 Tepper M (1997) Providing comprehensive sexual health care in spinal cord injury rehabilitation: implementation and evaluation of a new curriculum for health care professionals. *Sexuality and Disability.* **15**: 131–65.

17 Mann K, Weld Viscount P, Cogdon A *et al.* (1996) Multidisciplinary learning in continuing professional education: the Heart Health Nova Scotia experience. *Journal of Continuing Education in the Health Professions.* **16**: 50–60.

18 Nash A and Hoy A (1993) Terminal care in the community – an evaluation of residential workshops for general practitioner/district nurse teams. *Palliative Medicine.* **7**: 5–17.

19 Adamowski K, Dickinson G, Weitzman B *et al.* (1993) Sudden unexpected death in the emergency department: caring for the survivors. *Canadian Medical Association Journal.* **149**: 1445–51.

20 Cooke S, Chew G, Boggis C and Wakefield A (2003) 'I never realised that doctors were into feelings too': changing student perceptions through interprofessional education. *Learning in Health and Social Care.* **2**: 137–46.

21 Treadwell M, Frank L and Vichinsky E (2002) Using quality improvement strategies to enhance paediatric pain assessment. *International Journal for Quality in Health Care.* **14**: 39–47.

22 Dalton JA, Carlson J, Blau W *et al.* (2001) Documentation of pain assessment and treatment: how are we doing? *Pain Management Nursing.* **2**: 54–64.

23 Crawford M, Turnbull G and Wessely S (1998) Deliberate self harm assessment by accident and emergency staff – an intervention study. *Journal of Accident and Emergency Medicine.* **15**: 18–22.

24 Morey J, Simon R, Gregory DJ *et al.* (2002) Error reduction and performance improvement in the emergency department through formal teamwork training: evaluation results of the MedTeams project. *Health Services Research.* **37**: 1553–81.

25 Stein J and Brown H (1995) 'All in this together': an evaluation of joint training on the abuse of adults with learning disabilities. *Health and Social Care in the Community.* **3**: 205–14.

26 Cox S, Wilcock P and Young J (1999) Improving the repeat prescribing process in a busy general practice: a study using continuous quality improvement methodology. *Quality in Health Care.* **8**: 119–25.

27 Allison M and Toy P (1996) A quality improvement team on autologous and directed-donor blood availability. *Journal of Quality Improvement.* **22**: 801–10.

28 Ketola E, Sipilä R, Mäkelä M and Klockars M (2000) Quality improvement programme for cardiovascular disease risk factor recording in primary care. *Quality in Health Care.* **9**: 175–80.

29 Fraser S, Wilson T, Burch K *et al.* (2002) Using collaborative improvement in a single organisation: improving anticoagulant care. *International Journal of Health Care Quality Assurance.* **15**: 152–8.

30 Ponzer S, Hylin U, Kusoffsky A *et al.* (2004) Interprofessional training in the context of clinical practice: goals and students' perceptions on clinical education wards. *Medical Education.* **38**: 727–36.

31 Sully P (2002) Commitment to partnership: interdisciplinary initiatives in developing expert practice in the care of survivors of violence. *Nurse Education in Practice.* **2**: 92–8.

32 Barber G, Borders K, Holland B and Roberts K (1997) Life Span Forum: an interdisciplinary training experience. *Gerontology and Geriatrics Education.* **18**: 47–59.

33 Snyder B (1973) *Hidden Curriculum.* MIT Press, Boston, MA.

34 Margolis E (ed.) (2001) *The Hidden Curriculum in Higher Education.* Routledge, New York.

35 Freeth D, Hammick M, Barr H *et al.* (2002) *A Critical Review of Evaluations of Interprofessional Education.* Higher Education Academy Learning & Teaching Support Network for Health Sciences and Practice, London. (http://www.health.heacademy.ac.uk/publications/occasionalpaper/occasionalpaper02.pdf).

36 Hammick M, Freeth D, Koppel I *et al.* (2007) A best evidence systematic review of interprofessional education. *Medical Teacher.* **29**(8): 735–51.

37 Reeves S, Zwarenstein M, Goldman J *et al.* (2008) Interprofessional education: effects on professional practice and health care outcomes. *Cochrane Database of Systematic Reviews* 2008, Issue 1.

38 De Bere SR (2003) Evaluating the implications of complex interprofessional education for improvements in collaborative practice: a multidimensional model. *British Educational Research Journal.* **29**: 105–24.

39 Rogowski J, Horbar J, Plesk P *et al.* (2001) Economic implications of neonatal intensive care unit collaborative quality improvement. *Pediatrics.* **107**: 23–9.

40 Shafer M-A, Tebb K, Pantell R *et al.* (2002) Effect of a clinical practice improvement intervention on chlamydial screening among adolescent girls. *Journal of the American Medical Association.* **288**: 2846–52.

41 Thomas P (1994) *The Liverpool Primary Health Care Facilitation Project 1989–94*. Liverpool FHSA, Liverpool.

42 Dunbar J, Neufeld R, White H and Libow L (1996) Retrain, don't restrain: the educational intervention of the National Nursing Home Restraint Removal Project. *The Gerontologist.* **36**: 539–42.

43 Berman S, Miller C, Rosen C and Bicchieri S (2000) Assessment training and team functioning for treating children with disabilities. *Archives of Physical Medicine and Rehabilitation.* **81**: 628–33.

44 Walsh P, Garbs C, Goodwin M and Wolff E (1995) An impact evaluation of a VA geriatric team development program. *Gerontology and Geriatrics Education.* **15**(3): 19–35.

45 Robinson M and Cottrell D (2005) Health professionals in multi-disciplinary and multi-agency teams: changing professional practice. *Journal of Interprofessional Care.* **19**: 547–60.

46 White S and Featherstone B (2005) Communicating misunderstandings: multi-agency work as social practice. *Child and Family Social Work.* **10**: 207–16.

47 Dolmans DH, De Grave W, Wolfhagen IH and van der Vleuten CP (2005) Problem-based learning: future challenges for educational practice and research. *Medical Education.* **39**: 732–41.

48 Albanese M (2007) *Problem-based Learning.* Association for the Study of Medical Education, Edinburgh.

49 *Medical Education* (2003) Special issue containing a selection of papers addressing simulation in medical education. *Medical Education.* **37**(s1): 1–78.

50 Issenberg SB, McGaghie WC, Petrusa ER, Lee Gordon D and Scalese RJ (2005) Features and uses of high-fidelity medical simulations that lead to effective learning: a BEME systematic review. *Medical Teacher.* **27**: 10–28.

51 Kilminster S and Jolly B (2000) Effective supervision in clinical practice settings: a literature review. *Medical Education.* **34**: 827–40.

52 Launer J (2006) *Supervision, Mentoring and Coaching: one-to-one learning encounters in medical education.* Association for the Study of Medical Education, Edinburgh.

53 Sambunjak D, Straus SE and Marusic A (2006) Mentoring in academic medicine: a systematic review. *Journal of the American Medical Association.* **296**: 1103–15.

54 Dienst E and Byl N (1981) Evaluation of an educational program in health care teams. *Journal of Community Health.* **6**: 282–98.

55 Carpenter J (1995) Interprofessional education for medical and nursing students: evaluation of a programme. *Medical Education.* **29**: 265–72.

56 Mires G, Williams F, Harden R and Howie P (2001) The benefits of a multiprofessional education programme can be sustained. *Medical Teacher.* **23**: 300–4.

57 Fallsberg M and Wijma K (1999) Student attitudes towards the goals of an inter-professional training ward. *Medical Teacher.* **21**: 576–81.

58 Mu K, Chao C, Jensen G and Royeen C (2004) Effects of interprofessional rural training on students' perceptions of interprofessional health care services. *Journal of Allied Health.* **33**: 125–31.

59 Reeves S, Freeth D, McCrorie P and Perry D (2002) 'It teaches you what to expect in future…': interprofessional learning on a training ward for medical, nursing, occupational therapy and physiotherapy students. *Medical Education.* **36**: 337–44.

60 Knowles M, Holton E and Swanson R (1998) *The Adult Learner: the definitive classic in adult education and human resource development* (5e). Butterworth-Heinemann, Woburn, MA.

61 Kolb D (1984) *Experiential Learning: experience as the source of learning and development.* Prentice Hall, Englewood Cliffs, NJ.

62 Wenger E (1998) *Communities of Practice: learning, meaning and identity.* Cambridge University Press, Cambridge.

63 Engeström Y, Engeström R and Karkkainen M (1995) Polycontextuality and boundary crossing in expert cognition: learning and problem solving in complex work activities. *Learning and Instruction.* **5**: 319–36.

64 Engeström Y (2001) Expansive learning at work: toward an activity theoretical reconceptualization. *Journal of Education and Work.* **14**: 133–56.

65 Rogers C and Freiberg HJ (1994) *Freedom to Learn* (3e). Merrill, London.

66 Jarvis P (2005) *Towards a Comprehensive Theory of Human Learning.* RoutledgeFalmer, London.

67 Brookfield S (1986) *Understanding and Facilitating Adult Learning.* Jossey-Bass, San Francisco, CA.

68 Entwistle N and Ramsden P (1983) *Understanding Student Learning.* Croom Helm, London.

69 Marton F and Booth S (1997) *Learning and Awareness.* Lawrence Erlbaum Associates, Mahwah, NJ.

70 Schön D (1991) *The Reflective Practitioner: how professionals think in action.* Arena, Bury St Edmunds.

71 Eraut M (1994) *Developing Professional Knowledge and Competence.* Falmer Press, London.

72 Eraut M (2000) Non-formal learning, implicit learning and tacit knowledge in professional work. In: Coffield F (ed.) *The Necessity of Informal Learning.* Policy Press, Bristol.

73 Mezirow J (2000) *Learning as Transformation: critical perspectives on a theory in progress.* Jossey-Bass, San Francisco, CA.

74 Richardson J, Eysenck M and Piper D (1987) *Student Learning: research in education and cognitive psychology.* Society for Research in Higher Education & Open University Press, Milton Keynes.

75 Kaufman D and Mann K (2007) *Teaching and Learning in Medical Education: how theory can inform practice.* Association for the Study of Medical Education, Edinburgh.

76 Erricsson K, Krampe R and Tesch-Römer (1993) The role of deliberate practice in the acquisition of expert performance. *Psychological Review.* **100**: 363–406.

77 Healy A and Bourne L (eds) (1995) *Learning and Memory of Knowledge and Skills: durability and specificity.* Sage, Thousand Oaks, CA.

78 Engeström Y (1999) Expansive visibilization of work: an activity-theoretical perspective. *Computer Supported Cooperative Work.* **8**: 63–93.

79 Marton F and Säljö R (1976) On qualitative differences in learning: II Outcome as a function of the learner's conception of the task. *British Journal of Educational Psychology.* **46**: 115–27.

80 Prosser M and Trigwell K (1999) *Understanding Learning and Teaching: the experience of higher education.* Society for Research in Higher Education & Open University Press, Buckingham.

81 Ramsden P (1997) The context of learning in academic departments. In: Martin F, Housell D and Entwistle N (eds) *The Experience of Learning* (2e), pp. 1908–216. Scottish Academic Press, Edinburgh.

82 Entwistle N (1998) Approaches to learning and forms of understanding. In: Dart B and Boulton-Lewis G (eds) *Teaching and Learning in Higher Education*, pp. 72–101. Australian Council for Educational Research, Melbourne.

83 Gibbs G (1992) *Improving the Quality of Student Learning.* Technical & Educational Services, Bristol.

84 Entwistle N and Smith C (2002) Personal understanding and target understanding: mapping influences on the outcomes of learning. *British Journal of Educational Psychology.* **72**: 321–42.

85 Zimmerman B (1998) Developing self-fulfilling cycles of academic regulation: an analysis of exemplary instructional models. In: Schunk D and Zimmerman B (eds) *Self-regulated Learning: from teaching to self-regulated practice,* pp. 1–19. Guildford Press, New York.

86 Khal T and Cropley A (1986) Face-to-face versus distance learning: psychological consequences and practical implications. *Distance Education.* **7**: 38–49.

87 Laurillard D (2002) *Rethinking University Teaching: a conversational approach for the effective use of learning technologies* (2e). RoutledgeFalmer, London.

88 Jaramillo J (1996) Vygotsky's sociocultural theory and contributions to the development of constructivist curricula. *Education.* **117**: 133–40.

89 Hogan K and Pressley M (eds) (1997) *Scaffolding Student Learning: instructional approaches and issues.* Brookline Books, Brookline, MA.

90 Healy A, King C, Clawson D *et al.* (1995) Optimizing the long-term retention of skills. In: Healy A and Bourne L (eds) *Learning and Memory of Knowledge and Skills: durability and specificity,* pp. 1–29. Sage, Thousand Oaks, CA.

91 Prosser M (1987) The effects of cognitive structure and learning strategy on student achievement. In: Richardson J, Eysenck M and Piper DW (eds) *Student Learning: research in education and cognitive psychology,* pp. 29–38. Society for Research in Higher Education & Open University Press, Milton Keynes.

92 Bandura A (1986) *Social Foundations of Thought and Action: a social cognitive theory.* Cambridge Books, Englewood Cliffs, NJ.

93 Pask G and Scott B (1972) Learning strategies and individual competence. *International Journal of Man-Machine Studies.* **4**: 217–53.

94 Perry W (1970) *Forms of Intellectual and Ethical Development in the College Years: a scheme.* Holt, Rinehart & Winston, New York.

95 Perry G (1981) Cognitive and ethical growth: the making of meaning. In: Chickering A (ed.) *The Modern American College.* Jossey-Bass, San Francisco, CA.

96 Moon J (2000) *Reflection in Learning and Professional Development.* Kogan Page, London.

97 Johns C (2002) *Guided Reflection: advancing practice.* Blackwell, Oxford.

98 Irons A (2007) *Enhancing Learning through Formative Assessment and Feedback.* Routledge, Oxford.

99 Wood D (2007) *Formative Assessment.* Association for the Study of Medical Education, Edinburgh.

100 Grant J (2006) *Principles of Curriculum Design.* Association for the Study of Medical Education, Edinburgh.

101 Areskog N-H (1995) Multiprofessional education at the undergraduate level. In: Soothill K, Mackay L and Webb C (eds) *Interprofessional Relations in Health Care,* pp. 125–39. Edward Arnold, London.

102 Ker J, Mole L and Bradley P (2003) Early introduction to interprofessional learning: a simulated ward environment. *Medical Education.* **37**: 248–55.

103 Miller C, Woolf C and Mackintosh N (2006) *National Evaluation of Common Learning and AHP First Wave Sites.* Final Report (Department of Health Commission 0160050), University of Brighton (http://www.brighton.ac.uk/inam/research/projects/index.htm).

104 Bruner J (1977) *The Process of Education* (2e). Harvard University Press, Cambridge, MA.

105 Itano J, Williams J, Deaton M and Oishi N (1991) Impact of a student interdisciplinary oncology team project. *Journal of Cancer Education.* **6**: 219–26.

106 Kilminster S, Hale C, Lascelles M *et al.* (2004) Learning for real life: patient-focused interprofessional workshops offer added value. *Medical Education.* **38**: 717–26.

107 Dewey J (1933) *Experience and Education.* Heath, New York.

108 Freeth D and Chaput de Saintonge DM (2000) Helping medical students become good house officers: interprofessional learning in a skills centre. *Medical Teacher.* **22**: 392–8.

109 Madsen M, Gresh A, Petterson B and Taugher M (1988) An interdisciplinary clinic for neurologically impaired adults: a pilot project for educating students. *Journal of Allied Health.* **17**: 135–41.

110 Goodsman D and Moe E (2006) *Middle Years IPE: student study book.* City and Queen Mary Universities, London (http://www.ipecityqm.org.uk/downloads/AStudybook%20FINAL.pdf; accessed May 2007).

111 Steven A, Dickinson C and Pearson P (2007) Practice-based interprofessional education: looking into the black box. *Journal of Interprofessional Care.* **21**: 251–64.

112 Wahlström O and Sandén I (1998) Multiprofessional training at Linköping University: early experience. *Education for Health.* **11**: 225–31.

113 Hayward K (2005) Facilitating interdisciplinary practice through mobile service provision to the rural adult. *Geriatric Nursing.* **26**: 29–33.

114 Reeves S and Freeth D (2002) The London training ward: an innovative interprofessional learning initiative. *Journal of Interprofessional Care.* **16**: 41–52.

115 Hylin U, Nyholm H, Mattiasson A and Ponzer S (2007) Interprofessional training in clinical practice on a training ward for health care students: a two-year follow-up. *Journal of Interprofessional Care.* **21**: 277–88.

116 McCrorie P (2006) *Teaching and Leading Small Groups.* Association for the Study of Medical Education, Edinburgh.

117 Jaques D and Salmon G (2007) *Learning in Groups: a handbook for face -to-face and online environments* (4e). Routledge, Abingdon.

118 Light G and Cox R (2001) *Learning and Teaching in Higher Education: the reflective professional.* Paul Chapman, London.

119 Brockbank A and McGill I (1998) *Facilitating Reflective Learning in Higher Education.* Society for Research in Higher Education & Open University Press, Buckingham.

120 Savin-Baden M (2003) *Facilitating Problem-based Learning: illuminating perspectives.* Society for Research in Higher Education & Open University Press, Maidenhead.

121 Griffiths S (1999) Teaching and learning in small groups. In: Fry H, Ketteridge S and Marshall S (eds) *A Handbook for Teaching and Learning in Higher Education* (2e), pp. 91–104. Kogan Page, London.

122 Allport G (1979) *The Nature of Prejudice* (25e). Perseus Books, Cambridge, MA.

123 Hean S and Dickinson C (2005) The contact hypothesis: an exploration of its further potential in interprofessional education. *Journal of Interprofessional Care.* **19**: 480–91.

124 Salmon G (2004) *E-moderating: the key to teaching and learning online* (2e). RoutledgeFalmer, London.

125 McKendree J (2006) *eLearning*. Association for the Study of Medical Education, Edinburgh.

126 Amir Y (1969) Contact hypothesis in ethnic relations. *Psychological Bulletin.* **71**: 319–42.

127 Hewstone M and Brown R (1986) Contact is not enough: an intergroup perspective on the 'contact hypothesis'. In: Hewstone M and Brown R (eds) *Contact and Conflict in Intergroup Encounters*, pp. 1–44. Blackwell, Oxford.

128 Tajfel H (1981) *Human Groups and Social Categories*. Cambridge University Press, Cambridge.

129 Barnes D, Carpenter J and Dickinson C (2000) Interprofessional education for community mental health: attitudes to community care and professional stereotypes. *Social Work Education.* **19**: 565–83.

130 Hewstone M, Carpenter J, Franklin Stokes A and Routh D (1994) Intergroup contact between professional groups: two evaluation studies. *Journal of Community and Applied Social Psychology.* **4**: 347–63.

131 Carpenter J (1995) Doctors and nurses: stereotypes and stereotype change in interprofessional education. *Journal of Interprofessional Care.* **9**; 151–61.

132 Biggs J and Tang C (2007) *Teaching for Quality Learning at University* (3e). Open University Press, Maidenhead.

Further reading

Many of the other chapters in this book are valuable sources of additional reading to inform the development and delivery of interprofessional education (IPE), particularly:

Teaching and Learning in Medical Education: how theory can inform practice, David Kaufman and Karen Mann.

Principles of Curriculum Design, Janet Grant; *Teaching and Leading Small Groups*, Peter McCrorie

Good studies of IPE are dispersed across many journals, their location often reflecting the clinical setting for the IPE or the professional backgrounds of the authors. However, the most extensive single collection of papers about IPE – descriptions, evaluations and theoretical debate – can be found in the *Journal of Interprofessional Care* (http://www.informaworld.com).

This paper has not discussed the evaluation of IPE, although many of the studies cited ably demonstrate varied approaches to evaluating IPE selected according to context and the nature of the research questions. I have contributed to an extended discussion of evaluating IPE in Part III of Freeth D, Hammick M, Reeves S, Koppel and Barr H (2005) *Effective Interprofessional Education: development, delivery and evaluation*. Blackwell, Oxford.

The British Medical Association published a short information resource on IPE in 2006. It has several useful web links (http://www.bma.org.uk/ap.nsf/Content/ipe). The UK Centre for the Advancement of Interprofessional Education maintains a web site with important content and useful links (http://www.caipe.org.uk).

The Canadian Interprofessional Health Collaborative will keep you up to date with the burgeoning activity in Canada (http://www.cihc.ca).

The European Interprofessional Education Network is linking people and organisations in Greece, Finland, Hungary, Poland, Sweden, the UK and beyond to share ideas and IPE resources (http://www.eipen.org).

Work-based learning

Clare Morris and David Blaney

KEY MESSAGES

- The workplace is a fundamentally important site for learning in both undergraduate and postgraduate medical education.

- The erosion of time-served methods of apprenticeship creates challenges for those tasked with ensuring that healthcare professionals are appropriately trained to deliver safe, efficient and effective patient care.

- Insight into the theoretical concepts underpinning work-based learning reveals a range of tools and approaches that can be employed to 'revive' apprenticeship and support work-based learning.

- Faculty development for clinical teachers drawing on social theories of learning provides a way forward to enhance work-based learning in medical settings.

Introduction

Work is where we spend a considerable amount of our life and expend a great deal of physical and emotional energy. Work is essential to our well-being. Work is how many people define themselves, be it in relation to their role – 'I am a doctor' – or to their place of work – 'I work for the University of…'. For doctors, work and the workplace is where their professional learning is made real, where knowledge and skills are acquired, crafted and developed.

We all have different experiences of work and workplaces. We influence our workplace and it influences and shapes us. The workplace can be a nurturing environment where knowledge and skills are fostered, extended and developed through work activity and our interactions with others. Equally, it can be a dysfunctional environment that stifles creativity, dampens professional motivation and leads to psychological and physical ill health.(1,2)

In this chapter we explore the changing landscape of medical education, describe current conceptions of work-based learning and underpinning theoretical perspectives, and propose strategies to enhance work-based learning for medical students and trainees. Throughout, we acknowledge that the challenges faced by those involved in supporting work-based learning in medicine are equally relevant to those who work in dentistry, veterinary medicine, and other health and social care professions.

The Changing Landscape of Medical Education and Training

Medical education is undergoing a period of unprecedented and rapid change. In the UK, the number of 'stakeholders' with interests in, and influences over, education and training is growing, creating tensions within and across undergraduate and postgraduate sectors. Tensions arise between universities, who see their role as to promote academic excellence and produce world-class graduates, and the National Health Service, which requires trained staff to meet the current and future health needs of the population.(3) The UK is not unique in facing such challenges, with the reform of medical education in the US being described by Whitcomb(4) as 'the most serious challenge facing academic medicine's institutions', and others arguing that teaching and patient care have become subordinate to research and that the increased demand for productivity is eroding teaching time.(5)

Changes in clinical service organisation and delivery have resulted in patients spending less time in hospitals, which traditionally have been the main provider of work-based experiences for students and trainees. Concerns have been raised that 'healthcare as a business may threaten medicine as a calling', with clinical teachers being challenged to provide opportunities for learning through experience and practice.(6) In the UK, European working time regulations have contributed to the loss of 'firms', the traditional supervisory relationships that supported work-based learning. At the same time as increasing emphasis is being placed on the workplace as the site for education and training, concerns have been raised about graduate preparedness for practice. The outcomes of these changes mean that students and trainees compete for training time, patient contact and appropriate supervision.

Understanding Medical Education: Evidence, Theory and Practice. Edited by T Swanwick. © 2010 Association for the Study of Medical Education.

Finally, while work-based learning is seen as a fundamental aspect of education and training, its perceived status has been challenged by the privileges afforded to formal teaching. This is evidenced in protected teaching time, investment in formal teaching spaces and simulation resources within clinical environments, and investment in off-site development opportunities for trainees and their trainers. The danger of this is that work-based learning is marginalised and undervalued. Yet, as we argue in the next section, the curriculum of the workplace is fundamentally important to the development of future doctors.

The Current State of Work-based Learning in Medical Education

There is evidence to suggest that a significant proportion of medical graduates do not feel suitably prepared for clinical practice and have concerns about dealing with the day-to-day realities of working life, be it dealing with acutely ill patients, prescribing, managing their workload or being on call.(7–10) Significantly, additional challenges, such as understanding their role and boundaries, may only become evident in their first posts.(8) The reasons why some graduates feel unprepared are complex and span individual and organisational dimensions. However, the amount and nature of work-based experience undergraduates have and their opportunity to shadow first posts before commencing employment appears to increase their preparedness. Early experiences of the workplace were noted to have an impact on intended career pathways for half of those in the British Medical Association cohort study, with working conditions and work hours the main reasons cited for planned changes.(9) It is of concern that the number of graduates with a strong desire to practise medicine declines following these early work experiences.

The relevance and quality of work-based learning experiences have been called into question in a number of studies(11–17) and concerns are raised in the following areas:
- inadequate systems of structured educational appraisal(18)
- insufficient time available for teaching(19,20)
- insufficient outpatient experience(21–23)
- lack of involvement in clinical audit(23)
- too many educationally unproductive tasks(22)
- inadequate clinical supervision(16,24)
- poor induction(21)
- difficulty accessing study leave or library facilities(25,26)
- excessive and concentrated workload.(27)

There is little doubt that doctors in training value work-based learning experiences and seek opportunities to engage in work-based learning. They want a structured environment where work-based learning is valued, protected and appropriately supervised and supported. However, reform of healthcare, education and training, and threats to the time-served nature of training, is placing significant challenges on those in training and those who are charged with supporting and fostering their development in the workplace. A greater understanding of the nature of work-based learning and strategies is key to overcoming these challenges.

Learning and Work

In this section we review the dominant conceptions of work-based learning and the models commonly in use. This inevitably leads to a review of ideas of learning per se, which is important as these ideas shape the ways in which we engage with learners and the pedagogic practices we adopt. Scott(28) provides a thoughtful critique of curriculum theories, and drawing on Bernstein's model of curriculum as performance,(29) he identifies the following predominant elements in mainstream education:
- the strong focus on traditional forms of knowledge (discipline-based)
- distinctions between lower and higher domains of knowledge
- differentiation of learners and the curriculum (selection, differentiation)
- the teacher's role being to impart knowledge.(28)

While his critique focuses on schooling, there are parallels with professional education. In medicine, as with other health professions, the curriculum has been based on a model of technical rationality, where knowledge (in the mind of the learner) is 'applied' to the world of practice. Although this model has been challenged, it persists in the minds of many as the 'best' way to educate, leading to a continued focus on imitation and instruction as the primary tools of the teacher. However, Billet(30) and others(31,32) have argued that the tendency to compare work-based learning with formal learning, or to draw on formal models of learning in the workplace, is unhelpful. Responding to this, we examine existing and emerging notions of work-based learning and the potential to develop new approaches to professional education and training.

Formal, informal and non-formal learning
Medical education has tended to draw a distinction between 'formal' learning (medical school) and 'informal' learning (in the clinical work environment). Formal learning is typically characterised by timetables, aims and objectives, a defined curriculum and often progressive linear teaching and examinations.

In contrast, informal learning, usually in the workplace, has traditionally been less valued by teachers and students, viewed as haphazard and lacking any formal educational rigour, process or structure. As noted previously, these criticisms arise in part because work-based learning is compared with the process and pedagogy of formal learning rather than being viewed as having a pedagogy and process of its own.

Eraut(33) proposes a move away from the use of the term 'informal learning' to that of 'non-formal learning'. In so doing he proposes a typology of *non-formal* learning, focusing on the learner's intention to learn. *Implicit learning* is characterised by learning that takes place without any prior intention to learn by the learner, with the learner being unaware of the learning at the time. He contrasts this with *deliberative learning*, where the learner sets time aside to learn and approaches learning in a planned and purposeful way. Between these two points, Eraut describes *reactive learning*, which happens almost spontaneously as a result of situation and circumstance. While the learning is not consciously planned, learners recognise learning opportunities, are prepared for emergent learning opportunities and are likely to engage in brief, almost spontaneous reflection on learning events or experiences. This distinction is helpful when we consider ways to promote work-based learning, suggesting the possibility of explicitly recognising, responding to and valuing the learning that arises during everyday practice, and encouraging students and trainees to do the same.

Work-based learning

Work-based learning spans all stages of medical education and training, from early undergraduate years, through specialist training and, increasingly, continuing medical education. Boud and Solomon(34) have explored the place of work-based learning in professional education, noting that undergraduate courses now:

> acknowledge the workplace as a site of learning and as a source for making the curriculum more relevant. As such they are a signal of the blurring distinctions between the university and the workplace. (p. 34)

They go on to note that this 'blurring' signals the increasing legitimisation of learning outside formal academic contexts and argue that this creates both opportunities and challenges for students and trainees:

> Learning tasks are influenced by the nature of work and, in turn, work is influenced by the nature of the learning that occurs. The two are complementary. Learners are workers; workers are learners. They need to be able to manage both their roles. (p. 34)

This dual role is particularly striking in postgraduate training, where trainees are also employees and therefore have service as well as learning commitments. Seagraves(35) distinguishes three 'links' between work and learning:

- learning *for* work
- learning *at* work
- learning *from* work.

These semantic distinctions are important, signalling, albeit implicitly, different relationships between working and learning, and the intended purposes of that learning. The question that arises is whether, for example, the medical curriculum is designed or intended to enhance working practice or professional practice. In other words, is the learning undertaken for the benefit of the employer or the individual? To some extent, this depends on the perspective from which work is viewed.

Evans provides three perspectives that are of value in viewing work-based learning:

- industrial relations
- sociological
- social learning theory.(36)

Viewed from the *industrial relations* perspective, work is a contested activity, with constant tension between employee and employer over rights, obligations and the prevention or misuse of employee skills and labour. Work-based learning is driven by the needs of the workplace, rather than those within it, with access to further training and development opportunities being driven by desires to promote innovation or efficiency. Work-based learning is something employers control (e.g. study leave). For medical students and trainees this is visible in issues such as access to study leave, hours of work and rotas, and the emphasis on statutory training.

Viewed from the *sociological* perspective, however, work is more of a place of and for social interaction, socialisation and identity formation. Clearly this is of influence in the development of professional roles and identities, where interpersonal relationships, power, authority and status are all part of the dynamic of the workplace. In this context, how an individual trainee or student relates to others and how they are perceived by others may have a bearing on the types of learning experiences they are offered and the training they receive.(37) How work is perceived will have an effect on how an individual views and approaches work-based learning. Work involves professional activity but also demands of doctors, trainees and students additional duties, roles and responsibilities. Understanding this is central to work-based learning and, as we will argue later, is important if students and trainees wish to maximise their learning at work. The difficulty is that the privileging of, and overemphasis on, formal learning in undergraduate years may influence student and trainee ability to recognise the learning that is embedded in working activity.

The perspective of *social learning theory* will be addressed in the sections below, but any discussion of work-based learning in medicine would be incomplete without first a consideration of the centuries-old practice of apprenticeship.

Apprenticeship

At its most prosaic, an apprentice is someone who is paid by their employer to learn. But the apprentice–employer relationship has added complexities, and historical forms of apprenticeship have embraced learning at, for and from work, and provided opportunities for the apprentice to learn their craft through supervised practice.(38) Scott describes apprenticeship as a pedagogic approach where 'the learner is supported in their attempts to gain access to the culture of the society in which they are being educated'.(28) However, Dornan notes that traditional forms of apprenticeship are threatened by discontinuity of care (with decreased length of stay), over-specialisation of services, and staff and students living 'off site'.(39) Ideas of apprenticeship have been expanded, with the cognitive apprenticeship model – 'making thinking visible' – being of particular relevance to clinical teachers (*see* Box 5.1).

In keeping with the dominant paradigm of learning described earlier, traditional forms of apprenticeship have been focused on the instruction and development of the apprentice in the workplace. The focus is very much on the development of the individual, through engagement with the supervising expert. It does not accommodate the idea that the expert may learn from the apprentice and that the apprentice may in fact shape the practice in which they both engage. Contemporary views of apprenticeship, building on socio-cultural theories of learning, accommodate not only the reciprocal nature of learning between 'apprentice and master', but also the contributions made by others in the professional community. New formulations of apprenticeship are emerging that enable us to look beyond the novice–expert dualism and consider a social apprenticeship that much more actively recognises the contributions made by the wider community of the workplace.(42)

Theories of Social Learning

Theories of learning can be seen to sit within different educational schools of thought, from the behaviourist (learning through reinforcing), to the cognitive (learning through knowing) and the social (learning through becoming).

While behaviourist principles can be identified in skills-based teaching, cognitive models have long dominated the literature of medical education and training. Cognitive models align with the emphasis on analytic reasoning that has dominated medical educa-

BOX 5.1 How to: Adopt the practices of a cognitive apprenticeship

The cognitive apprenticeship model derives from traditional craft apprenticeship, but makes 'thinking visible'.(40) Collins *et al.*(41) identified six stages to their model, which can be readily adopted in work-based teaching and is particularly useful in teaching decision making, ethics, communication skills and other cognitively complex areas of professional practice.

Modelling: allow the learner to observe your practice in order to build up a conceptualisation of that practice.

Coaching: watch the learner practise, offering them guidance, critique and feedback.

Scaffolding: offer the learner more opportunities to practise, gradually and purposefully increasing complexity of the work undertaken while slowly fading out your input.

Articulation: use questioning and supervision time to encourage the learner to talk you through what they are doing, why and how, providing a rationale for the approaches taken.

Reflection: encourage the learner to consider his or her performance analytically and to compare it with that of the expert to identify ways to further enhance his or her own performance.

Exploration: provide opportunities for the learner to undertake new tasks and activities, prompting the learner to become independent in his or her activity and his or her thinking.

tion in the years following the Flexner report.(5) However, cognitive models, with their emphasis on the individual, have limitations when considering the complex nature of work-based learning. Attention is turning to social models of learning, and in particular socio-cultural theories of learning, as a way of illuminating ways in which students and trainees develop professional knowledge, skills, values and identities in the workplace.(43) In the following section, these differing perspectives on learning will be explored and their relevance to work-based learning considered.

Broadly speaking, behaviourism contests that learning is manifested by changes in behaviour, these changes being the result of stimuli that are external to the individual, that is, environmental factors. Hartley argues that the learning principles arising from the behaviourist school are focused on the importance of:

- learning by doing
- frequent practice in varied contexts
- reinforcement as a prime motivator
- the need to have clearly defined behavioural objectives that are communicated to the learner.(44)

These learning principles are readily observed in popular models of skills-based teaching in medicine and the rise of outcomes-based education. But however desirable the models may seem, they belie the complexity of the work-based and professional learning. The cognitive orientation to learning can be seen as a shift from behaviourists' focus on the external world to one that focuses on the internal world and changes in thinking.

Within the cognitive school, the focus shifts from the external to the internal world of learners. The focus is on the acquisition of knowledge and skills, be it as a result of input from a more able 'other' (through processes of transmission) or through engagement with one's own experiences (constructivism). Hager(45) refers to this as the standard paradigm of learning, which sees the 'best' type of learning as being:

- in individual minds
- propositional in nature
- expressible verbally or in writing
- transparent to the mind.

Constructivism, closely linked to the work of Jean Piaget, posits that meaning (or learning) is generated through human engagement with experience. As Scott and Palinscar note:

> Constructivists argue there is no such thing as ready-made knowledge; regardless of what a teacher does, learners construct their own knowledge. All learning (…) requires reinterpreting the information to be learnt or used in light of one's existing understandings and abilities.(46, p. 31)

Cognitive views on learning dominate medical education literature and practice. As Swanwick notes, the contested concepts of *andragogy*,(47) *experiential learning*(48) and *reflection*(49,50) have led to the almost wholesale adoption of portfolios, appraisal and personal development planning in all walks of medical education and training.(32) What is important to note here, however, is that these models present learning as essentially unmediated activity, which happens as a result of learner engagement with their own experiences. For example, Kolb's learning cycle of concrete experience, reflection, conceptualisation and experimentation(48) is abstracted from a social context and tells us little about the types of experience that may foster this cyclical process or the role of more expert practitioners in encouraging or supervising subsequent reflection, conceptualisation and experimentation. Lee *et al.*(51) note this emphasis on rational and cognitive aspects leads to work performance being 'conceived as thinking or reflection followed by application of the thinking or reflection'.(51) Central to these models is the individual learner's capacity to engage with an experience, reflect critically on it and deduce the lessons learnt that need to be applied to future activity. Cognitive perspectives of learning will tend to lead to an emphasis on instructional methods, with the importance of structure being stressed. The importance of building on prior knowledge is key, and so distinctions between individual learners are impor-

tant when planning teaching or supervision. Cognitive feedback (successes and failures) is an important dimension, providing learners with new information to assimilate and accommodate. However, cognitive models of learning are increasingly being called into question as an appropriate model for work-based learning in medicine.(31,32,52) Theories of learning that recognise and explicitly emphasise the social, participatory and context specific nature of learning are argued to be of greater relevance to complex practice that happens in teams and communities of workers and learners. Three of these – social cognitive theory, social constructivism and socio-cultural theories – will be considered in the next section.

Social theories of learning pay attention to both the inner and external worlds of learners, and the interaction between individuals and those around them is central to the process of meaning making. Each of the theoretical perspectives explored in the following section places different levels of emphasis on this interaction and the impact of the social elements on learning and practice. All offer valuable insights into the potential nature of work-based learning in medicine and suggest ways of working with students and trainees to foster learning.

Social cognitive theory

Social cognitive theory can be seen as a coming together or a bridging of the behaviourists' concern with external, environmental stimuli and the cognitive theorists' concern with the internal mind. Bandura proposed a model of learning to capture what he saw as the dynamic interplay between the personal, the cognitive and the environmental, which, combined, determine an individual's behaviour. He described this as *reciprocal determinism*(53; *see* Box 5.2).

Bandura also identified five fundamental human capabilities:

- *symbolising* (in order to give structure, meaning and continuity to their lives)

BOX 5.2 Reciprocal determinism in social cognitive theory

- *forethought* (planning for action, considering potential consequence of actions)
- *self-regulation* (through the positive and negative consequences that their behaviour produces)
- *self-reflection* (in relation to own functioning and self-efficacy)
- *vicarious learning* (through close observation of others).

It can be argued, therefore, that what people think, feel and believe will influence how they behave, with self-belief [also described as self-efficacy(54)] being an important determinant of motivation and achievement. The capability for vicarious learning has been argued to be an important element of role modelling in medicine and a powerful means of transmitting values, attitudes and patterns of behaviour, be it through imitation or identification.(55)

Role modelling is foregrounded in the medical education literature as a key process in professional development and enculturation, and Box 5.3 summarises some of the characteristics that 'good' role models are said to display. A recent review of the literature pertaining to 'good clinical teaching' notes the dominance of non-cognitive characteristics based on personal and relationship-based attributes.(56) It is unsurprising therefore that concerns have been raised about the erosion of role modelling through the demise of apprenticeship and the commercialisation of healthcare.(5,39) Despite the central importance ascribed to role modelling, its basis remains largely unexamined and considerable assumptions are made of its effectiveness.(55)

Social constructivism

In constructivist models the emphasis is on how the individual learner 'constructs' knowledge, that is, how the learner makes sense of new information and experiences provided by the teacher, the environment and their wider experience. Social constructivism goes one step further, emphasising the importance of social engagement in the learning process. In other words, learners make sense of new ideas and information by engaging with others, be it their teachers, their fellow students or others around them. An example of social constructivism at work in medical education would be (in its purest form) problem-based learning.

Vygotsky, who developed his theories of learning from observational studies of children interacting with adults, was a key contributor to social constructivism. He noted that children were more successful in learning tasks when they engaged with adults (a more knowledgeable 'other') than when they worked independently, arguing that learning awakens developmental processes that are able to operate only when the child is interacting with their peers and others in their environment.(59) This is significantly different from models of experiential learning explored above, which suggest that the provision of a learning experience itself leads to learning. Vygotsky drew attention to the concepts and tools teachers use to mediate the learning of another, stressing the importance of language (or shared talk) in the developmental process. Importantly, he introduced what has been described as a fundamentally new approach to the need to match learning to the learner's developmental stage, through the construct of the *zone of proximal development*.(46) This refers to what a learner can do with the support of a more knowledgeable other (be it their teacher or their peers) and is contrasted with their *zone of actual development*, or what they can do independently. Box 5.4 illustrates the ways in which Vygotsky's work can shape approaches to clinical teaching.

Social cognitive theory and constructivist approaches help us understand ways in which we might support student or trainee learning. However, even these models are limited in helping us better understand the complexity of work-based learning. Recent years have seen the development of socio-cultural theories of learning and these are explored now.

Socio-cultural learning

It has recently been argued that junior doctors learn by 'situated learning in communities of practice',(43) explicitly referring to the work of socio-cultural theorists and, in particular, the work of Lave and Wenger.(60,61) The evidence base supporting this assertion is explored in Box 5.5. Socio-cultural theories of learning have broad disciplinary origins and embrace a wide range of theoretical perspectives. However, it has been argued that they share some core tenets, these being that learning is:

- situated (shaped by the context in which it occurs)
- mediated (by a range of symbolic and conceptual tools)
- historically and culturally influenced.(62)

Social cultural theories have undoubtedly been influenced by Vygotsky's work (and others from the social-

---

BOX 5.3 How to: Be a good role model(55,57,58)

- Be positive about what you do
- Be enthusiastic, compassionate and open
- Analyse your own performance as a role model
- Model reflection and facilitate the reflections of others
- Articulate and discuss values
- Make the implicit more explicit
- Be learner-centred in your teaching
- Allow time for discussion and debrief
- Engage in personal and professional development activity
- Show respect to colleagues
- Work to improve workplace culture and values.

BOX 5.4 Focus on: Vygotsky

Consider the mediated nature of learning activity

Vygotsky drew attention to the 'tools' that we use to 'mediate' a learning experience, be it the language we use to explain or guide, or the tools we use to exemplify, such as handouts, paper cases, X-rays and patients-as-cases. This can help us look more purposefully at informal learning encounters, and recognise and make explicit the everyday tools and learning resources we use.

Identify learners' needs and learning potential

Vygotsky drew a distinction between what he termed the *zone of actual development* (what the learner can actually do unassisted) and the *zone of proximal development* (what the learner can do with some assistance or guidance). Learning is what takes place in the zone of proximal development, where we guide, assist, support and coach our learners. In working with students and trainees, therefore, it is important to recognise what they can do independently and then to work out how we can *scaffold* their learning so that they can move forward.

Engage 'more knowledgeable others' in the learning process

Vygotsky saw engagement with peers and others in the environment as an essential prerequisite for learning to take place. Recognising and valuing the contributions made by all members of the care team and the learners' peer group are essential to effective learning in the workplace.

BOX 5.5 Where's the evidence? Situated learning

Lave and Wenger developed their viewpoints on learning through ethnographic studies of traditional 'apprenticeships' as diverse as the apprenticeships of Yucatec midwives, Vai and Gola tailors, butchers, quartermasters and members of Alcoholics Anonymous.(60) From this work they developed ideas around situated learning and communities of practice, both of which have been influential on thinking about informal and work-based learning generally and, increasingly, in medical education specifically. Claims have been made for the value of drawing on their viewpoints when looking at work-based learning in medicine;(31,32,52,62–64) however, few studies have been undertaken to explicitly explore the extent to which their claims are true of medical education.

A qualitative study of medical student learning on clinical attachments supported the idea that attachments could be seen as times spent in communities of practice, albeit in a descriptive sense. The limits placed on student engagement in authentic work-based activity, the extent to which students and their teachers identify the learning resources embedded in this day-to-day activity and the hierarchical (and sometimes authoritarian) stance towards teaching and learning limited the extent to which this claim could be supported.(65) Likewise, a qualitative study of general practice training revealed that registrars may not be able to become full participants in the practices of a community, nor may they be able to access and engage with all of the community members to develop shared understandings of practice.(63) The work around preparedness of graduates for practice(7,8) and the limited nature of student engagement in authentic clinical activity(66) also questions the extent to which they are able to become full participants through legitimate peripheral participatory practices.

constructivism school), but they draw even greater attention to the wider context in which learning takes place, and the role of the wider community in which learners learn. They emphasise the historical context of practice, in other words they argue that in order for a student to understand workplace practices they need to have a sense of the history of those practices and how they have evolved over time. This gives support to the idea that it is important to recognise what has been successful in work-based learning in medicine and to find ways to ensure that these historically successful strategies can evolve to be equally successful in new times and contexts.

Socio-cultural theorists see the distinction between learning and working (or practice) as being artificial. They start from the assumption that learning is part and parcel of our everyday experience and practice. So, for example, when we talk to our colleagues about patients we are having difficulty with, or we 'think aloud' management options on the ward round, we

are engaged in both a working activity and a learning activity. Our understanding of each other, our patients and their illnesses is influenced by the conversations we have and this becomes part of the learning in the workplace. When we encounter a complex patient or a complex situation, we draw on the 'learning resources' around us (our peers, our seniors, other members of the healthcare team) to consider how to move forward. We might consult other types of resource such as internet search engines, but seldom do we immediately 'rush off to be taught' to address these issues. As students develop their practice, they are learning at the same time. Learning is therefore an everyday activity and is developed by joint participation. In other words, learning is 'situated' and collective, with a shift in emphasis from a focus on the individual learner or teacher to one that focuses on the 'team' or 'community'.

In recent years, the term 'community of practice' has been adopted by those in professional education and used, often uncritically, to capture a desire to foster collaborative working, be it face-to-face or online. However, its original use was much more specific and was to capture examples of situated learning in a range of 'apprenticeship systems' observed ethnographically by Lave and Wenger.(60) Their seminal text identifies a defining feature of learning in these contexts, that of legitimate peripheral participation, described as:

> a way to speak about the relations between newcomers and old-timers, and about activities, identities, artefacts and communities of knowledge and practice. It concerns the process by which newcomers become part of a community of practice. A person's intentions to learn are engaged and the meaning of learning is configured through the process of becoming a full participant in a socio-cultural practice.(60, p. 29)

Four key ideas emerge from their work, which have particular relevance to work-based learning in medicine and newly emerging models of apprenticeship:

- learning is part of social practice
- learning takes place in communities of practice
- learning takes place through legitimate peripheral participation
- language is a central part of practice.

We now explore these in more depth, first, *learning is part of social practice*. Every day at work we encounter new situations, new patients, new colleagues, trainees or students that lead us to question what we know, what we do, and how and why we do it. This is clearly a 'learning' situation, although we might not always label it as such. Second, *learning takes place in communities of practice*, which can be identified and defined by common expertise. The practice of a surgical team or the psychiatric outreach team demonstrates this in that their practice is effective because of the shared endeavour, the collective 'team think' that leads to successful outcomes. If we compare these two 'teams', while each contains doctors, nurses and healthcare professionals, they are clearly distinct in terms of the specialist work they do, the ways they do this and the 'cultures' of their practice (how they dress, how they talk to each other and their patients, etc.). Clearly, within medicine there are many distinct communities of practice, and students and trainees need to learn how to participate within them and indeed, across them. Third, *learning has a central defining process, that of 'legitimate peripheral participation'*, a process that enables the student to develop the expertise necessary to permit full access and participation in a community. When we delegate work to students and trainees we need to ensure it allows increasing engagement in 'real' work activity, from the periphery (e.g. scrubbing up to observe the surgical procedure) to more central core activity (e.g. leading the surgical procedure). It is important to note that the relationships described between 'newcomers' and 'old-timers' here are very different from the traditional hierarchical educational models of novice to expert. This is an important distinction as it recognises the valuable contributions students and trainees can make to shaping and developing practice and the impact they can have on the workplace. Finally, *language is a central part of practice*, not only in terms of learning from talk but rather in terms of learning to talk – a process of talking one's way into the expertise. For example, when students and trainees 'present cases', with implicit structures and cultures of doing so – 'Mrs Smith is a 55-year-old woman, who presented to A and E with a three-day history of…' – they are learning 'to talk' medicine and therefore learning medicine itself.

Socio-cultural perspectives on work-based learning clearly offer some theoretical and conceptual tools to allow researchers and practitioners to analyse important aspects of work-based learning. The emphasis on learning as being something that encompasses the processes of 'belong, becoming and identity', as well as meaning making,(61) encourages closer attention to what others have termed the hidden curriculum of medical education and training. However, Lave and Wenger's work has been criticised for its lack of attention to a number of important issues, namely:

- individual variations in accessing learning in the workplace(67)
- the ways in which 'old timers' continue to learn in the workplace(42)
- emotional dimensions of work-based learning(2)
- the role of formal learning opportunities for workers,(42,68)

Billett, in particular, argues the need to pay attention to the *invitational qualities* of the workplace, in terms of the ways in which the workplace provides and allows access to learning activities.(30,67) A concrete example can be seen in obstetrics and gynaecology attachments for medical students, where male students are likely to access fewer hands-on learning experience than female students due to patient preferences.(69) More subtle variations of opportunity may exist on the basis of 'qualities' attributed to students by staff. For example, more able students who express high levels of confidence, enthusiasm and interest in a specialty may access more learning opportunities than a shy or struggling student or one perceived to have limited insight into their own performance. In this latter case it may be that those who most need experience to develop confidence and competence are denied these experiences.(70) Despite these criticisms, social perspectives on learning can be seen as a way forward to understanding and therefore more effectively shaping the work-based learning opportunities offered to students and trainees.

Curriculum and Work-Based Learning: A Complex Relationship

In describing these different theoretical schools of thought, we have drawn out the ways in which work-based learning can be contrasted to more formal learning. The distinctiveness of work-based learning can also be highlighted in relation to the curriculum.

Traditional approaches to curriculum design, based in formal education, focus on the curriculum as transmission of a body of knowledge (e.g. paediatrics) or on the definition of desired end points and outcomes (e.g. a competent doctor). This is evident in the rise of outcomes and competency-based curriculum, which aligns to behaviourist and cognitive schools and derives from the work of Bobbit, Tyler and Popham.(71–73) The emphasis is on the clear delineation of specific knowledge, skills and attitudes, which are seen as measurable outputs of learning.

The risk with this model as a framework for work-based learning is that it assumes that all worthwhile attainments are visible and quantifiable,(28) that those external to the learner are best placed to identify what it is the learner needs and that learning itself is devalued with the emphasis on outcomes (to be signed off) rather than processes of learning,(74,75) The emphasis on competence, as opposed to excellence, has also been questioned in the UK following the wholesale introduction of work-based curriculum and assessment tools in postgraduate education.(3)

When we turn to social theories of learning, however, we are able to identify two other approaches that resonate with our understanding of work-based learning. The 'process curriculum', drawing on a social constructivist perspective, focuses on the construction of meaning and collaborative engagement. As Stenhouse argues:

> The superficialities of the disciplines may be taught by pure instruction, but the capacity to think within the disciplines can only be taught by inquiry.(76, p. 38)

A process-based curriculum places importance on the relationships between trainer and trainee and the outcome of their interaction. It is grounded in the individual experience of the trainee resulting from their clinical and professional experiences. A process curriculum assumes that trainers have experience and knowledge, that they understand their role and have a mature and internalised concept of what they are trying to achieve with the trainee. The content of the trainee's learning is to a great extent built on and derived from their experiences and is developed by promoting critical dialogue and thinking, reflecting both in and on outcomes and activity. In the process curriculum, both trainer and trainee seek to critically test knowledge, and the learning is continually adapted by both trainer and trainee. The consequence of such an approach is that learning outcomes can vary between trainees and are negotiable depending on the trainee's capability. But the purpose of the curriculum is to extend the trainee and to seek to maximise their potential rather than simply achieve competence. The learner is actively involved and manages the process of learning with the trainer, and the interaction and relationship with the trainer is central to this process.

The contrast between 'product' and 'process' models of curriculum lead us to consider the appropriateness of each *for* the workplace. However, socio-cultural theories of learning focus on the workplace and work *as* the curriculum; in other words, there is little separation between participation in working life and learning.(77) If the workplace is the curriculum, the challenge for those with educational roles in the workplace is to make the learning that can arise from working more explicit, and to ensure that learners are engaged in the process of seeking and accepting these opportunities to learn.

This is underlined by studies exploring the nature of work-based learning in clinical settings, which have emphasised the importance of:

- initiation processes to engage learners as part of the team(64)
- active involvement in patient care(66)
- access to conversations, coaching and feedback in order to foster professional thinking and skill development.(78)

Constraints may arise in terms of the number of 'learners' attached to a particular setting and the nature and scope of work activity undertaken by the team.(66) It is important to emphasise that if the workplace is the curriculum, the learning relationships to be developed must extend beyond those between individual learner and teacher to encompass the whole team.(31) More recent framings of apprenticeship(42,79) adopt these broader perspectives on learning and curriculum and identify the ways in which the workplace can both expand and restrict opportunities for learning.

Implications for the Clinical Teacher

The question reasonably arises: 'What does this all mean for an individual clinical or educational supervisor?' The direct implications can be summarised as follows.

1 Learning is part of everyday social practice
   Implication: we need to make learning opportunities explicit to our learners. We also need to make explicit specific workplace cultures and practices to help students and trainees 'make sense' of what they see, hear, sense and do.
2 Teams can be seen as 'communities of practice', which are identified and defined by their shared expertise
   Implication: we need to involve the whole team (community) in supporting student/trainee learning.

3 Novices become experts through participation in communities of practice
Implication: we need to consider the ways in which we can meaningfully involve our students/ trainees in workplace activity.

4 Workplaces do not always readily invite learners in and do not always offer equal opportunities to all learners(67)
Implication: we need to consider how we can create the right conditions for learning to take place in our workplace and to ensure certain students or groups of students/trainees are not inadvertently disadvantaged.

5 Horizontal learning is as important as vertical learning in the workplace(80)
Implication: we need to understand what our students/trainees already know (where they are coming from) and help them to use it to make sense of what they see, hear and do in the workplace.

6 'Talk' is a central part of practice – learners need to 'learn to talk their way into expertise' rather than just learn from the talk of an expert(60)
Implication: we need to find strategies to help our students and trainees talk themselves into the expertise, by using techniques such as 'thinking aloud' and case-based discussion.

7 Students and trainees learn from their entire setting
Implication: we need to be aware of the workplace climate and the effect this will have on trainees. This includes how staff relate to them and to each other, how staff are valued, and how they value their work and workplace.

8 Students require multiple learning experiences and learning methods
Implication: a balance needs to be found between the duration of attachments – sufficient to allow students to become immersed in the workplace – and providing enough attachments to give exposure to other workplaces and specialities.

9 Feedback to students and a sense of belonging are important in allowing them to feel confident and become active participants in the workplace
Implication: regular feedback is important and we need to provide trainees with increasing exposure to and involvement in workplace activities.

10 Learning in the workplace is an iterative process and trainees are active participants and can influence the workplace
Implication: we need to allow and value feedback from students and give them the opportunity to feed back their views and impressions of the workplace.

Challenges to Work-based Learning in Medical Education

As we hope we have illuminated, the workplace has the potential to be the central site for professional learning and development in both undergraduate and postgraduate years. However, it is important not to underestimate the potential barriers to effective work-based learning. Clearly there is an ongoing tension between working and learning, and the intensity of work for both trainers and trainees has a significant bearing on this. Trainees need opportunities to learn through working, but they also need to be released to access the formal aspects of their training and to have time to consider and discuss the learning that arises through engagement in work activity. The sheer number of learners in the workplace is also significant, and those with responsibility for organising training need to consider how to avoid the creation of learner hierarchies, which are at risk of favouring issues of seniority, power or status over learning need. The importance of organisational and work dynamics should not be overlooked.

The shortening and fragmentation of training has eroded time-served traditional apprenticeship models. However, the importance of the relationship between trainer and trainee continues to feature highly in studies of work-based learning in medicine. Developing safe and effective supervision strategies will be key, as will be the need to draw on new models of apprenticeship that value the relationships between and contributions of other members of the team. Finally, the rise of competency-based models of education, training and assessment brings a risk of a 'tick-box' mentality to training that must be challenged. The focus on process aspects of the curriculum will be fundamental to the ongoing development of trainees.

Throughout this chapter we have drawn attention to the ways in which conceptions of work-based learning can shape our practice, and the importance of a critical engagement with theoretical perspectives on learning, which can illuminate ways in which we can best support work-based learning in medicine. We have argued that social theories of learning in particular, which emphasise the social, participatory, mediated and context-specific aspects of learning, are best placed to support our activity. In the final section we will summarise the implications for those who organise, manage and deliver education and training in the medical workplace.

Developing and Promoting Work-based Learning

Implications for clinical teachers

Reviving apprenticeship demands a change of mindset from one that focuses on 'sitting at the master's feet' to one that focuses on the community, that is, a collective model of newcomers and old-timers working and learning together.(60,81) The named supervisor can assist this process by ensuring appropriate orientation to patient care and teamworking, and by highlighting

BOX 5.6 How to: Make the implicit 'explicit'

- Label the learning opportunities that arise spontaneously in day-to-day work.
- Signal expectations in terms of culture (dress code, ways of addressing members of the team and patients), practices (preferred ways of doing things and why) and participation.
- Encourage learners to articulate and discuss observed differences in culture and practice in different settings or specialties, and consider why these may occur.
- Be clear about the importance given to learning from work and set aside time to consider lessons learned (brief and debrief).
- Prime learners for observation and shadowing (using advanced organisers) making clear what it is possible to learn.
- Adopt the principles of 'articulation and reflection' in your approaches to clinical teaching cognitive apprenticeship.
- Talk about what you are role modelling and why.

opportunities to work and learn with all members of the team, including patients, carers and peers. Effective clinical teaching will involve planning for learning, which includes making sure that learners are open to the learning opportunities that arise through work.(33) The need to make the implicit 'explicit' arises as a key factor here (*see* Box 5.6).

A second shift of mindset may be from that of 'teacher' to 'facilitator of learning' to ensure that precious protected teaching time is not wasted. This will mean ensuring that you have a clear sense of the starting points of individual learners and that you have identified what they can do with the assistance of a more knowledgeable other, who may be one of their peers or another team member, rather than the named supervisor. Kilminster's guidance on effective supervision is particularly helpful here.(82)

The effective use of authentic, work-based assessments can be invaluable. Learners provided with appropriate support are able to access a broader range of working, and therefore learning, experiences. The emphasis on learning through participation with other team members allows the supervisor to be more targeted and effective with time set aside for teaching. Conceptualising this as time set aside for developmental conversations may help this process. The importance of shared talk, learning to talk and to articulate reasoning, cannot be overemphasised here. Launer's model of narrative-based supervision is flexible enough to encompass formal and informal supervision sessions as well as the skills needed to conduct case-based discussion more effectively.(83)

Implications for educational leaders and managers

Those charged with responsibility for overseeing the training of individuals (e.g. educational supervisors) or groups of trainees (e.g. directors of medical education, training programme organisers) can build on the strategies for clinical teachers highlighted above. Reconceptualising training as an opportunity for an 'expansive apprenticeship' leads to a closer consideration of the value of time spent in a range of clinical settings (albeit for relatively short periods compared with old) and the need to balance this with time 'out' for formal training and thinking time. Seeing induction as an opportunity to orientate learners to ways in which to make the most of the learning that happens in the workplace will be key. This will include:

- making explicit the value of learning through working
- supervision as an opportunity for developmental conversations
- work-based assessment as the key tool to identify learning needs and ensure regular and targeted feedback
- the cultural expectation of learning through teamwork.

Peer learning should be emphasised and explicitly valued, with the positive impact of mentoring relationships being explored. Interprofessional induction helps strengthen the value placed on working and learning in teams that go across professional boundaries.

Implications for faculty developers

Swanwick argues that the professionalisation of medical education, increased accountability and aspirations to excellence have heightened the attention being placed on faculty development in medicine.(84) In the UK, there is a growing expectation that all doctors who teach will undertake suitable training and be willing to demonstrate their competence to carry out their roles.(85–87) However, attention has been drawn to the organisational deterrents to engagement in faculty development(88) and it is worth noting that historically this activity has been based within medical schools (with the resulting emphasis on formal teaching) rather than the clinical workplace. If, as we have argued, a revival of medical apprenticeship requires shifts in mindset as well as practice, faculty development has the potential to be invaluable. Clearly there are some areas where developing teaching and assessing skills will be necessary. Norcini, for example, argues that faculty development is key to the successful use of assessment methods based on observation of routine encounters.(89) Faculty development that moves beyond a focus on teacher competence to a concern with the need to foster a critical dialogue between those who share responsibility for medical education and training is vital,(62,65,90) Faculty developers working with clinical teachers should be tasked with sharing insights into work-based learning that draw on social and participatory schools of thought rather than the cognitive models that dominate the formal educational arena. Approaches to faculty development that recognise the value of coaching, mentoring and peer observation of teaching will model the social and participatory aspects of learning through work and can be balanced with more traditional workshop-based activity focusing on skill rehearsal, dialogue and feedback.

Conclusion

The value and importance of work-based learning has never been clearer, nor the challenges faced greater. Reform of healthcare, medical education and training are eroding time-served approaches to training and demand a revival and creation of new models of apprenticeship. Conceptions of work-based learning, alongside a closer examination of educational theories and perspectives, may provide us with the tools to do this. While it will be important to hold on firmly to the time-honoured features of apprenticeship, rooted in a developmental relationship between trainer and trainee, there are opportunities to embrace opportunities for learning as active participants in patient care, supported by peers and colleagues within the communities in which we work and learn.

References

1 Firth-Cozens J (2006) A perspective on stress and depresssion. In: Cox J, King J, Hutchinson A and McAvoy P (eds) *Understanding Doctors' Performance*, pp. 22–37. Radcliffe Publishing, Oxford.
2 Turnbull S (ed.) (2000) The role of emotional in situated learning and communities of practice. Productive learning at work. Working Paper 59. Lancaster University Management School, University of Technology, Sydney, NSW.
3 Tooke J (2008) *Aspiring to Excellence: findings and recommendations of the Independent Inquiry into Modernising Medical Careers*. MMC Inquiry, London.
4 Whitcomb M (2003) Editorial. The most serious challenge facing academic medicine's insitutions. *Academic Medicine*. **78**: 1201–2.
5 Cooke M, Irby D, Sullivan W and Ludmerer K (2006) American medical education 100 years after the Flexner Report. *New England Journal of Medicine*. **355**: 1339–45.
6 Department of Health (2004) *Modernising Medical Careers – the next steps. The Future of Foundation, Specialist and General Practice Training Programmes*. DoH, London.
7 Goldacre M, Lambert T, Evans J and Turner J (2003) Preregistration house officers' views on whether their experience at medical school prepared them well for their jobs: national questionnaire survey. *British Medical Journal*. **328**: 1011–12.
8 Illing J, Davies C and Baldauf B (2008) *How Prepared Are Medical Graduates to Begin Practice. A Comparison of Three*

Diverse Medical Schools. Report to Education Committee. General Medical Council, London.
9 Unit HPaER (2008) *First Report of the BMA Cohort Study of 2006 Medical Graduates*. British Medical Association, London.
10 Cave J, Goldacre M, Lambert T *et al.* (2007) Newly qualified doctors' views about whether their medical school had trained them well: questionnaire surveys. *BMC Medical Education*. **7**: 38.
11 Bourne M and Paterson-Brown S (1999) Calman and the new deal – compromising doctor training and patient care. *Scottish Medical Journal*. **44**: 147–8.
12 Bruch G, Bahrami J and MacDonald R (1997) Training the SHO grade: how good is it? *British Journal of Hospital Medicine*. **57**: 565–8.
13 Cooke L and Hurlock S (1999) Education and training in the SHO grade a cohort study. *Medical Education*. **33**: 418–23.
14 Davis J, Tan K and Jenkins H (2000) The current status of SHO postgraduate education in a single region. *Medical Education*. **34**: 367–70.
15 Field A, Baker M and Williams J (2001) Formal education programmes for SHOs: comparison of experience in three hospital specialties. *Posgraduate Medical Journal*. **77**: 650–3.
16 Paice E (1998) Is the new deal compatible with good training? A survey of SHOs. *Hospital Medicine*. **59**: 72–4.
17 Pease R, Mitra A and Heymann T (1999) What the SHO really does. *Journal of the Royal College of Physicians of London*. **33**: 553–6.
18 Murphy D and Kelly M (2003) SHO formative assessment: an observational study. *Education for Primary Care*. **14**: 158–65.
19 Leverton T (2000) A method of assessment of hospital posts accredited for GP training. *Education for General Practice*. **11**: 405–11.
20 Rickenback M, Dunleavy J, Little P and Mullee N (1997) Impact of existing peer review visits needs to be increased. *British Medical Journal*. **314**: 1828–30.
21 Hand H (2000) Evaluation satisfaction with hospital training for general practice: a comparison of two surveys in East Anglia for the JCPTGP. *Education for General Practice*. **11**: 385–90.
22 Hand H and Adams M (1998) The development and reliability of the RCGP questionnaire for measuring SHO satisfaction with their hospital training. *British Journal of General Practice*. **48**: 1399–403.
23 Hand H, Shepstone L and Dawson H (2003) Judging the quality of SHO training: the work of the HRC of RCGP in England and Northern Ireland. *Education for Primary Care*. **14**: 18–24.
24 Grant J, Marsden P and King R (1989) SHOs and their training: personal characteristics and professional circumstances and perception of service and training. *British Medical Journal*. **299**: 1263–8.
25 Baker M and Spackling P (1994) The educational component of SHO posts: difference in perception of consultants and junior doctors. *Postgraduate Medical Journal*. **70**: 198–202.
26 Evans A (1997) Hospital component of GPVTS. *Journal of the Association of Course Organisers*. **3**: 46–9.
27 Wall D, Woodward D and Whitehouse A (2001) The development and use of a computerised evaluation for SHO posts in West Midlands Region. *Medical Teacher*. **23**: 24–8.
28 Scott D (2008) *Critical Essays on Major Curriculum Theorists*. Routledge, London.
29 Bernstein B (1996) *Pedagogy, Symbolic Control and Identity: theory, research and critique*. Taylor and Francis, London.

30 Billett S (2001) *Learning in the Workplace. Strategies for Effective Practice.* Allen and Unwin, Crows Nest, NSW.

31 Bleakley A (2006) Broadening conceptions of learning in medical education: the message from teamworking. *Medical Education.* **40**: 150–7.

32 Swanwick T (2005) Informal learning in postgraduate medical education: from cognitivism to 'culturism'. *Medical Education.* **39**: 859–65.

33 Eraut M (2000) Non-formal learning, implicit learning and tacit knowledge in professional work. In: Coffield F (ed.) *The Necessity of Informal Learning*, pp. 12–21. The Policy Press, Bristol.

34 Boud D and Solomon N (2003) *Work-based Learning. A New Higher Education?* The Society for Research into Higher Education, Open University Press, Buckingham.

35 Seagraves L and Boyd A (1996) *Supporting Learners in the Workplace: guidelines for learning advisers in small and medium sized companies.* University of Stirling, Stirling.

36 Evans K, Hodkinson P, Rainbird H and Unwin L (2006) *Improving Workplace Learning.* Routledge, Oxford.

37 Morris C (2000) Developing a pedagogy for doctors as teachers. Postcompulsory education. Unpublished manuscript available through the Institute of Education library.

38 Souster V and Jackson N (2003) Apprenticeship systems and work based learning. In: Burton J and Jackson N (eds) *Work-based Learning in Primary Care*, pp. 59–72. Radcliffe Publishing, Oxford.

39 Dornan T (2005) Osler, Flexner, apprenticeship and 'the new medical education'. *Journal of the Royal Society of Medicine.* **96**: 91–6.

40 Wooley N and Jarvis Y (2007) Situated cognition and cognitive apprenticeship: a model for teaching and learning clinical skills in a technologically rich and authentic learning environment. *Nurse Education Today.* **27**: 73–9.

41 Collins A, Brown J and Newman S (1989) Cognitive apprenticeship: teaching the crafts of reading, writing and mathematics. In: Resnick L (ed.) *Knowing, Learning, and Instruction: essays in honour of Robert Glaser*, pp. 453–94. Lawrence Erlbaum Associates, Hillsdale, NJ.

42 Fuller A and Unwin L (2006) Expansive and restrictive learning environments. In: Evans K, Hodkinson P, Rainbird H and Unwin L (eds) *Improving Workplace Learning*, pp. 27–48. Routledge, London.

43 Postgraduate Medical Education and Training Board (2008) *Educating Tomorrow's Doctors: future models of medical training; medical workforce shape and trainee expectations.* PMETB, London.

44 Hartley J (1998) *Learning and Studying. A Research Perspective.* Routledge, London.

45 Hager P (2004) The conceptualization and measurement of learning at work. In: Rainbird H, Fuller A and Munro A (eds) *Workplace Learning in Context*, pp. 242–58. Routledge, Oxford.

46 Scott S and Palinscar AS (2009) The influence of constructivism on teaching and learning in classrooms. In: Daniels H, Lauder H and Porter J (eds) *Knowledge, Values and Educational Policy: a critical perspective*, pp. 29–43. Routledge, London.

47 Knowles M (1973) *The Adult Learner. A Neglected Species.* Gulf Publishing, Houston, TX.

48 Kolb D (1984) *Experiential Learning.* Prentice Hall, Englewood Cliffs, NJ.

49 Schon D (1983) *The Reflective Practitioner: how professionals think in action.* Basic Books, New York.

50 Schon D (1987) *Educating the Reflective Practitioner: towards a new design for teaching and learning in the professions.* Jossey-Bass, San Fransisco, CA.

51 Lee T, Fuller A, Ashton D *et al.* (2004) Workplace learning: main themes and perspectives. Learning as work. Research Paper 2. University of Leicester, Centre for Labour Market Studies, Leicester.

52 Bleakley A (2002) Pre-registration house officers and ward-based learning: a 'new apprenticeship' model. *Medical Education.* **36**: 9–15.

53 Bandura A (1977) *Social Learning Theory.* Prentice-Hall, Englewood Cliffs, NJ.

54 Bandura A (1997) *Self-efficacy: the exercise of control.* WH Freeman, New York.

55 Kenny N, Mann K and MacLeod H (2003) Role modeling in physicians' professional formation: reconsidering an essential but untapped educational strategy. *Academic Medicine.* **78**: 1203–10.

56 Sutkin G, Wagner E, Harris I and Schiffer R (2008) What makes a good clinical teacher in medicine? A review of the literature. *Academic Medicine.* **83**: 452–66.

57 Cruess SR, Cruess RL and Steinert Y (2008) Role Modelling – making the most of a powerful teaching strategy. *British Medical Journal.* **336**: 718–21.

58 Paice E, Heard S and Moss F (2002) How important are role models in making good doctors? *British Medical Journal.* **325**: 707–10.

59 Vygotsky L (1978). In: Cole M, John-Steiner V, Scribner S and Souberman S (eds) *Mind in Society: the development of higher psychological processes.* Harvard University Press, Cambridge, MA.

60 Lave J and Wenger E (1991) *Situated Learning: legitimate peripheral participation.* Cambridge University Press, Cambridge.

61 Wenger E (1999) *Communities of Practice. Learning, Meaning and Identity.* Cambridge University Press, Cambridge.

62 Morris C (2009) Developing pedagogy for doctors-as-teachers: the role of activity theory. In: Daniels H, Lauder H and Porter J (eds) *Knowledge, Values and Educational Policy. A Critical Perspective*, pp. 273–81. Routledge, Oxford.

63 Cornford C and Carrington B (2006) A qualitative study of the experiences of training in general practice: a community of practice? *Journal of Education for Teaching.* **32**: 269–82.

64 Lyon P (2004) A model of teaching and learning in the operating theatre. *Medical Education.* **38**: 1278–87.

65 Morris C (2005) *Moving Beyond See One, Do One, Teach One: developing pedagogy for doctors as teachers.* Institute of Education, University of London, London.

66 Sheehan D, Wilkinson T and Billett S (2005) Interns' participation and learning in clinical environments in a New Zealand hospital. *Academic Medicine.* **80**: 302–8.

67 Billett S (2002) Toward a workplace pedagogy: guidance, participation and engagement. *Adult Education Quarterly.* **53**: 27–43.

68 Solomon N (1999) Culture and difference in workplace learning. In: Boud D and Garrick J (eds) *Understanding Learning at Work*, pp. 119–31. Routledge, London.

69 Higham J and Steer PJ (2004) Gender gap in undergraduate experience and performance in obstetrics and gynaecology: analysis of clinical experience logs. *British Medical Journal.* **328**: 142–3.

70 Wilkinson T and Harris P (2002) The transition out of medical school – a qualitative study of descriptions of borderline trainee interns. *Medical Education.* **39**: 466–71.

71 Bobbitt F (1918) *The Curriculum.* Houghton Miflin, Boston, MA.

72 Tyler R (1950) *Basic Principles of Curriculum and Instruction.* University of Chicago Press, Chicago, IL.

73 Popham WJ (1972) *An Evaluation Guidebook: a set of practical guidelines for the educational evaluator*. The Instructional Objectives Exchange, Los Angeles, CA.

74 Prideaux D (2004) Clarity of outcomes in medical education: do we know if it really makes a difference? *Medical Education*. **38**: 580–1.

75 Talbot M (2004) Outcomes-based teaching: 'monkey see, monkey do': a critique of the competency model in graduate medical education. *Medical Education*. **38**: 587–92.

76 Stenhouse L (1975) *An Introduction to Curriculum Research and Development*. Heinemann, London.

77 Billett S (2004) Learning through work. Workplace participatory practices. In: Rainbird H, Fuller A and Munro A (eds) *Workplace Learning in Context*, pp. 119–31. Routledge, London.

78 Dornan T, Boushuizen H, King N and Sherpbier A (2007) Experience-based learning: a model linking the processes and outcomes of medical students' workplace learning. *Medical Education*. **41**: 84–91.

79 Fuller A and Unwin L (2004) Expansive learning environments. Integrating organizational and personal development. In: Rainbird H, Fuller A and Munro A (eds) *Workplace Learning in Context*, pp. 126–4. Routledge, London.

80 Griffiths T and Guile D (2003) A connective model of learning: the implications for work process knowledge. *European Educational Research Journal*. **2**: 56–73.

81 Morris C (2010) Facilitating learning in the workplace. *British Journal of Hospital Medicine*. **71**(1): 48–50.

82 Kilminster S, Cottrell D, Grant J and Jolly B (2007) AMEE guide no. 27: effective educational and clinical supervision. *Medical Teacher*. **29**: 2–19.

83 Launer J (2006) *Supervision, Mentoring and Coaching: one-to-one learning encounters in medical education*. Association for the Study of Medical Education, Edinburgh.

84 Swanwick T (2008) See one, do one, then what? Faculty development in postgraduate medical education. *Postgraduate Medical Journal*. **84**: 339–43.

85 General Medical Council (2006) *Good Medical Practice*. GMC, London.

86 Postgraduate Medical Education and Training Board (2008) *Generic Standards for Training*. PMETB, London.

87 Department of Health (2008) *The Gold Guide: a reference guide for postgraduate specialty training in the UK*. DoH, London.

88 Steinert Y, McLeod P, Boillat M *et al.* (2009) Faculty Development: a 'field of dreams'? *Medical Education*. **43**: 42–9.

89 Norcini J (2007) *Workplace-based Assessment in Clinical Training*. Association for the Study of Medical Education, Edinburgh.

90 Morris C and McKimm J (2008) *Developing teachers: moving beyond teacher competence*. Paper presented at NET Conference, Cambridge, 2nd to 4th September, 2008.

Further Reading

Billett S (2001) *Learning in the Workplace: strategies for effective practice*. Allen and Unwin, Crows Nest, NSW.

Boud D and Solomon N (2003) *Work-based Learning. A New Higher Education?* The Society for Research into Higher Education & The Open University Press, Buckingham.

Evans K, Hodkinson P, Rainbird H and Unwin L (2006) *Improving Workplace Learning*. Routledge, Oxford.

Kilminster S, Cottrell D, Grant J and Jolly B (2007) AMEE guide no. 27: effective educational and clinical supervision. *Medical Teacher*. **29**: 2–19.

Lave J and Wenger E (2003) *Situated Learning. Legitimate Peripheral Participation*. Cambridge University Press, Cambridge.

Rainbird H, Fuller A and Munro A (2004) *Workplace Learning in Context*. Routledge, London.

Scott D (2008) *Critical Essays on Major Curriculum Theorists*. Routledge, London.

Wenger E (1998) *Communities of Practice. Learning, Meaning and Identity*. Cambridge University Press, Cambridge.

Learning medicine from the humanities

J Jill Gordon and H Martyn Evans

KEY MESSAGES

- Professional competence is enhanced when students are broadly educated; the humanities can foster personal and professional maturation by providing insights into the human experience of illness, disability and medical interventions.

- Despite the importance of the arts and humanities, their position within medical curricula tends to be precarious; educators need a clear and defensible view on teaching and learning medicine from the humanities.

- Philosophy, history and literature are key humanities disciplines and their relationship with medicine should

be part of the core curriculum; students should also have access to self-selected study modules suited to their particular interests.

- The processes involved in learning medicine from the humanities are as important as the course content.

- The humanities can often blend with other elements of the medical curriculum rather than being in direct competition. Teaching, assessment and evaluation should be aligned with each other and reflect the core values of the programme more generally.

- A rich supply of resources for teaching and learning is available.

Happy the person who has been able to understand the cause of things.
Virgil, Georgics: Book 2, Line 490.

Introduction

In developed societies, medical practice relies heavily on science and technology. Doctors have been accused of failing to care because the profession has lost sight of some fundamental elements of good doctoring.(1) The result has been harmful for both patients and the profession. In addition, it is now widely agreed that the overall cost of modern medicine is unsustainable,(2) even if no attempt is made to address the inequalities that exist within and between countries. Perhaps, it is suggested, doctors better versed in the medical humanities would help to redress the balance.

Medical students are typically motivated by a desire 'to understand the cause of things'. They usually enter medical school with the desire to study the biomedical sciences and the desire to use this knowledge to help others.(3) At the outset, students generally acknowledge that 'helping others' means more than simply solving medical problems and that curing is not equivalent to healing.(4) (When students are not immediately clear on the difference, the analogy of a burglary can be helpful. The police may track down the burglar and recover your possessions. This may 'cure' your material loss, but it will not guarantee your emotional recovery.) However, teaching and assessment in

medical school place strong emphasis on the medical sciences rather than on the medical humanities. Medical students also undergo socialisation in medical school; in particular, they observe that the doctors who deal with the broad philosophical and social challenges posed in primary care, mental health, rehabilitation, ageing and end-of-life care generally occupy the lower rungs of the medical hierarchy, while those who avoid the complex issues in medical care and focus on the technology tend to occupy the higher rungs.

The term 'medical humanities' was apparently coined by an Australian surgeon, Moore, in 1976. He described his approach to using literature in teaching undergraduate medical students at the University of Melbourne(5) as a way of understanding the human experience of health and illness and also as a way of exploring ethical issues in clinical practice.(6) At the same time, the University of La Plata in the Argentine Republic, among others, was making a specific commitment to the humanities, initially as a non-compulsory element.(7) While biomedicine focuses on 'objective' science, the medical humanities are distinguished by their concern with recording and interpreting the human experiences of illness, disability and medical intervention.(8) Students experience the medical humanities at the most basic level whenever they attend to patients' stories rather than simply extracting 'medically relevant' information, and whenever they themselves reflect on, and give expression to, their own and others' experiences of health, illness and care giving. In addition to these immediate experiences of the doctor–patient relationship, students can also access representations of illness, disability and medical intervention portrayed by others, for example, writers, historians, philosophers, artists and

Understanding Medical Education: Evidence, Theory and Practice.
Edited by T Swanwick. © 2010 Association for the Study of Medical Education.

musicians. These opportunities are arguably most important if students come from relatively narrow, culturally limited backgrounds with limited experience of the values, attitudes, needs and concerns of the majority of people. Although many medical schools now try to select students from broader backgrounds than has traditionally been the case, many students are still 'disadvantaged' by their material advantages when it comes to understanding other people's lives. The humanities can help such students to venture out into a less controlled and ordered world. Over the past 20 years, educational initiatives in medical humanities have flourished, albeit with a great deal more theoretical than empirical support. In 1984, the Hastings Center commissioned Cassell to write a paper on *The Place of the Humanities in Medicine*.(9) Cassell argued that in medicine there is 'an entire spectrum of functions that can be provided only by the humanities'. In the same year, Pellegrino outlined three particular uses for the humanities in medical education(10): 'they are vehicles for teaching the liberal arts, they convey a special kind of knowledge that liberates the imagination and they are sources of delectation for the human spirit' (p. 254).

Self(11) also describes the medical humanities in the US as being used for three purposes: 'cultural transmission', 'affective development' (with a focus on developing humanistic attitudes) and 'cognitive development' (with an emphasis on reasoning around scientific, social and moral issues).

Grant, who helped to make the medical humanities part of the core curriculum at the University of Auckland,(12) has set out four main arguments in favour of including the medical humanities:

- to increase understanding of the human condition
- to expose students to the critical analysis of ideas
- to make more allowance for individual differences
- to provide pockets of expertise and lifelong interests.

Our own view is that the medical humanities can play three complementary educational roles:

- to introduce the idea that the liberal arts can contribute to healthcare
- to extend the range of future doctors' sensitivities and insights into human experience in all its variety
- to deepen our understanding beyond merely biomedical interpretations of health and illness.

It is the second and third of these roles that have received most of the attention; the 'arts in health' movement has arguably less immediate relevance for the medical curriculum (Box 6.1).

Helping Students to Learn from the Humanities

Whether you are involved at undergraduate, postgraduate or continuing professional development level, your role may encompass

> **BOX 6.1 What can the humanities do for medical education?**
> - help learners (including medical students, junior doctors, more advanced trainees and established practitioners) to develop skills in interpreting their own experiences and the experiences of others
> - provide a wide range of opportunities for students to encounter and appreciate human diversity
> - help students to develop their own personal values
> - encourage medical students to take experience and subjectivity seriously
> - enable medical education to move from a technical training to a genuine university education
> - nourish a sense of wonder at embodied human nature and embodied consciousness, leading to medical that is, in its essence, reverential
> - helps students to appreciate the dangers of ignoring the lessons of history
> - help students to develop communication skills

- the design of all or part of a curriculum (integrated or discipline based, hospital or community oriented), organising a large or small group learning activity, etc.)
- curriculum content, perhaps in relation to your own particular discipline
- a specific interest and expertise in one or more of the medical humanities.

In this chapter we will focus on undergraduate and graduate-entry medical education, but the opportunities for extrapolation and adaptation to later levels of education and training should be clear.

Your background may be in medicine, other health sciences, the arts, humanities or social sciences, or a combination of these. Many doctors are amateurs in the best sense of the word. They maintain a deep love of the humanities, draw on particular disciplines for 'delectation' and use them to stretch themselves beyond the often dogmatic world of 'single best answers', which tend to characterise biomedicine. (Contrast these with HL Mencken's description of human problems: 'There is always an easy solution to every human problem – neat, plausible, and wrong.') They are often motivated to share their love of learning with medical students and junior doctors. This most frequently takes the form of stories about the achievements of medical scientists and practitioners over the ages; the discoveries and breakthrough moments. However, because of the demands of a typical medical career, very few doctors develop to a level of professional scholarship.

If you happen to be a professional humanities scholar, you may be accused of having insufficient 'street cred', of being too far removed from the realities of medical practice. If you make the mistake of offering too pointed a critique of biomedicine or of doctors, you may lose goodwill and end up talking to an empty room. Then again, if you are deferential and apologetic, you may find yourself largely ignored. Even the least gifted lecturer in physiology or pathology will command a certain amount of respect if there are to be questions in the exam, but the professional humanities scholar may have no such pulling power.

In 1976, while writing about technical/vocational education, Scally(13) made a plea to humanities teachers to enter the world of the student and not to simply stand outside and reject technology: 'A student should gain ... a vision of personal and social alternatives ... encouraging the awareness that there are other ways of living, other value structures, other social constructs besides the familiar' (p. 225).

Finding the Balance between the Science and the Art

In 2006, in the journal *Medical Education*, Weatherall wrote on science in the 20th-century medical curriculum.(14) He concluded the article with these words:

> as this essay was restricted to the role of science in medical education, it has not been possible to enlarge on how its teaching can be accommodated with the numerous other skills that have been introduced into the curriculum, including an over-liberal dose of the humanities, with the aim of humanising our doctors of the future. But when I see a surgeon poised over my abdomen with a knife, all that I ask is that he or she is a humble, self-critical professional whose biological and technical training has prepared their mind to cope with the infinite possibilities that lie beneath the skin, and that, when finished, they can communicate what they have done to my relatives in simple, kindly language; at that moment their skills at deciphering the arcane meanings of multiple-choice questions or their acquaintance, or lack of, with the late string quartets of Beethoven will not bother me too much. (p. 201)

The arguments are important since they are ones that you are likely to encounter. They can be summarised as follows:
- Science and the humanities must compete for curriculum time.
- I doubt that studying the humanities 'humanises' doctors.
- I would prefer a kind and competent surgeon to a highly sophisticated but incompetent one.

How to respond? You might wish to acknowledge that you would all share the same anxious desire, should the need arise, for access to a competent surgeon who is also humble and self-critical. Those qualities are fundamental if one is to avoid putting one's life into the care of someone who is insufficiently capable on the one hand and insufficiently risk averse on the other. In relation to the medical curriculum, the more helpful question to ask might be how to achieve the best educational outcomes in the time available, using the most relevant academic resources.

The argument that surgeons should always communicate in simple, kind language may evoke in you slightly uncomfortable memories of rather more paternalistic days. Better perhaps to wish for a surgeon with the insight into making an accurate judgement of individual needs and to respond appropriately.(15) You might mention that many doctors fail to elicit patients' complaints and concerns and comprehend little of the emotional and social limpact of the illness. Even worse, they fail to appreciate the adverse effects of their own well-intentioned behaviour on their patients.(16,17)

Perhaps you would also take the time to defend multiple-choice questions and poor Beethoven; there is, after all, evidence that well-constructed multiple-choice questions can indeed discriminate between candidates who know their science and those who do not,(18,19) and a shared love of the late string quartets of Beethoven may be deeply relevant for doctors who work in places such as the palliative care ward.(20) Finally, of course, you might wish to point out that competent surgeons do not need to be cultural philistines.

A medical school that offered an 'over-liberal dose of the humanities' would be bound to raise antibodies with some academic staff as well as with students. Do such curricula exist? What, we might wonder, is the right 'dose' of humanities? Is it wise to think of the humanities in the currency of teaching hours, with the implication that the humanities are taught in a discrete disciplinary 'slot'? If this were the case, would an average of an hour per week be too much, too little or just right? A review of 41 humanities programmes in North America and some international schools was provided by the journal *Academic Medicine* in 2003.(21) With only a few exceptions, most of the medical schools reported on modest, often elective programmes, with very limited hours of study. Few, if any, would offer as much as the equivalent of one hour per week.

We labour all of these points because you will face such challenges, even when the medical humanities component of your curriculum seems well embedded. Describing the position of the medical humanities as 'precarious', Friedman(22) argues that the humanities must be protected so that they can offer students different ways of analysing information, viewing the world and confronting dilemmas. The humanities raise issues that can help students confront questions about both their chosen field and their particular places within it. They do not need to compete with the biomedical sciences; each part of the curriculum needs to be assessed in terms of its intrinsic worth and its utility in the lives of students and graduates. However, if your curriculum does not currently provide any opportunities for students to learn medicine from the humanities, you may face the problem familiar to any who have tried it: 'It is easier to win a war then to change the medical curriculum by even one half hour'.(23)

Meeting Curricula Requirements

The UK General Medical Council's publication *Tomorrow's Doctors*(24) emphasises points of particular relevance to learning medicine from the humanities. The documents deal with

- qualities that are appropriate to future responsibilities
- a core curriculum supported by student-selected components
- skills of exploration, evaluation, integration and critical appraisal of evidence
- experience in a variety of clinical settings with early clinical experience
- up-to-date teaching and learning systems.

Qualities appropriate to future responsibilities

'A number of concepts from history, the social sciences and the humanities are central to understanding and internalizing professionalism'.(25) It has been argued that 'humanism' and 'professionalism' are qualities that must be taught and learnt,(26–28) but less acknowledged is the role of the learning environment.(29–31) There is ample evidence of the negative effects of inhumane environments in relation to the socialisation of medical students and junior doctors.(32) It is hard to imagine an educational or a working environment within which careful and genuine attention to the humanities would not help students and doctors avoid crossing over to the 'dark side' – the dehumanised working environment that causes the cynicism and despair portrayed in novels such as *The House of God*(33) and *Bodies*.(34) Contrast these examples with the enormously popular American television series *M.A.S.H.*, in which a supportive work environment is shown to help doctors to cope with even the most challenging medical situations. The difference is clearly due to the sympathy and humour with which *M.A.S.H.* portrayed the human experiences of illness and injury from the perspective of Hawkeye Pierce, the medical protagonist.

However, any attempt to force-feed professionalism using the humanities will serve only to discredit this approach, especially when it is done by non-medical teachers. Even students from humanities backgrounds who are trying to come to grips with the sheer volume of material to cover, in an undergraduate programme or during their specialty training, find themselves driven to ask, 'What's likely to be in the exams?' They will have little patience with 'irrelevant' subjects or topics that are seen as digressions from the 'core' of the programme. For this reason, many educators have

aimed to 'embed' the humanities(35) and to more clearly demonstrate their relevance(36) as more likely to appeal to learners. Poetry may not make 'better' doctors,(37) and it may not be a predictable way to teach ethics,(38) but if the resources drawn from the arts, humanities and social sciences are of high quality, they cannot help but 'liberate the imagination' and provide 'delectation for the human spirit',(39) both of which support the qualities that in turn support professional practice.

A core curriculum supported by student-selected components

'Student-selected components' have provided one way of challenging the rigidity of the traditional curriculum. Limiting the reach of a potentially inexhaustible core curriculum is a way of reducing rote learning and promoting deep understanding. Over the past 10 years, many accounts of humanities special study modules (in other countries, often called options or electives) have been published.(40–45) While these are generally received with enthusiasm by the students who volunteer, they have led to the understandable concern that the humanities might be relegated to parts of the curriculum that will be taken up only by this subgroup. A sensible compromise can be found in the identification of a medical humanities core (defined in terms of intellectual skills, rather than content) complemented by self-selected components, recognising that not all students will take the latter.

Emphasis on the skills of exploration, evaluation, integration and critical appraisal of evidence

If humanities students were required to undertake a course of study defined in terms of content alone, they would probably miss the benefits of a university education. What unites scholars across the arts and humanities is not the content of their studies, but the acquisition of intellectual skills. Whether graduating with a major in philosophy, history, literature, languages or a social science, humanities students are expected to be capable of rigorous and independent thought, to account for their decisions, and to be creative, imaginative and tolerant of ambiguity.

Unlike humanities students, who demonstrate these qualities through essay writing, medical students tend not to be required to write many essays; the introduction of reflective writing is a relatively new approach.(46) However, medical students and graduates do tend to participate in small group tutorials, especially if a course of study is problem or case based. Tutorials provide an ideal opportunity for students to share their experiences and refine their ideas and values; this is often overlooked as an example of learning medicine from the humanities. Deep learning(47) occurs when students learn to see things from different perspectives, discuss their ideas with others and apply knowledge in the real world.(43,48,49) These approaches respond directly to the General Medical Council's requirement for students to 'explore knowledge, and evaluate and integrate (bring together) evidence critically. The curriculum must motivate students and help them develop the skills for self-directed learning'(50) (p. 3). If you have responsibility for organising teaching and learning, then small group tutorials, appropriately facilitated, are the ideal way to achieve many of these goals. Small group discussions should help students to reflect on experience and to extend their insights by drawing on the humanities and social sciences. Many different ways of achieving the goal of reflective practice have been identified(51–54) and some of these may work well in your own situation.

Learning in a variety of settings and early clinical experience

Learning in a variety of settings has generally meant that, in addition to hospital-based experience, students now learn in general practices, community health facilities and patients' homes. These naturally introduce some of the complexities of context and relationships that are so often lost when patients are seen out of context, in a hospital bed. The humanities and social sciences can provide invaluable insights into the human experience of illness, disability and medical intervention in the patient's own setting. In addition, students can explore the roles of a broader range of health professionals, consider the operation of power structures and even participate in (or at the very least observe) inter-professional care. 'Poetry on rounds' was found to have a levelling effect(55) between attending physicians, house staff and medical students: 'Rounds became a time when the team shared not only medical knowledge but also life and emotional experiences' (p. 449).

Instead of feeling that they have little to offer, students can be encouraged to consider unfamiliarity as a gift, embodied in the Polish proverb 'the guest sees in one hour what the owner of the house does not see in a lifetime'. Seeing with a fresh eye is essential to remaining clinically alert over a professional lifetime, and students need explicit encouragement to do that, so that they are less likely to be socialised into accepting some of the less desirable aspects of the healthcare environment. Professional historians use this approach when they try to 'make the familiar strange' – to take nothing for granted.

Social history resources and fictional depictions of families can help medical students prepare for clinical attachments in patients' homes, hospitals, clinics and GP surgeries. Historical, philosophical, literary and artistic representations can be chosen to pique their interest without adding a large burden of additional study. You might invite beginning students to reflect on the difference between their way of seeing patients and the way an experienced clinician might see them.

Cultural competence is a relatively recent goal in medical education. It addresses the provision of appropriate healthcare when there are ethnic and cultural differences between patients, families and caregivers to consider. Kleinman and Benson,(56) who work at the interface between medicine and anthropology, have proposed an 'explanatory models' approach, which provides practical help for students. They aim 'to open clinicians to human communication and set their expert knowledge alongside (not over and above) the patient's own explanation and viewpoint'. They have outlined six steps that simultaneously illustrate the relevance of the humanities. Students should be able to:

- find out about [how] the patient's ethnicity relates to how she or he sees herself or himself and place within family, work and social networks
- evaluate what is at stake in terms of close relationships, material resources, religious commitments and even life itself
- reconstruct the patient's narrative in order to understand the meaning of the illness
- consider ongoing stresses and social supports
- examine culture in terms of its influence on clinical relationships, using critical self-reflection to explore, for example, the culture of biomedicine, 'including bias, inappropriate and excessive use of advanced technology interventions, and of course stereotyping' (p. 1675)
- reflect on the effects of attending to cultural difference – is it relevant and helpful for this patient in these circumstances?

Learners at all levels will find themselves revisiting these quite subtle and complex skills. In *The Spirit Catches You and You Fall Down*,(57) Anne Fadiman provides a powerful example of how well-intentioned care can go wrong. Her storied account of the healthcare system is a great educational resource. Greenhalgh(58) also gives examples of the power of stories to reduce the barrier of ethnic difference.

Narrative accounts of illness by real patients offer important learning opportunities.(59) Suitable patients are likely to have chronic conditions such as cystic fibrosis, diabetes, epilepsy or mental illnesses. They have an advantage over 'book learning' because students see and talk to them in a particular clinical context (whether at home, in a hospital ward, tutorial room or lecture theatre). Contextual factors make these experiences memorable; anyone who has organised such opportunities for students will be aware of the deep impression they can create. Most medical graduates can remember certain patients many decades after graduation, and one patient who describes the impact of a less-than-perfect encounter with the healthcare system may sometimes have a greater effect than statistical analyses of medical error.(58)

Up-to-date learning and teaching systems: integration and problem-based learning

The humanities can make sense of a medical curriculum by integrating all aspects of a patient's problem, avoiding the 'silo effect' that is typical of a traditional curriculum. Integration needs to be both vertical (pre-clinical and clinical) and horizontal (dealing with all aspects from the human perspective).

The approach is not new; in 1992, Almy *et al.*(60) reported on a course for fourth-year students which used a problem-based approach that demonstrated the relevance of the social sciences and humanities to clinical decision making. The course culminated in an assessment of individual students using a simulated patient with a complex management problem. Kirklin(61) describes the way in which the arts and humanities can be used to teach around a specific medical problem such as genetic disorders and therapies. At the University of Sydney, problem-based learning (PBL) cases are electronically linked to humanities resources in the form of poems, extracts from novels, artworks, history of medicine excerpts and music references (all with due attention to copyright law). There are dozens of connections that can be drawn: in Sydney, Shakespeare's sonnets accompany a PBL case on ageing; Degas's paintings accompany a case of rheumatoid arthritis (from which Degas suffered); a brief history of tobacco accompanies a case on smoking; and a reference to the Holocaust accompanies a case involving an elderly Dutch migrant. If your curriculum uses PBL, you may wish to identify resources that complement the cases your students study. Such resources bring convincingly drawn 'patients' to life and remind students that every real-life case occurs within a context from which the human experience of illness proceeds. If your medical school has created PBL cases using comic-book characters with demeaning nicknames, object and have them changed. It is not an amusing thing to do; it simply perpetuates the idea that patients are mere vehicles for interesting diseases. Students need to learn that the humanity they share with their patients(62) is just as important as the knowledge they bring to their service.

The *Journal of the American Medical Association* provides beautiful annotated examples from art as well as from the other humanities disciplines (see *Poetry and Medicine* and *A Piece of My Mind*). The Medical Humanities pages at the New York University School of Medicine (http://medhum.med.nyu.edu) provide resources and also links to other sites. In 2003, New York University published *Editors' Choices from the Literature, Arts and Medicine Database*(63) to celebrate its 10th anniversary. The Association of American Medical Colleges has produced selections from the journal *Academic Medicine* to commemorate 10 years of medicine and the arts.(64) The University of Pennsylvania has produced a CD-ROM on literature and medicine.(65) Radcliffe Publishing has produced a number of medical humanities titles (*see* Further reading section). Last but not least, students will respond to invitations to write and post their own compositions and book reviews, tasks that provide opportunities for their broader professional development.

A Curriculum for the Medical Humanities?

Macnaughton has described some of the ways in which students can learn medicine from the humanities.(66) Evans and Macnaughton(67) have asked, 'Is there, or could (should) there be, an agreed and coherent core curriculum for the study of medical humanities as such?' (p. 65). They suggest that the core curriculum should be guided by four principles:
- disciplinary openness
- humility in enquiry
- respect for subjectivity
- openness to a sense of wonder at embodied human nature.

The first three are, of course, applicable to all scholarship. The last one is especially important in medicine; wonder can often disappear under the weight of anxiety, sadness and the frustration that a doctor's life entails.

Not only is this a useful template against which to judge your own initiatives in medical humanities, it is also a prescription for the learning environment itself.(68) Philosophy, history and literature clearly provide a disciplinary core that meets all of these criteria, while social sciences (especially sociology and anthropology), art and music provide a 'second string' that meets some of them to some extent. Your own decision making about what to include will obviously take advantage of the local expertise available and the opportunities that arise. Not infrequently you will find other academics in a clinical, para-clinical or pre-clinical discipline, such as palliative care or infectious diseases, who will be enthusiastic collaborators (*see* Box 6.2).

BOX 6.2 A curriculum for the medical humanities

Philosophy

History of medicine

Literature

Narrative

Art and music

Spirituality

Philosophy

There is a tendency to assume that bioethics, now a distinct component of many medical curricula, is all that is required to 'cover' philosophy in a medical degree programme. However, philosophy of medicine, as an organised disciplinary strand, is much broader; its job is to ask questions about the questions that medicine asks.(69) It examines, for example, the phenomena of health and illness, the nature of the clinical encounter and many of the assumptions of modern medical practice. Because we are focusing on educating doctors and not humanities scholars, it is particularly important for students to see the point of 'studying philosophically' rather than 'studying philosophy'. Philosophy promotes logic and reasoning, and encourages the understanding of multiple perspectives.(70)

In the course of their studies, medical students learn to consider the human body of daily experience as a medical body, the object of scientific enquiry, standardised rather than individuated. The sense of mystery and the symbolic significance of the body can be lost quite easily if students come to consider it as merely a source of data on the physical status of a patient, and to consider it in terms of function alone.(69) However, the study of clinical medicine combines both universal and existential knowledge and can give concrete form to many of philosophy's traditional questions.

Louhiala(71) has described four different ways of approaching philosophy within a medical curriculum, only two of which he recommends:

- traditional lectures on philosophy without connection to medicine
- an academic philosophy of medicine course, as for philosophy students
- philosophy of medicine teaching related to the students' experiences
- full integration into the curriculum using, for example, PBL.

Traditional lectures, unconnected to medicine and with their content suited to philosophy rather than to medical courses, are unlikely to appeal to students. We know that the teaching needs to be related to students' experiences and that it is most effective when fully integrated. Louhiala suggests that the last approach may be too difficult, but in fact there are good examples. At Tampere University in Finland, a PBL block on medical knowledge and research provides an introduction to the philosophy of science.(72) At the University of Sydney the PBL cases have web links and discussion prompts. For example, concepts of illness are explored in a PBL case in which a patient is convinced that he has chronic fatigue syndrome.

History of medicine

George Santayana's warning that those who cannot learn from history are doomed to repeat it are particularly important for medicine. In the course of history, countless patients have suffered unnecessarily from inappropriate and even dangerous medical interventions.

Dufflin, author of *History of Medicine: a scandalously short introduction*,(73) argues that the study of history in relation to medicine can be used to

- foster critical thinking, or to instil scepticism about the content and durability of everything else students are taught in their professional training
- demonstrate that history is a research discipline, built on fascinating questions, rigorous methods and a wide variety of raw materials – a research discipline not unlike those in the clinical and basic sciences.

She has provided useful advice on the 'why', 'who', 'how' and 'what' of teaching medical students.(74) Confronted with a choice of physician historians or professional historians, her advice is to prefer expertise and to take whatever opportunities present themselves with respect to timing: with Year 1 students while medicine is still fresh; with Year 4 when it is less daunting. With respect to scheduling, 'Friday afternoons are suicidal. Instructors who agree to schedule their lessons in such a slot have participated in their own demise' (p. 159). The content is the least important consideration: 'As long as the information is accurate and relevant, the "what" does not matter as much as the "why," the "who" and the "how"'.

There are abundant resources for teaching in the history of medicine. Some are listed in the Further Reading section. Porter's legacy alone is substantial.(75–78)

Literature

Evans(79) suggests four medical educational 'goods' that literature supports:

- an education (as opposed to mere training)
- ethics and communication skills
- the development of personal values
- a sense of wonder at embodied human nature.

Medical curricula that include the arts and humanities often begin with literature. This is not surprising, given the range of forms: novels, poems, plays and non-fiction accounts of the experience of illness [so-called 'pathography'(80)], plus health providers' narratives, including reflective writing. To this list we can add film as an increasingly popular way of accessing the humanities.(81,82)

Others have promoted 'narrative medicine',(83,84) which is said to offer a way of understanding the medical history as the patient's story; 'narrative therapy' has grown out of this perspective.

William Osler often advised students and young doctors to intersperse their studies with reading in the humanities. One hundred years ago his recommended reading list included the Bible, Plutarch, Marcus Aurelius, Epictetus, Shakespeare, Montaigne, Miguel de Cervantes, Ralph Waldo Emerson and Oliver

Wendell Holmes. Given the choice, students are unlikely to select from this sample today and will often select films or modern novels and poetry that may be less familiar to an older generation. If you find yourself unable to outrun the avalanche of modern literature, it can be helpful to take advantage of students' choices to build your own collection.

An example of such a collection can be found in *Public Expectations and Physicians' Responsibilities: voices of medical humanities*.(85) Crellin draws largely from contemporary, mainly Canadian, sources, including film, poetry, patient narratives and even comic postcards.

In *The Moral of the Story: an anthology of ethics through literature*,(86) Singer and Singer provide excerpts from literary works that are both enjoyable and thought-provoking. Twenty-nine of their 79 authors were born in the 20th century. The book uses excerpts that question the nature of ethics, values and duties, racism and sexism, war and suicide, and so on. Literature used as a stimulus for teaching ethics raises particular issues. Wear and Aultman(87) found that some of their students were uncomfortable with literature that dealt with challenging social issues such as domestic violence, and Pickering has pointed out that using poetry, for instance to teach ethics, can have unpredictable results.(38) The underlying purpose of the exercise is to foster critical thinking, rather than inculcating a point of view, even in the well-intentioned goal of achieving 'professionalism'. Students are quick to react to perceived criticism of the profession while they are taking their first tentative steps towards acquiring a professional identity. This is one reason why team teaching, with a supportive humanities scholar and a clinician working together, is an important philosophical and practical consideration.

Special study modules remain the most popular means of including literature in the curriculum. Other approaches include the use of short excerpts that relate to clinical conditions being studied in a PBL or case-based curriculum. These can be used to provide a change of pace, for example, towards the end of a small group discussion. Shapiro *et al.*(88) introduced medicine-related poetry and prose to a Year 3 family medicine clerkship, using clinical notes in the 'SOAP' format (Subjective, Objective, Assessment, Plan) and into an end-of-clerkship Objective Structured Clinical Examination. Students were moderately interested, and felt that the experience had been positive in terms of encouraging empathic responses to patients.

Louis-Courvoisier and Wenger(54) have argued that the study of literature can help students to realise the extent to which their view of the world is context dependent and culturally shaped. 'Distancing' enables students to become aware that their point of view is only one of many alternative ways of seeing. They suggest that team teaching can overcome many of the difficulties that occur when literature is taught by

medical teachers who lack the professional expertise of the literary scholar, or of literary scholars who lack a deep understanding of the context of medical care. 'Team teaching entails numerous discussions and negotiations. It is a time-consuming process, but quite exciting because it is the result of a dynamic process and of a constructive confrontation rather than a mere juxtaposition of expertise' (p. 54). Because of the importance of role models in medicine, the admired clinician who gives critical endorsement to this approach and who can describe why they enjoy particular writers and films is likely to encourage students to read or view films with a discerning eye.

Narrative medicine

'Narrative medicine' has recently laid claim to a greater role in medical education(84) for the purpose of helping doctors to understand the different perspectives of doctors and patients.(89) Students are said to move towards narrative competence as they demonstrate 'the set of skills required to recognize, absorb, interpret and be moved by the stories one hears or reads. This competence requires a combination of textual skills (identifying a story's structure, adopting its multiple perspectives, recognising metaphors and allusions), creative skills (imagining many interpretations, building curiosity, inventing multiple endings), and affective skills (tolerating uncertainty as a story unfolds, entering the story's mood)'.(90) Greenhalgh and Hurwitz(91) describe the illness experience as a narrative embedded within a broader life narrative.

Is this really new or different? Are not these skills the 'bread and butter' of many communication skills training programmes? In a systematic review of such programmes, Gysels *et al.* found that not all of them include all the components of narrative medicine training. They concluded that 'learner-centred (communication training) programmes using several methods, combining a didactic component focusing on theoretical knowledge with practical rehearsal and constructive feedback from peers and skilled facilitators, proved to be very effective. Small groups encouraged more intensive participation'.(92, p. 366).

Clark and Mishler(93) have provided evidence of the practical utility of an approach that could be seen as related to narrative medicine. They present a comparative analysis of two clinical consultations and compare the successful storytelling exemplified by one with the constantly interrupted narrative in the other. The authors point out how focusing on the patients' attempts to tell a story can illuminate the exercise of authority in clinical encounters. The results from this research provide a powerful teaching tool. Many educators will be familiar with the use of video and/or audio recording to teach communication skills, but this chapter offers a detailed account of how stories are developed or suppressed. 'Attending to the patient's authorship of her/his story highlights the vicissitudes of authority in clinical encounters and the social transformation of illness in clinical relationships' (p. 368).

Equally useful for teaching communication is the rhetorical approach outlined by Lingard (94) and others. She points out that rhetoric is a science that can deepen understanding of communication and improve teaching, rather than relying on implicit, ad hoc teaching without a theoretical base. Books such as these are useful for staff development; clinical teachers will recognise the authentic contexts within which the research has taken place and see more clearly the benefits of the humanities in teaching and learning.

Your own curriculum may approach the skills described above using a range of teaching methods, without ever mentioning 'narrative competence'. What is important is that the teachers have a model or models to enable them to understand what they are trying to achieve when they teach communication skills.

Art and music

Some claims have been made for the role of the visual arts in learning and teaching. From an essentialist point of view, art education can be justified for the aesthetic experience alone,(78,95), while from an instrumentalist perspective, art education can be justified as a means of achieving curriculum goals, by sharpening students' powers of observation, for example.(95–97) Tapajos(95) points out the advantages of viewing a medical condition such as HIV/AIDS through a humanities lens; artistic representations of cancer have been a focal point for other initiatives, such as special study modules.(98)

There have been some published evaluations of the use of art and music to achieve curriculum goals; not surprisingly, these are all positive since positive outcome bias is probably just as applicable in medical humanities research as it is in clinical medicine.(99) While the evaluations themselves tend to be methodologically weak and/or to involve small numbers, the fact that such initiatives are part of a medical school curriculum contains an implicit message about what is valued in the curriculum, including student wellbeing. One student reporting on the Cornell experience(96) said, 'I found it to be a unique opportunity to interact with faculty on a non-medical level, and … would love to see it become a permanent programme at Cornell'. A more rigorous evaluation was carried out by Shapiro *et al.* in comparing the observation skills of a medical student group trained with clinical photographs and paper cases, and a group trained with art plus dance. Pattern recognition probably improved as a result of the first group's experience, but the second group thought that their emotional recognition, empathy, identification of story and narrative, and awareness of multiple perspectives had improved.(100) Dolev *et al.*(101) randomised first-year

students to a control or intervention group in which the students attended the Yale Centre for British Art for visual training as part of the general curriculum. The researchers found a modest, statistically significant improvement in observations skills in the intervention group and commented that this could be used as the basis for a continuing curriculum applicable to all physicians.

Family physicians participated in a workshop in Israel in which they discussed and wrote about artistic representations of suffering. Participants commented that this type of experience is rare.(102) At the University of California, San Francisco, interns are given the opportunity to use artistic expression through drawing, collage and mask making, which encourages reflection, and like other initiatives it has been well received.(103) These examples all provide ideas for educators looking for opportunities for the humanities. Kirklin *et al.* identified seven 'keys to success' based on their experience of a special study module that included art at University College London.(98)

They are:

- dedicated course coordinator
- enthusiastic tutors
- identification of students needing extra support
- flexibility to modify the course
- supportive environment
- opportunities for reflection and feedback
- individual feedback to students.

While educators claim a place for philosophy, bioethics, history, literature, art and so on, music has fewer advocates for a place in the core curriculum. However, at medical schools such as Dalhousie University in Canada,(104) strong advocacy at the highest levels has resulted in a programme that not only includes medical humanities in the curriculum, but also brings faculty together for musical performances as a means of strengthening the sense of belonging to a community of scholars (http://humanities. medicine.dal.ca).

Spirituality

The acceptance that good medical care requires a biopsychosocial or, perhaps more accurately, an 'existential' approach can lead to a discussion of the spiritual qualities that doctors need if they are to be able to respond to a range of different needs in their patients. Evans(105) suggests that doctors need to draw on 'a type of spiritual confidence that does not arise merely from a narrow scientific training; a spirit perhaps more dependent on ways of thinking, rather than content of thought; genuine education rather than training; development of personal qualities rather than acquired techniques; a completeness or fullness of human being' (p. 13). This type of 'spiritual confidence' should be distinguished from mere religious faith.

In the US, the Medical School Objectives Project(106) has defined learning objectives for spirituality. The American Association of Medical Colleges reported in a survey carried out in 2000 that approximately 70 medical schools were addressing spirituality in their curricula. By 2004, that number had reached 84.(107) Berlinger(108) from the Hastings Center has discussed the ethical implications of such courses, some of which are linked to developments in 'integrative' and 'complementary' medicine.(109,110) She points out some of the pitfalls of incorporating spirituality into the curriculum – for example, the fact that the research evidence linking spiritual and religious beliefs and practices to health and healing is very poor, that the practice of taking a 'spiritual history' from a patient is potentially intrusive and coercive, and that doctors who see themselves as healers may become overly impressed with their own mystique and regress to a less patient-centred and more paternalistic model of patient care.

Individual medical schools or training programmes should consider the extent to which spirituality needs to be singled out for special attention as opposed to being incorporated into a programme that emphasises respectful care and sensitivity to difference. Kleinman's work on the skills required to manage cultural difference,(56) outlined above, is equally relevant when applied to the different faiths and non-faiths that doctors and their patients hold.

Course Design and Assessment

Whether the medical humanities component of a curriculum is stand-alone or embedded, compulsory or voluntary, there are similar design questions to be addressed. By beginning with your curriculum goals in mind, you can try to ensure congruence between whatever type of programme you run and the assessment methods used (see Box 6.3).(48)

Consider assessment early. Do you have the resources and time to carry out both the learning activities and the related assessments? How practical are they? Will they survive the initial wave of enthusiasm?

BOX 6.3 How to: Implement a medical humanities curriculum

Questions for programme designers(3)

- Does our programme provide opportunities for students to reflect on their experiences? Do they have opportunities to explore the works of significant thinkers? Can our students interpret messages in different forms – literary, historical, artistic, musical, etc.? Can we ensure that they use language precisely, and that they can develop and defend a logical argument?

- How and when does our programme ensure that students encounter other sets of values and other experience of the world? How do we ensure that students can demonstrate their understanding of the subjective experiences of others? How are they required to provide evidence of, for example, 'cultural competence'?

- Does our programme foster independent thinking? Can our students articulate and defend their personal values? Can they describe their view of a morally good life? Can they use the resources of literature, philosophy, history etc., in achieving these goals?

- How do we ensure that students understand the respective contributions of the natural and human sciences to our understanding of the world? To what extent do we enable them to see that objective and subjective 'cures' need not be the same? Can they distinguish between disease and illness?

- How do we nourish, test for and demonstrate that students have acquired the generic skills associated with a university education – high-level reasoning, tolerance of ambiguity, creativity and imagination?

- How are students challenged to consider the 'why' versus the 'how'? Are they allowed to encouraged to tap onto their own aesthetic and emotional responses to human nature and its representation in the arts and humanities? Do they have opportunities to learn about the intellectual traditions of the range of cultures that they are likely to encounter? Do they have opportunities to see how patients and doctors share an awareness of our vulnerability, mortality and transcendence?

- Does our curriculum provide examples of the pitfalls of treating other human beings as means rather than as ends in themselves? What can we learn from the history of medical error both past and present? Do we equip students to understand how mistakes might be avoided in the future?

- How does my programme utilise insights, approaches and techniques derived from the humanities to help students to become more competent in communication? As well as demonstrating oral communication skills, are they required to demonstrate clear written communication? Is there a focus on the progressive development of these skills, using examples from the humanities?

If we are dealing with biomedical topics it is relatively easy to ask, 'How can we ensure that students have adequate knowledge of anatomy/physiology/pathology, etc., to progress safely to the next stage of learning?' This is not a question that can be applied to the humanities, and it is important for students to know that we are not trying to turn them into humanities scholars, but into more broadly educated doctors. We are therefore forced to acknowledge that humanities assessment cannot sample knowledge in a statistically defensible way, especially given the fact that both the cognitive and affective components of the humanities curriculum are important. However, when students are required to prepare a reflective essay, for example, not only does it challenge their higher-order skills, but it also indicates the value that the faculty places on this skill.

Take every opportunity to integrate the assessment into formats that are already being used for other parts of the curriculum. However, because of the different cognitive and affective requirements of assessments in biomedicine and the humanities, you may need to use a different approach, but keep it as simple as you can.

Essays and reflective diaries work well for many humanities subjects because they take time to draft, review and prepare for presentation, which are important skills for students to acquire and polish. Another approach that can work well is to assign topics for a group presentation and/or group poster. The process of preparing such a product requires students to consider other viewpoints around the topic. You might like to consider selecting a different theme each year, so students can compare their efforts and learn from one another. Your students should also be required to make a statement about the relative contribution of each group member, similar to that required of scholars submitting a paper to an academic journal (*see* Box 6.4).

Programme Evaluation and Research Opportunities

While attempts have been made to evaluate individual modules or complete strands or themes, evaluations are generally limited to feedback from surveys, questionnaires, individual interviews and focus groups to assess student satisfaction. Reports of feedback on special study modules usually acknowledge that students self-select into areas in which they have a particular interest, and only occasionally into areas in which they feel deficient.

Student feedback is essential for course correction and continuous quality improvement, which are dear to the hearts of educators who care about their courses. However, most enthusiastic teachers will elicit positive feedback, and this can lull one into a false sense of security concerning the impact of a course of study.

It is important to remember that such evaluations do not test the commonly proffered argument that the humanities make students and doctors more humane. This argument is often made in terms of questions that are presented rhetorically as 'How could one fail to respond to the lessons of history, or the magnificence of great literature or the insights of art or the cogency of the philosophical reasoning?', and so on. In reply, one could point out that our medical schools still graduate, year after year, a tiny number of students who are at risk for unprofessional behaviour. They may have participated in excellent programmes that incorporate the medical humanities, or they may not. However excellent their educational experience, it will not have been enough to change the values, beliefs, attitudes and behaviour of the psychopath or sociopath.

Leaving aside the minute number in this category, a more appropriate question would be whether the medical humanities are likely to provide fundamentally humane students with additional insights that are of value to themselves and of potential value to their patients. Theoretically, this question could be answered by a randomised controlled trial of sufficient size (a multi-centre trial perhaps), but one can imagine the practical challenges of randomisation within medical schools and the philosophical challenges of choosing outcome measures. In addition, such a trial would not answer two key questions concerning opportunity cost. The first can be formulated as the question 'Does any specific educational experience within a medical humanities course yield better outcomes than another?' (e.g. is a course on the history of medicine of greater value than a course on medicine and literature?). The second question is the one posed earlier by Weatherall concerning the relative importance of the humanities and the biomedical sciences for individual practitioners. Are insights into the history of medicine more important than knowing the detailed structure of, for example, cytokine receptors? The answer is, of course, 'It depends'. Because graduates follow so many different career paths, we can only look at individual students, and then only with the benefit of hindsight, after they have chosen their particular career paths. We are left, as is so often the case in medical education, with innumerable variables intertwined. This is not, however, a counsel of despair. Excellent research is being done on a small scale and the researchers deserve full credit for sourcing funds and carrying out interesting and innovative research projects on teaching, learning and assessment involving the humanities.

Creating the Right Environment

Through the biomedical sciences, students learn about how bodies function and malfunction. Through the humanities disciplines, students learn about how and

BOX 6.4 How to: Implement a medical humanities curriculum

Barriers and how to overcome them(4)

Barriers	Possible solutions
Power: Influential faculty, from the dean downwards, tend to be trained in the biomedical model that has both defined and served their careers; a different approach may engender anxiety and resistance.	Ensure that the dean and other influential people have been adequately briefed. Identify other potential supporters; form a faculty interest group. Describe how learning from the humanities will enrich both students and faculty; trial innovative approaches on a small scale and if the students feedback is positive, use it to help you to move forward.
Expertise: Faculties typically employ hundreds of biomedical scientists and very few scholars in the humanities and social sciences, and the latter group tends not to be in positions of leadership.	Foster faculty expertise by encouraging contributions to teaching. Make links with humanities departments and identify potential teaching exchanges. Scour research teams for humanities scholars engaged in interdisciplinary research: are they willing to contribute to the teaching programme?
Language: The language of the humanities is often unfamiliar and obscure; it can appear dismissive and derogatory in discussions of science and scientists.	Take account of the learning needs of the least humanities-oriented students. Use texts that take science seriously; avoid obscure language and hyper-critical humanities academicians. Use literary texts that show how the language of biomedicine can also be used to exclude others.
Objectivity: Medical science is concerned with reducing variables, achieving detachment and emphasising generalisability.	Highlight the limits of a purely scientific approach in the real world, especially with, for example, chronic illnesses. Use literature to illustrate the complexity of human experience. Distinguish the challenges of diagnosis from those of management.
Overcoming the problems of 'two cultures': Medicine focuses on health improvement and progress, minimising error and doubt, while the humanities investigate and celebrate uncertainty and ambiguity.	Demonstrate the utility of both approaches. Help students to see why scientific knowledge is always provisional; invite students to identify the inherent weaknesses and biases of scholarly activity. Communicate some of the lessons of history. Discuss the need for an 'illness service' and a 'health service'.
Competition for time in the curriculum: Medical curricula are typically crowded (and there is also competition between 'old' and 'new' biomedical subjects).	Look for opportunities for synergy: integrate the humanities with biomedical teaching, learning and assessment wherever possible. Look for opportunities to collaborate when new topics or courses are being developed. Stress the benefits for learning of a 'change of pace' between science and the humanities.
Values: Concerns are expressed about the status of personal and values.	Demonstrate to students that no human activity is value-neutral. Articulate the values of your medical school without forcing them onto students. Encourage open-minded debate.

why we think, feel and behave as we do; the humanities invite us to make sense of Socrates' observation that the unexamined life is not worth living. Much of the students' humanities-based knowledge is acquired in the same way that their non-medical fellows acquire it – through reading, reflecting, debating, discussing, listening and looking, as a part of everyday life. Without reflection we all live in a state of relative philosophical confusion and disorder.(111,112) In addition to the knowledge acquired as part of a broad education, doctors acquire insights through their privileged relationships with patients and families, and with society at large. The humanities can encourage students to trust their own aesthetic perceptions and judgements, a process that happens most readily when there is space for students to make personally relevant connections.

Medical teachers have the capacity to foster or neglect their students' personal and professional development alongside learning in the biomedical sciences.(68) Whether in primary, secondary, tertiary or post-tertiary learning, certain institutional factors consistently help students to achieve the twin goals of mastering the art and science of medicine. Here are just some of the characteristics of successful medical schools, against which you might like to compare your own organisation.

• To what extent do you have strong and effective leaders who value teaching and learning in both science and the humanities?

- Do you have competent teachers with respect to both humanities content and process?
- Do your courses encourage high levels of critical thinking, creativity, problem solving and teamwork?
- Does engagement with medical humanities foster a sense of belonging and pride and emphasise respect, tolerance, inclusion and diversity of views?
- Are all students required to master foundational knowledge and skills, acknowledging that some will go further with elective experiences?
- Is humanities teaching adequately resourced?
- Are assessment processes defensible?
- Are there good evaluation and monitoring systems in place?

Resources

Good ideas abound. There are now so many schools with interesting programmes running that it is impossible to describe them all. The 2003 issue of *Academic Medicine*(21) that attempted to cover a number of them is a good start. Once you access a web site for one of the schools that have committed to the medical humanities, you will find yourself in a rich maze of resources. At medical schools such as Dalhousie in Canada, strong advocacy at the highest levels has resulted in a programme that not only includes medical humanities in the curriculum, but also uses the arts and humanities to bring students and faculty together for musical performances, art competitions and to promote humanistic engagement.

Examples of interesting practice in the US can be found at the University of California, Irvine (http://www.meded.uci.edu/Medhum/index.html) and the University of Texas Medical Branch Institute for Medical Humanities. Medical humanities syllabi have also been listed on the New York University web site at http://medhum.med.nyu.edu/syllabi.html. Support for those engaged in teaching and curriculum development is also available from the Association for Medical Humanities (http://www.amh.ac.uk) in the UK and its sister association in Australia. Students with interests in medical humanities can be directed to web-based student discussions in the UK (http://medhum.blogspot.com) and the US (http://www.medhumanities.org).

While it is not possible to acknowledge all the resources available for teaching and learning in the humanities, it is even more daunting to try to list the philosophical, literary, historical, anthropological, sociological, artistic and musical resources that have the potential to open doors to the recording and interpreting of human experience in relation to illness, disability and medical care. We have not attempted to do

so. You and your colleagues will find your own favourites, especially those with local relevance.

Conclusion

When Virgil wrote the words with which we began our chapter, he was concerned with the science of agriculture. Small land owners in the second-century BC were being taken over by large farming 'companies' with access to slave labour – shades of the globalisation to come. Virgil was trying to restore a sense of balance – a sense that farming is not just about the 'bottom line', but also about the wise, scientifically based use of limited resources. All over the world, profit-driven agriculture is depleting vital food stocks on land and in the sea. Agriculture was, and is, potentially lifesaving, just as medicine is. Little wonder that the deep understanding of 'the cause of things' in any of the natural sciences gives rise to a particular kind of satisfaction.

It is sometimes tempting for medical students, selected to a large degree for their scientific ability, to focus on those areas of understanding over which they have the fullest mastery – physiology, pathology and so on. However, when biomedicine fails, as it must, they may be ill prepared to respond. It is not simply a question of how to learn medicine from the humanities; rather, it might be said that without the humanities medicine can never be truly learnt. The educator's task is to help students see how much wisdom, insight, support and comfort the humanities can provide for them and for their patients.

References

1 Irvine D (2003) *The Doctor's Tale: professionalism and public trust.* Radcliffe Publishing, Oxford.
2 Bodenheimer T (2005) High and rising health care costs. Part 3: the role of health care providers. *Annals of Internal Medicine.* **142**: 996–1002.
3 Vaglum P, Wiers-Jenssen J and Ekeberg O (1999) Motivation for medical school: the relationship to gender and specialty preferences in a nationwide sample. *Medical Education.* **33**: 236–42.
4 Greaves D (2004) *The Healing Tradition: reviving the soul of Western medicine.* Radcliffe Publishing, Oxford.
5 Moore A (1976) Medical humanities – a new medical adventure. *New England Journal of Medicine.* **295**: 1479–80.
6 Moore A (1977) Medical humanities: an aid to ethical discussions. *Journal of Medical Ethics.* **3**: 26–32.
7 Acuna LE (2000) Don't cry for us Argentinians: two decades of teaching medical humanities. *Medical Humanities.* **26**: 66–70.
8 Evans H and Greaves D (2002) 'Medical humanities' – what's in a name? *Medical Humanities.* **28**: 1–2.
9 Cassell E (1984) *The Place of the Humanities in Medicine.* The Hastings Center Institute of Society, Ethics and Life Sciences, New York.

10 Pellegrino E (1984) The humanities in medical education; entering the post-evangelical era. *Theoretical Medicine and Bioethics.* **5**: 253–66.

11 Self D (1993) The educational philosophies behind the medical humanities programs in the United States: an empirical assessment of three different approaches to humanistic medical education. *Theoretical Medicine.* **14**: 221–9.

12 Grant VJ (2002) Making room for medical humanities. *Medical Humanities.* **28**: 45–8.

13 Scally J (1976) Transvaluing: the humanities in a technical–vocational curriculum. *Journal of Higher Education.* **47**: 217–26.

14 Weatherall D (2006) Science in the undergraduate curriculum during the 20th century. *Medical Education.* **40**: 195–201.

15 Leydon G, Boulton M, Moynihan C *et al.* (2000) Cancer patients' information needs and information seeking behaviour: in depth interview study. *British Medical Journal.* **320**: 909–13.

16 Maguire P and Pitceathly C (2002) Key communication skills and how to acquire them. *British Medical Journal.* **325**: 697–700.

17 Helman C (2002) *Doctors and Patients: an anthology.* Radcliffe Publishing, Oxford.

18 Schuwirth L and van der Vleuten C (2003) Written assessment. In: ABC of teaching and learning in medicine. *British Medical Journal.* **326**: 643–5.

19 Corderre S, Harasym P, Mandin H and Fick G (2004) The impact of two multiple-choice question formats on the problem-solving strategies used by novices and experts. *BioMed Central – Medical Education.* **4**: 23.

20 Kuhl D (2002) *What Dying People Want: practice wisdom for the end of life.* Perseus Books, Cambridge, MA.

21 Dittrich L (2003) The humanities and medicine: reports of 41 US, Canadian and international programs: preface. *Academic Medicine.* **78**: 951–2.

22 Friedman LD (2002) The precarious position of the medical humanities in the medical school curriculum. *Academic Medicine.* **77**: 320–2.

23 Kamien M (1997) The reform of medical education. *Medical Journal of Australia.* **158**: 226–7.

24 General Medical Council (2009) *Tomorrow's Doctors.* GMC, London.

25 Ludmerer K (1999) *Time to Heal: American medical education from the turn of the century to the era of managed care.* Oxford University Press, New York.

26 Cruess R and Cruess S (1997) Teaching medicine as a profession in the service of healing. *Academic Medicine.* **72**: 941–52.

27 American Board of Internal Medicine Foundation (2002) Medical professionalism in the new millennium: a physician charter. *Annals of Internal Medicine.* **136**: 243–6.

28 Royal College of Physicians (2005) *Doctors in Society: medical professionalism in a changing world.* Report of a Working Party of the Royal College of Physicians of London. RCP, London.

29 Hafferty F (2006) Professionalism – the next wave. *New England Journal of Medicine.* **355**: 2151–2.

30 Gordon J and Lyon P (1998) As others see us: students' role models in medicine. *Medical Journal of Australia.* **169**: 103–5.

31 Turner L (2002) Medical facilities as moral worlds. *Medical Humanities.* **28**: 19–22.

32 Apker J and Eggly S (2004) Communicating professional identity in medical socialization: considering the ideological discourse of morning report. *Qualitative Health Research.* **14**: 411–29.

33 Shem S (1978) *The House of God.* Richard Marek Inc, New York.

34 Mercurio J (2002) *Bodies.* Jonathan Cape, London.

35 Gull SE (2005) Embedding the humanities into medical education. *Medical Education* **39**: 235–6.

36 Shapiro J and Lie D (2000) Using literature to help physician-learners understand and manage 'difficult' patients. *Academic Medicine.* **75**: 765–8.

37 Shapiro J and Rucker L (2003) Can poetry make better doctors? Teaching the humanities and arts to medical students and residents at the University of California, Irvine, College of Medicine. *Academic Medicine.* **78**: 953–7.

38 Pickering N (2000) The use of poetry in health care ethics education. *Medical Humanities.* **26**: 31–6.

39 Pellegrino E (1974) Medical practice and the humanities. *New England Journal of Medicine.* **290**: 1083–5.

40 Downie R, Hendry R, Macnaughton R and Smith B (1997) Humanizing medicine: a special study module. *Medical Education.* **31**: 276–80.

41 Meakin R and Kirklin D (2000) Humanities special studies modules: making better doctors or just happier ones? *Medical Humanities.* **26**: 49–50.

42 Weller K and Lempp H (2000) The visualization and modification of the body in art and medicine – how an innovative special study module explored the humanity of medicine. *Medical Education.* **34**: 951.

43 Kirklin D (2003) Responding to the implications of the genetics revolution for the education and training of doctors: a medical humanities approach. *Medical Education.* **37**: 168–73.

44 Lazarus PA and Rosslyn FM (2003) The arts in medicine: setting up and evaluating a new special study module at Leicester Warwick Medical School. *Medical Education.* **37**: 553–9.

45 Jacobson L, Grant A, Hood K *et al.* (2004) A literature and medicine special study module run by academics in general practice: two evaluations and the lessons learnt. *Medical Humanities.* **30**: 98–100.

46 Bolton G (2005) *Reflective Practice: writing and professional development.* Sage Publications, London.

47 Marton F and Saljo R (1976) On qualitative differences in learning 1: outcome and process. *British Journal of Educational Psychology.* **46**: 4–11.

48 Biggs J (2003) *Teaching for Quality Learning at University.* Open University Press, Buckingham.

49 Ramsden P and Watson D (2003) *Learning to Teach in Higher Education.* Routledge Falmer, London.

50 General Medical Council Education Committee (1993) *Tomorrow's Doctors: recommendations on undergraduate medical education.* GMC, London.

51 Shapiro J and Talbot Y (1991) Applying the concept of the reflective practitioner to understanding and teaching family medicine. *Family Medicine.* **23**: 450–6.

52 Blase J, Hekelman F and Rowe M (2000) Preceptors' use of reflection to teach in ambulatory settings: an exploratory study. *Academic Medicine.* **75**: 947–53.

53 Evans D (2001) Imagination and medical education. *Medical Humanities.* **27**: 30–4.

54 Louis-Courvoisier M and Wenger A (2005) How to make the most of history and literature in the teaching of medical humanities: the experience of the University of Geneva. *Medical Humanities.* **31**: 51–4.

55 Horowitz H (1996) Poetry on rounds: a model for the integration of humanities into residency training. *Lancet.* **347**: 447–9.

56 Kleinman A and Benson P (2006) Anthropology in the clinic: the problem of cultural competency and how to fix it. *Public Library of Science – Medicine*. **3**(10): 1673–6.

57 Fadiman A (1998) *The Spirit Catches You and You Fall Down*. Farrar, Strauss & Giroux, New York.

58 Greenhalgh T (2006) *What Seems to Be the Trouble? Stories of illness and healthcare*. The Nuffield Trust, London.

59 Spencer J, Blackmore D, Heard S *et al.* (2000) Patient-oriented learning: a review of the role of the patient in the education of medical students. *Medical Education*. **34**: 851–7.

60 Almy T, Colby K, Zubkoff M *et al.* (1992) Health, society and the physician: problem-based learning and the social sciences and humanities. *Annals of Internal Medicine*. **116**: 569–74.

61 Kirklin D (2003) Responding to the implications of the genetics revolution for the education and training of doctors: a medical humanities approach. *Medical Education*. **37**: 168–73.

62 Gaita R (2000) *A Common Humanity: thinking about love and truth and justice*. Routledge, London.

63 Aull FB (ed.) *Editor's Choices from the Literature, Arts and Medicine Database: 10th year anniversary*. New York University, New York.

64 Dittrich L (2001) *Ten Years of Medicine and the Arts: 100 selections from academic medicine*. Association of American Medical Colleges, Washington, DC.

65 Vannata J, Schleifer R and Crow S (2004) *Medicine and Humanistic Understanding: the significance of literature in medical practice [DVDROM]*. University of Pennsylvania Press, Philadelphia, PA.

66 Macnaughton J (2000) The humanities in medical education: context, outcome and structures. *Medical Humanities*. **26**: 23–30.

67 Evans H and Macnaughton R (2006) A 'core curriculum' for the medical humanities? *Medical Humanities*. **32**: 65–6.

68 Gordon J (2003) Fostering students' personal and professional development in medicine: a new framework for PPD. *Medical Education*. **37**: 341–9.

69 Evans M (2001) The medical body as philosophy's arena. *Theoretical Medicine and Bioethics*. **22**: 17–32.

70 Rudnick A (2004) An introductory course in philosophy of medicine. *Medical Humanities*. **30**: 54–6.

71 Louhiala P (2003) Philosophy for medical students – why, what, and how. *Medical Humanities*. **29**: 87–8.

72 Pasternack A (2005) Integration of medical humanities in a problem-based curriculum. Paper presented at Association of Medical Schools in Europe Annual Conference, University of Turku, Finland, September 4–6, 2005.

73 Dufflin J (1999) *History of Medicine: a scandalously short introduction*. University of Toronto Press, Toronto.

74 Dufflin J (1995) Infiltrating the curriculum: an integrative approach to history for medical students. *Journal of Medical Humanities*. **16**: 155–73.

75 Porter R (1998) *The Greatest Benefit to Mankind: a medical history of humanity*. WW Norton & Co, London.

76 Porter R (2002) The body. In: *Blood and Guts: a short history of medicine*. Allen Lane, London.

77 Porter R (2002) *Blood and Guts: a short history of medicine*. Allen Lane, London.

78 Porter R (ed.) (2006) *The Cambridge History of Medicine*. Cambridge University Press, Cambridge.

79 Evans M (2003) Roles for literature in medical education. *Advances in Psychiatric Treatment*. **9**: 380–5.

80 Hawkins A (1993) *Reconstructing Illness: studies in pathography*. Purdue University Press, West Lafayette, IN.

81 Friedman L (1995) See me, hear me: using film in health care classes. *Journal of Medical Humanities*. **16**: 223–8.

82 Lepicard E and Fridman K (2003) Medicine, cinema and culture: a workshop in medical humanities for clinical years. *Medical Education*. **37**: 1039–40.

83 Charon R, Banks JT, Connelly J *et al.* (1995) Literature and medicine: contributions to clinical practice. *Annals of Internal Medicine*. **122**: 599–606.

84 Charon R (2001) Narrative medicine: a model for empathy, reflection, profession, and trust. *Journal of the American Medical Association*. **286**: 1897–902.

85 Crellin J (2005) *Public Expectations and Physicians' Responsibilities: voices of medical humanities*. Radcliffe Publishing, Oxford.

86 Singer R and Singer P (2005) *The Moral of the Story*. Blackwell Publishing, Oxford.

87 Wear D and Aultman JM (2005) The limits of narrative: medical student resistance to confronting inequality and oppression in literature and beyond. *Medical Education*. **39**: 1056–65.

88 Shapiro J, Duke A, Boker J and Ahearn CS (2005) Just a spoonful of humanities makes the medicine go down: introducing literature into a family medicine clerkship. *Medical Education*. **39**: 605–12.

89 Toombs S (1992) *The Meaning of Illness: a phenomenological account of the different perspectives of physician and patient*. Kluwer, Boston, MA.

90 Charon R (2004) Narrative and medicine. *New England of Journal of Medicine*. **350**: 862–4.

91 Greenhalgh T and Hurwitz B (1999) Narrative based medicine: why study narrative? *British Medical Journal*. **318**: 48–50.

92 Gysels M, Richardson A and Higginson I (2004) Communication training for health professionals who care for patients with cancer: a systematic review of training methods. *Supportive Care in Cancer*. **13**: 356–66.

93 Clark JA and Mishler EG (1992) Attending to patients' stories: reframing the clinical task. *Sociology of Health & Illness*. **14**: 344–72.

94 Lingard L and Haber R (1999) Teaching and learning communication in medicine. *Academic Medicine*. **74**: 507–10.

95 Tapajos R (2003) HIV/AIDS in the visual arts: applying discipline-based art education (DBAE) to medical humanities. *Medical Education*. **37**: 563–70.

96 Bardes CL, Gillers D and Herman AE (2001) Learning to look: developing clinical observational skills at an art museum. *Medical Education*. **35**: 1157–61.

97 Elder N, Tobias B, Lucero-Criswell A and Goldenhar L (2006) The art of observation: impact of a family medicine and art museum partnership on student education. *Family Medicine*. **38**: 393–8.

98 Kirklin D, Meakin R, Singh S and Lloyd M (2000) Living with and dying from cancer: a humanities special study module. *Medical Humanities*. **26**: 51–4.

99 Easterbrook P, Berlin J, Gopalan R and Matthews D (1991) Publication bias in clinical research. *Lancet*. **337**: 867–72.

100 Shapiro J, Rucker L and Beck J (2006) Training the clinical eye and mind: using the arts to develop medical students' observational and pattern recognition skills. *Medical Education*. **40**: 263–8.

101 Dolev JC, Friedlaender LK and Braverman IM (2001) Use of fine art to enhance visual diagnostic skills. *Journal of the American Medical Association*. **286**: 1020–1.

102 Karkabi K and Cohen Castel O (2006) Deepening compassion through the mirror of painting. *Medical Education*. **40**: 462.

103 Rabow M (2003) Drawing on experience: physician artwork in a course on professional development. *Medical Education*. **37**: 1040–1.

104 Dalhousie University (2006) Humanities in Medicine: a program of the Division of Medical Humanities. Dalhousie University, Halifax, Nova Scotia.

105 Evans R (2003) Patient centred medicine: reason, emotion, and human spirit? Some philosophical reflections on being with patients. *Medical Humanities*. **29**: 8–14.

106 Anderson M, Cohen J, Hallock J *et al.* (1999) Learning objectives for medical student education – guidelines for medical schools. Report 1 of the Medical Schools Objectives Project. *Academic Medicine*. **74**: 13–18.

107 Fortin A and Barnett K (2004) Medical school curricula in spirituality and medicine. *Journal of the American Medical Association*. **291**: 2883.

108 Berlinger N (2004) Spirituality and medicine: idiot-proofing the discourse. *Journal of Medicine and Philosophy*. **29**: 681–95.

109 Ernst E, Cohen MH and Stone J (2004) Ethical problems arising in evidence based complementary and alternative medicine. *Journal of Medical Ethics*. **30**: 156–9.

110 Diamond J (2001) *Snake Oil and Other Preoccupations*. Vintage, London.

111 Weinstein A (2003) *A Scream Goes Through the House: what literature teaches us about life*. Random House, New York.

112 Magee B (1998) *Confessions of a Philosopher*. Phoenix, London.

Further Reading

Evans M and Finlay I (2000) *Medical Humanities*. BMJ Books, London.

Greenhalgh T (2005) *What Seems to Be the Trouble?* Radcliffe Publishing, Oxford.

Helman C (2002) *Doctors and Patients*. Radcliffe Publishing, Oxford.

Kirklin D and Richardson R (2001) *Medical Humanities: a practical introduction*. Royal College of Physicians, London.

Middleton J and Middleton E (2005) *Doctors and Paintings*. Radcliffe Publishing, Oxford.

Salinsky J (2002) *Medicine and Literature*. Radcliffe Publishing, Oxford.

Singer P and Singer R (2005) *The Moral of the Story*. Blackwell Publishing, Malden, MA.

Journal of Medical Humanities. Springer (http://springerlink.com/content/1041-3545).

Medical Humanities Review. University of Texas Medical Branch (http://www.utmb.edu/imh/publications.asp#journals).

Literature and Medicine. The Johns Hopkins University Press (http://www.press.jhu.edu/journals/literature_and_medicine).

Portfolios, personal development and reflective practice

John Pitts

KEY MESSAGES

- Portfolio-based learning has the potential to explore and develop an individual's professional practice.

- Portfolios embrace the professional artistry model of professional practice.

- Traditional approaches to assessment may be inappropriate for portfolios. In portfolio assessment, validity is more important than reliability and the reliability may be supplanted by the qualitative concept of trustworthiness.

- The expert judgement of the teacher will always be part of the assessment process, hence teacher development is essential.

- When assessment is used for regulatory high-stakes purposes, it should follow on from the formative processes that have enabled the professional to learn.

- Portfolios can be used as an acceptable and understandable method of professional accreditation and re-accreditation if traditional views and prejudices are set aside.

Rooted in the principles of experiential learning, portfolio-based learning is an approach that has the 'critical intellectual task of moving from a description of an experience to the identification of the learning derived from that experience and ultimately deciding what further education is required to fill in gaps revealed by the analysis of the described experience. It recognises the value and significance of past learning and experience for the individual; the ability of adults to learn and act autonomously; the centrality of reflection in the learning process; and the need for meaningful links to be made between experiences, learning opportunities and role requirements'.(1)

Although there may be many differences in purpose, structure and assessment requirements, certain key aspects are usually highlighted:
- the *experience* – what has happened, what has been done, seen, written, made, etc.
- the *learning* – the discovery that what has been recalled has significance for doing or changing things in the future
- the *evidence* – a demonstration of how the learning is being applied in a particular context
- *learning needs* – an identification of where it would be appropriate to go next

- *learning opportunities* – an educational action plan identifying ways in which learning needs might be met.(2)

A major characteristic is that the learner selects the contents, which may include a curriculum vitae, log books, case reports, critical incidents(3) and significant event auditing,(4) clinical data, written evaluations, audits, research projects, accounts of innovations, critical reading exercises and videotapes of performance. But it is important that the structure is not too rigid; a portfolio is a means to an end, not an end in itself. Throughout the rest of this chapter, the use of portfolios in medical education will be discussed under the three broad and interrelated headings of *contents*, *purposes* and *assessment*.

Contents of a Portfolio

The first challenge is to define what a portfolio is, or is not. At its widest, the term has been used to include course logs, dossiers, logbooks, training records and folders, and does not necessarily include the benefits and processes listed above. Such documents may exclude any evidence of reflection and self-analysis, and this has led to confusion in the understanding and evaluation of the portfolio approach.(5) Established definitions more clearly include those elements. For example, 'a purposeful collection of student work that exhibits the student's efforts, progress and achievements in one or more areas. The collection must

Understanding Medical Education: Evidence, Theory and Practice. Edited by T Swanwick. © 2010 Association for the Study of Medical Education.

include student participation in selecting contents, the criteria for selection, the criteria for judging merit and evidence of self-reflection'.(6)

Further definitions are 'a collection of evidence which demonstrates the continuing acquisition of knowledge, skills, attitudes, understanding and achievements…reflecting the current stages of development and activity of the individual'(7); and 'a professional development portfolio is a collection of material, made by a professional, that records and reflects on key events and processes in that professional's career'.(8) The latter definition is particularly noteworthy because of the inclusion of the term 'professional'. In terms of how material is collected and collated, Webb(9) outlined four portfolio models in common use. Each model structures the content in a different way. The four types are highlighted in Box 7.1.

Currently, the majority of portfolios in existence are paper-based, although audiotaped and videotaped material may be included where appropriate. Many organisations have developed 'off-the-shelf' portfolio formats, and there is a large growth in the use of electronic formats in both postgraduate and undergraduate medical education.(10–13) E-portfolios differ from paper-based ones in that there is generally a higher level of standardisation, and issues of mentoring and support and assessment processes present a challenge. In theory, it is possible for the contents of an e-portfolio to include video recordings and online assessments, so technological developments will offer increasing depth and scope. However, e-learning in this way does not appeal to everyone – a small-scale evaluation in UK primary care showed that only a minority completed what they had signed up for(14) – and careful implementation and training are, as with all portfolio-based approaches, vital. It is clear that the contents of a portfolio can vary greatly, both in terms of the material within, and from prescriptive to 'free range'. An important distinction can be made between inclusions that are *indirect*, that is, information *about* the writer, and *direct*, that is, created *by* the writer. This allows, for example, for the inclusion of performance data such as audit results *and* reflections and conclusions thereon.

Content, however, is ultimately dictated by purpose.

Purposes of Portfolios in Medicine and Nursing

There must be a clear reason for the existence of a portfolio. Some are used to record personal development and career progression, while others may be assessed for specific purposes such as the demonstration of a certain level of achievement. They range from personal documents held in privacy to a high-stakes assessment approach such as a 'final' examination.(15) Tomkinson(16) (Box 7.2) suggested a taxonomy for the development of portfolios where each characteristic represents a point at either end of a continuum.

BOX 7.1 Models of portfolios(9)

Shopping trolley

The portfolio is use to collect anything that could be seen as a vehicle to learning and the choice is limited only by what the student considers to be appropriate. There are rarely any linking strategies between components.

Toast rack

The portfolio contains a number of predetermined 'slots' that must be filled for each module of a programme, for example, action plans, reflective accounts of significant events, and skills checklists. Each component is formally assessed in isolation.

Cake mix

The parts of the portfolio are blended in that students are expected to provide evidence that they have achieved specified learning outcomes while on placement. The 'mixing' is provided by reflective commentaries addressing analytical criteria.

Spinal column

A series of competency statements form the central column of the portfolio and students collect evidence to demonstrate their achievement. One piece of evidence may be used against multiple statements.

BOX 7.2 A taxonomy for the development of portfolios(16)

Dimension of portfolio design	Possible characteristics	
Style	Descriptive	Reflective
Structure	Informal	Formal
Scope	Narrow (e.g. teaching activity)	Broad (e.g. all clinical and non-clinical activities)
Purpose	Developmental (formative)	Assessment (summative)
Confidentiality	Personal (closed)	Public (open)
Content	Focused (e.g. critical incidents)	Comprehensive (e.g. range of contexts and data)
Timing	Discrete	Continuous

BOX 7.3 Uses of portfolios
- Continuing professional development
- Enhanced learning
- Assessment
- Evaluation
- Certification and re-certification
- Career advancement

BOX 7.4 Where's the evidence? Themes from the literature

- There is growth in portfolio usage in healthcare education despite reservations and shortcomings.

- Portfolio users gain from the experience in their learning, understanding, concepts of 'empowerment' as adult learners and control over their learning, and in relationships with their teachers and tutors.

- The ability of portfolios to provide documentary evidence to demonstrate proficiency is held as a major strength.

- Benefits go beyond individuals. Teachers, departments and institutions all gain from the process and information gathered.

- In high-stakes assessment, reliability is seen as a problem, but rigour may be established through the adoption of qualitative paradigms.

- Users in all studies reports preconceptions of difficulty, uncertainty in what was expected and a lack of confidence in their ability to build the required portfolio.

Discussions between all parties involved about where on this continuum a portfolio should be situated can make explicit how and what should be achieved and expressed.

Within the published literature, six distinct, sometimes overlapping yet complementary, purposes can be identified (Box 7.3). We will explore these further in the following section. The evidence-base for portfolios in medical education is summarised in Box 7.4.

Continuing professional development

A substantial part of published literature refers to the use of portfolios in recording and demonstrating an individual's continuing professional development. In one study in UK nursing, an integrated system of professional development was established between a National Health Service trust hospital and a school of nursing and midwifery. This aimed to build a model of clinical supervision that developed standards for clinical competence that facilitated continuity in professional development throughout the practitioner's career. The collaboration between the two organisations ensured that the model reflected links between theory and practice, and encompassed the require-

ments of the UK Central Council for Nursing (UKCC) and the English National Board for Nursing, Midwifery and Health Visiting (ENB).(17) In the US, teaching portfolios for nurse educators have been used for both formative and summative purposes, and have been described as an effective solution to the dilemma of 'how to comprehensively present oneself as a teacher' (sic).(18) Building on this, two principal purposes for teaching portfolios were identified:

- to assist in the growth and development of the teacher
- to document teaching effectiveness for personnel reasons such as promotion and tenure.(19)

In medicine, a working party of the Royal College of General Practitioners(1) advocated a portfolio-based approach for continuing professional development for general practitioners. Following this, an autonomous learning project for a group of general practitioners (GPs), using the support of mentors, was piloted and found to be both acceptable and assessable through a checklist of quality of evidence,(20) an approach also used successfully with a group of newly established GPs attending a higher professional education course.(21) In general practice vocational training, groups of general practice registrars found portfolios to be of value in reminding, planning, tracking and encouraging reflection; as a route to exploring attitudes and values to stimulate feedback; as encouragement, not humiliation; and to act as a bridge from hospital practice to general practice.(22,23) As a means of recording continuing professional development for a group of GPs, completed portfolios were judged against efficiency (effort expended) and effectiveness (distance travelled), and satisfactory completion accredited for the postgraduate education allowance.(24) In a review of continuing professional development for GPs by the Chief Medical Officer in England, a practice-based portfolio – the practice professional development plan – was proposed(25) and broadly welcomed.(26) A project in Wales explored the potential for portfolios to enhance the learning of a group of GPs through 'professional dialogues'. Evaluation showed that there was strong support for portfolio-based learning; participants felt that their learning was very valuable, and attributed this in large part to the effect of the group.(27)

An evaluation of the use of an electronic portfolio for continuing professional development of consultant physicians in the UK demonstrated a high level of support in principle, although resource shortages limited its use.(28)

Enhanced learning

Another reason for using portfolios is to improve the effectiveness of learning. The use of portfolios as a strategy to support learner-centred learning in student nurses has also been studied.(29) Incorporating reflection on prior experiences, forward planning to meet course outcomes, critical incident analysis and a reflective journal, the portfolio was described as 'an attempt to enable the different knowledge bases of theory and practice to be bridged'. Its greatest gain was in the way the students moved from teacher dependency to self-direction. Presenting teaching accomplishments through a portfolio promoted self-reflection and a direction for improvement and advancement decisions.(30) At the start of the process, nurse educators felt lack of motivation, uncertainty as to what was expected, and anxiety about sharing personal thoughts and feelings. Peer assessment provided another source of concern, although the activity was ultimately seen as a positive experience, with both faculty and peer observers reporting having gained insight into each others' teaching practice and styles. After a situational analysis demonstrated a need for planned learning in an orthopaedic/trauma unit, an action research project explored whether portfolio preparation was itself developmental and if so, what factors influenced this.(31) The findings suggested that the process itself influenced development by acting as an initiator to reflection on experience.

In medicine, the educational effectiveness of prolonged community-based attachments for undergraduate medical students has been assessed using portfolios. Popular with both tutors and students, the educational achievements were rated as satisfactory or outstanding.(32) Reflective portfolios supported by a mentoring process have been used with success in Holland with undergraduate medical students.(33) In a group of registrars in general practice training, a portfolio-based approach worked well for some, but not all.(22) For those in favour, the portfolio became an important means of capturing the events of the training year to reflect on progress made and to define and set future learning needs. The authors concluded that in addition, this approach required considerable support and encouragement from the general practice trainers responsible for the registrars. Similarly, in an interview study, reflective practice was claimed as an outcome of a course for medical educators.(34)

However, for senior house officers in accident and emergency departments and an obstetric unit, using personal learning logs in the format of a controlled study did not increase learning in the study group.(35) The authors commented that the contents of the logs revealed great scope for learning, but few doctors documented the specific learning achieved, and that for the initiative to be successful, active participation from trained senior staff, protected time for learning and a 'more positive approach from all concerned' would be needed. The use of an electronic portfolio using a personal computer-based software program showed that users who agreed with the statement 'entering items of learning into my diary encourages me to think in terms of questions that guide my learn-

ing' recorded an attempt 'to modify their practice' as an outcome more often than those who disagreed with that statement.(36) An examination of the portfolios of medical teachers for 'reflectiveness' found good evidence,(37) yet concluded that set assignments could be too directive.(38)

Assessment
Formative assessment
Formative assessment, through feedback from teachers or peers, is a major benefit of portfolio learning. By providing the opportunity to review and reflect on progress, and through this, to reset objectives and goals, it is possible to monitor and shape learning. Beyond factual learning and recorded experience, reflection on issues behind events and situations allows and encourages the exploration and expression of assumptions, beliefs and values that underpin such experiences. Much of the published literature alludes to this, although details are sparse. The willingness of writers to commit to deeper expression is likely to be related to knowledge and trust of the mentor or supervisor.

In a study of undergraduates training in obstetrics and gynaecology, a structured portfolio was used to record practical procedures carried out and the individual reflections of students.(39) Group sessions tutored by consultants were also used as the basis for further reflections and the identification of future learning. The authors concluded that portfolios supported the development of complex skills, clarified learning goals and helped students to monitor their achievement. Currently in the UK, educational progress in postgraduate training (at every stage of training and in all specialties) is recorded and monitored through a portfolio-based approach.

The value of a portfolio approach in formative assessment is probably the least contentious application, because it is individually related, developmental and does not have to address the murky issue of robust judgement.

Summative assessment
The use of portfolios in summative assessment is still relatively untested. This is because of difficulties in addressing the issue of reliability, which is held as vitally important from the perspective of traditional assessment methodology and the prevailing positivist viewpoint, and the demonstration of a high level of 'trustworthiness' if a non-positivist viewpoint is taken. Generally speaking, portfolios have high face validity, but there are problems with reliability, relating to both content specificity and rater issues,(40,41) and deep suspicion in relation to the role of self-assessment.(42,43)

The medical school at the University of Dundee uses portfolio assessment in the final year examinations of medical students.(15) Evaluation of the first year of this process revealed strong support from staff and generally positive reactions from the students. The contents included clinical case reports and reflections thereon, practical procedure records, needs-based learning agreements, special study module assessment forms and reports, reports of an elective activity and a fourth-year assignment report. The assessment process comprised an initial grading followed by a session where four examiners (three internal, one external), working in pairs, reviewed each portfolio with the student. Conclusions from the evaluation were that portfolio building provided a bridge between formative and summative assessment, and a means of monitoring the progress of students. While concluding that portfolio assessment is a useful tool that provides a powerful approach to assessing a range of curricular outcomes not easily assessed by other methods, and may even provide a basis for a judgement on 'fitness to practise', there is a comment that 'attention must be paid to logistics with careful briefing of examiners and students'.

Using a checklist approach based on the five criteria of logical and coherent structure, level of critical reflection, level of actual or future skills development, use of documentary evidence and use of relevant literature, a summative assessment process for medical students produced a reliability of overall scores of 0.77 when two assessors jointly rated the portfolios,(44) thereby matching the 'best' objective tests. However, to reach similar levels of reliability in assessing GPs' learning plans, it has been calculated that five to eight assessors are required.(45) More recently, portfolios have been used successfully in the summative assessment of medical students at the University of Maastricht,(46) and here a purely qualitative methodology has been adopted, with the concept of *reliability* replaced with that of *trustworthiness*, a key issue in portfolio assessment that we will consider in more detail later.

Evaluation

Portfolios completed by learners offer an opportunity to judge the effects and effectiveness of the teaching and learning. In nursing, student nurse portfolios have been used to evaluate undergraduate nursing programmes. Portfolios represent a more realistic appraisal of what students are learning and allow validation of programme outcomes for both the institution and external agencies, as well as certification of competency. They also ensure that teachers know that their efforts have been effective and that intended learning has occurred. Overall, portfolios were seen as an opportunity to showcase a variety of work to demonstrate the attainment of professional competence and increase faculty–student collaboration and shared learning.(47)

In some fields of medicine, the gathering of evidence of 'quality of teaching' in the form of a teacher's

portfolio has been used.(48) The implementation of teaching portfolios for clinical teachers, while showing strong support from the academic leadership, revealed extraordinary pressures on staff to minimise engagement in teaching, an insufficient infrastructure to support documentation of educational quality, and conflicts between an external economic reward system and the valuing of teaching.(49) These authors concluded that there are significant challenges to those who chose academic medicine for its educational focus, and those who desired recognition and validation of those activities.

A log diary approach that encouraged medical students in internal medicine and community-based clerkship to record activities with patients and their teachers recorded both the use of time and the perceived quality of their teaching,(50) and a portfolio learning approach was used to provide individual evaluation of the teachers.(39)

Certification and re-certification

In many ways the same issues that confound and confuse portfolio use in summative assessments are relevant here. In any high-stakes assessment that can affect a person's livelihood and remuneration, there must be a high degree of trust that any judgement made is the 'right one'.

The UKCC(51) requires nurses 'to effectively demonstrate (sic) that they have taken action to maintain and develop professional knowledge and competence...to use a personal professional profile'. The ENB(52) similarly sees a professional portfolio as 'an essential part of the board's framework for continuing professional education'. Commenting on this, Jasper(53) stated that portfolio compilation had great potential provided that attempts were made to ensure its relevance to the practitioner and that a solid infrastructure of educational, managerial and financial support was in place.

In medicine in the UK, in order to fulfil the requirements of both annual appraisal and revalidation, all doctors are expected to maintain a 'folder' that includes an educational record, performance data, audit and evidence of effective communication with patients. These portfolios are structured according to areas defined by the General Medical Council in its publication *Good Medical Practice*.(54) These include good clinical care, maintaining good medical practice, relationships with patients, working with colleagues, teaching and training, research, probity and health.

Career advancement

Using a peer-reviewed portfolio as a basis for promotion in nursing has been described, where criteria that identify functioning as a role model, teaching colleagues and introducing change are used in a process of assessment by peer review.(55) Promotions via this 'clinical ladder system' were also accompanied by increases in salary. A summative evaluation of a baccalaureate programme for nurse development demonstrated that a portfolio approach represented a positive option for career development.(56) This was shown to reflect adult learning theory and provide maximum opportunity and flexibility for students to meet the leadership and management requirements of the course. The notion of a portfolio-based presentation at an annual appraisal as a means of moving away from the narrow areas of teaching, research and service towards the broader creative and reflective activities of the professional has been promoted,(18) and the potential for teaching portfolios as a means of provision of documentation for promotion and tenure purposes has also been identified.(19)

In the US, documentation of teaching accomplishments related to established criteria of effective teaching behaviour has been incorporated into a teaching portfolio and used in promotion, tenure and salary decisions about clinical medical staff. Beyond this, the university used the perceived quality of educational activity by means of the educators' portfolios to decide the distribution of funds between departments.(48) A survey of 134 medical schools in the US in 1994(57) revealed that 20% had a portfolio system in place, 8% were in the process of developing one and 21% were in discussion about it. Of those currently using this approach, the prime purpose was for supporting decisions of career promotion. A survey of all the medical schools in the US plus those in Canada three years later, showed that about half had a 'clinician-educator promotion track' based on an evaluation strategy that used a combination of awards, peer evaluations, learner evaluations and teaching portfolios. This formed the basis of promotion decisions for the majority of schools.(58)

Assessment through Portfolios

As an assessment instrument, portfolios have particular advantages, primarily stemming from the differences between a portfolio and a 'typical' examination situation, which is a pressurised and stressful time-limited event occurring at the end of a course or programme. Portfolios are not, intrinsically, an examination method, yet they can be used as a basis for assessment. Completing the portfolio over time allows for multiple attempts and opportunities, revision and reflection, and it can address multiple tasks and use many forms of data entry. Furthermore, portfolios offer the chance to continue to be both a record of personal development and a career log. They may be seen as an *authentic* assessment – one that looks at performance and practical application of theory.(23,59) The principal disadvantages stem from unfamiliarity, the effort involved and, in terms of assessment, the lack of evidence for supporting judgements that may be made.

Philosophical issues behind assessment

A fundamental issue with this relatively new (to medicine) approach to learning as an assessment method is the difficulty in making it fit with traditional views of an assessment process.(60) The paradox is that developing this to its full potential moves away from objective and standardised testing towards a subjective and non-standardised position.(61) To achieve high reliability means sacrificing individuality by constricting and controlling the format, and scoring according to some template or checklist. This thereby limits the greatest value of a portfolio to the individual, which is as a reflective tool – a personal account of professional practice that identifies and acknowledges both strengths and weaknesses. However, some authors have argued that in non-standardised assessments, reliability becomes less important.(48,62) In this area, it should be borne in mind that for many years there seems to have been little difficulty with the summative judgement of dissertations, theses, etc., or the selection of material for publication. Furthermore, much published work on portfolio assessment uses statistical methodology to assess inter-rater reliability that is inconsistent and open to challenge.(40) Kappa statistics are the most appropriate since they take into account chance agreement; they can be adapted to different numbers of assessors; different assessors can be used for different portfolios; and different numbers of assessors can be used for each portfolio.(63) Introducing the notion of external assessment alters learners' approaches to learning, which becomes directed towards the perceived purposes of the examination strategy.(64) How is this likely to influence what goes into a portfolio? Surely it will not be thought that identifying and displaying weaknesses will impress an examiner? Although perhaps now less rigidly interpreted than earlier, it may be that traditional psychometric views of reliability and validity are limiting more meaningful educational approaches.

Assessment approaches that attempt to measure the learning processes shown by portfolios require a different set of educational values that recognise the role of personal and professional judgements on the part of the learner. Reflective behaviour involves the practitioner investigating and seeking insights into their practice. It accepts the subjectivity of data and interpretations, and focuses on individual insights and development. It values creativity and, importantly, allows and understands the possibility of being wrong. Phillips(65)quoted Thomas Kuhn, who popularised the notion that inquirers always work within a paradigm or framework that determines the concepts that are used. He stated that in a sense, all inquirers are trapped within their own paradigms; they will judge certain things as being true (for them) that others will judge as being false (for them). This highlights the issue that assessors and their subjects carry, perhaps unwittingly, personal agendas into the assessment process that can lead to undue weightings and bias. Open discussions may go some way to improve reliability by making explicit the otherwise unstated assumptions, beliefs and values of the assessors.(66) While, in general, standardisation and structuring of assessment may improve reliability,(67) this may explain why traditionally high levels are not easily reached.

To explore this impasse, we need to consider the nature of reflective practice and what it means to practise as a professional.

Reflective Practice and Professional Development

Reflective practice

The term 'reflective practice' first appears in the work of Dewey,(68) and was expanded on in the 1980s by authors such as Schön.(69) Reflective practice has been defined as 'the process of internally examining and exploring an issue of concern, triggered by an experience, which creates and clarifies meaning in terms of self, and which results in a changed conceptual perspective'.(70) Schön(71) made a distinction between reflection-in-action and reflection-on-action, where the former is represented by 'questioning the assumptional structures of knowing-in-action' and thinking critically about 'the thinking that got us into this fix or this opportunity'.

Practical experience is at the centre of professional learning,(72) and it has been suggested that educational programmes should include reflective processes based on personal experiences.(73) Learning is the process of transforming experiences into knowledge, skills, attitudes and values, and as such has been represented graphically by means of experiential/learning cycles, for example, that of Kolb (Figure 7.1).(74)

Concrete experience, observations and reflections, formulation of abstract concepts and generalisations, and the testing of implications of concepts in new situations are the stations around this cyclical model. Jarvis(75) believed this to be oversimplistic, and devel-

oped a model that represents a more complex model of learning, suggesting nine possible responses to an experience, divisible into three categories, which include non-learning and non-reflective learning as well as reflective learning. Non-learning included responses such as presumption, where previous learnt experiences are trusted and comfortably taken for granted; non-consideration, where people are too busy or uncomfortable to explore further; and rejection, where the possibility of learning from an experience is rejected, sometimes, for example, through bias or bigotry. Non-reflective learning includes preconscious or incidental learning, the learning of repetitive or mechanical skills and memorisation. These might be detected when a portfolio is discussed through mentoring or an assessment process.

Most literature on experiential learning refers to learning from primary events, which are subjectively experienced. It is important to consider, and value, learning from secondary experiences of others, communicated in writing or verbally, by individuals or within groups. Within professions, such interactions within the community of practice represent a powerful means of learning not just about factual knowledge but about values, truths and meaning. This supports the inclusion of indirect data within a portfolio for reflection.

Sparks-Langer and Colton(76) suggested that there are three elements within reflection: cognition, critical thinking and narrative enquiry. Schön referred to these processes as *problem setting*, and believed that professional learning stems from continuous action and reflection on everyday problems. Such knowledge is often tacit and difficult to identify and analyse. Knowledge is constructed; as a professional reflects on an experience, they develop their own theoretical system. Ross(77) identified a series of steps in reflective thinking:

- recognising the nature of the problem
- responding by recognising similarities and differences to other consequences and implications of possible solution
- examining the intended and unintended consequences of the solution selected.

A similar approach is illustrated in Box 7.5.

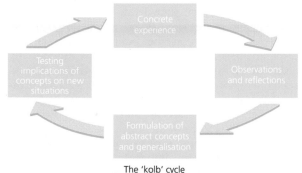

The 'kolb' cycle

Figure 7.1 Kolb's cycle of experiential learning.(78)

BOX 7.5 A model for reflective practice

- What was the nature of the problem?
- What were the consequences?
- How was it addressed?
- What was learned about (a) the problem and (b) myself?
- How will the same or a similar situation be addresses next time?

A key theme in reflection is an emphasis on a natural approach, where, in contrast to experiments and studies that control variables and aim for generalisable results, emphasis is given to meanings and interpretations to gain insights into practice and an appreciation of its complexity.

It is clear, therefore, that reflection is not a form of armchair relaxation best carried out alone. Assisting reflection by using colleagues, mentors and small groups, and writing down for preservation and future use, are valuable strategies that can be called upon. By reflecting on and theorising their practice, practitioners can make public, and therefore open to scrutiny and assessment, their processes of professional development.

Personal development in professional life

Learning in professional life, in the day-to-day reality of a professional's actual working practices, most importantly involves learning through reflection and conversations with peers. This establishes the important notion of a 'community of practice', a concept that will be discussed in more detail later. While there is potential for learning in any situation, the greatest source of learning is from other human beings, in particular peers and patients. Conversations around the interesting or unusual case, the problem shared that leads to the 'why don't you try…' form the very basis of peer group learning.

An increasing body of research has explored the situated character of human understanding and communication and examined the relationship between learning and the social situation in which it occurs,(78) regarding learning as a form of social co-participation, rather than the mere acquisition of knowledge. Conventional explanations see learning as the internalisation of knowledge, however acquired, leaving the nature of the learner, the world and its interrelationships outside and unconsidered. Situated learning has two perspectives.(79) The first implies an interactive and productive role for the skills acquired – the learner is not gaining a corpus of knowledge to be used at some later time, rather the skills to perform by actually engaging in the process under the modified conditions of *legitimate peripheral participation*.(78) This allows the learner to participate in the practice of an expert professional, but in a way limited by degree and responsibility. This term provides a way to speak about relationships, between newcomers and established practitioners, and activities and communities of practice. The process of joining to become a full participant is a socio-cultural process that subsumes the learning of knowledgeable skills.

The second perspective, in contrast to the view that learning occurs within the individual, is that learning takes place in a framework of participation, mediated by differences in perspective of the co-participants. It is the 'community' that learns. Whereas the learner, as an apprentice, may learn most, others learn as co-learners. The apprentices, therefore, cause changes in the larger community of practitioners. The community of practice itself contains a wide range of players, including, in addition to apprentices, young masters with apprentices themselves, as well as established practitioners who may be reaching the end of their careers. Interestingly, to sustain collaborative participation there must be conflicts between the forces that support the process of learning and those that oppose them. Within a professional group, this implies a collective grouping such as a professional organisation or trade union that stands up for the values and status of the group against what are perceived as external threats.

Learning in clinical practice moves through the stage of the novice, perhaps the medical student who 'observes', towards a notion of supervised practice, perhaps the junior doctor, who can call on a more senior member of staff if they are uncertain about how to proceed with a problem that is felt to be beyond their capability. Consequent learning is located in the increasing access of the learner to participatory roles in expert practice.(78) Even for established professionals, groups learn together through an often asymmetric co-participation in practice. Clinical practice is littered with tales told in conversations about difficulties and disasters, that is, significant events,(4) which can lead to reconsideration of practice, reflection and adaptive learning by the wider audience.

After a review of portfolio usage, an 'integrated proficiency-criterion framework' that linked levels of proficiency was proposed (novice, advanced beginner, competent), with outcome criteria in areas such as critical thinking, communication skills, therapeutic interventions, professional development, personal development and scholarship, allowing an assessment of an individual's overall competence.(80) This suggests that a process of maturation can be captured by means of a portfolio approach.

Professional knowledge

More light can be cast on the debate by considering the complex nature of professional knowledge. Eraut(81) divided professional knowledge into propositional, personal and process knowledge. While propositional knowledge resides in the public domain and is discipline-based, personal knowledge is individually acquired by experience. Process knowledge is represented as knowing how to conduct the various processes that contribute to professional action, including knowing how to access and use propositional knowledge.(81)

These may be best explored through a reflective approach. Among the implications for professional education and assessment are conclusions that are in direct opposition to the existing systems, as in reality any assessment of professional competence that fails to observe in some way the hidden aspect of one's expertise cannot be held to be valid.(82)

Professional practice

A further angle on the issue of assessment may be gained by considering the two models of professional practice described by Fish.(83) The first is the *technical-rational model*, which assumes that professional activity is a matter of technical performance, following a logical sequence as part of an efficient system. This values the technical aspects of the professional's work (measurable skills, performance and procedures that can be mastered) and logical systems and efficiency. This behavioural model assumes that professional activity consists of actions that are visible, observable and therefore amenable to measurement. The emphasis is on predetermined skills and procedures, and permanent and quantifiable propositional knowledge, and the process of measurement strives for objectivity. Fish argues that technical accountability has to be controlled by elaborate mechanisms of assessment, inspection, appraisal and accreditation, beneath which lies the view that professionals are not to be trusted – in other words, not fit to exercise professional judgement.

A second, alternative, view is the *professional artistry model*, which sees professional practice as an art. It stresses understanding rather than technical skills, and takes a holistic approach to skills and knowledge. Within a core knowledge of skills and routines it accepts that it is not possible to know everything, and sees open capacities and competencies that cannot be mastered as more valuable than closed ones that can, but are usually more trivial.(84) This model stresses investigation and reflection on practice, with the practitioner investigating and seeking insights into their practice. It accepts the essential subjectivity of data and any interpretations made, and focuses on individual insights and development. It accepts professional behaviour as self-regulating; beneath this model lies a view of professionals as deserving certain autonomy as a result of knowledge and moral responsibility. Its view about defining standards is that what is below standard is perfectly easily recognised when seen. There is no need for a complex 'schedule' of basic competence (which, unless very basic, will not be agreed upon by assessors), as it cannot take account of the unique practitioner in a unique practice.

An Interpretive Approach to Portfolio Assessment

If we accept the notion that portfolios are individual and subjective, how might an assessment process look? An assessor would need to see that the work within a portfolio is *valid*, showing what it claims to

show, and *sufficient*, detailed enough for an assessor to infer that learning has indeed taken place.(85) Along with the need for the work done to have been sufficiently recent, that is, *current*, to be meaningful, these constitute the degree of *authenticity* of the portfolio. The portfolio can be 'placed' in context on the continuum contained within a taxonomy of characteristics such as that of Tomkinson,(12) through discussions between the assessed and the assessors. This means that the purpose of the assessment is defined, overt and understood, and can be seen in relationship to where the learner is starting from and, at some point of judgement, how far the learner has travelled. Having ascertained the purpose, the choice of and responsibility for the contents can be devolved to the learner. This offers the opportunity for the individual, metaphorically, to talk about his or her practice and explore the beliefs and values involved. The source of evidence should be indicated; some will be direct (i.e. created by the learner), such as reflective accounts and audits, and some will be indirect (i.e. about the learner), such as performance statistics and correspondence. During the construction of the portfolio, collaboration with at least one other person will enhance development and provide feedback through assisted reflection and discussion.(86) Similarly, at the point at which an external judgement is required, discussions with and between the assessors allow opportunities for explanation, clarification and context setting. Merely taking part in the process is not sufficient. Assessors are, regardless of and independently of others, able to identify features that they take to be 'good practice' and areas with which they take issue. Discussion between two assessors, and perhaps also the writer of the portfolio, can enhance understanding and meaning such that the assessors can judge whether the writer is doing satisfactorily and exhibiting appropriate qualities and behaviours or, conversely, is not showing the learning and insights that they perhaps could. As a living instrument, the work in question can be revisited, reviewed, reconsidered, rewritten and re-submitted in the light of that conversation.

Over a predetermined period of time, learning needs identified can be recorded and incorporated into a 'learning contract'.(87,88) At subsequent review, fulfilment and completion of an agreement can be included within the assessment process.

Such a truly authentic approach would allow an individual's continuing professional development to be followed, encouraged and understood, perhaps over some considerable period of time, and values improvements made above deficiencies highlighted. Furthermore, a portfolio process avoids the philosophical trap of the 'false dualism' that forces one assessment approach to be taken to the exclusion of another. Taking a quantitative approach where appropriate, for example, for aspects of professional practice that are generalisable, and a qualitative one in areas that are

> **BOX 7.6 How to: Introduce a portfolio, successfully**
> - Be clear about the purpose of the portfolio
> - In design, consider together content, purpose and assessment
> - Understand the level of experience and maturity of the learner
> - Maintain the centrality of 'reflection on practice'
> - Base on individual professional practice
> - Provide clear instructions for use
> - Develop and implement a well-resourced training strategy
> - Provide institutional support and leadership

individual avoids this and places portfolio assessment within a model that focuses on the professional's progress as a developmental ideal (*see* Box 7.6).

Conclusions

The portfolio approach has many advantages, both theoretical and practical. At the beginning it allows individuals to define who and where they are, to take stock of their professional positions. Following reflective cycles of learning, disassembling and critically reconstructing their practice, drawing conclusions and planning learning are all in accord with theories of effective learning. The approach is congruent with the nature of professional knowledge, practice and how professionals learn, and represents a means of capturing the exercising of professional judgement. The process of writing represents a form of 'conversation with self' and is enhanced by reflective discussions with another person. It demonstrates *par excellence* the process of continuing professional development and provides a means of displaying this to another person, and the use of qualitative assessment approaches that are open and capable of being validated allows judgements to be made about the writer.

A portfolio approach has the potential to encourage, capture and record deep approaches to learning, through an active search for meaning, personal significance and linking to existing knowledge. Portfolios provide the opportunity for a reflective approach that allows experiences to be replayed and critically reconstructed in a way that identifies and highlights educational needs and thereby points the way for future learning. The philosophy is learner-centred; the learner takes responsibility for planning and demonstrating that learning has occurred. While initially the approach is often negatively influenced by attitudes related to uncertainty and unfamiliarity, it is clear that for many writers, portfolios can become an acceptable and often welcome form of recording continuing professional development and an assessment method that is seen as fair and transparent. Maintaining a portfolio throughout a career is a powerful means of demonstrating commitment, continued learning and career development.

It is likely that from a purely psychometric viewpoint, criticisms can be made of any existing method of portfolio assessment. The essentially subjective nature of a reflective portfolio represents a technical rationalist's nightmare, and their response might be to enforce such a degree of standardisation that reflective learning would be lost in the need to meet some standard of performance. However, from the professional artistry perspective, a portfolio has the potential to demonstrate the very essence of professionalism: capturing reflection, deliberation, insights and creativity. This requires some changes to our traditional ways of thinking.

Acknowledgement

Some of the material used in this chapter has previously been published in two articles by the author(89,90) in *Medical Teacher* and is reproduced here with permission.

References

1 Royal College of General Practitioners (1993) *Portfolio Based Learning in General Practice.* Royal College of General Practitioners, London.
2 Redman W (1994) *Portfolios for Development: a guide for trainers and managers.* Kogan–Page, London.
3 Flanagan J (1954) The critical incident technique. *Psychological Bulletin.* 51: 327–58.
4 Pringle M, Bradley C, Carmichael C et al. (1997) *Significant Event Auditing.* Royal College of General Practitioners, London.
5 Rees C (2005) The use (and abuse) of the term 'portfolio'. *Medical Education.* 39: 436.
6 Paulson F, Paulson P and Meyer C (1991) What makes a portfolio a portfolio? *Educational Leadership.* 48: 60–3.
7 Brown R (1992) *Portfolio Development and Profiling for Nurses.* Quay Publishing, Lancaster.
8 Hall D (1992) Professional development portfolios for teachers and lecturers. *British Journal of In-service Education.* 18: 81–6.
9 Webb C (2002) Models of portfolios. *Medical Education.* 36: 897–8.
10 Parboosingh J and McLaughlin R (1996) Learning portfolios: potential to assist health professionals with self directed learning. *Journal of Continuing Education in the Health Professions.* 16: 75–81.
11 Fung M, Walker M, Fung K, Temple L et al. (2000) An internet-based learning portfolio in resident education: the KOALA multicentre programme. *Medical Education.* 34: 474–9.
12 NHS Education Scotland (2006) Foundation programme portfolio (www.nhsdots.org/nhsdotsx/login.asp; accessed 10 October 2006).

13 NHS (2006) Appraisal toolkit (www.apraisals.nhs.uk; accessed 10 October 2006).

14 Dagley V and Berrington B (2005) Learning from an evaluation of an electronic portfolio to support general practitioners' personal development, planning, appraisal and revalidation. *Education for Primary Care.* **16**: 567–74.

15 Davis M, Ben-David M, Harden R *et al.* (2001) Portfolio assessment in medical students' final examinations. *Medical Teacher.* **23**: 357–66.

16 Tomkinson B (1997) *Towards a Taxonomy of Teaching Portfolios.* University of Manchester, Manchester.

17 Friedman S and Marr J (1995) A supervisory model of professional competence: a joint service/education initiative. *Nurse Education Today.* **15**: 239–44.

18 Melland H and Volden C (1996) Teaching portfolios for faculty evaluation. *Nurse Educator.* **21**: 35–8.

19 Oermann N (1999) Developing a teaching portfolio. *Journal of Professional Nursing.* **15**: 224–8.

20 Treasure W (1996) Portfolio-based learning pilot scheme for general practitioner principals in south-east Scotland. *Education for General Practice.* **7**: 249–54.

21 Pitts J and Vincent S (1995) A higher professional education course in Wessex – the first year. *Education for General Practice.* **6**: 157–62.

22 Snadden D, Thomas M, Griffin E and Hudson H (1996) Portfolio-based learning and general practice vocational training. *Medical Education.* **30**: 148–52.

23 Snadden D and Thomas M (1998) The use of portfolio learning in medical education. *Medical Teacher.* **20**: 192–9.

24 Challis M, Mathers N, Howe A and Field N (1997) Portfolio-based learning: continuing medical education for general practitioners – a mid-point evaluation. *Medical Education.* **31**: 22–6.

25 Calman K (1998) *A Review of Continuing Professional Development in Practice: a report to the Secretary of State from the Chief Medical Officer.* Department of Health, London.

26 Pitts J, Curtis A, While R and Holloway I (1999) Practice Professional Development Plans: general practitioners' perspectives on proposed changes in general practice education. *British Journal of General Practice.* **49**: 959–62.

27 Brigley S (2001) *Y Portffolio: the development of portfolio learning among groups of general practitioners in Wales.* University of Wales College of Medicine, Cardiff.

28 Dornan T, Carroll C and Parboosingh J (2002) An electronic learning portfolio for reflective continuing professional development. *Medical Education.* **36**: 767–9.

29 Jasper M (1995) The potential of the professional portfolio for nursing. *Journal of Clinical Nursing.* **4**: 249–55.

30 O'Mara L, Carpio B, Mallete C *et al.* (2000) Developing a teaching portfolio in nursing education: a reflection. *Nurse Educator.* **25**: 125–9.

31 Cayne J (1995) Portfolios as a developmental influence. *Journal of Advanced Nursing.* **21**: 395–405.

32 Grant J, Ramsey A and Bain J (1997) Community hospitals and general practice: extended attachments for students. *Medical Education.* **31**: 364–8.

33 Driessen E, Tartwijk J, Vermunt J and van der Vleuten C (2003) Use of portfolios in early undergraduate medical education. *Medical Teacher.* **25**: 18–23.

34 Beecher A, Lindemann J, Morzinski J and Simpson D (1997) Use of the educator's portfolio to stimulate reflective practice among medical educators. *Teaching and Learning in Medicine.* **9**: 56–9.

35 Kelly D and Murray T (1999) The development and evaluation of a personal learning log for senior house officers. *Medical Education.* **33**: 260–6.

36 Campbell C, Parboosingh J, Gondocz T *et al.* (1996) Study of the factors influencing the stimulus to learning recorded by physicians keeping a learning portfolio. *Journal of Continuing Education in the Health Professions.* **19**: 16–24.

37 Tigelaar D, Dolmans D, de Grave W *et al.* (2006) Portfolio as a tool to stimulate teachers reflections. *Medical Teacher.* **28**: 277–82.

38 Tigelaar D, Dolmans D, de Grave W *et al.* (2006) Participants' opinions on the usefulness of a teaching portfolio. *Medical Education.* **40**: 371–8.

39 Lonka K, Slotte V, Halttunen M *et al.* (2001) Portfolios as a learning tool in obstetrics and gynaecology undergraduate training. *Medical Education.* **35**: 1125–30.

40 Pitts J, Coles C and Thomas P (1999) Educational portfolios in the assessment of general practice trainers: reliability of assessors. *Medical Education.* **33**: 515–20.

41 Roberts C (2002) Portfolio-based assessments in medical education: are they valid and reliable for summative purposes? *Medical Education.* **36**: 899–900.

42 Gordon MJ (1991) A review of the validity and accuracy of self-assessments in health professions training. *Academic Medicine.* **66**: 762–9.

43 McKinstry B and Evans A (2006) Self-assessment or self-delusion? *Education for Primary Care.* **17**: 432–5.

44 Rees C and Sheard C (2004) The reliability of assessment criteria for undergraduate medical students' communication skills portfolios: the Nottingham experience. *Medical Education.* **38**: 138–44.

45 Roberts C, Cromarty I, Crossley J and Jolly B (2006) The reliability and validity of a matrix to assess the completed reflective personal development plans of general practitioners. *Medical Education.* **40**: 363–70.

46 Driessen E, van Tartwijk J, Overeem K *et al.* (2005) Conditions for successful reflective use of portfolios in undergraduate medical education. *Medical Education.* **39**: 214–20.

47 Karlowicz K (2000) The value of student portfolios to evaluate undergraduate nursing programmes. *Nurse Educator.* **25**: 82–7.

48 Speer A and Elnicki D (1999) Assessing the quality of teaching. *American Journal of Medicine.* **106**: 381–3.

49 Lee L, Froh R and Petrusa E (1997) Assessing the implementation of teaching portfolios in the academic medical center. In: Scherpbier A, van der Vleuten CPM, Rethans JJ and van der Steeg AFW (eds) *Advances in Medical Education.* Kluwer Academic Publishers, Dordrecht.

50 Murray E, Alderman P, Coppola W *et al.* (2001) What do students actually do on an internal medicine clerkship? A log diary study. *Medical Education.* **35**: 1101–7.

51 United Kingdom Central Council for Nursing (1994) *The Future of Professional Practice. The Council's Standard for Education and Practice Following Registration.* UKCC, London.

52 English National Board (1991) *Professional Portfolio.* ENB, London.

53 Jasper M (1995) The portfolio workbook as a strategy for student-centred learning. *Nurse Education Today.* **15**: 446–51.

54 General Medical Council (2001) *Good Medical Practice.* GMC, London.

55 Deckert B (1990) Reach for excellence – a clinical ladder promotion system. *Journal of the American Nursing Association.* **17**: 296–8.

56 Oechsle L, Volden C and Lambeth S (1990) Portfolios and RNs: an evaluation. *Journal of Nursing Education.* **29**: 54–9.

57 Simpson D, Morzinski J, Beecher A and Lindemann J (1994) Meeting the challenge to document teaching accomplishments: the educator's portfolio. *Teaching and Learning in Medicine.* **6**: 203–6.

58 Beasley B, Wright S, Cofrancesco J *et al.* (1997) Promotion criteria for clinician educators in the United States and Canada. *Journal of the American Medical Association.* **278**: 723–8.

59 Newmann F (1990) Higher order thinking in teaching social studies: a rationale for the assessment of classroom thoughtfulness. *Journal of Curriculum Studies.* **22**: 41–56.

60 Schuwirth L and van der Vleuten C (2006) A plea for new psychometric models in educational assessment. *Medical Education.* **40**: 296–300.

61 Pitts J and Coles C (2003) The challenge of non-standardised assessment of professionals – the need for a paradigm shift. *Education for Primary Care.* **14**: 397–405.

62 Moss P (1994) Can there be validity without reliability? *Educational Researcher.* **23**: 5–12.

63 Davis M and Fleiss J (1982) Measuring agreement for multinomial data. *Biometrics.* **38**: 1047–51.

64 Newble D and Jaeger K (1983) The effects of assessments and examinations on the learning of medical students. *Medical Education.* **17**: 165–71.

65 Phillips D (1990) Subjectivity and objectivity: an objective enquiry. In: Eisner E and Peshkin A (eds) *Qualitative Enquiry in Education – the continuing debate.* Teachers College Press, New York.

66 Pitts J, Coles C, Thomas P and Smith F (2002) Enhancing reliability in portfolio assessment: discussions between assessors. *Medical Teacher.* **24**: 197–201.

67 Van der Vleuten C (1996) The assessment of professional competence: developments, research and practical implications. *Advances in Health Sciences Education.* **1**: 41–67.

68 Dewey J (1933) *How We Think: a restatement of the relation between reflective thinking to the educative process.* DC Heath, London.

69 Schön D (1983) *The Reflective Practitioner.* Jossey-Bass, San Francisco, CA.

70 Boyd E and Fales A (1983) Reflective learning: key to learning from experience. *Journal of Humanistic Psychology.* **23**: 99–117.

71 Schön D (1987) *Educating the Reflective Practitioner.* Jossey-Bass, San Francisco, CA.

72 Bines H and Watson D (1992) *Developing Professional Education.* Open University Press, Milton Keynes.

73 Boud D and Walker D (1993) Barriers to reflection on experience. In: Boud D, Cohen R and Walker D (eds) *Using Experience for Learning*, pp. 73–86. Open University Press, Milton Keynes.

74 Kolb D and Fry R (1975) Towards an applied theory of experiential learning. In: Cooper C (ed.) *Theories of Group Practices.* John Wiley and Sons, London.

75 Jarvis P (1987) *Adult Learning in the Social Context.* Croom Helm, London.

76 Sparks-Langer G and Colton A (1991) Synthesis of research on teachers' reflective learning. *Educational Leadership.* **48**: 37–44.

77 Ross D (1990) Programmatic structures for the preparation of reflective teachers. In: Clift R, Houston W and Pugach M (eds) *Encouraging Reflective Practice in Education.* Teachers College Press, New York.

78 Lave J and Wenger E (1991) *Situated Learning: legitimate peripheral participation.* Cambridge University Press, Cambridge.

79 Hanks W (1991) Foreword. In: Lave J and Wenger E. *Situated Learning: legitimate peripheral participation*, pp. 13–24. Cambridge University Press, Cambridge.

80 Wenzel L, Briggs K and Puryear B (1998) Portfolio: authentic assessment in the age of the curriculum revolution. *Journal of Nursing Education.* **37**: 208–12.

81 Eraut M (1994) *Developing Professional Knowledge and Competence.* Falmer Press, London.

82 Coles C (2000) *Credentialing through the Natural Processes of Continuing Professional Development: what more do we need?* American Board of Medical Specialties, Chicago.

83 Fish D (1991) But can you prove it? Quality assurance and the reflective practitioner. *Assessment and Evaluation in Higher Education.* **16**: 22–36.

84 Passmore J (1989) *The Philosophy of Teaching.* Duckworth Press, London.

85 Simosko S (1991) *APL: a practical guide for professionals.* Kogan-Page, London.

86 Woodward H (1998) Reflective journals and portfolios: learning through assessment. *Assessment and Evaluation in Higher Education.* **23**: 415–23.

87 Solomon P (1992) Learning contracts in clinical education: evaluation by clinical supervisors. *Medical Teacher.* **14**: 205–10.

88 Martenson D and Schwab P (1993) Learning through mutual commitment: broadening the concept of learning contracts. *Medical Teacher.* **15**: 11–15.

89 Pitts J, Coles C and Thomas P (2001) Enhancing reliability in portfolio assessment: shaping the portfolio. *Medical Teacher.* **23**: 351–6.

90 Pitts J, Coles C, Thomas P and Smith F (2002) Enhancing reliability in portfolio assessment: discussion between assessors. *Medical Teacher.* **24**: 197–201.

Further Reading

Ben-David M, Davis M, Harden R, Howie P, Ker J and Pippard M (2001) AMEE guide no. 24: portfolios as a method of student assessment. *Medical Teacher.* **23**: 535–51.

Challis M (1999) AMEE guide no. 11: portfolio-based learning and assessment in medical education. *Medical Teacher.* **22**: 370–86.

Klenowski V (2002) *Developing Portfolios for Learning and Assessment. Processes and Principles.* RoutledgeFalmer, London.

Supervision, mentoring and coaching

John Launer

KEY MESSAGES

- Supervision and one-to-one support occurs throughout medical education and the medical career cycle. It often forms the most important part of professional learning and acts as the foundation of reflective practice. It may play an essential part in motivating and retaining practitioners, and in preventing stress and burnout.

- One-to-one supervision can take a variety of forms and names, including clinical supervision, educational supervision, mentoring and coaching. The boundaries between these activities are often unclear. Terminology can be confusing, but definitions are probably less important than understanding what is going on and why.

- All one-to-one supervision contains an element of professional development and an element of performance monitoring or standard setting. These elements may be present either implicitly or explicitly. The emphasis on one or the other will vary greatly, depending on the circumstances.

- There are three principal types of focus for supervision: clinical cases, the wider contexts of these cases (e.g. professional networks) and career choices. Sometimes the focus will move around between these.

- One-to-one supervision can occur formally or informally; on an obligatory basis or a voluntary one; and in a hierarchical relationship or between peers. It can take place as part of management, training, remediation or routine professional work.

- Whatever its form or context, good supervision depends on identical skills. These include affirmation, emotional attunement, awareness of external requirements and standards, and ability to question and challenge people appropriately.

- Skills for supervision can be taught and learned. These include the use of questions designed to help learners extend their understanding without raising excessive anxiety.

Introduction

Traditionally, medicine has been an area where the emphasis has been on didactic training rather than facilitated learning. The reasons for this are fairly obvious. Doctors need to acquire, and to keep acquiring, tremendous amounts of factual knowledge and practical skills. In social terms, medicine has had a hierarchical internal structure, alongside a high external status. As a reflection of this, the chief mode of medical school teaching has traditionally been the ward round: a male consultant in a suit addressing and interrogating a group of medical students in short white coats, in the presence of a silent and supine patient.

In spite of this, most doctors can probably remember one-to-one encounters and relationships from every stage of their undergraduate and postgraduate careers that helped or influenced them. Such supervision, coaching or mentorship – although never formally named as such – may have been the most important part of their learning. For those who have always provided it, particularly junior hospital doctors in the case of teaching medical students, it may have been one of the most gratifying parts of their work.

Approaches to teaching and learning in medical careers are now undergoing a transformation in many places. This is bringing one-to-one activities such as supervision and mentoring to the fore in two ways. First, the kinds of encounter that are taking place within medicine and medical education are often different from how they might have been in the past. They are likely to be more informal and dialogical in style, and perhaps more tentative as well. They may also go beyond informational input, and involve discursive and wide-ranging consideration of cases and work issues. They are therefore coming closer to the notion of 'bringing forth' understanding. Second, the structures within which such one-to-one support takes place are likely to be less 'ad hoc' and more organised or rigorous. Thus, in an increasing number of settings, one-to-one support is being placed at the centre of professional learning. In the UK, for example, these now include

- tutorials for trainee general practitioners (GPs)(1)
- training for foundation year doctors and speciality training grades(2,3)
- appraisal of doctors(4)

Understanding Medical Education: Evidence, Theory and Practice. Edited by T Swanwick. © 2010 Association for the Study of Medical Education.

- mentoring for hospital consultants or GPs(5)
- executive coaching for senior doctors(6)
- remedial work done under the aegis of departments of postgraduate medical education (known as deaneries in the UK).(7)

The factors that have led to such changes are many, but the following are probably the most significant:

- Education in many professional fields has undergone widespread change, with an emphasis on adult learning as opposed to traditional pedagogy, and on reflective practice rather than on the acquisition of facts.(8–10)
- Social developments have made both patients and learners less deferent in many societies and therefore less likely to accept authoritative or directive instruction without question or challenge; 'patient-centred' and 'learner-centred' styles are becoming the norm.(11)
- Doctors now work more closely with other professionals such as nurses, social workers, psychologists and psychotherapists, who have all established one-to-one supervision as the mainstay of their basic training and continuing professional development.(12–16)
- There is an increasing need for lifelong learning in medicine, and this has led to some loss of the boundary between initial training and continuous professional development, including work-based learning.(17–19)
- Many doctors have a greater awareness of medical ethics and new areas of exploration, such as complexity,(20) social constructionism,(21) whole systems approaches(22) and narrative.(23) They are therefore aware that any clinical case may be amenable to multiple interpretations and possible solutions.
- Political influences in many countries have put quality, performance, clinical governance and patient-centred care permanently on the medical agenda, and these in turn have all required doctors to be more open about their failings and uncertainties, and more amenable to discussion of their competencies.(24)

Although there is still far less of a tradition of organised, regular, one-to-one pedagogy within medicine than in some other professions, the situation is changing rapidly. It is now possible that one-to-one support may become the mainstay of basic training and lifelong learning in the medical profession, although much still needs to be done for this to happen.

What Does Supervision Mean?

There are many definitions of one-to-one learning activities such as supervision, mentoring and coaching. Different authors take different approaches, largely according to their own professional backgrounds, experience and agendas. Some use the terms supervision and clinical supervision interchangeably. Others introduce phrases or hybrid terms of their own such as 'learning support'(25) or 'coach-mentoring'.(26) It is easy to get bogged down in semantics and lose sight of the important principles. This section attempts to cut through the jargon and focus on what matters in one-to-one support.

The origin of the term 'supervision' is from professions outside medicine. It has been used for many years in the mental health world and nursing to mean regular, structured, extended encounters aimed at reflecting on casework.(27) Over time, people in these professions and more widely have come to take a far wider view of its meaning, suggesting that it should cover any encounter that provides support in a clinical context, whether this is formal or informal, hierarchical or non-hierarchical, and part of a training programme or outside one. Butterworth, for example, offers this very inclusive definition from a nursing perspective: 'an exchange between professionals to enable the development of professional skills'.(28) Burton and Launer, looking at primary care, define it as 'facilitated learning in relation to live practical issues'.(29) Clark *et al.* have suggested that supervision should be considered an umbrella term, covering all one-to-one professional encounters and thus including mentoring and coaching, as well as activities that include an element of management, training, assessment or remediation.(30)

In this paper, the term 'supervision' is used in this wider sense to cover all one-to-one encounters aimed at promoting competence and reflective practice, including mentoring and coaching. Box 8.1 outlines

---

BOX 8.1 Should doctors use the word supervision?

Within medicine, people often cannot hear the words 'clinical supervision' or 'supervision' without feeling it involves mainly instruction. Many doctors say they would sometimes prefer an alternative term: 'case discussion', 'clinical case analysis' and so on. In spite of this, there are good reasons to promote both the word and the concept of supervision in the wide sense that is now understood in other fields. This usage connects doctors with the richness of thinking about supervision that has gone on in these fields, especially in nursing and the mental health professions. It also enables people to identify the many encounters in medicine that have an element of supervision in them, although they may not be named as such. Over time, this may help to promote an enhanced culture of supervision within medicine, not just within training, but throughout professional life.

Supervision can focus on either development or performance or both, depending on the context and the agreed relationship between supervisor and supervisee. Some supervision is entirely about development (e.g. mentoring); in other cases it is entirely about performance (e.g. remedial supervision). In most cases the circles overlap to a greater or lesser extent.

Figure 8.1 The two faces of supervision.

the argument in favour of doctors adopting the term in this way, to cover the entire range of one-to-one encounters.

One cause for controversy is whether supervision is principally about professional development or about monitoring and standard setting. This may arise from the inherent ambiguity in the English word 'supervision' itself; some people automatically assume it to mean 'looking after someone', while others understand it to mean 'looking over someone's shoulder'. As the word is used in both senses, both colloquially and within education, it is probably best to acknowledge that the word can carry either meaning, or both, depending on the speaker and the context. Again, that is the approach adopted in this paper.

In practical terms, it may be useful to think of supervision in terms of two overlapping circles labelled 'development' and 'performance' (*see* Figure 8.1). On some occasions, the focus will be entirely on personal and professional development. The supervisor will be more or less able to take performance standards for granted. This occurs, for example, where a doctor is helping an experienced and proficient colleague to think through a highly complex case and consider a range of different management options. On other occasions, supervision has to move almost entirely towards directive teaching. This may happen, for example, when a supervisee presents a case for discussion but exposes a huge ignorance of basic knowledge in doing so.

In both these extremes, however, it is clear that supervision will always pay attention to both development and performance to some extent. Even when two experienced peers are discussing a case, both colleagues will assume certain norms that define the options that are worth considering – even if the norms remain unspoken during the supervision itself. Similarly, the supervisor who pulls up a poor trainee on the facts is still working within a framework of development and aiming at an eventual relationship where standards can be assumed.

What Is Supervision For?

It is generally helpful to make a distinction between supervision and related activities on the one hand, and straightforward didactic training on the other. (The particular case of educational supervision, which can lie somewhere between the two, is discussed below.) While training addresses the high ground of facts, figures, rules and guidelines, supervision in all its forms addresses the 'swampy lowlands' of everyday practice(9): the uncomfortable, inconvenient realities that professionals face all the time. They are realities for which the textbook never quite seems to have the answer, and which never exactly correspond to any case that the practitioner has seen before. For students, such cases may initially seem rare. As professionals advance in their careers, they may become more frequent rather than less; curiosity and courage have increased with experience; and problems that were previously disguised or withheld appear.

There is an inseparable connection between supervision and reflective practice. One way of looking at this is to regard supervision as an intelligent conversation with a colleague about a case or issue, and reflective practice as an intelligent conversation with oneself.(31) Supervision nurtures reflective practice, while reflective practice in turn leads to a thirst for supervision in all its forms. The same can be said in connection with team discussion, which may or may not be present in the workplace as a regular activity and as an attitude of mind.

Not surprisingly, the same transferable skills operate in relation to consultations with patients, good supervision with colleagues and effective team discussion. These include careful listening, the formation of credible hypotheses, and the construction of helpful and challenging questions. All these skills enhance critical thinking and, as such, generate a vision in the workplace that is 'open and malleable, not closed and fixed'.(8)

The relationship between reflective practice, supervision, team discussion and the learning work place is symbolised in Figure 8.2.

One useful set of concepts to help understand the different purposes of supervision is the one provided by Proctor.(32) She regards supervision as having three aspects: 'normative', 'formative' and 'restorative'. The normative aspect is what links supervision to the 'world out there', where there are standards to meet and rules to be followed. The formative aspect is what helps supervisees to develop. The restorative aspect is what sustains colleagues in their jobs. Each of these aspects may come to the fore or remain in the background, according to the context and the circumstances.

Looking specifically at formal professional supervision, Morton-Cooper and Palmer list its purposes as follows:(25)

Figure 8.2 The learning organisation.

- as a defence against feelings of disorientation, disillusionment and burnout.
- as a framework for clarifying human values.
- as a way of recovering meaning in our social relationships.
- as a means of providing skill rehearsal and access to appropriate role models in the workplace (both personally and collegially).
- as a device for evaluating and disseminating best practice in healthcare.
- as a way of acquiring 'emotional literacy to deal constructively with our emotions in a mutually beneficial way'.

Although supervision is generally understood as a very different concept from clinical governance, there is an argument for regarding supervision as an important means of putting governance into action. While guidelines, protocols, audits and other tools may provide an external framework for acceptable practice, supervision can be thought of as a collective activity through which professionals refine and develop their own personal practice. In other words, it is a regulatory activity, but one of continual mutual regulation.

One aspect of supervision that is vital but often understated is that of imagination. As with research supervision in an academic context, supervision in a clinical setting can at times (and in some hands) be a very dull affair, but it also has the potential to inspire people to perform at their best, and to go to places clinically and professionally that they may never have been able to reach otherwise.

Box 8.2 covers the issue of evidence and evaluation in relation to supervision, mentoring and coaching.

Cases, Contexts, Careers: the Three Domains Covered by Supervision

Cases

Most supervision takes place mainly in order to address cases, namely the everyday work that profes-

BOX 8.2 Where's the evidence: Is supervision effective?

In terms of effectiveness, there are several studies from professions such as nursing showing that recipients place a high value on supervision, mentoring and coaching for what they bring about in terms of general well-being, knowledge, confidence, morale, understanding, self-awareness, job satisfaction and professional endurance.(33–37) There are also studies showing benefits to those who offer mentoring to their organisations.(38) However, there are few, if any, studies showing a direct relationship between the presence of supervision, or its quality, and its effects on patient satisfaction or patient outcome. There are a number of reasons for this, including the difficulty of assessing the clinical efficacy of any complex educational intervention with may variables involved.(39) There is clearly a need to develop methodologies that will allow researchers to establish what difference it makes to patients for clinicians to have regular supervision or other forms of one-to-one support, and which approaches to supervision seem to make the most difference.(40) In this connection, some writers have questioned the assumption that supervision automatically enhances good practice, and they have suggested that it can also sometimes lead to collusion and complacency.(5,41) It can also be limited by poor supervision skills, bad matching, intrusive management or other obstacles.

sionals undertake. These cases may be approached from the point of view of straightforward technical case management, for example, what is good practice or best practice. Far more commonly, however, cases needing supervision raise issues far broader than this. For example,

- when there is no one easy answer
- ethical issues
- complex comorbidity
- when it is unclear when to stop investigations or treatment
- 'grey area' cases, for example, somatisation, frequent attenders, chronic fatigue, irritable bowel
- complaints, distressed families, angry patients, unlikeable patients.

In all cases like these, discussion of the technical or pragmatic options that may be available is inseparable from what has been called 'emotional work', that is, the processing of difficult emotions attached to the case. This may involve a simple discharge of negative feelings, or it may require something more complex and skilled, depending on the capacities of both supervisor and supervisee: a careful analysis of why particular feelings have arisen and what information this provides in respect of the dynamics of the case and the doctor–patient relationship.

Contexts

Most supervision in medicine relates to the content of cases only, because the working context is itself quite unproblematic. However, sometimes this is not the case. Even at the best of times, careful case management can depend on trying to achieve coherence among the professionals rather than simply trying to identify the right treatment for the patient. In reality, a great deal of discussion of context arises naturally in supervision. In postgraduate medical education, it is rare to have an intelligent discussion about any case without at some point having to consider how the professional network is functioning, and whether it is supporting or hindering practitioners in their work. Similarly, formal or informal case discussions among experienced hospital doctors will regularly address issues such as professional or inter-professional rivalries and problems concerning communication, money, politics or power. In addition, much supervision addresses difficulties in relation to roles and boundaries, for example, the extent and limits of what patients can legitimately expect from clinicians and what colleagues or team members can legitimately expect from each other.

Careers

While specific discussions aimed at clarifying the client's career goals and choices do sometimes take place, it is probably much more common for these to be addressed incidentally in the course of discussions about cases or network issues. For example, a clinical case may well bring certain learning needs to light and raise issues about whether the client should undertake further training to improve their level of skill. Similarly, supervision in relation to a difficulty in the workplace may lead to the question 'Is this any longer the right workplace for the supervisee?' The case of professional appraisal is interesting in this respect. Although it is not often considered a form of supervision or mentoring, professional appraisal does offer similar opportunities by creating a space where clients can reflect on their competencies, learning needs and future aspirations.(42) However, there are clearly conflicts when appraisal is linked with professional revalidation or re-accreditation and some have argued that supervision and mentoring cannot be combined with anything that has regulatory implications.(43) Figure 8.3 highlights the inter-relationship of these three supervisory 'domains'.

Types of Supervision

This section describes some of the commonest types of supervision, with examples of each type. The typology used here is adapted from Clark *et al.*(30)

Informal supervision

Informal supervision takes the form of opportunistic exchanges that are generally short and arise spontane-

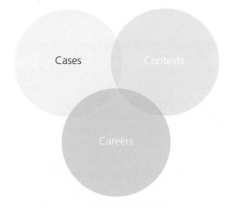

Figure 8.3 The three domains of supervision.

ously in the context of everyday work. Typical examples are chats over coffee, in the corridor or in the operating theatre changing room. There is often a risk that informal supervision will merely take the form of swapping anecdotes or will reinforce banal or stereotypical practice. However, colleagues who work well together and respect each other may be able to provide excellent and challenging supervision even in brief moments snatched from the hurly-burly of everyday work. In many circumstances, such supervision 'on the hoof' provides the mainstay of much postgraduate learning and support, whether or not this is explicitly noticed or acknowledged. While formal supervision is usually given by someone more experienced, informal supervision can come from all sorts of people, including juniors, spouses, clerical staff and even hairdressers. Sometimes the most imaginative supervision that doctors ever receive comes spontaneously and unexpectedly from people outside the medical profession.(29) Some have argued that other personal experiences, including reading novels and poetry, seeing films and operas, or walks in the countryside, are among opportunities for 'self-supervision', since they may provide the conditions for processing the thoughts and emotions that arise from everyday work (*see* Box 8.3).

Clinical supervision

Clinical supervision is the commonest form of supervision in most medical settings. It consists of the day-to-day discussion of clinical cases and their management, and any issues arising from this. It may take a variety of forms from very brief discussions on ward rounds or in clinics, to more extended and reflective discussions of complex cases or options for clinical management. In a training context, clinical supervision may overlap with didactic training, particularly where case discussions reveal gaps in knowledge or skills. Even here, however, a conversational approach based on questioning is often more effective than giving advice since this will help to establish the supervisee's

Dr K was working late one evening in her family practice when a new patient arrived without an advance appointment. The patient had a complicated and long-standing problem of back pain. He demanded a full clinical assessment and immediate referral to an orthopaedic surgeon. Dr K felt pressurised. She responded by telling the patient very firmly about the appointment system in the practice and by insisting that he must return for a booked appointment with full details of all his previous tests and medication. Later, before locking up her office, Dr K talked to her receptionist and expressed her frustration at patients like this, and how she hated having to behave 'like a police officer'. The receptionist remarked that Dr K would probably have handled the patient more carefully if he had come in the morning when she was less tired. The comment led Dr K to realise that she had probably been too harsh with the man, who may have been pressurising her because his pain was so bad. She also felt she should have carried out at least a basic examination to rule out any serious pathology.

existing ideas and promote independent thinking. It will also ensure that any advice that is needed is pitched at the right level.

Doctors do not generally use the term 'clinical supervision' for case discussions taking place beyond the training years. Nevertheless, much clinical supervision does take place between peers or within teams, although it may not necessarily be labelled as such. Typical forms of this include case review meetings, primary care team meetings and phone calls to colleagues to seek expert advice or an independent view of a problem. Many established doctors, particularly those working in isolation, express a wish for more regular or systematic opportunities to discuss cases than their work patterns may allow.

Educational supervision

Educational supervision is regular supervision taking place in the context of a recognised training in order to establish learning needs and review progress. It is most common in the pre-registration years, and also between registration and gaining certification in a specialty. Arguably, this is the most complex and challenging form of supervision since the educational supervisor has to fulfil many overlapping and (in some situations) conflicting roles. As well as facilitating learning, the supervisor has a responsibility to assess the supervisee's performance while the supervision is taking place, or by formal means at a later date.

In the UK, the concept and practice of educational supervision has come to the fore with the introduction of 'Modernising Medical Careers'.(44) This involves a national curriculum for all doctors in training grades. Educational supervisors play a key role in this. Their tasks include

- setting learning objectives
- establishing a learning contract
- assisting the supervisee in maintaining a learning portfolio
- coordinating the supervisee's educational experience and graded exposure to casework
- offering opportunities for case-based discussion
- offering career guidance
- undertaking appraisal
- carrying out assessment
- producing reports.

Educational supervisors are also more likely to have to offer pastoral care at times, particularly for students and trainees who are going through crises in their personal lives or careers.

An educational supervisor may or may not take on the task of day-to-day clinical supervision. In general practice, for example, it is highly likely that one and the same person will do both jobs. On a programme of hospital training, by contrast, it may be preferable to have a single skilled and trained educator assigned to a trainee as an educational supervisor for the duration of the programme, while the day-to-day clinical supervision is carried out by clinicians working with the trainee at any given time. This is especially the case when trainees rotate through a number of different specialties and where an educational supervisor could not possibly have the skills to offer case-based discussion across the whole range of work. When this kind of arrangement is in place, it is essential to have close coordination between all the people involved, to prevent people working at cross-purposes or giving conflicting messages to the trainee. It also makes sense to link the approval of training placements to the quality of the supervision arrangements on offer.(45) This is particularly important because research has shown that the quality of the supervisory relationship is the key to effective supervision in medical settings.(46)

In all educational supervision, there is a tension between assessment and supervision. Trainees may feel that their performance is being judged covertly under the guise of a supportive discussion or that their qualifications and careers may depend on what they say in apparently innocent discussions. Equally, it is hard for educators to stop themselves from being influenced by how trainees present themselves in the course of day-to-day exchanges about casework. Because of this, it is important to remain aware of the two different contexts and be willing to address this difference transparently. When real concerns arise about a trainee's competence, it is fairer and more effective to say so, to set explicit targets, with a clear timetable and (if necessary) an explanation of possible sanctions (*see* Box 8.4).

Dr K is the educational supervisor for Alan T, a doctor who qualified 18 months ago. As a paediatrician, Dr K is also the clinical supervisor while Alan is working on the children's ward. Over the past few weeks, there have been several children on the ward who are possible victims of physical abuse by their parents. Dr K has been concerned about Alan's apparently simplistic and judgemental attitude towards the problem: he seems to believe that the only desirable solution in every case is adoption outside the family. Dr K arranges for Alan to spend some time with the child and the family mental health team, seeing them do therapeutic work with parents who have abused their children but have also (in many cases) themselves been victims of abuse in the past. He also fixes up for Alan to attend a case conference, in which some of the complexities of a particular case are examined. He uses their regular education supervision sessions to review what Alan has learnt and to discuss how he might record this in a reflective piece of writing for his learning portfolio.

Dr L has had a considerable number of complaints from patients. His local health board has referred him to an agency that specialises in assessing and helping doctors whose performance is causing concern. The agency has carried out an occupational psychology assessment, some tests of Dr L's knowledge and skills, and a review of selected case notes. On the basis of this, they have found that Dr L has particular difficulty managing 'grey area' cases that involve vague somatic symptoms with low-grade depression. He tends to dismiss such patients, putting them on antidepressants straight away without first doing adequate investigations. The agency has now assigned Dr L a remedial supervisor who has sat in on some of his surgeries and reviewed some video records of his consultations. The supervisor has now held a series of meetings with Dr L to go through some cases systematically and challenge him on his approach and attitude, in order to help him attain an acceptable level of practice.

Remedial supervision

Remedial supervision is a form of supervision that takes place when a regulatory agency has formally determined that there are concerns about someone's performance. This can only happen if the agency has the authority to assess performance and prescribe the supervision as a proposed remedy.

Remedial supervision takes place within a framework of assessments and reports. Essentially, remedial supervision is a type of educational supervision where the context is one of prescribed retraining rather than basic training undertaken on a voluntary basis (*see* Box 8.5).

Professional supervision

Professional supervision consists of regular, extended one-to-one meetings between established practitioners, mainly to discuss specific cases. It is particularly common in professions such as counselling and psychotherapy, where it is generally a requirement of continuing professional practice. Such supervision is often devoted to reflection on the emotions provoked by these cases, and on the information that these emotions represent.(47) In the context of medicine (with the exception of psychiatry and a small number of GPs) such supervision is uncommon. Professional supervision is usually, although not always, delivered by experienced members of the same profession. However, it is reasonably common for senior mental health professionals such as psychologists to offer supervision to members of other professions, including doctors and nurses. Depending on the cases being discussed, and their context, the supervisor's lack of

Dr J, a psychiatrist, goes to an experienced psychotherapist colleague once a month to discuss cases that are causing him concern. His last supervision session was taken up with an account of a patient he is seeing regularly, who has made several suicide attempts. This session was spent examining Dr J's feelings of helplessness in relation to his patient's behaviour, and also his sense of personal responsibility for her. His supervisor helped him to understand how he was picking up the patient's own feelings of helplessness, and touched gently on memories of a family member who had committed suicide some years previously in spite of psychological help. They also looked at how Dr J could help the patient understand that others did feel responsible for her and care for her, in spite of her fixed belief that nobody ever did.

specific technical knowledge may or may not matter (*see* Box 8.6).

Managerial supervision

Managerial supervision is supervision carried out by someone with direct management responsibility for the supervisee. This may or may not take place within an educational framework (e.g. nurse training) and may or may not involve explicit assessment. In some of the non-medical literature, anything involving clinical line management or direct accountability in employment terms is explicitly disqualified as a form of supervision. Within medicine, this is probably unrealistic. It probably makes sense to regard managerial

BOX 8.7 Managerial supervision: an example

Ms B, a community nurse, was seeing a woman who caused her concern because of how depressed she seemed. The woman came from Thailand, had been married only a year and had just had twins. She seemed cowed by her European husband, who clearly expected her to keep the house immaculate in spite of having two new babies. Ms B had never come across a family situation like this and she felt insufficiently trained to know what to do. She took the case to her regular meeting with her nurse manager. The manager spent nearly an hour with her exploring all the different issues in the case. These included the risk of serious puerperal depression, the demands of twins, the cultural and age differences between the parents, homesickness and isolation, and the difference in perception between the nurse and the husband. Through the meeting with her manager, Ms B came to realise that she could make things worse by trying to 'rescue' the woman from her husband and that she needed to build up his trust instead. She also came away from the discussion with a range of options in her mind. These included a joint visit with the doctor, putting the mother in touch with the local twins' club and exploring to see if there were any other Thai mothers in the locality who might be willing to make contact with the woman.

BOX 8.8 Mentoring: an example

Since attaining her first hospital consultant post three years ago, Dr M has had meetings every few months with an experienced doctor she met when she was in training. She has used these meetings to discuss the inevitable difficulties she has had in adjusting to life not just as a newly qualified radiologist, but also as a team leader, a manager and (most recently) a new mother. Over the past two or three mentoring sessions, the same theme has come up repeatedly: the feeling that her male consultant colleagues are paternalistic and sexist. At her most recent session her mentor simply asked her, 'Are you really just asking my permission to get out?' Dr M felt enormous relief at being asked the question. She realised that she did indeed want to move on, but had feared her mentor would be critical of her for leaving her first senior post so soon.

BOX 8.9 Coaching: an example

Dr T, a gastroenterologist, was recently promoted from medical director of his hospital to chief executive. As a result, he has decided to give up most of his clinical work except for a small private endoscopy practice, and to concentrate on his management role. He is paying to see a coach from a private consultancy organisation to help him develop his new professional identity. Quite a few of his fortnightly coaching sessions have been spent examining how he can keep his trusting relationships with his medical colleagues at the hospital (some of whom have been his friends for many years) while also behaving equitably and responsibly in relation to all the other staff groups at the hospital, including nurses, technicians, non-clinical staff and manual workers.

supervision as an inevitability in some circumstances (*see* Box 8.7).

Mentoring

Mentoring is usually understood as guidance and support offered by a more experienced colleague,(48–50) although there are also descriptions of peer mentoring or co-mentoring.(51) Mentoring may be either informal or formal. Where it is informal, it may have arisen naturally between colleagues and may not even be described as mentoring except in retrospect. Where offered as part of a formal scheme, mentoring is often wide ranging, covering not just clinical work but professional relationships and career plans as well. Although it should not be confused with counselling, life-cycle issues such as family events will quite often come into the picture. It is often an entirely private encounter, with total confidentiality given and expected on both sides. Virtually all the literature concerning mentoring includes the assumption, implicitly or explicitly, that the arrangement is both voluntary and confidential, although agencies funding mentors may want to know in general terms that their clients are finding it useful (*see* Box 8.8).

Coaching

Coaching is a form of supervision that has been defined as 'unlocking a person's potential to maximise their own performance'.(52) The coaching relationship, like mentoring, is a voluntary and confidential one. Unlike mentoring, however, there may be a focus on a limited number of tasks or just one important task, for example, leadership. A useful analogy here is with sports coaching, where the client already has an advanced degree of proficiency and the coach, who may or may not be an exponent of the sport, helps the client to work towards further excellence. However, even the word 'coaching' can be somewhat confusing since it is also used colloquially when someone needs extra help (e.g. 'she needs specific coaching in how to talk to patients'). Recently, the term has come more into vogue within medicine, either within the context of 'life coaching'(53) to help people achieve personal and career fulfilment, or in a more general sense to describe any one-to-one learning relationship that does not involve management or assessment. It is too early to say whether this terminology will catch on in preference to the term 'supervision' as used in a broad sense here (*see* Box 8.9).

The types of supervision listed here are not exhaustive or mutually exclusive. Among the huge variety of learning encounters that occur in medicine, there will be many that only loosely fit any of the categories described here, while other encounters may include aspects of several types of supervision, or shift between them from moment to moment. Clark *et al.* have suggested that it is less important to achieve consensus on terms than to ask the following questions in relation to any supervision activity.(30)

- Who is asking for this to be done?
- What do they want, and why?
- Do they know what the supervisor does and does not offer?
- Will the client be attending voluntarily?
- Is anyone expecting specific outcomes, should they be and, if so, what?
- Who is paying whom, and do all the parties know this?
- Who is reporting to whom, about what, exactly when, and do all the parties know this?
- Is everyone agreed on the terms being used, and on their meaning?

Similarly, Proctor has proposed that 'What the role relationship is called is probably unimportant in practice … The roles, responsibilities and rights need to be identified from the beginning, and to be discussed, made real and reviewed.'(54)

Conceptual Frameworks for Supervision

There is no single conceptual framework that is universally recognised within the world of supervision and mentorship. Different writers use – or assume – frameworks that draw on various fields, including psychoanalysis,(55–57) systemic psychotherapy,(58–60) Rogerian counselling,(61) neuro-linguistic programming(62) and learning theory, with a particular emphasis on authorities such as Schon(10) and Kolb.(63) Some explicitly address learning styles or personality types.(64,65) Many writers have adapted the work of educational theorists in order to construct models that fit the professional context of supervision. One useful model based on learning theory comes from Proctor,(32) drawing on Wackman *et al.*(66) This suggests that learners move continually through a cycle from 'unconscious incompetence' through 'conscious incompetence' to 'conscious competence' and finally 'unconscious competence'. In other words, supervision invites people to consider how they may be avoiding more adventurous areas of practice, and to explore these – at first tentatively, then as a matter of course – until they are ready to extend themselves even further (*see* Figure 8.4).

Certain themes arise again and again in the supervision literature, suggesting that there is a consensus

Figure 8.4 The supervision cycle.

around particular ideas that cross theoretical boundaries. These themes include the following:

- Supervision should be about enabling, empowerment and sustaining human values.
- Supervisors may need at different times to take on a variety of roles, including guide, advisor, role model, sponsor, teacher and facilitator.
- Supervision needs to pay attention to the personal, professional and relational aspects of the work.
- Supervisors always have to bear in mind three separate 'clients': the supervisee, the patient and the organisation or agency.
- Supervision needs to address the complexity and uniqueness of the problems brought, in order to generate solutions or options that are the best fit.
- Supervision is an interactional process. To be effective, it depends on emotional attunement, mutual trust and usually an evolving relationship between supervisor and supervisee.

In keeping with the modern emphasis on narratives and their importance, a number of writers have suggested that supervision is inherently a narrative-making activity.(67,68) The role of the supervisor is therefore to elicit an existing narrative of 'the problem' as it is currently understood, and to question the supervisee in such a way that a new understanding emerges, in the form of a different narrative in which 'the problem' is either lessened or has dissolved. One advantage of using this approach in a medical context is that it places less emphasis on eliciting emotion and more on 'bringing forth new stories'. Many doctors without specific training in psychotherapy or counselling find it more comfortable and more appropriate to take such a narrative-based approach, rather than adopting a technique that is centred on the direct examination of emotions or on learning theory. In addition, a narrative-based technique allows the technical and factual content of cases to be integrated into the evolving story that the supervisee brings (*see* Box 8.10).

BOX 8.10 Focus on: Narrative-based supervision

In the context of training GPs to carry out effective supervision, I have developed a simple theoretical framework for a narrative-based approach, summarised as 'the seven Cs'.(23)

1 *Conversation.* Wherever possible, supervision should aim to resolve problems through the conversation itself rather then through giving advice.

2 *Curiosity.* The best stance for the supervisor is one of curiosity: establishing what the supervisees already know and what options they have already thought of, or want to explore further.

3 *Contexts.* It is often more important to discover the contexts for a problem rather than focusing on the content. These contexts include the patient's and the supervisee's beliefs, values and preference, and the needs and pressures of the organisation.

4 *Complexity.* Most problems brought to supervision are inherently complex, involving many levels of difficulty or intersecting difficulties. Supervision mainly offers opportunities for supervisees to enrich their understanding of what is going on, in order to find a way forward. It rarely helps by finding a 'quick fix'.

5 *Creativity.* Supervision requires imagination and risk taking on both sides.

6 *Caution.* It also requires respect and circumspection: operating within the limits of the supervisee's capacity to tolerate anxiety, while not avoiding the challenge within those limits.

7 *Care.* Most of all, supervision requires attentiveness and positive regard.

BOX 8.11 How to: Do effective supervision(69)

- The supervisor is not considered to be in a position of authority over the supervisee, except where this is clearly required by the context (e.g. in training contexts).
- Wherever possible, the supervisor's role is to help the supervisee reflect and expand the problem they are presenting in a non-judgemental way.
- The supervisor should offer advice only when this is specifically requested by the supervisee.
- The supervisor needs to pay close attention to the words used by the supervisee and to pursue their meaning.
- Wherever possible, the supervisor should ask questions rather than offer interpretations.
- Each question should, wherever possible, be based on the response to the previous question.
- The supervisor should note non-verbal cues and body language and use this to help frame subsequent questions at the right level of challenge.
- The supervisor will necessarily base their questions on their own knowledge and experience but needs to be wary of making assumptions and imposing these on the supervisee, unless this is necessary for medical safety.
- The conversation does not at first set out to explore the supervisee's feelings, although their emotional response may become an important factor to consider.
- The skill of the supervisor often involves working 'on the cusp', offering enough challenge to the supervisee to help in the exploration of new ideas, but not so much that the supervisee becomes excessively defensive or anxious.
- It is not necessarily expected that the conversation will lead directly to any solution, but may simply help shift the dilemma or case narrative in a more helpful way for the supervisee.

A set of operational 'rules' for effective supervision, based on this narrative approach, appears in Box 8.11. The rules are generic: they can be used or adapted for a wide range and variety of supervision encounters, both formal and informal. They can also be used in the context of consultations; indeed, it has been suggested that consultations are really just about providing supervision for the patient. Self-evidently, guidelines such as these cannot be transferred simplistically from the written page to everyday practice. They are the starting points for a spiral learning process that may involve both formal and informal training, as well as sustained reflective practice in conversational skills.

Common Tensions in Supervision

As with any human relationship, supervision and related activities are subject to particular tensions. The ones most commonly experienced by practitioners and cited in the literature are:

- facilitation versus training
- the needs of the client versus the needs of the organisation
- affirmation versus challenge.

This section addresses each of these tensions in turn.

Facilitation versus training

In a technical specialty such as medicine, supervisors may have an overriding wish to bring out the best in their supervisees, and yet at the same time will be aware of the need for a secure basis of knowledge and skills. There are certain facts that any practitioner needs to know. These may be scientific facts that are fairly solid and indisputable (such as how to tell the difference between herpes simplex and shingles), or they may be pragmatic facts because there is a professional of political consensus about them (such as guidelines on smoking cessation). There is little point in trying to 'bring forth' such knowledge where it is absent. On the other hand, there is always the risk that supervisors will be tempted to remain in a didactic, knowledge-imparting mode even when this is unhelpful. For example, teaching about the safe use of antidepressants can easily slide into direct advice about prescribing them in a case where it might be more helpful to widen the discussion into areas such as the patient's social circumstances. Supervisees can put pressure on their supervisors, consciously or unconsciously, to offer a quick fix. Supervisors therefore need to offer clear signposting for areas of professional certainty (e.g. the correct doses of drugs) and areas of considerable uncertainty (e.g. the wider contexts of case management).

The client versus the organisation

In some circumstances the tension between the client's needs and those of the organisation can be almost entirely ignored, for example, in a voluntary arrangement for peer supervision or mentorship undertaken between two experienced and competent colleagues. However, in many circumstances organisational needs, spoken or unspoken, will be present. In one sense, the organisation and regulatory bodies can be a proxy for the needs of the patient, in so far as they exist to ensure acceptable standards of practice. At the same time, there may be situations where the reverse tension exists, for example, where the supervision client believes that they are pursuing the interests of the patient in the face of oppressive restrictions from the agency, including financial or bureaucratic ones. Supervisors and mentors who are employed by the organisation concerned therefore have to manage a fine line between loyalty to the client and loyalty to the organisation. Trust and transparency are needed to negotiate this kind of tension.

Affirmation and challenge

The core tension in any form of supervision is the extent to which the supervisor sets out to support, or challenge the client. Every supervisor or mentor wants their clients to feel good about themselves. Equally, every supervisor wants (or should want) clients to be capable of change and to develop as far as their potential will allow. Much of the skill of supervision depends on a capacity to go just beyond the 'comfort zone'. This involves offering enough challenge to the supervisee to help in the exploration of new ideas and new possibilities, but not so much that the supervisee becomes excessively anxious, defensive or deskilled. It may also involve fine judgement as to whether the context permits some careful exploration of personal issues

that may be impeding professional performance. Like the skill of consulting with patients who may be anxious or fearful, this is not something that can be learned from books or articles. It depends on a gradual, sometimes lifelong, acquisition of the capacity to calibrate every utterance with the exact circumstances and with the wishes and needs of the client.

Raising the Profile of Supervision: Changing the Culture of Medicine

There are no simple prescriptions for promoting a culture change within medicine involving greater emphasis on supervision. Proctor in particular has emphasised the great importance of every profession and discipline discovering its own approach to supervision; while general principles can be transferred from one profession to another, each will also have its own demands, its own established ways of working and its own supervision needs.(32) Readers will no doubt be able to call to mind some imaginative and creative examples of incremental change in this direction within a variety of medical settings and specialties, including medical schools.(70) Such examples will often involve individual doctors taking the initiative to move from traditional forms of learning (such as lectures, conventional ward rounds or team meetings mainly devoted to administrative matters) towards more enlightened and engaging types of learning approach involving one-to-one reflection.

Conclusions

Medical work is not just about scientific facts. It requires practitioners to apply scientific knowledge in the context of individual lives and complex human systems. It crosses many domains of knowledge, including the social and interpersonal. Doctors are exposed constantly to risks, including stress, alienation, over-involvement, automatic behaviour and burnout. Other professions have rightly recognised that they need organised support as professional oxygen in order to sustain reflective practice in the face of such risks. The medical profession has until now been in the paradoxical position of needing as much of this oxygen as any other group of clinicians (if not more) but generally getting less.

To practise reflectively, doctors need emotional and intellectual trust, so that they can reflect frankly on their own work and learn continually without feeling overexposed or under excessive scrutiny. Activities such as supervision, mentoring and coaching provide opportunities for them to examine their own work safely and effectively, based on their everyday professional experience, and in a way that complements other forms of education and training.

Doctors are always pulled in two directions. On the one hand, there is a clear need for concrete facts, explicit guidelines and consistent policies – in other words, for certainty. On the other hand, there is also the need for practitioners to gain in confidence and in wisdom, and to be able to grapple with the complex, multidimensional problems that they encounter with an ever-increasing level of understanding, sophistication and adventurousness – in other words, for the management of uncertainty. Supervision, mentoring and coaching have the capacity to ensure that medical practice rises consistently above the uninspired, the routine and the automatic. They are often what is needed in order to transform excellence in theory into excellence in action.

There are compelling reasons why the profile of supervision and related activities in medicine should now be raised greatly. These include the increasing complexity of the work, and of the demands placed on practitioners. They also include the pressures placed on doctors by patients, governments and society, and the need to maintain a medical workforce that is well motivated. The challenge of promoting effective methods of supervision, mentoring and coaching among doctors, and of training a generation of competent supervisors, may be one of the most important and exciting projects now facing medical educators.(71,72)

Acknowledgements

Many colleagues made helpful comments on an earlier draft of this work. I particularly want to thank Dr Jonathan Burton, Dr Julie Draper, Dr Helen Halpern, Dr Gareth Holsgrove, Dr Tim Swanwick and Prof. Frank Smith.

References

1 Gray R (2001) A framework for looking at the trainer/registrar tutorial in general practice. *Education for General Practice.* **12**: 153–62.
2 NHS Modernising Medical Careers (2005) Curriculum for the foundation years in postgraduate education and training. Department of Health, London.
3 NHS Modernising Medical Careers (2008) *A Reference Guide for Postgraduate Speciality Training in the UK: The Gold Guide (2e).* Department of Health, London. (http://www.mmc.nhs.uk/pdf/Gold%20Guide%202008%20-%20FINAL.pdf; accessed 13 February 2009)
4 School of Health and Related Research (ScHARR) Appraisal for GPs (http://www.dh.gov.uk/assetRoot/04/03/47/75/04034775.pdf; accessed 13 February 2009).
5 Garrett-Harris R and Garvey B (2005) *Towards a Framework for Mentoring in the NHS.* Mentoring and Coaching Research Unit, Faculty of Organisation and Management, Sheffield Hallam University, Sheffield.
6 Beecham B, Dammers J and van Zwanenberg T (2004) Leadership coaching for general practitioners. *Education for Primary Care.* **15**: 579–83.
7 Bowden R and Schofield J (2004) Work based learning and poor performance. In: Burton J and Jackson N (eds) *Work Based Learning in Primary Care.* Radcliffe Publishing, Oxford.
8 Brookfield S (1987) *Developing Critical Thinkers: challenging adults to explore alternative ways of thinking and acting.* Open University Press, Milton Keynes.
9 Schon D (1983) *The Reflective Practitioner: how professionals think in action.* Temple Smith, London.
10 Schon D (1987) *Educating the Reflective Practitioner: towards a new design for teaching and learning in the professions.* Basic Books, New York.
11 Stewart M, Brown J, Weston W *et al.* (2004) *Patient-centred Medicine: transforming the clinical method (2e).* Radcliffe Publishing, Oxford.
12 Bishop V (ed.) (1988) *Clinical Supervision in Practice, Some Questions, Answers and Guidelines.* Macmillan, London.
13 Bond M and Holland S (1998) *Skills of Clinical Supervision for Nurses.* Open University Press, Buckingham.
14 Cutcliffe J, Butterworth T and Proctor B (2001) *Fundamental Themes in Clinical Supervision.* Routledge, London.
15 Hawkins P and Shohet R (eds) (1989) *Supervision in the Helping Professions.* Open University Press, Milton Keynes.
16 RCN Institute (2000) *Realising Clinical Effectiveness and Clinical Governance through Clinical Supervision.* Radcliffe Medical Press, Oxford.
17 Boud D and Solomon N (eds) *Work-based Learning: a new higher education.* Open University Press, Buckingham.
18 Department of Health (2001) *Working Together, Learning Together: a framework for lifelong learning.* Department of Health, London.
19 Burton J and Jackson N (eds) (2004) *Work Based Learning in Primary Care.* Radcliffe Publishing, Oxford.
20 Steinberg D (2005) *Complexity in Healthcare and the Language of Consultation.* Radcliffe Publishing, Oxford.
21 Lupton D (1994) *Medicine as Culture: illness, disease and the body in Western societies.* Sage, London.
22 Thomas P (2006) *Integrating Primary Care: leading, managing, facilitating.* Radcliffe Publishing, Oxford.
23 Launer J (2002) *Narrative-based Primary Care: a practical guide.* Radcliffe Medical Press, Oxford.
24 Department of Health (2004) *Modernising Medical Careers: the next steps: the future shape of foundation specialist and general practice training programmes.* Department of Health, London.
25 Morton-Cooper A and Palmer A (eds) (2000) *Mentorship, Preceptorship and Clinical Supervision: a guide to professional support roles in clinical practice (2e).* Blackwell, Oxford.
26 Foster-Turner J (2006) *Coaching and Mentoring in Health and Social Care.* Radcliffe Publishing, Oxford.
27 Scaife J (2001) *Supervision in Mental Health Professions: a practitioner's guide.* Brunner Routledge, Hove.
28 Butterworth T (1992) Clinical supervision as an emerging idea in nursing. In: Butterworth T and Faugier J (eds) *Clinical Supervision and Mentorship in Nursing.* Stanley Thornes, Cheltenham.
29 Burton J and Launer J (eds) (2003) *Supervision and Support in Primary Care.* Radcliffe Medical Press, Oxford.
30 Clark P, Jamieson A, Launer J *et al.* (2006) Intending to be a supervisor, mentor or coach: which, what for and why? *Education for Primary Care.* **17**: 109–16.

31 Launer J (2003) Practice, supervision, consultancy and appraisal: a continuum of learning. *British Journal of General Practice.* **53**: 662–5.

32 Proctor B (2001) Training for the supervision attitude, skills and intention. In: Cutcliffe J, Butterworth T and Proctor B (eds) *Fundamental Themes in Clinical Supervision.* Routledge, London.

33 Begat I, Severinsson E and Berggren I (1997) Implementation of clinical supervision in a medical department: nurses' views of the effects. *Journal of Clinical Nursing.* **6**: 389–94.

34 Butterworth T, Bishop V and Carson J (1996) First steps towards evaluating clinical supervision in nursing and health visiting. I. Theory, policy and practice development: a review. *Journal of Clinical Nursing.* **5**: 127–32.

35 Hallberg I, Hansson U and Axelsson K (1994) Satisfaction with nursing care and work during a year of clinical supervision and individualised care: comparison between two wards for the care of severely demented patients. *Journal of Nursing Management.* **1**: 296–307.

36 Kelly B, Long A and McKenna H (2001) Clinical supervision: personal and professional development or the nursing novelty of the 1990s? In: Cutcliffe J, Butterworth T and Proctor B (eds) *Fundamental Themes in Clinical Supervision.* Routledge, London.

37 Winstanley J (2001) Developing methods for evaluating clinical supervision. In: Cutcliffe J, Butterworth T and Proctor B (eds) *Fundamental Themes in Clinical Supervision.* Routledge, London.

38 Garvey B and Garrett-Harris R (2005) *The Benefits of Mentoring: a literature review.* Sheffield Hallam University, Mentoring and Coaching Research Unit, Sheffield.

39 Feltham C (2000) Counselling supervision: baselines, problems and possibilities. In: Lawton B and Feltham C (eds) *Taking Supervision Forward: enquiries and trends in counselling and psychotherapy.* Sage, London.

40 Kilminster SM and Jolly BC (2000) Effective supervision in clinical practice settings: a literature review. *Medical Education.* **24**: 827–40.

41 Kirkpatrick D (1967) Evaluation of training. In: Craig R and Bittel I (eds) *Training and Development Handbook.* McGraw-Hill, New York.

42 Pringle M (2003) Re-evaluating revalidation and appraisal. *British Journal of General Practice.* **53**: 437–8.

43 Bulstrode C and Hunt V (2000) What is mentoring? *Lancet.* **356**: 178–8.

44 NHS Modernising Medical Careers (2009) Modernising medical careers. Department of Health, London (http://www.mmc.nhs.uk/default.aspx; accessed 13 February 2009).

45 PMETB (2009) *Generic Standards for Training.* PMETB, London (http://www.pmetb.org.uk/index.php?id=gst; accessed 13 February 2009).

46 Cottrell D, Kilminster S, Jolly B and Grant J (2002) What is effective supervision and how does it happen? A critical incident study. *Medical Education.* **36**: 1042–9.

47 Shipton G (ed.) (1997) *Supervision of Psychotherapy and Counselling: making a place to think.* Open University Press, Buckingham.

48 Freeman R (1998) *Mentoring in General Practice.* Butterworth-Heinemann, Oxford.

49 Gupta R and Lingam S (2000) *Mentoring for Doctors and Dentists.* Blackwell, Oxford.

50 Department of Health (2004) *Mentoring for Doctors: signposts to current practice for career grade doctors.* Department of Health, Doctors' Forum, London.

51 Sackin P, Barnett M, Eastaugh A and Paxton P (1997) Peer supported learning. *British Journal of General Practice.* **47**: 67–8.

52 Whitmore J (1996) *Coaching for Performance.* Nicholas Brierley, London.

53 Kersley S (2006) *Prescription for Change: for doctors who want a life (2e).* Radcliffe Publishing, Oxford.

54 Proctor B (2000) Postscript. In: Morton-Cooper A and Palmer A (eds) *Mentorship, Preceptorship and Clinical Supervision: a guide to professional support roles in clinical practice (2e).* Blackwell, Oxford.

55 Casement P (1988) *On Learning from the Patient.* Routledge, London.

56 Obholzer A, Roberts V (eds) (1994) *The Unconscious at Work: individual and organisational stress in the human services.* Routledge, London.

57 Salinsky J and Sackin P (eds) (2000) *What Are You Feeling Doctor? Identifying and avoiding defensive patterns in the consultation.* Radcliffe Medical Press, Oxford.

58 Burnham J (1993) Systemic supervision. The evolution of reflexivity in the context of the supervising relationship. *Human Systems* **4**: 349–81.

59 Todd T and Storm C (eds) (1997) *The Complete Systemic Supervisor: contexts, philosophy and pragmatics.* Allyn and Bacon, London.

60 Campbell B and Mason B (2002) *Perspectives on Supervision.* Karnac, London.

61 Patterson C (1997) Client centred supervision. In: Watkins C (ed.) *Handbook of Psychotherapy Supervision.* John Wiley, New York.

62 Claridge M-T and Lewis T (2005) *Coaching for Effective Learning.* Radcliffe Publishing, Oxford.

63 Kolb D (1984) *Experiential Learning.* Prentice Hall, Englewood Cliffs, NJ.

64 Honey P and Mumford A (1992) *Manual of Learning Styles.* Honey, Maidenhead.

65 Houghton A and Allen J (2005) Understanding personality type: doctor–patient communication. *BMJ Career Focus.* **330**: 36–7.

66 Wackman DB, Miller S and Nunnally EW (1976) *Student Workbook: increasing awareness and communication skills.* Interpersonal Communication Programmes, Minneapolis, MN.

67 Benner P, Tanner C and Chesla C (1986) *Expertise in Nursing Practice – caring, clinical judgment and ethics.* Springer, New York.

68 Launer J (2003) A narrative based approach to primary care supervision. In: Burton J and Launer J (eds) *Supervision and Support in Primary Care.* Radcliffe Medical Press, Oxford.

69 Launer J and Halpern H (2006) Reflective practice in clinical supervision: an approach to promoting clinical supervision amongst general practitioners. *Workbased Learning in Primary Care.* **4**: 629–32.

70 Driessen E, van Tartwijk J, Overeem K *et al.* (2005) Student learning: conditions for successful reflective use of portfolios in undergraduate education. *Medical Education.* **39**: 1230–5.

71 Bennett J, Gardener B and James F (2001) Implementing clinical supervision in an NHS community trust: sharing the vision. In: Cutcliffe J, Butterworth T and Proctor B (eds) *Fundamental Themes in Clinical Supervision.* Routledge, London.

72 Launer J (2004) Training GP educators in clinical supervision. *Workbased Learning in Primary Care.* **2**: 366–9.

Teaching and leading small groups

Peter McCrorie

KEY MESSAGES

- Always consider whether a session can better be run in small groups.
- Plan the session carefully in plenty of time.
- Vary the session plan according to the size of the group and the venue.
- For large groups (≈ 30) run the session in workshop format, by splitting the group into four or five smaller groups.
- Consider which format is most appropriate for the group task.
- Include a range of formats in any one session, recognising that active learning is likely to be more successful than passive learning.

- Consider your own role in the group process; remember that being the group leader is only one of several options.
- Remember the importance of maintaining good group dynamics.
- Deal with issues as and when they arise, bearing in mind that it is often better to let the group address the issues themselves.
- Take care not to overstep boundaries and destroy good working relationships.

Introduction

Two people give a lecture on a medical topic. One is charismatic and inspirational. He holds the audience in his hands – they are on the edge of their seats throughout the lecture. He does not use notes, illustrates his talk with a few well-chosen photos and uses the traditional 'talk and chalk' approach. He regularly wins the 'best lecturer' prize.

Contrast this with the second lecturer – a very dry and serious speaker, who has carefully prepared every word he intends to use, uses a myriad of PowerPoint slides, each laden with detailed information, and who whips each slide away before his audience has had a chance to get down the half of what he says.

Now imagine that each sets an examination question based on his lecture. Which question do you think the students would perform better in?

In fact, they would get higher marks in the second, less charismatic, lecturer's question. Why? Because in order to make any sense of his lecture, the students would have made a beeline for their textbooks and this self-directed learning would have enabled them to learn and retain the information more effectively. While the first lecture was stunning at the time, the students would have assumed they would remember every word of it several weeks later and therefore would not have bothered reading around the subject – an approach that would let them down on the day.

The conclusion from the above is that an active, self-directed approach is likely to have a much greater impact on a student's learning than passive, lecture-based learning. Lectures should be used sparingly and for broad overviews, summaries and difficult topics. Sadly, only about 5% of what is taught in lectures is actually retained and too many people use lectures for imparting large quantities of detailed information that could easily be picked up, and more effectively, by reading a textbook. (See Chapter 10 for more on lectures and lecturing.)

Learning in small groups is a sort of halfway house involving active learning, or more precisely, interactive learning. But here the direction of learning is determined by the group as a whole, rather than individually, as in self-directed learning. Group learning can be a most rewarding and effective experience at all stages in a medical career – undergraduate, postgraduate and throughout years of continuing professional development. Too many people still consider that unless material is passed on from professor to student or consultant to trainee in a formal lecture, it would not be learnt properly. This chapter aims to challenge that assumption and to provide some ideas and suggestions, backed up by educational theory and the available evidence, for getting the most out of the small group learning experience.

Understanding Medical Education: Evidence, Theory and Practice.
Edited by T Swanwick. © 2010 Association for the Study of Medical Education.

The Learner Experience

If you were to ask a group of medical graduates to relate their personal experiences of small group work in their undergraduate course or postgraduate training, their responses would vary considerably. But the two factors most likely to underpin their accounts would probably relate to *tutor variability* and *curriculum philosophy*.

A *tutor* who creates a relaxed atmosphere, who keeps the group focused on the task in hand, who deals effectively with group dynamics, who allows the learners to take ownership of their learning and who helps make the process an effective, yet enjoyable, experience will produce strongly positive and enthusiastic responses. On the other hand, a tutor who talks all the time, who does not encourage group participation, who belittles learners who answer questions incorrectly, who has clear favourites in the group and who creates an atmosphere where one is frightened to open one's mouth does an extreme disservice to education.

A traditional *curriculum*, heavily dependent on imparting information through lectures, where students or trainees are seen as an inconvenience and a hindrance to research and their clinical practice, rather than as a benefit and an opportunity to mould and influence the future medical workforce, and where time spent by large numbers of tutors on small group teaching is perceived as an ineffective use of staff time, is likely to be received unfavourably. A progressive university or postgraduate team that values its students, believes in active learning, encourages small group teaching and trains its staff in the art of facilitation of learning will undoubtedly invoke a positive response.

At the postgraduate level, lectures are of even less value than at the undergraduate level, yet they are used just as frequently. Trainees gain far more from small group teaching sessions and on-the-job training than from, for instance, revision courses for passing membership exams. In the UK, primary care has tended to lead the way with its long-established one-to-one training relationship and regular group-based release courses, but effective education and training is also possible in secondary care and Bulstrode and Hunt,[1] in their training manual *Educating Consultants*, offer a number of very constructive suggestions for running on-the-job training that allow consultants to carry out effective education while at the same time maintaining their clinical practice load. And the training need not be one to one. It is common practice to train senior doctors, junior doctors and medical students at the same time. Bedside teaching is an example of this, but sadly such sessions are often still run in an inappropriate and humiliating way. The effectiveness of bedside teaching is discussed by Jolly in his book entitled *Bedside Manners*.[2]

De Villiers *et al.*,[3] in a report of an evaluation of a continuing professional development programme for primary care medical practitioners in South Africa, suggest that the following aspects should be incorporated into the design of small group activities to make them effective. Namely that they should:

- build on prior knowledge and experience
- relate to the perceived learning needs of the participants
- involve active learning
- be focused on problems
- be immediately applicable to practice
- involve cycles of action–reflection
- allow the acquisition of technical skills.

Steinert[4] researched medical students' perceptions of small group teaching in a Canadian medical school. Her conclusions at the undergraduate level were not a million miles away from de Villiers' findings at the postgraduate level viz that small groups should include:

- effective small group tutors
- a positive group atmosphere
- active student participation and group interaction
- adherence to small group goals
- clinical relevance and integration
- cases that promote thinking and problem solving.

The inefficiency argument is often used by those opposed to small group teaching. Twenty-five tutors spending two to three hours working with students in small groups of eight is clearly less efficient than one lecturer talking to 200 students all at once – but only in terms of delivery of material. Efficiency does not just take account of the delivery of *teaching*; what the students *learn* is what matters. I return to the point made earlier, that the taught curriculum is not the same as the learnt curriculum. Through small group discussion, much more is retained, especially if the learning is contextualised, for example, in case scenarios. In terms of efficiency of learning, small group work wins hands down. More particularly, small group work encourages critical thinking, which, although not impossible, is less common in lectures. *See* Box 9.1.

What Constitutes a Small Group?

The ideal size of a small group is probably around seven or eight. If the group is smaller, it becomes too threatening, the synergistic effect – the collective knowledge of the group being greater than the sum of the knowledge of each member of the group – is reduced and the interaction is less successful. If the number increases above eight, some learners can get by without fully participating, or without joining in at all, and others are less able to get their voice heard because the size of the group deters them from expressing their point of view. For problem-based learning (PBL), the size of the tutorial group rarely exceeds eight

**BOX 9.1 Where's the evidence:
Does small group work encourage
critical thinking?**

Most of the research around small group work relates
specifically to problem-based learning (PBL) – a
specialised form of small group learning discussed in
detail in Chapter 3. The nature of courses structured
around PBL is such that small group work, and the
subsequent self-directed learning, is the main vehicle by
which students gain information, with lectures
contributing relatively little to students' knowledge
acquisition. This is in contrast to courses where lectures
and other forms of didactic teaching provide the main
source of information for students, and where small
group teaching is really an adjunct to their learning.
Tiwari *et al.*(5) have compared the effects of these two
course styles on the development of students' critical
thinking. They found that PBL students had
significantly higher levels of critical thinking (measured
using the California Critical Thinking Disposition
Inventory(6)) compared with students on a
predominantly lecture-based course. Furthermore, they
continued to have higher scores for two years
afterwards. Similar conclusions have emerged from a
variety of other sources.(7–9)

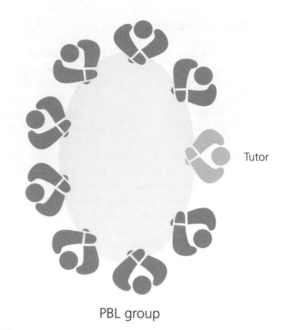

PBL group

Figure 9.1 Seating arrangement for a problem-based learning
(PBL) tutorial.

Housekeeping

Before embarking on small group teaching, some
thought needs to be given to the environmental
arrangements. It seems obvious to say it, but the first
requirement is to hold the session in an appropriately
sized room. What is appropriate depends on the
number of learners participating. Consideration
should also be given to heating, lighting and temperature control in the room, all of which are the unique
responsibility of the group leader.

For a group of eight or so undertaking PBL or some
similar activity, a room with a table in it, preferably
round or oval-shaped and big enough for all to sit
around it comfortably – including the tutor, who
should be part of the group and not outside it – is ideal
(*see* Figure 9.1). The walls of the room should be lined
with whiteboards or flip charts for students to write
and draw on.

For a session where argument is more important
than capturing information, for example, an ethical
debate, then a circle of chairs is all that is required (*see*
Figure 9.2).

The positioning of the tutor is important. To maximise the effectiveness of the process, the tutor should be
in the group, rather than *separate* from it. Sitting in a
circle has two advantages:
• everyone in the circle is equal
• everyone has eye contact with each other.
This arrangement also suits the role of the tutor as
facilitator.

For larger groups, the workshop format is the
method of choice and hence the room has to be larger

– the process would simply fall apart were there any
more in the group. Norman(10) recently carried out an
email survey of a cross-section of medical schools
around the world using PBL, asking about the size of
group they felt was appropriate, and eight turned out
to be the norm. Peters(11) cites academic evidence that
supports his own findings that the optimum size of a
group is somewhere between 5 and 10.

Some medical schools are so short of willing and
able teachers that they operate small groups of 20 or
more. This can still be successful, however, if the larger
group is run in workshop format, where the whole
group is given a task to carry out in smaller subgroups
of seven or eight. Here, one facilitator handles several
groups. Many postgraduate training courses are run
this way.

Group size is probably less important than what the
group actually does. The purist view of small group
teaching is that it must be learner-centred, with all
students joining in free discussion of a particular topic.
Some teaching may indeed take place in small groups
but sit outside this definition. The seminar is a case in
point, where invited speakers present on a topic about
which they are passionate. The seminar has its place
in a university – particularly at the Bachelor of Science
or Masters level – but is invariably teacher-centred,
with any discussion taking the form of questions and
answers.

Even within the confines of our working definition,
a wide range of styles of small group work exists, and
many of these are discussed later.

Tutor

Discussion circle

Figure 9.2 Seating arrangement for a group discussion.

Cafeteria style

Figure 9.3 Seating arrangement for a workshop.

and laid out in cafeteria style (several round tables with chairs round them, laid out like a cafeteria; *see* Figure 9.3). There needs to be space at the front of the room for the tutor, PowerPoint and/or overhead projector facilities (including an accessible power source), and whiteboard(s) that everyone can see. Ideally, each group should have a flip chart as well. Again, if there is no requirement for a table, then several circles of chairs will suffice.

Positioning of the tutor is different for a workshop. Plenary sessions are commonly part of a workshop, usually at the beginning to introduce the topic or task, and at the end to take feedback from the groups and summarise what has been achieved. Since the tutor needs to be able to engage everyone together, he or she needs to stand or be seated at the front of the class for these plenaries. But for the rest of the session, the tutor's job is to go round the groups to check how they are getting on.

The Role of the Tutor

The tutor can adopt a range of roles depending on the nature of the small group session. Rudduck(12) suggests that tutors can have four differing roles:

- the instructor, who is there to impart information to the students
- the devil's advocate, who intentionally adopts a controversial view in order to stimulate discussion
- the neutral chair, who literally chairs the discussion but expresses no strong opinions
- the consultant, who is not part of the group, but is there for the students to ask questions.

To these roles, I would add a fifth:

- the facilitator, similar to the neutral chair, but with more of a guiding role, for example, asking the group open-ended questions to facilitate their progress with the task in hand. The facilitator need not be the chair of the group – this role might fall to a student.

Tutors may adopt any or all of the above roles during the course of a small group teaching session. They may begin the session in instructor mode, defining the task for the students. During the rest of the session, they may adopt a more facilitatory role, at times prompting discussion by playing the role of the devil's advocate or taking up a chairing role. If the students get stuck, they may even take on the role of expert to allow them to move on (not in PBL, of course, where the tutor must reflect any questions back to the group and encourage them to research the answers for themselves).

Richmond(13) defines more specific roles for tutors, which he refers to as 'strategic interventions':

- to start and finish group discussion by outlining the group task, summarising the group's or groups' achievements and conclusions, and setting further learning activities
- to maintain the flow of content, for example, by preventing sidetracking and keeping the group(s) focused on the task
- to manage group dynamics by encouraging the shy or bored student(s) and by handling the dominant, aggressive, offensive or nuisance student(s)
- to facilitate goal achievement through open questioning, making suggestions and checking group understanding
- to manage the group environment by keeping an eye on the time and dealing with any distractions (e.g. noise, insufficient flip-chart paper, pens running dry, heating).

According to Brown,(14) tutors need a range of skills in order to make a success of small group teaching. These include questioning, listening, reinforcing, reacting, summarising and leadership. But the *real* skill, one that Brown refers to as a *super skill*, is the skill of knowing when to use which skill.

Getting Started

The first time the tutor meets with a new group of students or trainees is always exciting. Is it going to be the group from heaven or the group from hell? Often, the first encounter is the defining moment for the group. How the tutor handles the opening small group teaching session may establish the atmosphere for the sessions that follow.

The group members may or may not know each other. At the start of the course they almost certainly would not, but even later on, particularly in undergraduate curricula, because of the trend to have large numbers of students on courses they may still not know every other person on the course. Ice-breakers have a useful role here – ways of introducing strangers, trying to relax the group and getting group members to interact with each other.

There are many ice-breakers in common use – some simple, some elaborate. A standard technique is to ask the group members to pair up and talk to someone they do not know. Their task is to learn something about their partners and report it back to the group. This exercise works better if the task is fairly specific, and in addition to their partners' names and brief biographical details, participants may be asked to report back on the most interesting place their partners have visited, something unusual that they have done in their life or something they have done of which they are proud. Participants could also be asked to imagine themselves as a musical instrument or a vehicle or a colour, and to describe which most closely matches their character – all of which can be quite revealing!

An example of a more complex ice-breaker, which needs a bit of time, is to divide the group into two teams, which have to compete with each other to build a bridge of specific dimensions and requirements out of Lego bricks in a specified time. The dimensions and rules they have to adhere to make this a hard task, but it enables the tutor to observe how each member of the team behaves under pressure. It also provides an opportunity for discussing people's behaviour at the end of the exercise, and seeing how each team worked. Such exercises or games are common on off-campus postgraduate training courses.

Having got the group talking, the next thing to do is set the ground rules. This is a really important activity and should never be omitted. It is essential that the group itself comes up with the ground rules – they must not be imposed by the tutor. Box 9.2 shows examples of ground rules that my own undergraduate students have come up with.

Probably the most important ground rule is to do with valuing each other's contribution. That way a relaxed atmosphere is created where no one is embarrassed about saying something stupid. Humiliation must be avoided at all costs.

> **BOX 9.2 Examples of ground rules for small groups**
> - Turn up punctually
> - Finish on time
> - Do not talk over each other
> - Do not interrupt
> - Value each person's contribution
> - Respect each other's viewpoint
> - Turn off mobile phone
> - Turn up prepared
> - Join in the discussion
> - Keep personal issues outside
> - Maintain confidentiality within the group

Techniques to Use in Small Groups

Following on from the ice-breaker, a good technique to get a group engaged in the topic under discussion is known as snowballing. The students are given a question, for example, 'How might cystic fibrosis affect the life of a 15-year-old young man?', and asked to think about it individually, without conferring with anyone else. After five minutes, the students are asked to pair up with another student and discuss their thoughts with each other. After another 5 minutes, the pairs are invited to join with another pair and all four students continue their discussion. Two sets of fours then compare notes and so on. The process is called snowballing because of its resemblance to a snowball rolling down a hill, gathering more and more snow and getting bigger and bigger in size. The big advantage of this technique is that everyone has to participate, even the most reticent of students. By allowing time for them to gather their own thoughts and then share these thoughts with one other, it gives even the shyest student confidence to speak. A variation on snowballing is called jigsaw groups, where the participants divide into small groups and discuss an issue. After a period, the groups reform into new groups, with each of the new groups containing one member of each of the old groups, thereby maximising the mix of participants (*see* Figure 9.4).

Brainstorming is another widely used technique. Again, learners are given something to think about (e.g. possible diagnoses for a patient who presents with lower back pain). One group member acts as scribe and writes all the suggestions from the group – in this case possible diagnoses – on a whiteboard. Absolutely everything is written up, no matter how unlikely the suggestion may be. No one is allowed to make any value judgements on the suggestions at this stage. It is followed by reflective analysis of what has

First 10-minute discussion		

```
1  2  3        1  2  3        1  2  3
4  5  6        4  5  6        4  5  6



1  2  3        1  2  3        1  2  3
4  5  6        4  5  6        4  5  6
```

Second 10-minute discussion		

```
1  1  1        2  2  2        3  3  3
1  1  1        2  2  2        3  3  3



4  4  4        5  5  5        6  6  6
4  4  4        5  5  5        6  6  6
```

Jigsaw groups

Figure 9.4 How jigsaw groups work.

been written up, where items are prioritised, grouped together or removed altogether.

A third introductory technique involves the use of buzz groups. This technique is more generally used in lectures, but can also be used in small groups if the group becomes stuck in its thinking. The tutor who senses an impasse can interrupt the discussion and throw in a question for the group to ponder in pairs or threes, to help the members get back on track. If students are struggling to understand respiratory acidosis for instance, the tutor might ask them to discuss in pairs what the role of the kidney is in maintaining pH or what blood buffers exist. When this technique is used in lectures, there is a loud 'buzz' as members of the audience start talking with their neighbours – hence the name.

Further on in the life of the learning group, a number of other techniques may be used.

Simply chairing a discussion – or, better still, getting one of the group members to do so – works well when there is more than one perspective about an issue, such as a genuine ethical dilemma like abortion, animal experimentation or euthanasia. Occasionally with moral and ethical arguments, the tutor may need to step in to clarify matters of fact, such as primary legislation, case law or professional guidelines – an example of the tutor acting as a consultant or expert. A more imaginative and hands-off approach to such issues would be to get the students to set up a formal debate, with students primed to speak for or against a particular motion such as 'This house believes that patients with coronary artery disease, who continue to smoke after they have been repeatedly counselled about the dangers of smoking, should be refused heart bypass surgery'. The advantage here is that the relevant factual elements to the discussion are prepared in advance.

A variation of the discussion group is called lineups. The tutor makes a controversial statement, such as 'Doctors should be allowed to hasten the death of old people who have a terminal illness'. The tutor identifies a point in one corner of the room where everyone who strongly agrees with the statement should stand. Another point is identified, as far away as possible, where those who strongly disagree should stand. The rest of the group members have to line up somewhere between the two points, according to how much they agree or disagree with the statement. The participants have to talk to the others in the line and argue their point of view. The tutors, and indeed the participants, get an immediate view of the spread of participants' opinions on the topic. If the line-up is carried out at the beginning and the end of a session, the tutor can gauge if there has been a change of opinion after the session has been run and the participants are better informed.

There are a number of variations on the discussion approach to small group teaching. Some of these are less than satisfactory, however. One approach used frequently in postgraduate medical education is the journal club. Staff are asked to present their comments on recent papers in the medical literature. This works well, provided the topic is of direct relevance to everyone and there is plenty of opportunity for discussion. It is less successful at the undergraduate level, where it is more usual to run the session along the lines of a syndicate presentation, where a topic such as diabetes is subdivided into several subtopics (e.g. mechanism of action of insulin, diabetic ketoacidosis, clinical presentation of diabetes, treatment of diabetes) and each of these subtopics is given to a student or pair of students to research. They then all report back at the next tutorial. The problem with both of these methods is that the presentations become mini-lectures, are frequently delivered in an uninspiring manner and, frankly, bore the pants off everyone. Discussion is limited because only the chosen few have researched the topic, and then only the subtopic they were allocated. Unless everyone researches everything, the only people who join in the discussion are those who researched the topic and the tutor!

Another old favourite at the undergraduate level is the post-lecture tutorial. This is another disaster site. Most students come unprepared and have not read up around the lecture topic (indeed they may not even have attended the lecture or may be blissfully unaware what lecture topic is being discussed). Many students see it as an opportunity to listen to a rerun of the original lecture, which is what it often turns into, particularly if the tutor gets monosyllabic responses to the questions they ask to try to stimulate the students. There is really only one solution to this – ensure that students are given a self-directed learning exercise to prepare *before* the tutorial. A good example would be to give them a detailed case study to read up, with some questions attached for them to research, for example, a case history of a patient with a peptic ulcer, followed by a series of questions on, for instance, medical imaging, regulation of intestinal pH, *Helicobacter pylori*, drug treatment and dietary advice. In this way, the students know what the topic of the tutorial is, have done their homework, and therefore feel able to join in the discussion and get a lot more out of the whole exercise.

The use of triggers provides an ideal springboard for a tutorial. The tutor can design a whole session around one or more of these. They are commonly used when running sessions in the workshop format. At the beginning of the session, after a brief introduction, the tutor hands out a trigger. A trigger is simply a tool to get the discussion started. They might take various forms. For example:

- an electrocardiogram (ECG) strip from a patient with ventricular fibrillation – to stimulate a discussion about cardiac muscle, the sinoatrial node, ECGs, arrythmias, defibrillation
- a photomicrograph showing neoplastic growth changes to stimulate discussion about the appearance of cancerous tissue, the characteristics of cancer cells, metastasis
- a chest X-ray showing a pneumothorax to stimulate discussion about X-rays, pleura of the lungs, pneumothorax – its causes, presentation and treatment
- an audiogram from a patient with age-related and noise-related hearing loss to stimulate discussion about the anatomy of the ear, the hearing mechanism, sensorineural hearing loss, audiometry, Rinne and Weber's tests
- a copy of *Good Medical Practice* to stimulate discussion on what constitutes a good standard of practice and patient care, professionalism, working with colleagues and probity
- an anonymised or mock-up of a patient record for students to discuss record keeping in the context of a particular case
- a photograph of a patient with an obvious goitre and exophthalmos to stimulate discussion around the thyroid gland, thyroid disorders including clinical signs, symptoms and treatment
- a photograph of a man in a wheelchair playing with a young child to stimulate discussion around disability, psychosocial sequelae of chronic illness, social care, child care, single-parent families
- a family pedigree, showing the distribution of a genetic disorder such as haemophilia to trigger a discussion on genes and patterns of inheritance
- a video showing, for example, a doctor explaining to a couple that their baby has Down's syndrome
- a paper, or excerpts from a paper, showing some statistical data, in order to get the students talking about *P*-values or odds ratios or randomised control trials.

In PBL, a paper-based case scenario would normally act as the trigger and there are two main variants of this: one where the case is presented in the form of a short summary; the other where the case is much longer, and is released in stages by the tutor (presentation, history, examination findings, investigations, treatment, patient progress, outcome). The former is generally used for school leavers, the latter for graduates. The tutor has rather different roles in the two versions. In short-case PBL tutorials, the students take turns at being chair of the group and the tutor is passive, intervening only to ask the odd question to stimulate discussion or to keep the group on track. In the long, progressive-release version of PBL, the tutor acts as the chair, moves the group along when their discussion has come to a halt and occasionally asks specific, programmed questions. Both styles of PBL are student-centred and produce deep and high-level discussions, particularly with graduate students.

PBL is covered in more detail in Chapter 3.

Role play also uses a trigger. Students are given a scenario to act out, for example, taking a headache history, explaining a medication regime for eczema or breaking bad news about a cervical smear result. Professional actors are often employed to simulate real patients and students can try out their clinical communication skills in a safe environment. If the students are video-recorded as well, they can study their communication attempts in their own time and work on improving their technique before encountering the real thing. This technique works well at the postgraduate level too, especially with doctors who have been identified as having a communication problem. Watching your own performance can be very revealing and informative. Discussing your performance, captured on videotape, with a trained communication skills expert, is invaluable and always leads to improvement. The secret is to have enough insight and be brave enough to do it in the first place.

Clinical skills are also taught in small groups, but rather than using a trigger, the clinician will demonstrate the skill to the group before letting them have a go. One commonly used technique takes place in four stages:

- the tutor demonstrates the skill in silence
- the tutor runs through it again, but explains the rationale behind the technique at the same time
- the students then talk the tutor through the technique
- finally, a volunteer student runs through the technique without tutor intervention.

The Balint group(15,16) is a special kind of group activity undertaken mainly by general practitioners (GPs), although increasingly patients, and even students, are becoming involved. Michael Balint was a Hungarian psychoanalyst who worked extensively with UK GPs in helping them to understand the psychology behind the doctor–patient relationship. He set up discussion groups with GPs to allow them to share their personal experiences of specific problems or dilemmas that had arisen in their practice. A modern-day Balint group consists of a handful of GPs, who meet on a regular basis, often with a psychoanalyst and sometimes with one or more patients, to discuss specific issues concerning patients arising from their daily practice. The presenting clinician brings to the group cases that have given cause for thought. The purpose of the group is to increase understanding of the doctor–patient relationship, not to find solutions to the patient's problem. Discomfort or distress in the doctor are not ignored, but are worked through in the context of the needs and problems of the patient rather than of the doctor. Balint group members find the benefit gained by sharing their experiences far outweighs any pain they may feel as a result of the experience. Balint groups are not for everyone and should not to be entered into lightly.

Another type of group activity used in the postgraduate arena is the action learning set. An action learning set is a group of six to eight people who meet regularly to help each other learn from their experiences. The set is not a team, since its focus is on the actions of the individuals within it rather than on a shared set of work objectives. Sets are usually facilitated by a set adviser whose responsibility is to create a suitable learning environment by encouraging, challenging and focusing on learning. Action learning is based on the concept of learning by reflection on experience. It is underpinned by the cycle of experiential learning,(17) as shown in Figure 9.5, where the stages of reflection and generalisation are worked through with the members of the set.

The action learning approach was first developed by Revans.(18) Each participant works on a project or task over the life of the set (which may be a few weeks, or spread over several months). The set decides on its

Figure 9.5 The 'Kolb' cycle.

own way of working, but usually a meeting involves participants taking turns to present their project to the set.

This will normally involve:

- an update of progress on actions from the last meeting
- a discussion about current issues or problems
- an agreement on actions for the future.

Participants work with the presenter, by listening and questioning, to help them decide what actions to take. This kind of group is useful for individuals working on an educational or research project largely on their own.

Group Dynamics

Before considering the role of the tutor in addressing issues of poor group dynamics, it is worthwhile taking a look at how a group evolves during its lifetime. Tuckman(19) has summarised it into four stages, which have been further interpreted by Walton(20) and Mulholland.(21)

Forming
The participants get to know each other, form alliances and establish themselves. The tutor must ensure they are introduced to each other.

Norming
The participants set the ground rules for working as a group. Being unfamiliar with what is expected of them can lead to some uncertainty and insecurity at this point. The tutor may need to explain the way the tutorials are to be run to alleviate anxiety at this point.

Storming
The group begins to function. Individuals adopt the roles with which they feel comfortable. One might be a leader; another good at initiating conversation; a third might be skilled at asking probing questions; a fourth might be good at clarifying and explaining; another might be good at keeping the team together, coming to the rescue of anyone who appears lost, frustrated or angry; one or two may simply be good

listeners and may only contribute to the process when they have something to say. There is the potential for a good deal of friction during this stage while the group is sorting itself out. The tutor needs to keep a careful watch on the group members, identifying problems and trying to relieve tensions. If the participants are mature enough, they may be able to address their own issues as a group. This is to be encouraged. The less the tutor gets involved the better. Such a group skill takes time to develop and the tutor will undoubtedly need to facilitate the process initially.

Performing

This is the position every group should aim for. Essentially the group has settled down and is functioning well. The group members are comfortable with their roles. There is a good atmosphere within the group and the goals of each tutorial are generally accomplished through successful collaboration. The tutor can now relax.

Unfortunately, some groups never achieve this state. This is usually due to one or two personality clashes and the odd difficult student. If the group cannot sort itself out, the tutor must act. Otherwise participants and tutor will dread meeting up for tutorials and attendance will fall off.

Adjourning

This is the final stage of working in groups. The lifetime of the group has run out and members move on to join new groups. This phase is a mixture of celebration and sadness (or relief, in the case of an unsuccessful group). A good group will look back over its achievements and reflect on each other's contribution, on lessons learnt, on what worked well and what could have been done better.

This process of reflection can be formalised and the tutor can help the group debrief itself in a structured way. One process that works quite well is carried out in two stages. First, the group rates itself as a whole against set criteria. The criteria depend on the nature and purpose of the small group work, but might include attendance and punctuality, preparedness for the sessions, adequacy of input into the sessions and behaviour towards each other within each session. Having established a group rating for each criterion, the members of the group then rate themselves against the group rating. Everyone shares their scores and a discussion ensues. A good group will recognise individual's strengths and weaknesses, will be constructively critical, and will try to be supportive and encouraging to the more self-effacing members of the group. A good group will also not shirk its responsibility to address issues arising from individuals who are lacking in insight as to their own behaviour. Often, as a result of this kind of caring, inward reflection, change does take place when the member moves on to their next group (Box 9.3).

BOX 9.3 Focus on: Discussion in small groups

Visschers-Pleijers *et al.*(22) have carried out an analysis of verbal interactions in tutorial groups. They have subdivided these interactions into five types:

- exploratory questioning – exchanging ideas, critical exchange of ideas
- cumulative reasoning – uncritical accumulation of information
- handling conflicts about knowledge – discussion of contradictory information; arguments and counter-arguments
- procedural interactions – conversations relating to process matters
- off task/irrelevant interactions – general asides; discussion about the weather

Most of the interactions (about 80%) were learning oriented, demonstrating the high task involvement of the group and confirming the findings of De Grave *et al.*(23)

The Interprofessional Group

Interprofessional learning is considered important at both the undergraduate and the postgraduate level (see Chapter 4 for a full discussion).(24) Healthcare is all about working in teams and it is sensible therefore to have regular joint educational training throughout the continuum of learning. The key to interprofessional education is that it should relate to real practice and should not be contrived just so that the box can be ticked for the next accreditation visit. Furthermore, interprofessional education does not require the participation of *all* the professions at each session – only those for whom it is appropriate.

Interprofessional team meetings are common at the postgraduate level, interprofessional training less so although both acute and primary care trusts provide programmes of training sessions for their staff. Quite a few of these are interprofessional, although they tend to be for large numbers, rather than small groups. Training in leadership and management for senior staff is less likely to be profession-specific and often follows the workshop format.

At the undergraduate level, certainly in the UK, there is only a small amount of useful interprofessional education taking place. What there is takes a variety of forms, ranging from a common foundation term with shared PBL, lectures and anatomy sessions,(25) shared clinical skills training,(26,27) a simulated ward environment for junior medical and nursing students,(28) and an interprofessional training ward(29–31) to regular joint interprofessional sessions spread over a number of years.(32) Apart from the lectures and the anatomy sessions, most of this involves small group work.

The skills training described,(26,27) involved final-year medical students with newly qualified staff nurses and took place in an interprofessional clinical skills centre. The programme was based around a developing patient scenario, which was pertinent to the participants' area of practice. Each session was led by an experienced nurse lecturer and doctor, supported by specialist contributors. The style of learning was participative, with small interprofessional groups addressing a range of patient management issues. In this way, relevant clinical and communication skills were integrated within the context of holistic patient care. This short exposure to interprofessional learning appears to have been highly effective.

The interprofessional training ward takes small group learning in the context of simulation even further. Here, final-year nurses, physiotherapists, occupational therapists and medical students look after a small ward.(29–31) They work shifts, carry out all ward duties, work extensively with each other and learn about each other's professions while at the same time building up their uniprofessional skills. Handover from one shift to another is key to the learning process. This provides students with an excellent preparation for working on the wards when they graduate, and is again popular with most students.

Undergraduate or postgraduate, the issues around interprofessional learning are the same and revolve around group relations (*see* Bion in the Further reading section). There is a strong hierarchical culture, which pervades all areas of the health service. When people from different professions find themselves being trained together, there is a tendency to adopt these hierarchical roles. Even at the undergraduate level, medical students, physiotherapists, occupational therapists and nurses all have different entry requirements, and immediately a barrier exists. Of course, that is one of the aims of interprofessional education – to break down such barriers. Another aim is for the members of one profession to have a clear understanding of the roles of the other healthcare professionals. Putting these two aims together leads to the third, overarching, aim – to learn how to work in teams, thereby leading to a more efficient and effective health service. Small group learning in interprofessional groups is one way to help achieve this last aim.

For an inter-professional group, good facilitation is essential. If the guidance described for any small group work activity is followed, the majority of problems will soon disappear. Setting clear ground rules and ensuring that the group adheres to them is vital – particularly the rule about valuing everyone's input. In addition, the topic or activity needs to be inclusive, that is appropriate for all professions present. The learning needs of the students or trainees must be taken into account as they will not be the same for all professions. Where they *are* the same, then joint interprofessional learning is more likely to succeed.

Dealing with Difficult Group Members

Dealing with difficult group members is a key role of the tutor running small group teaching sessions. Box 9.4 provides a list of common problems encountered, and regular group leaders will recognise them all. It is not the purpose of this chapter to provide suggestions for dealing with *each* form of aberrant behaviour – for a full discussion of this topic read Tiberius's excellent book *Small Group Teaching: a trouble shooters guide*.(33) One general point, however: wherever possible, the group should sort out its own problems. This is liable to be much more effective in the long term than the tutor taking control, which often leads to resentment. The tutor's role here is to raise the group's awareness of the issue. One way of doing this is to say 'Let's take time out for a minute. Is everyone happy the way the group is working? Does anyone want to make a comment about the group process?' Then stand back and watch the sparks fly!

Of course, this is not always appropriate, nor does it always work. In such circumstances, the group leader has to step in. Sometimes issues have to be addressed in the presence of the group; at other times

---

BOX 9.4 Challenging learners

- the dominant learner
- the arrogant learner – the know it all
- the learner who wants to be the centre of attention all the time
- the aggressive or argumentative learner
- the offensive and rude learner
- the politically incorrect learner
- the flirtatious learner
- the joke-a-minute learner
- the garrulous learner
- the disengaged learner
- the bored learner
- the learner who relies on everyone else to do the work
- the lazy learner
- the shy learner
- the delicate, tearful learner
- the over-dependent learner
- the constantly late learner
- the frequently ill learner
- the mentally disturbed learner

the leader needs to address the issue outside the group, for example, in the case of a learner who is clearly upset, or one who has failed to respond to everything the tutor has tried in the session. Failure to address group dynamics by one means or another can be very harmful, not just for that particular group, but for future groups. The issue will rarely go away of its own accord and often gets worse and worse if nothing is done about it. No matter how difficult or painful it is, the tutor has a responsibility to sort matters out.

Here are some ideas.

The dominant group member

People can dominate discussions for a number of reasons:
- they simply know a lot
- they think they know a lot – but are frequently wrong
- they like to be the centre of attention and are showing off
- they want to impress the tutor, or their girlfriend/boyfriend
- they enjoy teaching others and are keen to share their knowledge
- they feel that someone has to start the ball rolling, as no one else seems to want to.

If dominating group members are allowed to continue, the group will get really angry, the shy group members will disappear into their shells and people will either switch off or drop out. Often the dominant member can contribute successfully to a group and does actually have some really useful information to bring. The secret is to reduce their input while not causing offence.

Sometimes group members realise that they have a tendency to dominate and readily accept being told to keep quiet. Not many have such insight, and one suggestion for dealing with those who do not is to give them a specific task to do, for example, acting as scribe for the rest of the group. Make sure, however, that they do put up the group's ideas on the whiteboard, and not just their own interpretation. Another technique is to ask them to discuss a particular point and let them have their say, but next time invite someone else to start the ball rolling. Seating can also play a key role. If the tutor sits opposite the dominant student, then that student has the eye of the tutor for the whole session. On the other hand, if the dominant student sits *beside* the tutor, interaction is significantly reduced and the tutor's eye catches other students much more readily. The use of the sweeping hand gesture directed at the dominant student can sometimes be effective – the held-up hand is saying 'Hang on a minute. I want to hear contributions from other students.' Indeed, sometimes the tutor has to speak these very words aloud. If none of this works, then a word outside the session is necessary, explaining how valuable the individual's contribution is, but how it is important to give *everyone* a chance to be heard.

The reticent group member

The converse of the above is the reticent group member. Again there are many reasons for this:
- they *are* innately shy
- they are upset or worried about something going on in their lives
- they are in a bad mood
- they are upset with someone in the group
- they have not done any work for the session
- they do not know anything about the topic
- they are completely out of their depth
- they are very tired
- they are very bored
- they have lost their motivation to be a doctor
- they are ill or depressed.

Some of these are most definitely not in the group tutor's remit to deal with, particularly the last one. Ill or depressed group members need to be seen by qualified practitioners – GPs, occupational health physicians or student counsellors. Under no circumstances should the small group learning tutor attempt to address such issues. Other issues may need to be taken up with the learner's personal tutor, trainer or educational supervisor.

The group leader's role is to encourage the individual concerned to seek help from the appropriate person, and to help identify who that person might be.

But dealing with a genuinely shy, or work-shy, learner is down to the tutor of the small group session. The former needs to be subtly encouraged to join in. Snowballing and buzz groups work quite well, since the learner does not have to speak in front of the whole group. Like the dominant group member, giving the shy individual a task to do, such as being scribe, works well. They are responding to the rest of the group's ideas, a role they are comfortable with. Pointing a finger at them and asking them a direct question is likely to send them deeper into their shell. Humiliating them in any way, for instance by laughing at their answers, is hugely counterproductive. Getting them to comment on something that they are almost certain to know might work, but sometimes the shy person simply needs to be left alone for a while, particularly if the reason for their non-involvement is transitory.

As to the work-shy, usually peer pressure takes care of this, but if not, then a quiet word outside the group is the solution. If a student is really out of his or her depth, this is a more serious situation and needs reporting to the appropriate member of staff responsible for academic progress, so that they can consider whether some form of remediation would help.

The flirtatious, 'jokey' or offensive group member

These are definitely examples of when the tutor should get the *group* to deal with the issue. One way is to get the group to take time out from the session and ask them if everyone is comfortable with the atmosphere in the group, or with the behaviour of everyone in the group. Usually someone is heartily sick of it and says so. If this does not do the trick, the tutor should speak to the student out of hearing of the group. They should be very firm with them.

The late or absent group member

Groups can get really angry with perpetually late or absent group members and usually make their feelings on the matter quite clear. Starting the group later to accommodate the perpetually late learner is not an option. The only possible exception to this is the person who has *genuine* problems getting in for, say, a 9 a.m. start – perhaps for child care reasons or finishing off a ward round. If they really are unable to change their arrangements, then the issue should be taken up with the group right at the beginning, when forming the ground rules.

Persistent absence is a course or programme attendance issue, even if this is due to illness. The learner may, as a result, be held back and the school or postgraduate dean may refuse to sign them off or award credits. These are issues of professionalism, and unprofessional behaviour must be addressed when it first appears, not left to smoulder until it is too late to help learners amend their behaviour.

And there is one other essential ground rule, particularly at the undergraduate level: if a person is unable to attend a session for whatever reason – planned or last-minute – they must inform the tutor prior to their absence, or as soon after as is possible. If the tutor is unavailable, then they must inform someone in the group. In the era of mobile phones, there really is no excuse for not adhering to this policy.

The over-dependent group member

Here, the tutor has to learn to keep a distance from that individual and must take great care not to overindulge him or her. Some people are good at manipulating vulnerable members of staff for their own ends – another instance when the person concerned should be seated out of the sightline of the tutor.

Exploring Boundaries

Before taking charge of a small group, it is essential to be trained in the art of facilitation. Usually such training will itself take the form of a workshop in which an experienced facilitator demonstrates how to facilitate a small group by example. The facilitator is likely to cover the issues described in this chapter. The training session is likely to include some consideration about handling difficult group members and may also include some consideration about interpersonal boundaries – boundaries for the students, and boundaries for the staff. Boxes 9.5–9.8 depict four scenarios

BOX 9.5 Case A

Stephen is tutor to a group in which Tom and Sarah are students. Tom is a likeable but dominant member of the group who has strong knowledge that he likes to demonstrate to the group. Sarah is a student who comes from an arts background and is not confident about her ability. During a session, Tom begins (as always) to tell the group about his understanding of the learning issues. Stephen stops Tom briefly, and asks everyone if they understand what Tom is describing. The group nods, apart from Sarah, who replies 'This is all over my head, but don't worry about me. I just don't have the basic knowledge to join in this conversation. I'll catch up one day I'm sure.' Tom continues his feedback and Sarah immerses herself in a textbook. Stephen is sympathetic to Sarah but does not want the group to get behind. He believes that it is important that the group finishes its work in the time allocated and never allows the session to run over. Anyway, he has a lecture to give immediately after the session.

BOX 9.6 Case B

Hannah is a student in Rebecca's group. Hannah is a lively and strong character who has said quite openly that she 'wears her heart on her sleeve'. During a tutorial that focuses on lung cancer, Hannah spends a lot of time describing very emotionally how her grandmother died from lung cancer last year. As learning issues are written up on the board, Hannah says that she does not think she will 'be able to do many of these as it's all too close to home for me'. Later in the tutorial, Hannah suddenly begins to cry and says 'its all too much for me', and runs out of the tutorial in tears. Rebecca follows her and is out of the room for about 20 minutes.

BOX 9.7 Case C

Claire has been a student in Maria's group for several weeks. She is known to be struggling with the course and is open about a number of personal problems that she says are 'affecting her work'. Maria is concerned about Claire and has become something of a confidante to her. At various points in tutorials, Maria has mouthed the words 'are you okay?' to Claire. Maria has offered to talk to Claire 'any time' about her difficulties and Claire has taken to staying behind after teaching sessions to chat to Maria.

that illustrate some situations that may arise for group leaders. There are no comments on these scenarios. They are presented for the reader to think about whether the tutor's response was appropriate.

> **BOX 9.8** Case D
>
> Mike is a student in Hardeep's group. Mike is an extremely confident and able student who is a lively and enthusiastic contributor to the group. At the start of the tutorial Hardeep asks the group how their week has been. Most members of the group make comments about how useful they have found the lectures so far and how they have enjoyed their GP visits. Mike adds, looking at Hardeep, 'The content of that Asian guy's session was crap. I could hardly make out one word he said.' Later, when the students are presented with the first page of a new problem, Hardeep asks them to identify its key features. The front cover to the week's problem shows a picture of a young woman in some distress. Mike says, 'Well, she's blonde, about 20 and far too skinny. Not my type at all. She's probably gay anyway!' The group dissolve into laughter. Hardeep joins in.

Frequently Asked Questions

How long should a small group teaching session last?

There is no simple answer to this. Everyone's attention span is limited. The key is to vary the activities on a regular basis. This is easy in a workshop format, but in, for instance, a PBL session, students may be incarcerated in a window-less room engaged in more or less the same activity for up to three hours. In any lengthy session, it is essential to build in a reasonable break for rest and refreshment. In summary, a session should last between 45 minutes and 3 hours, depending on the activity. The less the students are engaged in active learning, the shorter the session has to be.

Many postgraduate workshops last all day, sometimes they are spread over two or three days, or even a week, for example, for residential training courses. All-day workshops must be split into manageable chunks, separated by frequent refreshment breaks. Week-long courses should include at least a half day of relaxation.

How often should groups be changed?

In undergraduate education, a group should generally remain together for something between a term and a year. It is important for students to learn to mix and establish new teams. Groups that function well never want to change; groups that function poorly cannot wait to change. A term is probably a good compromise.

In postgraduate education, for example, day-release courses in vocational GP training schemes, or Balint groups, it is important to maintain as much continuity as possible, and groups should stay together for their natural lifetime (welcoming newcomers as appropriate).

Should learners who do not get on be swapped into other groups?

As far as medical students are concerned, absolutely not – under any circumstances. Doctors have to work in teams for the rest of their lives. These teams may not always function ideally. There may be personality clashes, jealousy, rivalry, too many chiefs and too few Indians – but they still have to work as a team. The sooner they learn to find a way to get on with people they do not like, the better they will function when it really matters.

In postgraduate education, doctors know their own needs (unfortunately not always) and are free to attend whatever courses they feel they will gain the most from. Continuing professional development is a requirement for all healthcare professionals, but apart from essential updating of skills, for example, resuscitation and life-support courses, few courses are compulsory and most are one-offs. Apart from GPs and psychiatrists, doctors therefore do not tend to attend regular workshops with the same people, although they do meet together as teams all the time. Instead, doctors tend to create their own 'clubs' and meet up frequently at conferences. Rarely, these national or international meetings involve small group work, consisting mainly of hundreds of usually fairly dire presentations.

Do I need to be an expert on a topic to run a small group?

It depends. For PBL, there is some evidence that the best tutors are those who are expert facilitators, but that it helps to have knowledge expertise as well.(34,35) Knowledge experts who have no skills of facilitation and who turn each PBL session into a question-and-answer session, or worse still, a mini-lecture, make poor tutors, as do those who do not even have the excuse of being knowledge experts and who are unable to grasp the principles of PBL (and indeed scorn the whole approach to learning). But for other small group activities, such as a seminar or workshop, and for most postgraduate teaching, where the tutor has more input, knowledge expertise is indeed necessary, again alongside the skills of small group facilitation.

Can a group survive with a series of different facilitators?

Generally, continuity of group leader is important, although rarely is an undergraduate tutor available to take every session in a term because of other commitments. One solution to this is to have paired tutors, so that when one is absent, the other can take over.

In the case of, say, a series of small group sessions covering a range of specialist topics, such as in day-release workshops for junior doctors, then it is actually desirable to have different tutors because specialist medical expertise is required. The problem then is that the group never really has the time to develop a meaningful relationship with each tutor, because they are with them for such a short time. The group may get beyond the forming stage, but the tutor rarely does. There are two solutions to this: reduce the number of guest tutors; or maintain continuity through the use of a regular co-facilitator.

Is there such a thing as a floating facilitator?

In fact, that is exactly what a workshop facilitator does. But the question is more to do with a single facilitator looking after more than one group simultaneously, where the groups are not located in the same space but, for example, in nearby rooms. This is rather like the consultant surgeon keeping an eye on his trainees in adjacent operating theatres – common enough practice, but is it *good* practice? Usually this kind of multi-group facilitation only happens because of tutor shortages, and is aimed at making economies. The economies are really perceived economies rather than actual economies, because they only take into account savings in staff time and not quality of student learning. The learning experience is unlikely to be beneficial to the student (although sharing one good tutor is undoubtedly better than being tutored by two separate bad tutors). For multi-group facilitation to work, the activities being undertaken by each group must be task-based, with the tutor popping in now and again to check on group progress. Again, in the postgraduate arena, where the learners are often more committed and motivated, groups can be left to get on with the task by themselves for a while, which leads in nicely to the next frequently asked question.

Do groups need a facilitator at all?

Again, the answer is that it depends. Students in the early stages of their course undoubtedly need a facilitator around. Partly this is simply because they do not know what to do, and partly for reassurance that they are learning what they are supposed to be learning. 'Will it come up in the exam?' is a question frequently asked of tutors. As students develop and become more mature, the need for a tutor is reduced. Such students can facilitate their own groups. Once they are let loose on the wards, students revert to Stage One again and need a bit of mollycoddling and guidance.

Postgraduate groups can survive without a tutor if the purpose of the small group session is clear. They may then appoint a chair from within the group and get on with the task in hand.

Summary

Learning in small groups can be very productive, if at times challenging. Not everyone enjoys the process, particularly if the group is dysfunctional. Here, the skills of the facilitator are put to the greatest test, although there are guidelines for handling difficult group members, which are touched on here and elsewhere. A poor facilitator can jeopardise the success of even the best of groups, however – through bullying, humiliating, patronising, prejudicial or over-didactic behaviour. A good facilitator can help the group to achieve a high standard of learning, by encouraging active learning and reflective thinking, by questioning and challenging, and by setting a good example. The most successful groups are tutored by people who are good at facilitation, and not necessarily those who have subject expertise.

Small group learning is particularly successful if the facilitator adopts a variety of techniques during sessions. Workshops, which often last a morning or afternoon, must be split up into a range of activities – discussion, role play, debate, exercises using triggers, watching videos, practising skills, observing demonstrations, problem solving, question-and-answer sessions, presentations – the list is endless.

Facilitation expertise does not grow on trees. People who are brilliant teachers do not necessarily make good facilitators, because they may find it hard to get out of the information-giving mode in which they excel. Group facilitation should never be forced on such people. It is more sensible to recognise their skills and make use of them in the more didactic elements of a course, leaving facilitation to those who are good at it. Would that life were that simple …

References

1 Bulstrode CJK and Hunt VL (1997) *Educating Consultants.* SUMIT, Oxford.
2 Jolly BC (1994) *Bedside Manners: teaching in the hospital setting.* Universitaire Pers Maastricht, Maastricht.
3 De Villiers M, Bresick G and Mash B (2003) The value of small group learning: an evaluation of an innovative CPD programme for primary care medical practitioners. *Medical Education.* 37: 815–21.
4 Steinert Y (2004) Student perceptions of effective small group teaching. *Medical Education.* 38: 286–93.
5 Tiwari A, Lai P, So M and Yuen K (2006) A comparison of the effects of problem-based learning and lecturing on the development of students' critical thinking. *Medical Education.* 40: 547–54.
6 Facione NC, Facione PA and Sanchez CA (1994) Critical thinking disposition as a measure of competent clinical judgement: the development of the Californian Critical Thinking Disposition Inventory. *Journal of Nursing Education.* 33: 345–50.
7 Barrows HS (1986) A taxonomy of problem-based learning methods. *Medical Education.* 20: 481–6.
8 Engel CE (1997) Not just a method but a way of learning. In: Boud D and Feletti G (eds) *The Challenge of Problem-based Learning* (2e), pp. 17–27. Kogan Page, London.
9 Kamin CS, O'Sullivan PS, Younger M and Deterding R (2001) Measuring critical thinking in problem-based learning discourse. *Teaching & Learning in Medicine.* 13: 27–35.

10 Norman GR (2006) Personal communication.

11 Peters T (1995) *In Search of Excellence: lessons from America's best-run companies*. Harper Collins Business, London.

12 Rudduck J (1979) Learning to teach through discussion. Centre for Applied Research in Education occasional publications no. 8. University of East Anglia, Norwich.

13 Richmond DE (1984) Improving the effectiveness of small-group learning with strategic intervention. *Medical Teacher*. **6**: 138–45.

14 Brown G (1982) How to improve small group teaching in medicine. In: Cox KR and Ewan CE (eds) *The Medical Teacher*, pp. 70–78. Churchill Livingstone, Edinburgh.

15 Balint M (1957) *The Doctor, His Patient and the Illness*. Churchill Livingstone, Edinburgh. [1964, reprinted 1986].

16 Balint E and Norell J (eds) (1983) *Six Minutes for the Patient: interaction in general practice consultations*. Tavistock Publications, London.

17 Kolb DA (1984) *Experiential Learning: experience as the source of learning and development*. Prentice Hall, Englewood Cliffs, NJ.

18 Revans R (1982) *The Origins and Growth of Action Learning*. Chartwell Bratt, Bromley.

19 Tuckman BW (1965) Development sequence in small groups. *Psychological Bulletin*. **63**: 384–99.

20 Walton HJ (1997) *Small Group Methods in Medical Teaching*. ASME medical education booklet no. 1. Association for the Study of Medical Education, Edinburgh.

21 Mulholland H (1994) Teaching small groups: facilitating learning. *Hospital Update*. **20**: 382–4.

22 Visschers-Pleijers AJSF, Dolmans DHJ, de Lang BA *et al.* (2006) Analysis of verbal interactions in tutorial groups: a process study. *Medical Education*. **40**: 129–37.

23 De Grave WS, Boshuizen HPA and Schmidt HG (1996) Problem-based learning: cognitive and metacognitive processes during problem analysis. *Instructional Science*. **24**: 321–41.

24 Molyneaux J (2001) Interprofessional teamworking: what makes teams work well? *Journal of Interprofessional Care*. **15**: 29–35.

25 Mitchell BS, McCrorie P and Sedgwick P (2004) Student attitudes towards anatomy teaching and learning in a multiprofessional context. *Medical Education*. **38**: 737–48.

26 Freeth D and Nicol M (1998) Learning clinical skills: an interprofessional approach. *Nurse Education Today*. **18**: 455–61.

27 Tucker K, Wakefield A, Boggis C *et al.* (2003) Learning together: clinical skills teaching for medical and nursing students. *Medical Education*. **37**: 630–37.

28 Ker J, Mole L and Bradley P (2003) Early introduction to interprofessional learning: a simulated ward environment. *Medical Education*. **37**: 248–55.

29 Areskog N (1994) Multiprofessional education at the undergraduate level – the Linköping model. *Journal of Interprofessional Care*. **8**: 279–82.

30 Reeves S, Freeth D, McCrorie P and Perry D (2002) 'It teaches you what to expect in future …': interprofessional learning on a training ward for medical, nursing, occupational therapy and physiotherapy students. *Medical Education*. **36**: 337–44.

31 Kirk A, Parish K and Buckingham I (2006) Interprofessional education – the benefits and drawbacks of an interprofessional training ward. Paper presented at the 12th International Ottawa Conference on Clinical Competence, New York, 20–24 May.

32 O'Halloran C, Hean S, Humphris D and Macleod-Clark J (2006) Developing common learning: the New Generation Project undergraduate curriculum model. *Journal of Interprofessional Care*. **20**: 12–28.

33 Tiberius RG (1990) *Small Group Teaching: a trouble-shooting guide*. Ontario Institute for Studies in Education Press, Toronto.

34 Barrows HS (1988) *The Tutorial Process* (2e). Southern Illinois University School of Medicine, Springfield, IL.

35 Schmidt HG, van der Arend A, Moust JHC *et al.* (1993) Influence of tutors' subject-matter expertise on student effort and achievement in problem based learning. *Academic Medicine*. **68**: 784–91.

Further Reading

Bion WR (1952) Group dynamics: a review. *International Journal of Psycho-Analysis*. **33**: 235–47. [Reprinted in: Klein M, Heimann P and Money-Kyrle R (eds) (1955) *New Directions in Psychoanalysis*, pp. 440–77. Tavistock Publications, London; Bion (1961), pp. 141–91].

Bion WR (1961) *Experiences in Groups*. Tavistock Publications, London.

Campkin M (1986) Is there a place for Balint in vocational training? *Journal of the Association of Course Organizers*. **1**: 100–104

Dennick R and Exley K (2004) *Small Group Teaching: tutorials, seminars and beyond*. Routledge, Abingdon.

Habeshaw S, Habeshaw T and Gibbs G (1988) *53 Interesting Things To Do in Your Seminars and Tutorials*. Technical & Educational Services, Bristol.

Jacques D (2000) *Learning in Groups: a handbook for improving group work* (3e). Kogan Page, London.

Jacques D (2003) Teaching small groups. *British Medical Journal*. **326**: 492–4.

Lee A and Higgs J (1988) How to help students learn in small groups. In: Cox KR and Ewan CE (eds) *The Medical Teacher* (2e), pp. 37–47. Churchill Livingstone, Edinburgh.

McGill I and Beaty L (1995) *Action Learning, a Guide for Professional, Management & Educational Development* (2e). Kogan Page, London.

Newble D and Cannon R (2001) Chapter 3: Teaching in small groups. In *A Handbook for Medical Teachers*, (4e) pp. 39–54. Kluwer Academic Publishers, Dordrecht.

Norman GR and Schmidt HG (2000) Effectiveness of problem-based learning curricula: theory, practice and paper darts. *Medical Education*. **34**: 721–8.

Weinstein K (1995) *Action Learning: a journey in discovery and development*. Harper Collins, London.

Westberg J and Jason H (1996) *Fostering Learning in Small Groups*. Springer Publishing Company, New York.

Lectures and large groups

Andrew Long and Bridget Lock

KEY MESSAGES

- Lectures continue to be one of the main methods of knowledge transmission in both undergraduate and postgraduate education, despite evidence to suggest that they have little impact on 'deep' learning.

- A better understanding by lecturers of the limitations of the human memory, and the ability of the learner to be able to concentrate over an extended period of time, could lead to lectures becoming more effective learning opportunities.

- A well-structured lecture with explicit learning objectives, defined contextual relationships and linkage of theory to experience is more likely to maximise the learning opportunity for those attending the lecture.

- Preparation by those attending the lecture as well as those organising and speaking will enhance the educational experience.

- Lectures provide a focus for the 'community of learners', offering opportunities for extended learning and professional conversations that can serve to widen debate and offer knowledge-sharing opportunities for all participants.

- Interactivity during lectures is an important adjunct to allow questioning and engagement of the learners, which is likely to improve the learning experience.

- A range of different techniques may be employed to engage larger groups in constructive learning processes that lead to better concentration and sustained enjoyment for all participants.

- Visual aids, used wisely, enhance the quality of the spoken word and improve the experience for most learners.

Some people talk in their sleep. Lecturers talk while other people sleep.

Albert Camus

Introduction

Traditional lectures, during which information is imparted to a passively receptive audience, have been the mainstay of undergraduate and postgraduate education for centuries, but there is an increasing body of evidence questioning the place of this style of learning in medical education. Only a small percentage of the information delivered during a lecture is retained, and often what is told does not equate to what is learnt.(1) Despite this widely recognised fact, most undergraduate courses continue to have a significant lecture component within their curricula and practising clinicians continue to choose to attend lecture-based meetings at the local, national and international level as part of their professional development. This suggests that even in the information-rich 21st century lectures still have a place.(2) The challenge is to reconcile the inherent educational problems of the lecture format with the expressed need of the professional community for

this activity and to use valuable professional time productively.

This chapter explores the difficulties of the lecture format from both theoretical and educational perspectives and aims to offer practical solutions on how the organisation and delivery of lectures can be adapted to effectively meet the educational needs of clinicians of both current and future generations. As with much of this volume, although the focus for this chapter is on medical education, the messages within it apply equally well across the healthcare professions.

Clinical Knowledge

Clinicians require what has been termed *propositional* knowledge to inform their practice.(3) Such knowledge is available in the public domain and provides a shared theoretical and practical base for the profession's activities. Propositional knowledge is available from published sources – journals, textbooks, the Internet – or educational programmes, examinations and courses, and an experienced doctor can easily find and acquire the necessary facts. But the complex professional activity of clinical practice cannot be described by a simple algorithmic processing of data alone, as it requires an amalgam of propositional, practical, situational, technical and *personal* experiential knowledge applied to each new situation to make

Understanding Medical Education: Evidence, Theory and Practice.
Edited by T Swanwick. © 2010 Association for the Study of Medical Education. ISBN 978-1-4051-9680-2.

a justifiable, informed clinical judgement.(4) Each new piece of knowledge that comes the clinician's way is judged in relation to its applicability to the context of everyday practice.(5)

Developing knowledge that is useful to practice is a professional duty.(6) Knowledge to inform clinical decision making is derived from a number of sources, including reflection on the variance of actual to expected outcome.(7) It is the unexpected that can yield the most benefit to an individual's fund of experiential knowledge, and the capacity to manage uncertainty and the unexpected is a hallmark of a professional.(8) Solitary reflection is important in developing practice but in itself is not sufficient. Like medicine itself, professional learning is a social activity. If lectures, for instance, are to be of any worth, they need to be valued by the community of learners, and they also need to offer an insight into the context in which the knowledge was generated,(9) its place within accepted wisdom and how it fits into or serves to modify current practice. The presentation must be delivered in a manner that can be readily assimilated by clinicians and drawn on when required for clinical practice.(10)

Communities of Practice

Deeply embedded in the medical profession is the concept of specialisation and the development of expertise for both a broad aspect of practice and the opportunity to sub-specialise into smaller divisions. Each of the subspecialties may be viewed as communities of practice, united by a professional activity, focusing on a particular area of expertise.(11) Each member of the community holds a professional duty to engage in continuing professional development. This includes both learning and teaching of specialist professional knowledge in its widest sense, and assessment of the value of new information for patients through questioning of, and deliberation on, emerging research knowledge within a 'safe' professional grouping. By engaging in debate about practice, the scale of import of new and current research can be determined.

New entrants to the community have to learn the tradition and knowledge of the profession for its continuity. Working within the professional community and engaging in conversation about the work of the community enables situated learning and allows limited participation of newcomers.(12) A professional works in dialogue with a patient but develops the expertise that professionals need to draw on for practice within their professional community, with all the multiple interrelationships and opportunities for learning that membership implies. Through these 'professional' conversations, the professional then learns to 'walk-the-walk' and 'talk-the-talk' of professional practice.(13)

Communities of practice have cognitive benefits too. By researching a case alone, a doctor can only have a unique view of a piece of information attained in whatever form. However, this may not be a sufficient depth of knowledge to practise safely. It is too limited in its range of viewpoints to gauge its value when the doctor is required to make a clinical judgement. A critical collaborative review of research knowledge or an overview of a subject will reveal the flaws in an argument and allow the identification of strengths or weaknesses of new research and due interpretation in the context of accepted practice. In-depth enquiry and group discussion through questioning can bring fallacies to light. The larger the number and variety of experiences among discussants, the better the insight into the value of a piece of information.

In order to deliberate, communities have to meet, and although teleconferencing and web-based discussion forums are now readily available, the interaction and opportunities for learning can be rather one-dimensional. However, if the community is to assemble, then learning needs to be facilitated, and this requires some structure and planning. A lecture or large group can provide this opportunity.

Lectures and Learning

Within a community of practice a range of educational activity can occur, with the method of learning varying according to the nature of the subject matter. A balance of all types of educational activity is needed as one style of learning does not suit all.(14) Bligh has usefully summarised the evidence that provides the basis for the continuance of lectures as a useful instructional method.(15) It is suggested that lecture is at least as effective as any other method for transmitting information. However, while lectures can provide a new insight into a difficult subject matter, and provoke thought and debate, there is little evidence to suggest that they have any role in modifying behaviour or values, or in inspiring interest. On the contrary, lectures have the potential to induce a sense of complacency in the recipient, as they take notes in the ill-founded belief that this information can be recalled from memory when needed. Alternatively, and perhaps even more dangerously, lectures may engender a sense of inadequacy and impotence as listeners are overwhelmed by the volume of information for which they have no context and can develop no new understanding. In this instance, they will have no opportunity to situate the initial information with present knowledge before more complex ideas are delivered, and may be left disheartened and disengaged.

If the purpose of a given learning event is the presentation of new information, a review of new developments in an area of study, or merely to highlight some

BOX 10.1 Where's the evidence: Attention and recall

During the course of an hour-long lecture:

- attention is at its height during the first 10–20 minutes and the final five minutes(27)
- the most note taking occurs during the first 10 minutes(28)
- only 42% of the key points of a lecture can be recalled immediately afterwards
- this drops to 20% within one week

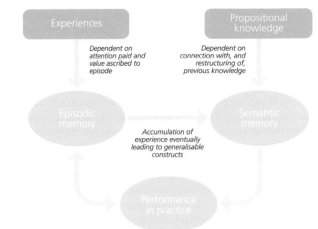

Figure 10.1 Memory, learning and performance. Source: Eraut(19).

key issues, then a lecture format may be appropriate. If this is the case then the manner of presentation should aid learning, and how this task is approached depends on an understanding of how learning occurs from a psychological and physiological perspective.

Memory, learning and performance

Theories of how memory is laid down and knowledge retrieved for later use offer some insight into how a presenter might support his or her audience in their learning. As words are heard and understood they are assimilated into working or short-term memory through the recognition of patterns and context. Without context, the information is forgotten if not learnt through immediate repetition. To secure the information into long-term memory, coding must occur.(16) Long-term memory is thought to have two components: an *episodic* memory for events and a *semantic* recall for symbols, that is, words or numbers.(17) Episodic memory makes multiple associations or links with events, sequences, sounds, smells or sights over time. Recall is dependent on the importance of the event and on developed connections to other pieces of retained knowledge in its many forms (Box 10.1). Something heard may literally 'strike a chord' in relation to a patient seen or event experienced. Filing, or coding, episodes into long-term memory is personal, dependent on the attention paid and the value ascribed to the episode by the individual, as well as to how it connects with other previously retained knowledge.(18) Semantic memory relies on the classification and structuring of concepts built from individual experience. This takes time, and without adequate time to construct links and formulate code, information will not be assimilated into long-term memory and is subsequently discarded from short-term memory. The relationship between learning memory and professional performance is summarised in Figure 10.1.

Limits to learning

Key to all this is that there is both a physiological *rate limit* to the system (too fast a delivery and the mechanism of retention is overwhelmed) and a physiological

capacity to the system (overload of information will lead to a lack of capacity for retention). The capacity of the system relies on a fully engaged concentration generated by motivation for the learning task in hand.

The presenter should heed these physical limitations and take care not to swamp the memory with too much information delivered too fast or exceed reasonable concentration limits. Some tactics can be adopted to enhance memory, for example, providing the description of an event, setting memorable context or assisting in the development of relevant connections or anchors.(20) Lecturers must offer an opportunity for questioning at reasonable time intervals, enabling listeners to check their construction of knowledge and reveal and correct misunderstandings. As little is recalled after 20 minutes of uninterrupted concentration,(21) introducing variety in presentation every 15–20 minutes will aid learning (Figure 10.2). A listener needs an opportunity to participate or question to avoid misinterpretation and incorrect integration into existing knowledge. The marked decline in attention after 15 minutes might offer the opportunity for a brief anecdote illustrating the principles described by the lecture. This will act to embed the delivered ideas in the narrative component of the listener's long-term memory, complementing information stored in conceptual or semantic memory.(22)

Figure 10.2 Audience concentration during standard lecture with and without interaction. Source: Higher Education Academy Engineering Subject Centre(24).

Worse still, Bligh describes processes that may result in memory *loss*: *retroactive* and *proactive* interference.(15) The former relates to when there is a requirement to learn a new series of facts shortly after committing the first set to short-term memory, such as in successive lectures. The latter is where memorising the first set of facts interferes with remembering the second set. Presenters therefore need to take account of both the volume and the concordance of the subject matter presented. It is also relevant to note that there is a beneficial effect in repetition, which has the opposite effect of interference and tends to consolidate learning, although if learning has not taken place the first time (i.e. the listener did not understand), then repetition has no additional benefit.

This has necessarily been a simplified description of a dynamic and complex process, but viewing a presentation from the perspective of the learner's capability to assimilate new information may assist lecturers in structuring their presentation to facilitate, rather than inhibit, learning. Useful learning occurs when the learner makes connections with pre-existing knowledge and can anchor new knowledge to previous concepts.(20) A context for information is also needed both for understanding and for recall. The level of understanding will depend on the listener's level of expertise; those that already have core knowledge will find their knowledge base enhanced in a different way to a naive listener. Similarly, a generalist in a field may enlarge his or her range of expertise. Each listener will have personal levels of depth and breadth of understanding related to past experience and motivation for learning. What is learnt depends on knowledge of the range of the subject; old information may become obsolete or be viewed with different importance, and new information develops and finds a place. But this will only be of use in patient care if the learner has the internal connections to draw out the information when needed and put it into practice (Box 10.1).

Lecturing and listening

Lecturing, then, offers an opportunity for a student or a practitioner to establish where the new information sits in his or her present knowledge. The resultant new knowledge will be unique to the learner as it is the result of selective attention and engaged interest, and the product of the learner's active efforts to relate new knowledge to pre-existing concepts.

The listener has social responsibilities as a participant and needs to be more than a passive recipient of information. The lecturer has offered his or her view, but the use remains the prerogative and responsibility of the recipients as they integrate what they hear into their established knowledge and in doing so have the opportunity to reshape it.(23) Before a lecture is delivered, the listeners should take a little time to prepare, even if it is only to ask himself or herself, 'What do I know of this subject?' and call to the front of his or her

consciousness his or her present understanding. It is not unreasonable for the listeners to challenge themselves, or the arguments of the lecturer, as this level of mental engagement facilitates the active process of learning, develops additional connections and aids coding into long-term memory. The role of active listening also involves noting problems of understanding for questioning at an appropriate opportunity.

Until this point, it has been implied that the deliverer is always 'the expert' and that the recipient is always a novice to the subject. This is not necessarily the case. In most national and international settings, research workers with expertise in a localised area of knowledge will present their ideas to an audience with profound experience in their field for adjudication of its value to present knowledge. In contrast, at the local level, a young doctor may present a difficult case for debate by a group of experienced doctors to advance his own clinical judgement through public deliberation on practice. An experienced teacher may lay out the framework of a topic for first-year undergraduate medical students in the morning and listen to a visiting professor discourse on a specialist subject in the afternoon. These are examples of a community of professional educational practice where the roles taken by participants vary, depending on the educational purpose of the activity. What is learnt by listeners and deliverers will vary with circumstance, but the teachers may learn as much or more than the learners. In some roles, what is learnt may demonstrate an individual's need for help in developing clinical understanding. This is a different purpose from the transmission of information in a didactic fashion. The organisers of the meeting and the presenters need to take heed of underpinning theory to enable effective learning to occur, especially the time for discussion. And it is to the organisation and delivery of effective lectures that we turn next.

Putting Theory into Practice

Organisational aspects

Lectures have the advantage of economy of scale, but to be cost-effective they must succeed in their primary purpose. At all levels of education the number of individuals that can be 'taught' by a single lecturer is increased by the use of this format. The more 'students' that can be taught by a single 'teacher' the better the return on investment, and as academic staff are relatively expensive and in short supply, this seems to make good economic sense. It is not often the case that those responsible for managing the budgets within organisations are charged with considering the value of the intervention for the recipient.

Organisers need to make sure that there is clear guidance for chair, speakers and listeners well in advance of the event. Electronic support for dialogue must be efficient and enabling of debate. A chairman must facilitate intelligently. At large gatherings, participants need time and information about the presentations on offer to enable choice of learning. Résumés of the presentation help recall at a later date and enable concentration during a delivery as listeners are not distracted by the need to scribble and can listen for understanding, annotating as they wish.

Since lectures form the backbone of most major conferences at the postgraduate level, often attended by thousands of delegates, many of whom have attained high levels of educational qualifications, it must be perceived by those attending that the lectures are of personal value. It would appear that those who attend voluntarily, as part of an educational plan, expect to be educated and are therefore prepared to engage with the educational process. There are, of course, a multitude of reasons why delegates choose to attend conferences, and it will be a little different for each of them.

If we assume that most people who attend lectures are motivated to do so, then it offers an opportunity to enhance learning. The critical need is to ensure that those who attend remain engaged during the lecture as there is evidence to suggest that not all who attend are equal in terms of their ability to learn in a primarily auditory fashion;[25] their ability to work at the same pace; their high-volume memory capacity; their basic knowledge required for the lecture; and their note-taking ability.[26] At least part of the solution is to ensure that lecture techniques are optimised to accommodate the principles of learning discussed previously.

The public role of each participant should be clear for each educational activity. The lecturer should present and the audience should inquire for understanding. It is entirely inappropriate for a member of the audience to stand and offer a discourse of their own or interrogate the presenter. In some circumstances, however, the audience may become the teachers as they are invited to give a view of the weighting of the value of information. Explicit guidance must be offered to audience and presenters before the event, and signals for role changes must be made clear by the nominated chair to ensure the rules of the game are observed. Without guidance, the event becomes meaningless shambles to everybody's dissatisfaction because the activity will not fulfil its purpose.

Building the community

Delivering the content is not the only purpose of a lecture. A secondary function can be viewed as the essential creation of community links and exchange of clinical knowledge. The essential 'informal space' created by refreshment breaks offers the opportunity for attendees to engage in networking and community building. Collaborative learning is at the centre of developing communities of practice and credit needs to be given to the discussion that takes place between engaged learners united by a common goal and establishing virtual relationships where the focus is on the exchange of ideas and information.[11]

Providing adequate time, space and comfortable surroundings aids reflection on what has been heard. This can be offered within an informal setting or as more formal groups. The latter may benefit from a facilitator and a published summary, but the spontaneity of the former may be of considerable benefit to an individual's understanding. The development of extensive memory connections is enhanced by early revisiting of the material covered during dialogue with other participants. The provision of an unthreatening and intellectually stimulating learning environment is key to the success of both the formal and the informal educational event.

Developments in information technology and the ability to engage in a number of different modes of online learning have been challenges to the existing lecture format. A move towards transforming lectures and similar large-group settings to make them more academically and socially interactive is a welcome development. If teachers truly understand the limitations and potential of this teaching methodology, then there is an opportunity to significantly enhance learning.

Preparation

The most important part of any successful lecture is the preparation. The audience to whom the talk is to be given should be taken into account, and the lecturer should ask the course leader or conference organiser about the context and type of talk expected. Poor preparation may compromise whole teaching programmes and has led to many courses being poorly valued by either the recipient or the deliverer. If the assumption is made that each episode offers a unique educational event that will never be repeated and that its value will be enhanced by the contribution of the lecturer and the audience, then it is likely to be successful, enjoyable and well received. It is a fundamental principle of educational and professional practice that all participants should treat one an other with respect and courtesy. To do other than prepare for an educational event is discourteous.

Most lecturers who are asked to present on undergraduate courses or at international and national meetings are informed many months in advance, and it is common practice to start preparation of thought processes and development of ideas in debate with others a long time before the presentation. There is often a temptation to 'rehash' a previous lecture that has been well received. However, if the talk is not tailored to the specific context, it will be discordant and uncomfortable for both the recipients and the deliverer. This should be avoided as it does not show due regard for the new audience that will be receiving the talk, nor for the organisers of the meeting who have invited the lecturer. There are a number of valuable texts on how to present at meetings (*see* Further reading section), and many offer a wide range of 'hints and tips' for use by anyone, from novice to expert.

Brown and Manogue(29) outline a model that demonstrates the method by which the recipients of a lecture learn from the event. It is based on work from Baddeley,(30) which identified modes of information processing and their effect on human memory, and confirmed much of previous observational work undertaken by previous authors.(31) It suggests that there is a dynamic relationship between the lecturer and his or her audience that has a direct effect on the way the lecture is delivered. Four components seem to contribute to making lectures more effective:

- *intentions* of the lecturer *and* the recipient
- *transmission*, including both verbal and non-verbal messages
- *receipt* of key messages by the learner
- *output*, in terms of both the immediate response of the recipient and the ability of the learner to store information in short-term memory, transfer to long-term memory and effect changes in attitudes and behaviour.

The authors suggest that it is this reciprocity that makes it so difficult to convert lectures entirely to an electronic medium. Encouraging interaction is then essential to good learning but this may be denied to a live audience when programmers curtail discussion time in order to provide more speakers, or a lecturer, desperate to impart more facts, overruns into question time so denying the audience the opportunity to fully understand the speaker's reasoning through debate.

The principle of 'more is not always better' is useful to consider. As we have established, this simply overloads the long-term memory. Getting value from the activity in terms of its contribution to understanding and learning is more useful than documenting large volumes of talks. Professionals travel long distances to meet since they perceive the value of debate to professional practice and the ability to understand the information proffered.

There is a strong association between subject knowledge and competence in teaching.(29) But the most effective teaching is also underpinned by an insight into the knowledge and level of understanding of the audience. It is essential to successful lecturing to prepare the talk by taking into account the diversity of the stages of learning of the audience, and to structure the talk accordingly. The enthusiasm of the lecturer for their subject matter is a prime motivator in the interest level generated in the listeners, promoting engagement with the topic and encouraging a positive approach to learning. Therefore an in-depth knowledge and extended level of interest on behalf of the lecturer is much more likely to have a beneficial outcome for the student wrestling with understanding

new facts and concepts because they are much more likely to be explained in relatively simple terms.

One of the cardinal rules of lecturing is the requirement to set objectives. These should be stated early on in the presentation and repeated as often as necessary to optimise learning. It may also be necessary for the lecturer to try and understand what the student is feeling and how this affects the belief in the subject matter that the lecturer inspires. The outcome from the learning event should be the product of the understanding and feeling, which should aid interpretation and the ability to process information and store it in memory. This is helped by visual and auditory imagery, which aids recall from deeply stored memories. Too much detail and content within lectures blunts learning(15) – detail can be learnt from texts. Students most value explanation supported by a structure and framework on which to build concepts of learning.

It is therefore apparent that a lecturer needs to prepare an outline that fits the purpose before adding the content. If the lecturer can identify a clear path through the duration of their talk, it is highly likely they will convey that structure to the listener. A sense of order in the presentation of facts will aid learning as it will prevent the audience from having to make cognitive leaps in order to follow the train of thought – another possible source of interference in learning (*see* Box 10.2).

BOX 10.2 How to: Structure a lecture

Approximate timing of the performance is important to ensure understanding and maximum recall of the lecture content. Understanding of the human mind and memory offers a rationale for action about which a more detailed discussion is to be found in the text. Here is some guidance (and a rationale) for structuring a traditional hour-long lecture:

- 5 minutes: Introduction and scoping
  sets minds
- 5 minutes: Ascertain knowledge base question
  engages mind and memory
- 15 minutes: Delivery
  just enough new information – at just the right speed
- 10 minutes: Question and discussion
  set connections in long-term memory
- 15 minutes: Delivery
  check volume and speed of delivery
- 5 minutes: Questions
  consolidate connections
- 5 minutes: Summary and close
  pull it together

Content

The main danger for the lecturer is to try and cover too much in a single presentation. Too much information can cause a number of serious problems that may adversely affect learning. First, there is a temptation to increase the pace of delivery in order to include all the subject matter. Audiovisual aids become either too crowded or too numerous, and there is inadequate time for the learner to grasp the essential facts, add some context and transfer to note form. To compensate for the last factor, many lecturers produce printouts of the slides from their talk. This may lead to students attending, collecting the handout and leaving before the talk starts (or even more cynically, getting someone else to collect the paperwork). These actions deny the participants the most useful portion of the lecture: the interaction with the lecturer and the learning community.

It therefore makes sense for the lecturer to identify the key messages they wish to deliver, ensure this material is covered and fits into a logical structure and then enhance it with information that cannot be gleaned from written sources, such as practical examples, personal experience and expert insight. All participants, at any stage of learning, gain added value from examples that demonstrate the theory put into practice, harnessing episodic memory and encouraging contextual understanding.(32) It is often useful to introduce controversial or challenging components at key points during the presentation to excite (possibly flagging) interest and engage the attention of the participants. Experienced and skilful lecturers might allow (or even plan) some deviation from their 'script' if they feel it is likely to enhance understanding, and it might be worth identifying in advance such detours and possible variance in reaching the desired endpoint.

The content should be put into a structure that allows the learner to follow clearly the thought trains that underpin the delivery. This generally includes

- an *introduction*, which should be designed to capture the interest of even the most disaffected participant and provide some explanation of the context and importance of the subject matter
- the *body* of the presentation, which contains the facts that are to be presented
- the *conclusion*, where the main points should be emphasised and summarised.

Style

The style of lecturing relates in part to the experience, level of confidence and comfort of the lecturer, and in part to the type of presentation, the audience and the subject matter being covered. It also appears that there is considerable variation in lecturing style across cultures and academic disciplines,(33) which may reflect the different volume of material being delivered and affect the speed of delivery. Lecture styles do seem to have generational differences, perhaps reflecting learners' needs, or possibly because lecturers and institutions are becoming more aware of the limitations of their medium and adjusting style to match the evidence relating to effectiveness of lectures in general. Certainly, a move to a more participatory style has introduced a cultural shift – from a lecturer-centred to a learner-centred teaching event.

Dudley-Evans and Johns(34) identified three distinct lecturing styles that seem to be contributory to, or inhibitive of, interactivity during the lecture. The traditional *reading* style, where the lecturer sticks closely to a script, which is often pre-rehearsed, offers the least opportunity for interaction, is least conducive to learning and is probably obsolete in 21st-century informed society as the knowledge conveyed is best read from source. This style is often adopted by lecturers who lack confidence, either in themselves or in their material. It has been observed that this style offers the greatest opportunity of being 'the process whereby a lecturer's notes are transferred to a student notebook without the need for mental effort on anybody's part'. This type of lecture is more likely to be delivered in a monotonous fashion and may be less well understood by those for whom the language in which it is delivered is not their first language.(35) This style also encourages more monologues and less dialogue.

The second style of lecturing described is the *conversational* style, where the lecturer speaks more informally, either without notes or from a notation format rather than a script. It is helpful if the lecturer encourages discussion at regular intervals to check that learning is taking place. This more informal style encourages interaction and offers a more explanatory approach within lectures, and the tonal expression tends to have a more beneficial effect in engaging the learner. The additive effect of engagement facilitates learning by pacing to encourage physiological retention. The lecturer is generally more relaxed and less rigid in the lecture content. This style seems to be the most predominant in all areas of higher education.

The third lecturing style involves the lecturer taking a role as a performer. The *rhetorical* style is characterised by frequent digressions and asides. It is much more akin to daily conversation and implies a much greater sense of informality between the lecturer and the listener. The style is very interactive; the structure is less rigid and requires a great deal of confidence on the part of the speaker. The tempo of the lecture is much more upbeat, with a wide range of tonal variance, and it is often the style that is entertained when lectures are being video-taped, emphasising the function of the lecturer as a performer. It is, of course, the case that during a single lecture or study course, combinations of styles might be employed and use of audiovisual aids might well predetermine the style and content of the lecture.

Brown and Bakhtar(36) have taken a different approach to describing lecturing styles based on the characteristics of the individual lecturers. They describe that *oral presenters*, who tend to use no visual aids, are less likely to rely on notes and tend not to provide lecture notes. The *visual presenter*, on the other hand, tends to make full use of all media to aid explanation and uses diagrams and structures to help the student to understand. They are likely to use full notes and will offer more time to students during the lecture. The *exemplary performer* uses a wide range of techniques and is generally very confident in their presentation, offering students a highly structured approach and setting clear learning objectives. *Eclectic performers* also use a variety of techniques, including humour, but lack confidence and tend to be more disorganised, often digressing from the main content of the lecture, whereas the *amorphous talker* is very confident but ill-prepared, vague and less likely to consider the structure or objectives of their lecture.

Understanding the strengths and weaknesses of these lecturing styles is essential for the lecturer wishing to complement the learning process for the recipient and develop their own style. Careful thought in planning and preparing each lecture with due regard for the knowledge base of the audience, the agreed learning objectives and the time frame for presentation will avoid the novice lecturer falling into a style that fails to meet the needs of the audience.

Aids to lecturing

Visual aids can significantly enhance lecturing and add an extra dimension when explaining or describing difficult or complex inter-relationships. However, they can also be an unnecessary distraction, illegible and incomprehensible, and serve no purpose in aiding learning.(37) Therefore, if aids are used, they should complement the subject and the context being taught, add rather than subtract from the aural presentation, be instantly understandable and used appropriately.

The chalkboard and chalk as a teaching methodology, although still used in some parts of the world, has now been largely superseded by the whiteboard or flip-chart and coloured marker pens. This ancient technology has been updated in recent times by adding functionality such as the ability to electronically project, record and print written scripts, together with the use of magnetic strips and other highlighting techniques. When used appropriately it can be an extremely effective teaching aid, although it is generally more appropriate for smaller rather than large groups. However, its use requires careful thought and preparation to maximise its potential, as it is easy to produce a messy and even more confusing display if the contents are produced in an unstructured fashion. Its use is generally more suited to the conversational or rhetorical style of presentation, as there is more informality, and it can be used in a fashion where ideas are built

up throughout the duration of the lecture. It requires the lecturer to turn away from their audience, which results in some loss of interaction and the ability to gauge audience response. However, this medium can be used to encourage learner participation and engagement with the subject matter.

Thought should be given to both the colours and nature of the medium being used. The lecturer's handwriting is key to effective delivery, and complex diagrams should be planned well in advance. It is always best to start and finish with a clean board, and care should be taken that the marker pens used on whiteboards are water-soluble.

The overhead projector (OHP) became the medium that initially threatened the chalkboard as the premier teaching medium. The ability for the lecturer to face the audience while writing, the 'build' capacity where layered overheads could be interlaced to provide a structured diagram and the potential to prepare 'acetates' in advance were significant advantages in favour of the OHP. Once again this medium can prove to be as fallible as other media with their reliance on intact power supply, functioning bulbs and transparencies with colours that are visible and text that does not smudge. The OHP also offers the temptation to photocopy small text and complex diagrams onto transparencies in the hope that they will be comprehensible. There is continuing debate about the benefits of displaying each part of the screen sequentially or whether the whole screen should be displayed at the same time so that the observer is not constantly trying to guess what will be revealed next. Like all use of audiovisual media, in the hands of an expert they will enhance a good presentation, and for novice lecturers they provide the opportunity for additional clarity of presentation with relatively few technical demands provided the medium is used wisely.

The major change in the use of audiovisual aids for lecturing came with the Microsoft dominance of the world of personal computing and the introduction of 'bundled' Office software, which included PowerPoint. Before this, the 35-mm slide dominated significant educational events and was the recommended media for important talks prepared at any level, from local presentations to international meetings. Slides were generally difficult to prepare, expensive to produce and inflexible to change. The advent of widespread use of PowerPoint brought its own challenges as it became the accepted standard; however, the ability to transport talks easily was limited by disk capacity. Now the increased availability and relative cheapness of USB memory sticks has meant that almost any size of talk can be accommodated and changes can be made easily at any time before the start of the presentation.

The full functionality of PowerPoint is rarely utilised. However, it now dominates the audiovisual league table and is largely accepted as the international standard. There are many texts that offer sound advice on the best use of this media (*see* Further reading section), and it is not intended to replicate the information here. However, it is reasonable to review some of the strengths and weaknesses of this technology. The ability of PowerPoint to produce a full range of slides, outlines, lecture notes and handouts makes producing lecture material relatively easy, and talks can be translated from computer-projected slides to transparencies for projection on an OHP or even into web-based annotated presentations as part of a virtual learning environment. Nearly all lecture theatres, classrooms and auditoriums have PC projection equipment installed, and the relatively low cost of portable projectors and laptop computers has made this an increasingly affordable and transportable means of providing highly professional presentations in almost any venue.

All types of audiovisual aid have the ability to be abused, and generally the higher the degree of technological dependence, the higher the risk for the presenter. While the 'hard' technology has become increasingly reliable, the temptation for the lecturer to extend the limits of safety to achieve dazzling effects has sometimes overshadowed the message that is being promoted. PowerPoint comes with a range of colourful backgrounds, artistic fonts and highly sophisticated 'build' and 'transition' effects, complete with sound. There is the ability to add in video clips to enhance and extend the range of demonstrable material, and sometimes the technology becomes overwhelmed almost as much as the audience. Evidence suggests that increasing volume of images and competing inputs might challenge the ability of the learner to store the information being transmitted in their short-term memory.(38) It has also been clearly demonstrated(39) that students' perception of the images they are shown is highly variable, and it is often necessary for the lecturer to pause a presentation to emphasise a point or check that there is consensus on the material presented at that time.

There is little doubt that emerging technologies will make audiovisual media even more exciting in the future. The ability to provide images of 'virtual reality', the ability to video-conference across large distances and the possibility of widely distributed networks with interactive functionality introduces opportunities that are restricted only by the imagination of the presenter. However, it should always be remembered that the key objective is the imparting of information and any medium that clouds the message being presented is harmful, both for the learner and for the reputation of the speaker (*see* Box 10.3).

Delivery

The final and perhaps the most important aspect of lecturing is the presentation itself. Once the talk has been prepared, taking into account aspects of style, content and audiovisual aids, it is the lecturer's responsibility to convey his or her message clearly. This in

---

BOX 10.3 How to: Design a PowerPoint presentation

- Ensure that PowerPoint is the best format for the type of talk you are giving and the audience you are addressing.
- Use background colours and contrasting text that will be seen well – white or yellow on a blue background project well under most circumstances.
- Try to use the same font throughout and a type size that will be easily visible.
- Using bold type or text 'shadowing' can improve the legibility, and the use of bold, italics or underlining may serve to enhance key points.
- Don't overcrowd the slides – as a general rule there should be no more than seven words per line and seven lines of text per slide.
- Use 'exciting' slide transition and slide 'build' with caution – listeners might become more interested in the action on the slide rather than the message you wish to convey, although dynamic build sequence can enhance the message.
- Break up blocks of solid text with pictures, cartoons or photographs. Visual images can serve to imbed messages into long-term memory.
- Exercise caution with the use of graphics – try to use only simple graphs and tables that do not have too much information or require too much explanation.
- Running video clips from within presentations can produce spectacular results but is fraught with technical risks.
- It is best not to read the text from the slide but allow the audience to read the slide contents and talk around the key points raised.
- As a general rule allow one minute per slide – too many slides might lead to your talk overrunning, which will not be popular with the chairman or audience.
- Use an introduction slide to explain the structure of your talk and a summary slide of your conclusions – 'tell them what you are going to tell them; tell them; tell them what you have told them'.
- Practise your talks with a friendly audience so you can judge timing, content and presentation style.

---

itself requires some forethought and preparation no matter how experienced or skilled the lecturer. Much depends on the familiarity of the presenter with the group and the venue for the talk, but it is all too easy to become complacent, which in itself may prejudice an excellent presentation.

It is essential that the lecturer arrives at the venue in plenty of time to prepare themselves and (if appropriate) the group to whom they are presenting. Depending on the media being used, it will be necessary to check equipment, both for correct functionality and for ease of use, to gain familiarity with the mode of operation and to enable the presenter to feel comfortable. It may offer an opportunity to start a process of engagement with the learners, to check assumed knowledge levels and to demonstrate appropriate intent to ensure that learning opportunities are maximised.

When the presentation starts, the expert lecturer will take clues from the audience to judge the pace of the talk and the degree of detail required. The importance of maintaining eye contact with the recipients cannot be overemphasised, and interpretation of body language and non-verbal clues about their well-being and receptivity is learnt over a period of time. The novice lecturer might wish to gauge audience response by asking questions or inviting responses. Timing is very important and the risk of preparing and expecting too much has already been emphasised. All the evidence suggests that the more enthusiastic the presenter, the better prepared the presentation and the simpler the message, the more likely it is to be understood and to have a positive impact. The use of handouts as an aid to both clarity and retention is discussed in Box 10.4.

Beyond lecturing

Learning in all environments can be improved if learners are actively involved in the process, are expected to develop knowledge, receive feedback on their work and feel part of a community of learning. The organisation of a lecture can be adapted to increase its effectiveness in the light of new concepts of effective learning. Provided lecturers understand the context of the lecture and are prepared to try and establish the baseline knowledge of the audience, agree and set objectives from the lecture, and retain the interest of the listener by using interactive elements, they can be very useful educational events. Furthermore, the organisers should ensure that topics presented are current (and perhaps controversial) and that lecturers are selected for their presentation abilities, including their ability to engage with the audience, as well as their knowledge and experience. Structuring the programme to allow frequent breaks at roughly 20-minute intervals and encouraging participants to take notes, ask relevant questions and interact with other learners all helps to build the community of practice facilitating the development of collaborative professional working and learning.

A range of other techniques may be used to engage learners and create an environment of 'active learning' during the lecture. The Further reading section includes a book entitled *53 Interesting Things to Do in Your Lectures*, which includes a wide range of hints and tips designed to stimulate the interest of students and increase the enjoyment and effectiveness of lectures. *Cinemeducation. A comprehensive guide to using film in medical education* also includes a number of ideas on how commercial film clips may be used to liven up an

BOX 10.4 How to: Use handouts effectively

- Think clearly about the purpose of the handout – simple regurgitation of the PowerPoint presentation is easy to do but does not necessarily aid learning.
- Handouts may be the most effective way of conveying key, complex information and diagrammatic representations that need detailed explanation.
- Consider the audience to which you are talking and design the handout to suit the learning needs of those attending.
- An 'outline' handout may be just a one-page summary of the contents of the lecture with key references.
- Providing electronic 'hot links' and references within handouts will offer the opportunity for those attending the talk to undertake further reading at a later date.
- 'Skeletal notes', which contain a set of the lecture notes with pieces of information missing, might be valuable in maintaining attention, adding some interaction to the lecture and thereby enhancing learning.
- If you choose to provide printouts of a PowerPoint presentation remove unnecessary slides and use the format that best conveys the information required with minimum wasted paper (three slides or six slides per sheet).
- Consider whether you wish to provide handouts before the talk so participants can use them for note taking or distribute them after the talk so attention is not distracted during the presentation.
- Using a handout to set tasks or raise controversial issue for discussion may facilitate small group work within the lecture or provide material for 'break-out' groups following the talk.
- Handouts might be used to provide personal background information before a lecture to ensure commonality of knowledge across a whole group.
- It might be easier to make handouts available electronically after a talk, thereby reducing paper wastage and maximising the capability to provide electronic links for further information.

Source: Bligh(15) (Chapter 10, p.148)

otherwise dull subject and aid learning by providing a contextual basis for the subject of the lecture through the provision of examples. A range of other relatively simple techniques may also be used to break up a lecture and ensure audience participation.

Questioning

This is the simplest of interactive lecturing techniques, but often the most valuable. Individuals within large groups might potentially feel threatened, and this often leads to migration to the back row if there is a fear that questions will be asked and knowledge gaps identified. The wise lecturer, however, will judge the 'educational climate' and introduce this technique in a fashion that is non-threatening, such as through the use of humour to lighten the inevitable tension when questions are introduced. A simple 'show of hands' might provide the answer, and anonymised 'audience response' keypads are becoming ever more affordable. As a general rule, questions should be 'open' rather than 'closed' (yes/no answers), and used wisely, this technique will identify the level of group knowledge, enable planning of future direction and offer the opportunity for fears and concerns to be addressed. Allow plenty of time for responses, giving the audience time to think; if responses are poor, try rephrasing the question rather than offering an answer.

Buzz groups

While most traditional lecturers try to discourage talking between students attending lectures, an alternative approach is to recognise that this is likely to happen anyway and will encourage interchange of ideas at appropriate intervals. The concept is to set a task for groups of two or more students to discuss at regular intervals. The task can be related to the preceding section of the lecture or a controversial issue raised, or (perhaps even braver) it can provide the opportunity for the learners to 'shape' the next section of the lecture. The challenge is always to regain the interest of the students, but the task should include a requirement for selected feedback to the rest of the audience to maximise group learning.

Brainstorming

This is a method widely used in commerce and can be used by teachers to test group knowledge or discuss areas where there are likely to be a range of viewpoints. The lecturer invites answers to a question or problem from the audience, and it is important to emphasise that each contribution will be treated with equal importance and should be written down without further comment. The list of answers will then form the basis for a discussion with the audience and should lead naturally to the next part of the talk.

Snowballing

This aptly describes a process where each individual member of the audience is invited to work alone on a problem or issue for a couple of minutes, then share with their neighbour for a similar length of time, the two of them generating a discussion which they then share with another pair, and so on. This process can be time-consuming so it generally suits smaller groups, and enough time should be included to get useful feedback from all the groups before the lecture continues or comes to an end.

Nominal group technique

For some groups and suitable subject material, it may prove desirable to divide the audience into smaller groups with a set task. This particular technique gives all group members the right to express any opinion without challenge. All the group contributions are written down by a nominated group leader and time is then given for elucidation, explanation and challenge to the ideas raised. At this point similar items can either be aggregated if they are very similar, or disaggregated if a group's members feel they are materially different. After this period of discussion the group members are invited to vote for the issues raised, identifying their perceived importance, and the key issues are then fed back to the wider audience.

Evidence suggests that interactive lectures promote understanding in the audience rather than simply encouraging fact retention.(40) Interactivity also offers the opportunity for lecturers to check assumptions and participants to feel included, engenders collective learning and aids retention of learning through facilitating different learning styles and empowering the audience in the learning process.

Conclusion

Lectures will continue to hold a useful place among the methods of learning that may be included in the educational toolbox of medical educators. They will remain the bedrock for most professional and interprofessional educational meetings at the local, national and international level. However, to be effective, they must be employed judiciously with a clearly thought-through purpose for the presenter and the audience. The manner of delivery and the aids used must be carefully tailored to facilitate effective learning, giving due responsibility equally to the organisers, the lecturer and the audience, recognising the limitations of human physiology and taking heed of the capabilities and needs of the audience. Preparation for each unique learning event is essential and due regard should be given to the opportunity for those attending to continue discussion during refreshment breaks, sharing knowledge and good practice and continuing to build the community of learning. Due consideration should be given to the place of interactive learning, and lecturers might learn a great deal if they are required to sit through their own lectures, a learning opportunity that is now freely available through the use of modern digital recording techniques.

References

1 Dunkin MJ (1983) A review of research on lecturing. *Higher Education Research and Development.* **2**: 63–78.

2 Charlton BG (2006) Lectures are an effective learning method because they exploit human nature to improve learning. *Medical Hypotheses.* **67**: 1261–5.

3 Fish D and de Cossart L (2003) *Cultivating a Thinking Surgeon: new perspectives on clinical teaching, learning and assessment.* tfm Publishing, Shifnal, Shropshire.

4 Ashcroft RE (2004) Current epistemological problems in evidence based medicine. *Journal of Medical Ethics.* **30**: 131–5.

5 Dewey J (1938) *Experience and Education.* Macmillan, New York.

6 General Medical Council (1995) *Duties of a Doctor.* GMC, London.

7 Schön DA (1983) *The Reflective Practitioner: how professionals think in action.* Basic Books, New York.

8 Schön DA (1987) *Educating the Reflective Practitioner: towards a new design for teaching and learning in the professions.* Jossey-Bass, San Francisco, CA.

9 Eraut M (1994) *Developing Professional Knowledge and Competence.* Routledge Falmer, London.

10 Benner P (1984) *From Novice to Expert: excellence and power in clinical nursing practice.* Addison-Wesley, London.

11 Wenger E (1998) Communities of practice: learning as a social system. *Systems Thinker* (http://www.co-i-l.com/coil/knowledge-garden/cop/lss.shtml; accessed 27 July 2007).

12 Lave J and Wenger E (1991) *Situated Learning: legitimate peripheral participation.* Cambridge University Press, Cambridge.

13 Swanwick T (2005) Informal learning in postgraduate medical education: from cognitivism to 'culturism'. *Medical Education.* **39**: 859–65.

14 Stenhouse L (1975) *An Introduction to Curriculum Research and Development.* Heinemann, London.

15 Bligh DA (2000) *What's the Use of Lectures?* Jossey-Bass, San Francisco, CA.

16 Entwistle NJ (1988) *Styles of Learning and Teaching.* David Fulton, London.

17 Tulving E (1972) Episodic and semantic memory. In: Tulving E and Donaldson W (eds) *Organisation of Memory,* pp. 381–403. Academic Press, London.

18 Neisser U (1976) *Cognition and Reality.* Freeman, San Francisco, CA.

19 Eraut M (2000) Non-formal learning and tacit knowledge in professional work. *British Journal of Educational Psychology.* **70**: 113–36.

20 Ausubel DP (1968) *Educational Psychology: a cognitive view.* Holt, Reinehart and Winston, Austin, TX.

21 Stuart J and Rutherford RJD (1978) Medical student concentration during lectures. *Lancet.* **2**: 514–16.

22 Ellis AW and Young AW (1988) *Human Cognitive Neuropsychology.* Erlbaum, Hillsdale, NJ.

23 Biggs J (1999) *Teaching for Quality Learning at University.* Open University Press, Buckingham.

24 Higher Education Academy Engineering Subject Centre: guide to lecturing (http://www.heacademy.ac.uk/resources/detail/SNAS/snas_854).

25 Baddeley A (1992) Working memory. *Science.* **255**: 556–9.

26 Kiewra K (1988) Cognitive aspects of autonomous note taking: control processes, learning strategies, and prior knowledge. *EducationalPsychologist.* **3**: 39–56.

27 Verner C and Dickinson G (1967) The lecture: an analysis and review of research. *Adult Education.* **17**: 85–100.

28 Gardiner L (1994) Redesigning higher education: producing dramatic gains in student learning. George Washington University, Washington, DC. ASHE-ERIC Higher Education Report No. 7 www.ntlf.com/html/lib/bib/94-7dig.htm (accessed 1 August 2007).

29 Brown G and Manogue M (2001) AMEE Medical Education Guide No. 22: Refreshing lecturing: a guide for lecturers. *Medical Teacher.* **23**: 231–44.

30 Baddeley A (1996) *Your Memory: a user's guide.* Penguin, Harmondsworth.

31 Strodt-Lopez B (1991) Tying it all in: asides in university lectures. *Applied Linguistics.* **12**: 117–40.

32 Tulving E (2002) Episodic memory: from mind to brain. *Annual Review of Psychologychology.* **53**: 1–25.

33 Nesi H (2001) A corpus-based analysis of academic lectures across disciplines. In: Cotterill J and Ife A (eds) *Language across Boundaries,* pp. 201–18. BAAL in Association with Continuum Press, London.

34 Dudley-Evans A and Johns T (1981) A team teaching approach to lecture comprehension for overseas students. In: *The Teaching of Listening Comprehension,* pp. 30–46. ELT Documents Special. The British Council, London.

35 Chaudron C and Richards JC (1986) The effect of discourse markers on the comprehension of lectures. *Applied Linguistics.* **7**: 113–27.

36 Brown GA and Bakhtar M (1987) Styles of lecturing: a study and its implications. *Research Papers in Education.* **3**: 131–53.

37 Norvig P (2003) PowerPoint: shot with its own bullets. *Lancet.* **362**: 343–4.

38 Baddeley A (1996) *Human Memory: theory and practice.* Erlbaum, Hillsdale, NJ.

39 Abercrombie MLJ (1960) *The Anatomy of Judgment: concerning the processes of perception, communication, and reasoning.* Hutchinson, London.

40 The Higher Education Academy Social Policy and Social Work (SWAP) website (http://www.swap.ac.uk/learning/interactive1.asp; accessed 16 January 2007).

Further Reading

Alexander M, Lenahan P and Pavlov A (eds) (2005) *Cinemeducation. A comprehensive guide to using film in medical education.* Radcliffe, Oxford.

Bligh DA (2000) *What's the Use of Lectures?* Jossey-Bass, San Francisco, CA.

Brown G and Manogue M (2001) AMEE Medical Education Guide No. 22: Refreshing lecturing: a guide for lecturers. *Medical Teacher.* **23**: 231–44.

Cantillon P, Hutchinson L and Wood D (eds) (2003) *ABC of Learning and Teaching in Medicine.* BMJ Publishing, London.

Gibbs G, Habeshaw S and Habeshaw T (2000) *53 Interesting Things to Do in Your Lectures.* Cromwell Press, Trowbridge.

Hall G (ed.) (2007) *How to Present at Meetings.* Blackwell, Oxford.

Higher Education Academy Engineering Subject Centre Guide to lecturing (http://www.heacademy.ac.uk/resources/detail/SNAS/snas_854; accessed 16 January 2007).

Midmer D (2003) Presentation Magic. *BMJ Careers.* **326**: S120.

Newble D and Cannon R (1983) *A Handbook for Clinical Teachers.* MTP Press, London.

e-Learning

Jean McKendree

KEY MESSAGES

- Effective e-learning, or learning by using technology appropriately in various contexts, should be viewed as a curriculum design issue and not just use of a set of tools. Technologies are tools, not teachers.

- Blended learning, combining online and face-to-face teaching, is the most common approach to incorporating e-learning in medical schools.

- Using technologies effectively requires knowledge of how people learn, how to design interactions with the tools and how to evaluate best use given the desired learning outcomes.

Introduction

Read the following quotes and guess which words fill the blanks. The answers are to be found below,* but no cheating!

> My judgment is that the _____ can do its part; that it is a perfectly legitimate and satisfactory way for distribution; that it would carry more genius to the common child than he has ever had or ever possibly could have …(1)

> _____ _____ have all the vital ability to influence and improve education that the printing press had five hundred years ago.(2)

> There is no limit on imagination. Thus there is no limitation on how you can use _____ _____ to communicate effectively with your class. Just as science is opening new vistas for mankind, _____ _____ is opening new doors for teaching.†

Claims about the ability of technology to transform teaching and learning are obviously not new. The latest emergent technology is invariably heralded as the 'killer' invention that will make learning effortless. Most recently, claims have been made that using computers and the Internet, an educational strategy often called e-learning, will recreate learning and even obliterate the need for teachers, schools and formal education:

> … the computer, and particularly, its future development, will change 'children's relationship with knowledge' producing a revolution comparable to that of the 'advent of printing and writing'.(4)

*Answers: radio, motion pictures, overhead projection.
†The quotes were collected and cited in an article in *Phi Delta Kappan International*.(3) Used with permission.

Understanding Medical Education: Evidence, Theory and Practice.
Edited by T Swanwick. © 2010 Association for the Study of Medical Education.

> In the new economy, where mindcraft replaces handicraft as the main form of work, HL [hyperlearning] makes obsolete the teaching, testing, and failure on which academic credentialism rests.(5)

Such effusive pronouncements are usually followed by a period of backlash and criticism attacking the enthusiasts and calling for a return to basic, traditional teaching, whatever that is conceived to be at the time. The aim of this chapter is to steer a course through this sea of hyperbole to find a safe harbour for those who are interested in using e-learning, but would like to anchor it on the rocks of research evidence and shared best practice.

Technologies on their own will not alter the fundamental fact that learning a discipline such as medicine always requires considerable effort on the part of students and teachers. However, there is evidence that technology can enhance teaching and learning, when used thoughtfully and appropriately. This guide outlines such approaches based on available research on using new (and not so new) computer technologies effectively. There are some references to examples and web sites in the text and at the end of the publication, but these have been kept brief deliberately, as there is no guarantee that the links will be there when you look for them – one pitfall of the Internet as a learning resource.

Computer-based Teaching‡

The term 'electronic learning' or e-learning is currently used in a variety of ways. Sometimes it refers to

‡Some portions of the section on computer-based teaching packages were written by the author for the Higher Academy Subject Centre for Medicine, Dentistry and Veterinary Medicine web site and have been adapted here with permission.

learning in which some content or activity is delivered via computers in any way, sometimes to learning content from the Internet and sometimes to using a virtual learning environment (VLE). For the purposes of this chapter, I use the term e-learning to refer to any computer-aided approaches, although this use of the term is waning and the Internet and VLE meanings are becoming more common. However, as many of the concepts apply to the wider scope, I will first cover non-internet-based learning approaches, as much of the fundamental research on effective learning with computers has been done in these areas.

So, does electronic or computer-based learning 'work'? There are so many different types of and approaches to e-learning that it is almost impossible to give a simple 'yes or no' answer to this question. Instead, I will break it down a bit into some different kinds of materials and look at some key research evidence.

Hypertext or Online Reading Resources

Hypertext, or electronically linked, non-linear text, began being used seriously in the late 1980s when HyperCard became available on the Macintosh computer, although the basic concept was outlined by Vannevar Bush in 1945(6) and the term 'hypertext' was coined by Ted Nelson in 1963.(7) Early hypertexts tended to be tightly constructed, stand-alone programmes, rather like electronic textbooks. With the advent of the Internet, this type of resource varies now from online books, to packages of organised and inter-related materials, to random collections of text studded with links to pages all over the world.

Here I shall look only at the hypertext resources that have been designed with teaching in mind and consist mostly of text, perhaps with images, animations and videos. Do these facilitate learning? Does a textbook? The answer to both is, of course, 'yes', but only if the person reading the material pays attention and engages at a deep level. A great deal of research has shown that people who read material actively, that is, asking questions as they go, stopping to summarise points, taking notes, anticipating what the author will write next, can learn effectively from either online or paper texts.(8)

Such learning depends not only on the learner, but also on the quality of the resource. Just as some books are not very good, some web pages are not very useful. What is *not* effective is to put up a large amount of poorly structured, fragmented material with no guidance about what is intended to be learnt from it or how to approach learning.(9) Studies of hypertexts show that comprehension from large, complex, hyperlinked materials is generally poorer than from a well-structured book with the same information, and that readers tend not to see all the available information – in effect they get lost in hyperspace.(10)

However, well-designed hypertext can be useful for learning when it makes explicit the connections between chunks of information in the domain (*see* Box 11.1). Navigating hypertext links can give the learner a clearer idea of the way that the information fits together in the domain to form a coherent whole. Some possible ways this can be accomplished is to design hypertexts around goal-oriented tasks, such as answering questions as they read, or by constructing a *concept map*(11) which explicitly displays the relationships between different sections of a hypertext. A good example of such an approach is the Visual Thesaurus at http://www.visualthesaurus.com.

Computer-aided Learning

Often e-learning software packages, particularly on CD-ROM, but increasingly web-based, have not only textual and pictorial information, but interactive exercises as well. This type of package is referred to as, variously, computer-aided learning, computer-based tutorials or training, computer-assisted instruction or simply courseware. Many such packages have self-assessment questions included as students work through the software. Given equivalent amounts of time, students using these types of package that more or less reproduce a textbook – with perhaps some animations and assessment questions – generally learn at a very similar level to the level they would learn at if they were using a textbook, and they often enjoy using the software packages more than they enjoy using textbooks. A screenshot of a typical computer-aided learning package is shown in Figure 11.1.

In some computer-aided learning packages, the student is presented with structured exercises empha-

The Retina: an annotated diagram

Retinal Ganglion Cells

Retinal ganglion cells form the third and final stage of the neural chain in the retina, conveying the results of retinal processing to higher visual centres.

They receive input from bipolar cells and thus combine the responses of several receptors, some of which have an excitatory influence, while others have an inhibitory effect.

Retinal ganglion cells also receive input from amacrine cells, which function to turn them off during prolonged, unchanging stimulation.

Figure 11.1 Example of a computer-assisted learning software screen.(12) Used with permission.

sising repeated practice of an increasing skill, often until a certain criterion is met. This was the fundamental idea behind BF Skinner's *Teaching Machines* in the late 1950s,(13) and more recently in *Integrated Learning Systems* used in many UK schools. A typical example would be a software that lets children practise addition and subtraction skills. Such programs have also been used to help students in the health professions become proficient at dosage calculations, radiograph interpretation, electrocardiogram lead placement and other skills that benefit from extended practice.

This type of 'drill-and-practice' software is sometimes maligned as being proscriptive, unimaginative and old-fashioned. However, when used appropriately, it can teach fundamental skills very effectively.

Using technology to practise basic skills can be highly effective according to a large body of data and a long history of use.(14) Students usually learn more, and learn more rapidly, in courses that use computer-assisted instruction (CAI). This has been shown to be the case across all subject areas, from pre-school to higher education, and in both regular and special education classes. Fletcher *et al*.(15) report that in the military, where emphasis is on short and efficient training time, the use of CAI can cut training time by one-third. CAI can also be more cost-effective than additional tutoring, reduced class size or increased instruction time to attain equivalent educational gains.(16)

While this kind of e-learning can indeed lead to better mastery procedures that lend themselves to repeated practice, research has shown that spaced exposure is very important – 10 minutes per day three to four times a week is more effective than 30–40

minutes at one go.(17) This is a finding backed up by decades of psychological research on learning in general – and which dictates against cramming for exams, too.

Again, the exercises need to be well designed. This crucial issue of instructional design is important in all forms of teaching, of course, and is one that is all too frequently ignored. Another reason for the effective learning seen in these systems is the delivery of instantaneous feedback. Feedback is critical for all learning, but immediate feedback is especially effective when basic skills are involved, where practising incorrectly can cause a wrong method to become engrained and difficult to change.(18)

Simulations

A giant step up in complexity from these practical exercise-based systems is simulation. In simulation, a student must work through an exercise of some sort, but one that exemplifies much of the complexity of a real-world situation. Simulations may or may not involve instructional feedback; the problems may be highly complex or relatively simple. In all of these, the goal is for the student to actually *apply* knowledge in order to solve the problem or resolve the situation in an environment that attempts to capture at least some of the important features of the real world.

These types of programme can lead to very effective learning if they capture the critical characteristics of the situation the student is intended to be learning. It

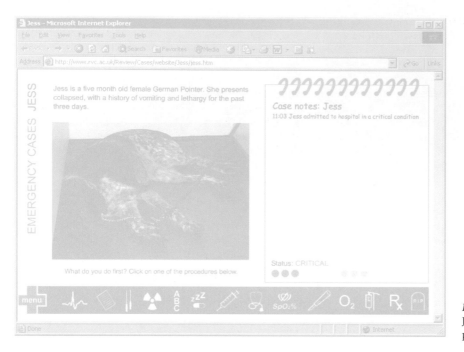

Figure 11.2 Example simulation: Jess the dog.(20) Used with permission.

is fairly obvious, and there is plenty of supporting evidence, that high-fidelity (and highly expensive) simulators such as those used for teaching airplane pilots or surgeons can be effective.

Less high-fidelity e-learning simulations can also teach students effectively when they emphasise the reasoning and knowledge underlying the concepts being taught. For example, BGuILE(19) simulates the activities of collecting and analysing data to learn about variation and microevolution using the example of finches from the Galapagos Islands. Figure 11.2 shows Jess the dog, from the Royal Veterinary College (follow the web link listed on page 162), as an example of a web-based, structured simulation requiring application of knowledge. Regrettably, I have not yet managed to save Jess.

However, with such simulations there can be a problem with students becoming proficient at playing the 'game' without learning the underlying lessons. The Sim-series, such as SimCity, SimLife and now SimUniversity, are highly sophisticated and complex programmes in which players design and manipulate parameters of various systems and undoubtedly they can help students to learn something about the concepts being simulated. Sometimes, though, students learn to run the simulations with a high degree of skill, but learn nothing about the underlying concepts that were the intended learning target.(21)

It is critical to combine relatively unstructured simulations such as this with discussions of the concepts they are intended to illustrate and specific tasks or assessments in order to best promote learning. Any exercise using concrete examples, electronic or not, can benefit from being explicitly framed in the larger domain to promote a grasp of abstract concepts.(22) Indeed, to be effective, the e-learning approaches discussed in this publication should always be embedded and framed in an educational environment that includes activities, discussion and reflection – this 'learning conversation' is designed to be conducive to promoting effective learning.

The range of available simulation equipment and the effective design and use of simulation is covered in detail in Chapter 12.

Intelligent Tutoring Systems

In the 1980s, researchers began to develop electronic tutoring systems based on cognitive models built up from observations of the actual learning processes used by students, rather than by simply structuring material based on textbooks or how designers think students might best learn. By modelling what a good student would do, these 'intelligent tutors' can dynamically track the progress of students as they apply their knowledge to problems, give context-sensitive feedback and model common errors that students make in order to present problems in a sequence optimised for each learner and offer specific advice on areas to review.

Studies of these tutors for algebra, geometry, statistics, physics and programming found that students could learn material in one-half to one-third of the time needed in traditional classrooms, perform 15–25% better on assessments and perform 50–100% better on complex problem solving in the domain. These types of tutor also seem to benefit weaker students the most.(23)

These results are undoubtedly due to a combination of factors: focused practice, instant feedback, strong instructional design based on detailed models of learning, and well-integrated supporting materials (including the teacher) to enhance conceptual learning. However, these tutors have been designed for procedural problems – areas in which there are exercises that can be set and worked through in a reasonably standard way – and they are expensive and time-consuming to build, so can only really be created for domains in which curriculum goals are not likely to change rapidly. Nevertheless, this is a very effective approach that could be explored further in the future in medical education, perhaps for teaching in such areas as informatics, evidence-based practice, routine diagnosis, radiological interpretation or pharmacological procedures in which extended practice on a range of problems is useful for developing well-honed skills, and expert pattern recognition. One example of a tutor of some relevance to medicine is the genetics tutor currently being piloted at Carnegie Mellon University (*see* web links on page 162).

Learning Styles and e-Learning

There is an intuitive appeal to the popular idea that multimedia or interactive computer-based courseware may be effective because it caters to different learning styles. While this may be true, evidence is very mixed and the area is controversial. One difficulty is that there are many different meanings of 'learning style' and many different instruments to measure it. A systematic review of learning style studies(24) found over 70 different measures being used in the literature, only a handful of which had been researched sufficiently to make sound judgements about reliability or predictive validity.

There is also variation in the underlying assumptions about where learning style differences might originate. The measures found in the review suggested three sources of learning style variation: constitutional, ability and instructional preferences.

The *constitutional* measures, implying an innate or fixed trait, tend to be tied either to sensory modality (e.g. visual, kinaesthetic or auditory) or to a stable personality measure. The review concluded that there was no reliable evidence that matching teaching either to adult learners' measured sensory preference or to their personality measure aided learning. In fact, some studies cited suggested that pictorial materials helped *all* learners, no matter what their self-reported preference, and may have had the biggest benefit for those labelled as 'verbal' by the learning style instruments.

Nevertheless, there is evidence that presenting information in more than one modality may help all learners, no matter what their particular score on any given measure.(25) The 'dual-code' theory(26) that originated in the 1970s indicates that presenting information in multiple ways allows learners to integrate knowledge by having multiple representations and links, so that assimilation with existing knowledge is stronger and therefore recall is improved.

Ability measures of learning style are those that consider that learners have relatively stable, if not fixed, abilities that direct their learning preferences and are not likely to change (e.g. convergent-divergent thinking, focusing-scanning). Again, there is inconclusive evidence that matching teaching and learning styles promotes better learning, but another confounding factor is that these measures tend to be correlated with various measures of aptitude,(24) and thus may simply be reflecting variations in general intelligence rather than a 'learning style' in the usual sense of equally effective but different approaches to learning. There is much debate here whether instruction should match the students' abilities or should create a mismatch in order to encourage adoption of a wider range of approaches to learning.

The final category of learning style addresses *instructional* preferences or approaches to study. These tend to emphasise that students have preferences about approaches to learning, but these may be flexible depending on context and motivation. In fact, the evidence is that good learners are 'versatile': able to adapt their approach to what needs to be learnt and the amount of time available to do so. Probably one of the best known researchers in this area currently is Noel Entwistle, who has evolved the Approaches to Study Skills Inventory for Students (ASSIST) over the past 30 years.(27) The ASSIST instrument gives an indication of whether students tend to be deep, strategic or shallow learners. Entwistle discusses the difference between a student's *style*, which is the preferred approach to learning, and *strategy*, which is the approach adopted at any given time according to the perceived demands of the task at hand.

Briefly, surface learners have an extrinsic motivation for learning: earning a high mark, fear of failure. Typically, this results in an emphasis on rote learning and a focus on getting through assessments. Deep learners have more intrinsic motivations: curiosity, commitment to the subject. They will make more of an attempt to analyse new knowledge, derive general principles and seek understanding, rather than learning just enough to pass exams. Strategic learners use a combination of strategies. They become adept at choosing study methods based on the cues they have picked up as to what type of work will result in the best outcomes for the given curriculum. Some studies have shown that medical school students, often the very good ones, tend to start out as deep learners, but may move towards being strategic, probably due to the heavy demands of a typical course plus the traditional emphasis on summative, knowledge-based assessments. In fact, strategic learning has a significant positive correlation with final marks,(28) so in the current climate, this may be the best strategy for students to adopt.

In the end, students will adopt what is suggested by the teaching – surface learning will emerge under time pressure and examinations that stress factual learning; deep learning emerges via extended activities, student–student interaction, learning conversations and perhaps problem-based learning.(29)

So what can we conclude about the relationship between these various style measures and e-learning? The lack of strong evidence for matching preferred style to presentation of learning content does not necessarily mean it is not useful, but this is a complex and contested area. While the debate rumbles on, it is best to design materials using as many of the modes of presentation as are appropriate to the domain, which may also tend to allow more flexibility in use, according to student needs. For instance, using text with an audio transcription that can be turned on or off will allow better access for students with limited sight, while the audio can be turned off for students who lack access to broadband networks and want the text only, or who can read faster than they can listen.

It is also the case that learning style measures can be useful as tools to generate a discussion with students about their own learning processes. Students often find these scales very interesting and can learn important lessons by working through one (it does not really matter which one) and then comparing their results with those of other students. This often demonstrates that people do not all choose to approach learning in the same way, which can be a useful insight for students and may help smooth tensions, for instance in a problem-based learning group in which people prefer to approach the learning along different paths.

Workplace-based Learning and Continuing Professional Development

In the previous sections, the emphasis has been on *e-learning* in a formal course of instruction, particularly in an undergraduate medical curriculum. Of course, doctors are learning informally and formally throughout their careers, in the workplace and through a process of continuing professional development (CPD). Increasingly, these established practitioners depend on technology for supporting this learning.

Some online resources offer easily accessible and quickly updated sources of information, such as the electronic British National Formulary (http://www. bnf.org), and the Merck Manuals (http://www.merck. com/pubs). While these are not e-learning tools per se, such resources begin to blur the lines between reference books and professional development tools. For instance, all general practitioners (GPs) in the UK now use computers in consultations, and many will regu-

larly consult systems such as GP Notebook (http:// www.gpnotebook.co.uk), an online reference database that also offers GPTracker, a service that tracks the information that the doctor has looked up and records it for use as evidence of educational activity during the year. The GP can then add personal notes and record their learning needs in the electronic record. Such integrated educational resources and planning tools are becoming more commonplace in practices worldwide.

Such 'just-in-time' learning, what Eraut(30) refers to as 'opportunistic' or 'reactive' learning, is where much new knowledge is encountered once doctors are practising. The danger with this approach is that such knowledge may remain tacit or disconnected from other knowledge and perhaps difficult to recall or apply in future. To be most fruitful, such informally encountered knowledge must be integrated with other experiences and eventually become more generalised so that it is not tied to a single context or incident. Time for reflection is needed to assimilate and clarify information, and turn such reactive learning encounters into more usable knowledge. Portfolio-based tools, such as the log book developed by the Royal College of Surgeons (http://www.elogbook.org/), are intended to promote this type of reflection on experience in a professional context.

Online CPD, a more formal approach to work-based learning, is becoming more commonplace. Some courses involve timetabled modules with online tutor support such as Medical Law for Medical Professionals (*see* web links on page 163). Some can be started at any time, but offer interactions with other students and tutors during a specified time period, as in the MDcme courses from Canada. Some offer modules that can be worked through at any time, with self-assessment questions at the end, which carry CPD credit, such as those offered by the American Medical Association.

Virtual Learning Environments

The term e-learning is often used to refer to the use of a *virtual* or *managed* learning environment. These systems are not actually learning technologies themselves, in terms of being the content to be learned, but they provide a framework or infrastructure into which materials are placed and in which activities take place. They are part of a larger learning environment, in the way that classrooms, computers networks and libraries are in a university. Just as these physical facilities need to be planned to be effective for students, so the choice and use of a virtual learning environment needs planning and support to be usefully implemented.

In general, although the terminology is still evolving, a VLE refers to the teaching and administrative tools available in a system, while a managed learning environment also includes tools such as those for admissions, finance and enrolment at an institutional level. You may also find these called Enterprise systems, which generally refers to very large, commercial VLEs intended to manage and integrate data from many institutional information sources. This section will refer to VLEs, because it concentrates on those tools that directly affect the tutors and students in a medical course. It does not go into any great detail about specific VLEs, since they are evolving constantly. For those who want to know more about systems, a number of web sites are listed in the Web links section at the end of the publication. The example screenshots are from the system used at Hull York Medical School, which happens to be Blackboard™, but this is not intended to be an endorsement, simply a convenience.

Blended Learning

There is a common misunderstanding that e-learning via a VLE implies that the course is a distance-learning course, that is, one in which the learner is at a location geographically distant from the tutors and never sees them face to face. There are some courses like this delivered using VLEs, such as those from the Open University (www.open.ac.uk), but VLEs are actually much more commonly used as one aspect of a course in which students meet regularly with

tutors and other students, sometimes in an otherwise relatively traditional course. This use of VLEs combined with face-to-face teaching is called *blended learning.*

The crucial aspect of blended learning is to think very hard about which aspects of a course are well supported by a VLE and which are best supported face to face, or in other ways. The next section reviews some of the current uses for VLEs in medical schools.

Tasks and Activities in Virtual Learning Environments

In the early days of the Web and VLEs, many course instructors simply put up all their lecture notes and PowerPoint presentations electronically and did nothing more. The VLE certainly can be a useful repository for *content* such as presentations, especially those with colour images that may best be viewed on a screen rather than on a small, black-and-white printout. Such content areas can be very useful for student revision by gathering the resources from each year into a single, readily accessible area, and they can help to manage content in the curriculum by timing the release of items, providing rapid updates of documents and allowing access to commonly used items such as student forms. The screenshot in Figure 11.3 shows a content area in which a radiograph appears as part of

Figure 11.3 Example of content in a virtual learning environment.(31) Screenshot from Hull York Medical School Blackboard™ VLE, copyright HYMS 2006.

a consultation with a 'virtual patient' and the VLE has posted an announcement for the students to review it for the next problem-based learning session.

There is an increasing number of repositories of useful electronic teaching resources being shared among institutions. They contain a variety of types of content, such as images, videos, short interactive exercises and self-assessment questions. These content items are often called *reuseable learning objects*. The concept behind this growing area is that objects can be designed to be downloaded and used flexibly in the local VLE by tutors in the context of their own curriculum, rather then having a large amount of fixed content such as most of the computer-aided learning packages discussed previously.

Another very common use of VLEs is to deliver assessment, either formative (that does not feed into an official assessment for the course) or summative (that is part of the official assessment). Most VLEs come with tools to write common types of questions such as multiple choice, extended matching, fill in the blank and true/false. Testing tools allow flexible administration, such as having tests appear and disappear either at a specified time or when a student has completed another activity satisfactorily, allowing students to have one or multiple attempts, presenting randomised questions, and marking automatically and entering the marks into an online gradebook. Also, many VLEs allow seamless integration of external online assessment packages such as Questionmark Perception™, which is widely used for both formative and summative exams (Box 11.2).

One of the more recent developments in VLEs is *ePortfolios.* While these tools are still developing, most allow students to organise and annotate any any materials they have online, including essays, personal statements, feedback collected from tutors, images, or any other item that might feed into a portfolio and is available electronically. Usually students can submit material to a specified tutor for marking and feedback, and the tutor mark will automatically be recorded in the online gradebook in the VLE. Some portfolio tools also allow students to sign up for tutorial sessions and record the agreed outcomes of such meetings, keep learning diaries, link evidence to specific learning outcomes for personal development planning or reaccreditation, or build an online curriculum vitae. The student can manage the content, so that material can be kept private, made public or permission granted to specified people only. These tools are currently changing and developing rapidly. Information on one such project, the FDTL4 ePortfolio, can be found at http://www.eportfolios.ac.uk/.

Perhaps most interestingly, VLEs are widely used to facilitate different types of communication. Email, of course, is used widely by students and tutors, and discussion lists and chat rooms were around long before the appearance of VLEs. But a VLE can pull

BOX 11.2 Focus on: Computer-based assessment

Computer-based assessment is a major area that in increasing in sophistication and use. Chapter 14 covers this in greater detail, but a few of the possibilities and advantages will be mentioned here.

Of course, one major reason for using computer-based testing is the opportunity for automated scoring and immediate feedback to students. In the past, test items have been limited to easily scored question types such as multiple choice, true-false and matching. Recently, however, researchers have made progress in automated scoring of essays using Latent Semantic Analysis.(32)

Because computer can monitor a student's performance in real time, it is possible for a system to adapt the test to the ability and level of the student. In sequential testing, a short test is given to all candidates. If the calculated confidence interval shows that a student has clearly passed or clearly failed, those students do not have to continue. For those students for whom there is still uncertainty, more test items can be presented until a judgement can be made or the system runs out of test items.

Computer-adaptive testing is similar in concept, but here the system begins by presenting all candidates with a test item that has been judged to be moderately difficult. If the student answers correctly, a more difficult item is presented; if the candidate answers incorrectly, an easier one is given. Using this method, the relative competence of the candidate can be gauged and the system can suggest areas where further study should be considered.

together different methods and allow students and tutors to choose the most appropriate methods for the moment.

Probably the most widely used communication tool in most VLEs is the *asynchronous threaded discussion forum.* These tools allow learners or tutors to log in at any time, read contributions by others and respond without the need for anyone else to be using the tool at the same time. Figure 11.4 is a screenshot showing an example of one such forum.

In this example, a student posted a question about confidence intervals and a list of the headings of responses by other students appears at the bottom of the screen. In this case, the students themselves answered the question satisfactorily, possibly more quickly than a tutor would have done. Tutors should monitor the discussions regularly to make sure that the information is correct, but often it is the case that students are perfectly capable of answering the questions. This can be a very important factor in promoting the acceptance by students of their peers as a 'learning resource' and can reduce the attitude that only lecturers are acceptable as sources of help.

Figure 11.4 Example of an asynchronous discussion forum in a virtual learning environment.(31) Screenshot from Hull York Medical School Blackboard™ VLE, copyright HYMS 2006.

Discussion forums can be useful for allowing tutors or students to post and discuss questions and debate issues. An important aspect of using these forums, however, is to establish rules for using the forum, sometimes called 'netiquette'. Generally, these are commonsense guidelines, such as keeping to the topic, being courteous, using appropriate language and not writing huge amounts. It is a good idea for somebody with some authority to monitor forums in case something gets out of hand or posts need to be removed for whatever reason.

An important factor in using discussion forums effectively, particularly if you want to include student discussion as an official component of the course, is defining specific tasks to get students started. It is seldom sufficient to simply say 'Discuss the course here'. Often, the first task in a course is for students to post a short introduction about themselves in order to learn how to use the forum. The tutor may then post a specific question for discussion or may assign students to summarise a reading and post a question. Such discussion areas can be very effective as learning tools if used as an integral part of the course, just as face-to-face discussion can be a very useful pedagogical intervention.(22)

And finally, while perhaps not as pedagogically interesting, VLEs can be very useful for administration and management functions, such as submitting and time-stamping assignments, signing up for student electives, sending group emails and posting reminders or urgent announcements. Some have been used to release official exam results: after authenticating via their system login, students are allowed to see final marks in the gradebook.

Figure 11.5(33) shows the results from a survey of 51 UK medical, dental and veterinary schools summarising the different uses of their VLEs. It is apparent that schools choose to use these tools in different ways, adapting and selecting them based on their own curriculum needs.

New Developments

New technologies that could be integrated into e-learning frameworks are constantly being introduced. This section mentions just a few such new developments with pointers to some examples of use. However, the basic principle is still the same: why are you using these in the context of your curriculum? Do not feel the need to cave in to students demanding the latest 'whizzy' technology unless there is a good reason to do so and adequate expertise and support are available. Having said that, often the students themselves may be a source of such expertise and may help schools develop innovative uses of these new tools.

As with many e-learning tools, some of the newly emerging ones emphasise communication among learners. *Wikis* are an example of shared writing spaces that can be used to encourage sharing of information and support for group writing. Probably one of the best known examples of a wiki is Wikipedia, a shared and constantly evolving encyclopaedia to which anyone can contribute.

Figure 11.5 Use of virtual learning environments in UK medical schools.(33) ©University of Bristol.

The definition of a Wiki from Wikipedia is:

A **wiki** <wee-kee> or <wick-ey>) is a type of website that allows anyone visiting the site to add, to remove, or otherwise to edit all content, very quickly and easily. … This ease of interaction and operation makes a wiki an effective tool for collaborative writing.

A related type of web site is a web-log or *blog*. These are web sites where new pages or entries can be entered easily without knowing HTML or web page authoring software, like wikis. However, contributions to blogs are generally restricted to the owner or a chosen group of members. They are similar to a discussion forum, but are generally organised as pages of text rather than threads or hierarchies, as is typical of a discussion forum.

Many blogs are used as online diaries or journals and could be used for medical students to keep personal or public notes for a portfolio. Many VLEs now supply wiki or blog tools, or stand-alone versions can be used.

Podcasting has grown out of the technology used for the Apple iPod to download and play music. In a typical podcast, audio or video is downloaded and can be played either while the listener is logged on to the internet or stored for later. This method is being used in some courses for storing lectures for students to review. This is very similar to earlier methods for storing radio broadcasts, for instance for listeners to retrieve later. The difference is mainly the underlying software to define and automatically download the content to a mobile audio or video device. Some VLEs are beginning to incorporate tools for creating and distributing podcasts.

Mobile learning, sometimes called M-learning or nomadic learning, refers to learning in which the student is using a mobile device such as a phone, hand-held personal computer (PC), personal digital assistant or tablet PC. While this is very similar to e-learning with VLEs, the primary difference is the ability to 'carry the learning' so that resources are at hand wherever they might be needed. Also, information can be 'beamed' to a device when it is detected, to deliver information at the most appropriate time and place. This is done in some museums(34) and city tours, as well as to attract people's attention with advertisements as they walk by shops. This type of mobile resource is also becoming more common in schools and hospitals for accessing information such as formularies, filling in common forms and recording other information, as well as for learning purposes.

Conclusions

So what is e-learning? Currently, the term tends to be used in a very techno-centric way, with definitions built around descriptions of the types of hardware and software used in teaching and learning. However, views are starting to change and conceptualisations of e-learning are becoming less about delivery and more about the more interaction with the learner. A recent research review(35) proposes a new definition:

e-Learning is the capability required of a learner/user in order that they can manage their own learning … , using technology as appropriate to context, sector and task.

In essence, this captures the main argument of this publication: e-learning technologies by themselves are tools, not teachers. Too often, e-learning resources are left isolated from the rest of the educational experience. Decades of research on technology-supported learning has shown that this approach is not the most effective means for using these tools and the key is to use these tools when and if appropriate with thought given as to how to integrate them into the curriculum and help students and tutors become proficient and discerning users. In a recent systematic review of high-fidelity simulators in medical education,(36) most of the factors that were critical for effective learning were true not just for simulators, but for all technology-based tools, and indeed all effective learning. These factors, adapted slightly to refer more generally to e-learning, include:

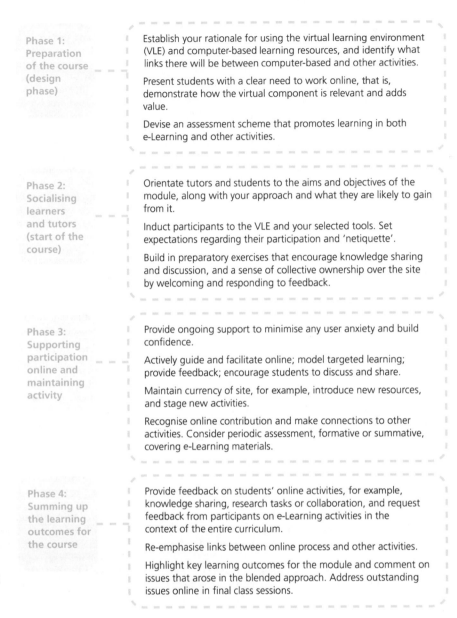

Phase 1:
Preparation of the course (design phase)

Establish your rationale for using the virtual learning environment (VLE) and computer-based learning resources, and identify what links there will be between computer-based and other activities.

Present students with a clear need to work online, that is, demonstrate how the virtual component is relevant and adds value.

Devise an assessment scheme that promotes learning in both e-Learning and other activities.

Phase 2:
Socialising learners and tutors (start of the course)

Orientate tutors and students to the aims and objectives of the module, along with your approach and what they are likely to gain from it.

Induct participants to the VLE and your selected tools. Set expectations regarding their participation and 'netiquette'.

Build in preparatory exercises that encourage knowledge sharing and discussion, and a sense of collective ownership over the site by welcoming and responding to feedback.

Phase 3:
Supporting participation online and maintaining activity

Provide ongoing support to minimise any user anxiety and build confidence.

Actively guide and facilitate online; model targeted learning; provide feedback; encourage students to discuss and share.

Maintain currency of site, for example, introduce new resources, and stage new activities.

Recognise online contribution and make connections to other activities. Consider periodic assessment, formative or summative, covering e-Learning materials.

Phase 4:
Summing up the learning outcomes for the course

Provide feedback on students' online activities, for example, knowledge sharing, research tasks or collaboration, and request feedback from participants on e-Learning activities in the context of the entire curriculum.

Re-emphasise links between online process and other activities.

Highlight key learning outcomes for the module and comment on issues that arose in the blended approach. Address outstanding issues online in final class sessions.

Figure 11.6 A framework for designing and delivering blended e-learning.(37) Used with permission.

- curriculum integration: integration of [e-learning]-based exercises into the standard medical school or postgraduate educational curriculum is an essential feature of their effective use
- providing feedback: educational feedback is the most important feature of [e-learning]-based medical education
- individualised learning: the importance of having … educational experiences where learners are active participants, not passive bystanders
- defined outcomes: clearly stated goals with tangible outcome[s] … will more likely lead to [effective learning].

Figure 11.6 encapsulates some of these principles and summarises a framework for designing and using VLEs and associated computer-based learning resources in a blended model of e-learning. The key is to create a resource that is useful to the students and to keep it relevant and current in order to make the most effective use of your educational environment.

References

1 Robinson J (1931) Broadcasting to the schools of a city. In: Levering T (ed.) *Radio and Education*, pp. 91–2. University of Chicago Press, Chicago.

2 Hoban C (1942) *Focus on Learning: motion pictures in the school.* American Council on Education, Washington, DC, p. 4.

3 Baines L (1997) Future schlock: using fabricated data and politically correct platitudes in the name of education reform. *Phi Delta Kappan International.* **78**(7): 492–8.

4 Murphy E (1996) Review of Seymour Paper. The children's machine: rethinking school in the age of the computer (http://www.cdli.ca/~elmurphy/emurphy/papert.html; accessed 31 March 2010).

5 Perelman LJ (1992) *School's Out: hyperlearning, the new technology, and the end of education*. William Morrow, New York.

6 Bush V (1945) As we may think. *Atlantic Monthly*. **176**(1): 101–8 (http://www.theatlantic.com/magazine/archive/1969/12/as-we-may-think/3881/).

7 Nelson TH (1965) Complex information processing: a file structure for the complex, the changing and the indeterminate. Proceedings of the Association for Computing Machinery 20th Annual Conference, pp. 84–100. Available from the ACM Digital Library (http://portal.acm.org/dl.cfm).

8 Kintsch W (1998) *Comprehension: a paradigm for cognition*. Cambridge University Press, Cambridge.

9 McKendree J, Reader W and Hammond N (1995) The homeopathic fallacy in learning from hypertext. *Interactions*. **2**(3): 74–82.

10 Charney D (1994) The impact of hypertext on processes of reading and writing. In: Hillgoss S and Selfe C (eds) *Literacy and Computers*, pp. 238–63. Modern Language Association, New York.

11 Novak J (1998) *Learning, Creating, and Using Knowledge: concept maps as facilitative tools in schools and corporations*. Lawrence Erlbaum Associates, NJ.

12 From PsyCLE © University of York for the TLTP PsyCLE Consortium.

13 Skinner BF (1958) *Teaching Machines. Science*. **128**: 969–77.

14 Kulik JA (1994) Meta-analytic studies of findings on computer-based instruction. In: Baker EL and O'Neil Jr HF (eds) *Technology Assessment in Education and Training*. Lawrence Erlbaum Associates, NJ.

15 Fletcher JD, Hawley DE and Piele PK (1990) Costs, effects, and utility of microcomputer assisted instruction in the classroom. *American Educational Research Journal*. **27**: 783–806.

16 Kosakowski J (1998) *The Benefits of Information Technology*. ERIC Digest, Report ED420302 1998-06-00, Washington, DC. (http://www.eric.ed.gov/ERICWebPortal/contentdelivery/servlet/ERICServlet?accno=ED420302; accessed 31 March 2010).

17 Underwood J, Cavendish S, Dowling S, Fogelman K and Lawson T (1996) Are integrated learning systems effective learning support tools? *Computers and Education*. **26**(1–3): 33–40.

18 McKendree J (1990) Effective feedback content for tutoring complex skills. *Human-Computer Interaction*. **5**: 381–413.

19 Reiser BJ, Tabak I, Sandoval WA, Smith B, Steinmuller F and Leone TJ (2001) BGuILE: strategic and conceptual scaffolds for scientific inquiry in biology classrooms. In: Carver SM and Klahr D (eds) *Cognition and Instruction: twenty five years of progress*. Lawrence Erlbaum Associates, NJ.

20 From Emergency Case Simulator © Royal Veterinary College 2006.

21 Turkle S (1997) *Life on the Screen: identity in the age of the internet*. Simon & Schuster, New York.

22 McKendree J (2002) The role of discussion in learning. Paper presented at Association for Medical Education in Europe conference, 29th August to 1st September 2002, Lisbon, Portugal. Full paper available from the author.

23 Koedinger KR (2001) Cognitive tutors as modeling tool and instructional model. In: Forbus KD and Feltovich PJ (eds) *Smart Machines in Education: the coming revolution in educational technology*, pp. 145–68. AAAI/MIT Press, Menlo Park, CA.

24 Coffield F, Moseley D, Hall E and Ecclestone K (2004) Learning styles and pedagogy in post-16 learning: a systematic and critical review. Report for Learning and Skills Research Centre. (https://crm.lsnlearning.org.uk/user/order.aspx?code=041543; accessed 31 March 2010).

25 Mayer RE and Sims VK (1994) For whom is a picture worth a thousand words? Extensions of a dual-coding theory of multimedia learning. *Journal of Educational Psychology*. **86**(3): 389–401.

26 Paivio A (1971) *Imagery and Verbal Processes*. Holt, Rinehart and Winston, New York.

27 Entwistle N. Contrasting perspectives on learning. In: Marton F, Hounsell D and Entwistle N (2005) *The Experience of Learning: implications for teaching and studying in higher education* (3e), pp. 3–22. University of Edinburgh, Centre for Teaching, Learning and Assessment, Edinburgh.

28 Ferguson E, James D and Madeley L (2002) Factors associated with success in medical school: systematic review of the literature. *British Medical Journal*. **324**: 952–7.

29 Dochy F, Segers M, Van den Bossche P and Gijbels D (2003) Effects of problem-based learning: a meta-analysis. *Learning and Instruction*. **13**(5): 533–68.

30 Eraut M (2000) Non-formal learning and tacit knowledge in professional work. *British Journal of Educational Psychology*. **70**: 113–36.

31 Hull York Medical School Blackboard™ VLE, copyright HYMS 2006

32 Landauer TK, Laham D and Foltz P (2003) Automatic essay assessment. *Assessment in Education: Principles, Policy and Practice*. **10**(3): 295–308.

33 Cook J (2005) Review of virtual learning environments in UK medical, dental and veterinary education. Newcastle: Subject Centre For Medicine, Dentistry And Veterinary Medicine. Report 6.

34 Bellotti F, Berta C, de Gloria A and Margarone M (2002) User testing a hypermedia tour guide. *Pervasive Computing IEEE*. **1**(2): 33–41.

35 Coultas J, Luckin R and du Boulay B (2004) How compelling is the evidence for the effectiveness of e-Learning in the post-16 sector? Consultation Paper. Eduserv Expert Seminar. (http://www.reveel.sussex.ac.uk/files/ConsultES204.pdf; accessed 16 April 2006).

36 Issenberg SB, McGaghie WC, Petrusa ER, Gordon DL and Scalese RJ (2005) Features and uses of high-fidelity medical simulations that lead to effective learning: a BEME systematic review. *Medical Teacher*. **27**(1): 10–28.

37 Adapted from *Planning Your Blended Module*, eLearning Development Team, University of York © 2005.

Web Links to Further Information

Courseware

EURCA: http://www.eurca.org/list_res.asp?CatID=All

Genetics Tutor: http://www.cs.cmu.edu/~genetics/index.html

Jess the dog, Royal Veterinary College emergency case simulations: http://www.rvc.ac.uk/Review/Cases/website/Jess/jess.htm

Other Royal Veterinary College examples: http://www.rvc.ac.uk/Review/

Pharma-CAL-ogy: http://www.pharmacalogy.com/

Software for the pharmaceutical and healthcare industry: http://www.coacs.com/software/published_titles/default.htm

Content repositories

Biomed Image Archive: http://library.hud.ac.uk/wiki/Bristol_
Biomedical_Image_Archive

Bioscience Image Bank: http://www.bioscience.heacademy.ac.
uk/imagebank/

EDINA online resources: http://edina.ac.uk/index.shtml

Education Media Online: http://www.emol.ac.uk/

Microbiology resources: http://www.microbelibrary.org/

Trauma images: http://www.trauma.org/imagebank/
imagebank.html

Online continuing professional development web sites

AMA CME Online, online modules with self-assessments: http://
www.ama-cmeonline.com/

Medical Law for Medical Professionals: http://www.law.ed.ac.
uk/distanceLearning/ecpd/medical-ethics-consent-law.htm

MDcme Canada, variety of modules offered for CME credit:
http://www.mdcme.ca

Virtual learning environments and other online tools

Only a few of many such systems are listed here. This list is not
intended to be an endorsement.

Blackboard: http://www.blackboard.com

FDTL4 ePortfolio Project: http://www.eportfolios.ac.uk/

EduTools (useful site with tools for comparing course management systems, e-learning policies at many (American) universities and online student support services tools): http://www.
edutools.info

Moodle: http://moodle.org

Sakai: http://www.sakaiproject.org

Questionmark Perception (information on this assessment tool –
not a VLE, but often used with them): http://www.qmark.
com/uk/home.htm

Questionmark Sample Tests: http://www.questionmark.com/
us/tryitout_college_university.htm

Wikipedia: http://www.wikipedia.org

Further Reading

Approaches and Study Skills Inventory for Students. The instrument is available for those who would like to try it out: http://
www.etl.tla.ed.ac.uk//questionnaires/ASSIST.pdf

Concept Mapping. Summary of concept mapping theory and
tools: http://www.cocon.com/observetory/conceptmap-
pingvs1.htm

e-Learning Reviews. Provides concise reviews of publications on
research in e-learning: http://www.eLearning-reviews.org/

Innovative Practice with eLearning. JISC report on using mobile
and wireless technologies with case studies: http://www.jisc.
ac.uk/eli_practice.html

UCISA Report: surveys from March 2001, March 2003, March
2005 and March 2008 for higher education in the UK: http://
www.ucisa.ac.uk/groups/ssg/asg/surveys.aspx

Higher Education Academy eLearning Resources: http://www.
heacademy.ac.uk/resources

Simulation in medical education

Jean Ker and Paul Bradley

KEY MESSAGES

- Simulation is a powerful learning tool when learning outcomes are clearly defined.
- Simulation should be integrated within the curriculum.
- Simulation provides a safe, learner-centred educational method.
- Debriefing and feedback are essential components of any learning experience.
- The authenticity required should relate to the learning context of the simulation.

- The development of expertise in performing clinical procedures to accepted standards requires 'deliberate' practice.
- Research into simulation should focus on appropriateness, effectiveness, the context and transfer into practice.
- Simulation cannot replace clinical experience but may be a valuable tool in preparing clinicians for practice.

Introduction

This is an exciting time to be involved in simulation, as with an increasing emphasis on patient safety,(1,2), simulation is becoming an essential component of most medical education and training programmes.(3,4) This chapter introduces the reader to the potential of simulation in medical education and in doing so covers four key areas:

- definitions and classifications
- application of educational theories
- the role of debriefing and feedback
- practical applications.

As research into simulation has hitherto been limited – often to descriptive, low-level evaluation(5) – we will try to provide a balanced overview of the field and consider the theoretical underpinnings of simulation, in the hope that this will point the way towards areas for further research.

A Brief Historical Perspective

Simulation has been around for centuries in many areas of human endeavour.(6) Simulators in healthcare learning date back as far as 18th-century France when Madame Du Coudray used her foetal model and pelvis to train midwives.(7) The modern movement in simulation training coincided with developments of the part task trainer. Resusci Anne led the way in stand-

ardising resuscitation training by making available a simple, low-cost, practical and effective manikin.(8) Sim-One, a higher fidelity human patient simulator, was developed by Abrahamson at the University of Southern to help novice anaesthetists develop skills in inserting endotracheal tubes.(9,10) Since then anaesthesia has been at the forefront of simulator development. The 1980s saw the development of the Gainesville Anaesthetic Simulator(11) and the Comprehensive Anaesthesia Simulation Environment (CASE).(12) The CASE group linked the simulator to a programme on anaesthesia crisis resource management,(13,14) which was the start of many disciplines using simulation for learning both technical and non-technical skills.(15,16) Barrows introduced simulated patients, providing learners with a controlled, staged experience of simulated practice.(17) Following recent technological developments, computer-assisted simulation, virtual reality and the use of haptics (tactile sensations) have been added to the simulation armamentarium.

What Is 'Simulation'?

The narrow, popularist view of simulation is that of advanced technologies recreating the clinical experience, such as those found in virtual reality and advanced computer-controlled human patient simulators. But simulation does not focus exclusively on technical or psychomotor performance; it encompasses a broad perspective, incorporating both cognitive and affective domains. Simulation may involve a wide range of techniques and approaches applicable to learners at all levels of seniority, from novice to expert, one of the major underlying drivers being to develop safe healthcare practitioners (*see* Figure 12.1).

Understanding Medical Education: Evidence, Theory and Practice.
Edited by T Swanwick. © 2010 Association for the Study of Medical Education.

Figure 12.1 The simulation continuum.

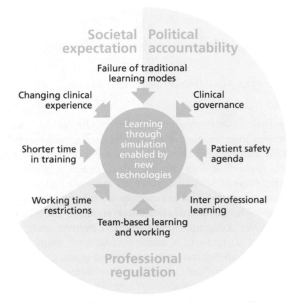

Figure 12.2 Drivers for the development of simulation.(6)

Simulation is not therefore dependent on high (or low) technology, nor is it confined to interactions with people or models, physical or virtual; it could just as easily be a paper-based activity. Neither is simulation restricted to a particular setting and set of clinical skills, and simulation centres are not exclusive venues for this activity.

Why Use Simulation?

A number of societal, political, clinical and educational influences have driven the development of simulation over the past 40 years (*see* Figure 12.2).

Patients remain important participants in medical education, although they are no longer unquestioning.(18,19) There is now an expectation that learners and practitioners will have been prepared, to an acceptable level, for their sphere of practice before being let loose on patients.(20,21) Furthermore, changes in healthcare delivery have resulted in fewer opportunities for students to learn from a breadth of real patients,(22) and the changing roles of other healthcare professionals have also reduced learning opportunities in practice.(23–25)

To Err Is Human(26) and *An Organisation with a Memory*(27) increased our awareness of clinical adverse events and their underlying causes. The patient safety agenda and clinical governance requirements for standards of practice can, in part, be addressed through prior exposure, using simulation to prepare for rare and unexpected events.(28) Simulation can help educate staff in defined processes in a realistic healthcare context with defined and assessed outcomes. It can improve patient care through team-based approaches,(29–36) and aid the development of non-technical skills.(2–4,37–39)

Safe technical skills can also be enhanced and standardised using simulation. New diagnostic and therapeutic technologies, for example, endoscopy and minimally invasive surgery, have revolutionised clinical practice, but they have also imposed a requirement for safe, effective training for both trainee and established practitioners.(40–46) New interventional techniques can be pioneered through simulation.

Worldwide, there have been major changes in medical education, both undergraduate and postgraduate, which recognise the need to incorporate all aspects of a doctor's practice, including knowledge, skills and expected attitudes, within an outcomes-based framework.(47–53) The defined outcomes of competency-based curricula lend themselves well to a simulation approach. With more emphasis on the cost-effectiveness of clinical care and a reduction in working times, clinical teaching has been squeezed, with learners receiving less time on direct bedside teaching.(54–56) There has also been significant evidence of the failure of traditional serendipitous approaches to skills acquisition across a wide range of core skills.(57–65) The traditional apprenticeship model in this context is no longer effective, and simulation offers a feasible alternative for learning procedural skills(66) and the opportunity to rehearse performance in complex integrated scenarios in a safe, protected, learner-centred simulated clinical setting.(31,67,68)

Assessment and monitoring of both non-technical and technical skills can also be delivered in educationally supportive clinical skills and simulation centres.(69–73) Behaviours observed in a simulated environment can provide a prediction of how professionals will behave in the reality of practice.(74) A more extensive list of potential applications is listed in Box 12.1.

Fidelity of Simulation

Meller developed a classification scheme for a medical simulation with four components(75):
- the patient and/or disease process
- the procedure, test or equipment
- the physician or other practitioners (learner)
- the expert practitioner (teacher)

- Routine learning and rehearsal of clinical and communication skills at all levels
- Routine basic training of individuals and teams
- Practice of complex clinical situations
- Training of teams in crisis resource management
- Rehearsal of serious and/or rare events
- Rehearsal of planned, novel or infrequent interventions
- Induction into new clinical environments and use of equipment
- Design and testing of new clinical equipment
- Performance assessment of staff at all levels
- Refresher training of staff at all levels

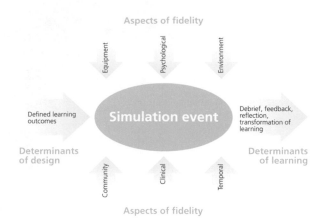

Figure 12.3 Factors influencing simulation fidelity.

BOX 12.2 Fidelity

Miller(76)

- Psychological – degree to which the skills or skill in real task are captured in the simulated task.
- Physical or engineering – degree to which the device or environment replicates the physical characteristics of the real environment

Rehmann(77)

- Equipment fidelity – relates to the degree to which the simulator duplicates reality.
- Environmental fidelity – concerns the extent to which the simulator duplicates the visual and other sensory clues.
- Psychological fidelity – concerns the degree of reality perceived by the trainee or student.

technical sophistication. However, hi- or lo-fidelity relates to more than advanced technology and simulation authenticity should be considered in relation to the real world and community of practice. Such classifications of fidelity do not fully embrace all the determinants of realism relating to a defined simulation event. The fidelity of simulation required for teaching a novice venepuncture is very different from that needed to recreate a multi-professional team in the throes of an operating theatre-based crisis. Contextual fidelity, which has both clinical and temporal components, is a very important consideration. Our own model, which describes simulation not as a task, but as an event influenced by a number of factors relating to fidelity, is shown in Figure 12.3.

Classification of Simulators and Simulations

A range of simulators and types of simulation event are used in medical education (*see* Box 12.3), and in this section we will review those in common use.(26,80) An extensive list of available simulators is available at http://www.pennstatehershey.org/web/simlab/home.

Part-task trainers

Part-task trainers (PTTs) are often used to teach and learn psychomotor, procedural and technical skills. They are used to develop mastery of these skills in an educational setting. As well as lo-fidelity trainers, for example venepuncture arms, PTTs also include highly sophisticated computerised human patient simulators such as Harvey and Simulator K.(81,82)

Taking venepuncture as an example, with a PTT (and a little imagination) the tutor can incorporate clear demonstration of communication skills, health and safety issues (including patient identification, clinical hygiene, hand washing, safe disposal of sharps and clinical waste, and use of universal precautions),

However, an analysis that looks at the fidelity of the simulation, the simulator and the component parts is probably more meaningful. Simulation can be viewed as a continuum that runs from low to high levels of fidelity and from low to high levels of authenticity, dependent on the learners and learning context. (*see* Box 12.2).

Fidelity is the extent to which the appearance or/and behaviour of the simulation or simulator matches the appearance and behaviour of the real system.(78) Miller(76) made the distinction between two different types of fidelity: psychological and physical. Rehmann further expanded physical fidelity to incorporate equipment and environmental fidelity.(77) This typology is, of course, based on the trainer's perspective. The required overall fidelity configuration is best determined by intended learning outcomes.(79)

Simulation has also been classified as high (hi) or low (lo) fidelity, traditionally related to the level of

BOX 12.3 Classification of simulators

Simulator type	Examples
Part-task trainers	Venepuncture arms, arterial arms Male and female pelvic models Skin and tissue jigs for injection and suture practice
Computer-based systems	Emergency medicine (Microsim, Laerdal) Anesoft – range of modules including anaesthesia simulator, haemodynamic simulator, critical care and bioterrorism
Virtual reality and haptic systems	
Precision placement	Venepuncture trainer IV Cannulation
Simple manipulation	Endoscopy trainer Ultrasound trainer
Complex manipulation	Minimally invasive surgery Complex surgical procedures
Integrated simulators	
Instructor-driven simulators	SimMan
Model-driven simulators	METI (Medical Education Technologies Inc adult and paediatric simulators)
Simulated patients	
Simulated environments	Simulated wards, operating rooms, intensive care, etc.

Adapted from Kneebone(80) and Maran and Glavin(29)

completion of documentation, labelling of specimens, safe handling of specimens, and proper handling and despatch to ensure the best-quality specimens arrive at the laboratory. Therefore, even for this relatively low level of skill, a fairly sophisticated set-up and performance may be required, placing the learning in the context in which it will eventually be applied.(31,83)

Computer-based systems

There have been significant developments in computer-based simulations. Learners are provided with interfaces that allow them to interact with materials relating to basic sciences, which can be staged and can progress at the student's own pace. These programs ensure learners receive relevant feedback to reinforce their learning.

A number of programs have been produced that include sophisticated physiological models. Some also provide feedback on the decision-making ability and performance of the user; in the case of Laerdal's MicroSim suite, it can be used to reinforce an emergency care curriculum.

Virtual reality and haptic systems

Virtual reality generates images representative of objects or environments with which the user interacts and which respond to those actions. Haptic systems provide the kinaesthetic and tactile sensation. These two approaches may be combined to provide training in basic skills such as venepuncture, and more sophisticated skills such as endoscopic, laparoscopic and endovascular procedures. Such simulation systems can also generate user data, which can be presented subsequently as detailed feedback on performance and maintained as an ongoing record.

Integrated simulator models

Integrated simulators combine a whole- or part-body manikin with a computer that controls the model's physiology and the output to monitors showing graphic displays. The observed clinical vital signs and the electrical readouts can be controlled and altered in response to interventions and therapies initiated by the users interacting with the manikin. The capabilities of modern integrated simulators are extensive, encompassing the life-like representation of body parts and functions, to generating realistic monitoring data such as electrocardiography and pulse oximetry, and providing a hi-fidelity mans of rehearsing a range of procedures such as the insertion of a chest drain or urinary catheters.

Integrated simulators are divided into two subgroups: model and instructor driven.

Also called hi-fidelity simulators, model-driven simulators are built around physiological and pharmacological models that directly control the manikin's responses to intervention and treatments. Examples include the highly sophisticated METI (Medical

Education Technologies Inc) adult and paediatric simulators, which have up to 100 changeable physiological parameters to recreate accurate patient responses to illness and therapies. Hi-fidelity simulators usually require dedicated facilities, faculty and specialised technical support.

Instructor-driven or intermediate fidelity simulators respond to instructor intervention, either directly via the computer keyboard or via a pre-written computer algorithm. They are less resource intensive than hi-fidelity simulators and are widely used by skills and simulation centres.

Simulated patients

The terms 'standardised patient' and 'simulated patient' are often used interchangeably. Barrows defined a simulated patient as 'a well person trained to simulate a patient's illness in a standardized way'.(17) Here the emphasis is on the simulation of reality, and there is now widespread use of simulated patients in medical education in teaching, learning and assessment. Simulated patients may be usefully involved in the teaching of a number of domains, including communication and consultation skills, physical examination, non-invasive procedural skills and the assessment of professionalism. There is also a special group that provides learners with opportunities to undertake male and female genital and digital rectal examination, and female breast examination. These people are trained and give the learners feedback on all aspects of their performance.(84–86)

Simulated patients need training and considerable organisation in relation to matching simulated patient training needs to scripts and in timetabling simulated patients for both training sessions and student/learner training programme and needs. This can be even more complex when simulated patients are required to provide feedback to students or to participate in assessment or complex healthcare scenarios when simulated patient training may require more than one session. A database can be used to manage the bank of simulated patients effectively.(67) There will also need to be considerable investment in time and resources, and the financial costs may be high, particularly if your simulated patients are professional actors.

Script development for simulated patient exercises can be used to support wider learning outcomes beyond the simulation and immediate learning goals. Inevitably, however, there are some physical signs and situations that cannot be simulated and such patients can in no way substitute for direct clinical experience (*see* Box 12.4).

Simulated environments

The development of clinical skills and simulation centres provides varying degrees of recreation of the clinical setting in a protected environment.(70,87–89) Within these venues, application of contextual fidelity

---

> **BOX 12.4 Focus on: 'Patients' in simulation**
>
> Standardised patient: A person with a particular history and/or physical signs, trained to present them in a consistent manner for the purposes of teaching or assessment.
>
> Simulated patient: A person without a history or physical signs who is trained to portray a role and/or mimic particular physical signs for the purposes of teaching or assessment.
>
> Real patient: A person with minimal training who consents to present his or her history and findings for the purposes of teaching or assessment.
>
> Lay educator/patient teacher/expert patient/patient instructor: A patient with a particular condition who has been trained to provide facilitation, feedback and assessment about their condition and its history and findings.
>
> Role-play patient: The recreation of a patient role or event by a learner or teacher.

> **BOX 12.5 The range of simulated settings**
>
> - Generic teaching and learning rooms
> - Consultation rooms
> - Simulated ward
> - Operating theatre, including anaesthetic room, scrub area and recovery room
> - Emergency department cubicles and resuscitation area
> - High dependency and intensive care areas
> - Domestic settings
> - Roadside and motor vehicle

---

enables the suspension of disbelief and facilitates transfer to the real world. It might be argued that real clinical settings are better places for learning; however, the disruption of normal clinical activity and the distraction of peripheral events may prevent the required learning. One advantage of a dedicated facility is access to additional educational and audio-visual resources (*see* Boxes 12.5 and 12.6).

The Theoretical Basis of Simulation

A number of theories of learning and instruction underpin the design and delivery of the simulated clinical experience, and these can be used not only to affirm educational credibility but also to develop appropriate research questions. What follows is a short description of the major relevant educational theories,

BOX 12.6 How to: Design a simulation event

Gaba analysed simulation events in 11 dimensions.(90) These provide a way of approaching the design and delivery, ensuring all aspects are aligned for maximum benefit. We have adapted his approach and condensed these considerations under three 'Ps': purpose, process and participants.

Purpose is an essential consideration for any learning programme as identification of intended outcomes ensures that the learning is integral to the overall curricular programme.

Process relates to the reality factor; whether this is computer, real patients (RP), part-task trainers (PTT), simulated patients (SP), virtual reality (VR), replicated clinical environment (RCE) or the actual clinical environment (ACE). The reality factor is crucial to the process and needs to be judged in relation to both the purpose and the participants. Often the focus is on too much realism, which can distract from the purpose of the event in the first place.

Participants should be considered carefully. Are the right people present and is the simulation at the right level for the healthcare professional concerned? Simulation can provide excellent inter-professional learning opportunities.

with examples of their relevance to simulation. For a more detailed exposition of some of the educational theories described, see Chapter 2 by Kaufman and Mann.

Behaviourism

Behaviourism(91,92) ignores the 'black box' of the mind and describes a model in which a stimulus is used to produce a response that may be 'rewarded' or 'punished' to reinforce or weaken the response through a process known as 'conditioning'. Knowledge is therefore seen as a repertoire of behaviours. Neo-behaviourists, such as Bandura,(93) also point out that a reciprocal determinism exists between the behaviour, the environment and a number of personal factors, such as personality, affect and knowledge.

In simulation training, feedback is used extensively to bring about new behaviours. Simulation also permits 'over-learning' as a means of making such behaviours automatic. An example of such a behaviourist approach in simulation is the 'skills and drills' of resuscitation training to which we are all exposed throughout our undergraduate and postgraduate career.(94,95)

Cognitivism

Cognitivism, as expounded by Piaget(96) and Bruner,(97) posits that learners develop new ideas, constructs, hypotheses and decisions based on their interaction with the world and their own prior knowledge as an internal mental process. Learning is assimilated (the experience fits into the existing structure and adds to the body of examples) or accommodated (the experience does not fit the existing structure, which must be changed to incorporate the new knowledge) into a cognitive structure that gives meaning and organisation to the knowledge.

In the context of simulation, the tutor can help facilitate the learners' learning by establishing their preconceptions, presenting a cognitive conflict, drawing attention to the discrepancy between learners' expectation and experience of the event, asking questions and engaging in dialogue to prepare the learners to be receptive to new ideas, teaching the new ideas and drawing attention to the way in which they are better than the learners' previous knowledge structures.

Social constructivism

Based on the work of Vygovsky,(98) social constructivism emphasises social interaction as the means of learning. Language and culture are considered central to human intellectual development and how the world is perceived. Knowledge is co-constructed as a social phenomenon.

The tutor can work collaboratively to support ('scaffold') the learner's development and in time remove such support to encourage independence. Through, for example, discussion of salient points and problems arising, the tutor mediates social interactions. Constructivism requires the learning environment to be safe, where ridicule or embarrassment will not follow mistakes and, by extrapolation, patients would not be at risk.

Situated learning and cognitive apprenticeship

Lave and Wegner(99) introduced the term 'legitimate peripheral participation', describing the position of learners within a community of practice. The learning is described as a product of the activity, culture and context (the social interaction within the workplace). As a learner moves from the periphery towards the centre, they become more actively involved and socialised (accepting beliefs and behaviours) and take on more senior and expert roles. This process is often not deliberate but evolutionary.

In a related model, Collins *et al.*(100) developed the concept of the cognitive apprenticeship, where the processes of the task are identified and made visible; abstract tasks are situated in the context of authentic settings; situations are varied to emphasise commonalities; and transfer of learning is promoted, that is, through a process of

- modelling
- coaching
- scaffolding
- articulation

- reflection
- exploration/transferability.

The cognitive apprenticeship approach can be used in the teaching of a practical skill prior to its integration, application and transfer to the clinical environment, whereas situated learning is the more appropriate paradigm in the workplace environment where a junior learner would increasingly become part of the team during a clinical attachment and their learning would benefit from that socialisation.(101)

Experiential learning

Although criticised as an oversimplification with a weak theoretical basis, experiential learning, as defined by Kolb,(102) provides a useful model for simulation training (*see* Figure 12.2). Experience provides the main motivation for learning and new knowledge is established from reflection. The model of learning from experience includes concrete experience (apprehension) and abstract conceptualisation (comprehension) as means of perceiving experience, and critical reflection (intension) and active experimentation (extension) as means of transforming the experience.

Engaging learners in a healthcare exercise using simulation provides both the realism relevant to the learner's experience and the time in which to analyse and interpret different potential scenarios and their outcomes. The experiential learning process using simulation techniques allows learners to reflect critically on how they felt during the exercise. They can then begin to formulate concepts and hypotheses concerning the experience through discussion and individual reflection. Further experimentation with newly formed concepts and experiences can then lead to further reflection on experimentation. In this way, simulation provides a safe opportunity to experience healthcare, again without compromising patients.(103,104)

Reflective and transformative learning

Reflection-in-action (thinking on your feet) and reflection-on-action (evaluating after the event) are key concepts in the work of Schön.(105,106) Reflection-in-action occurs during an event; little time is given or available and recall of reflection might be limited, but prior experiences and knowledge are drawn upon and applied (almost experimentally) within the content of an unfolding situation, adding to the wealth of experiences already in place. Reflection-on-action is more indirect and formalised; writings, recording and other recall may be used to analyse an event, actions and outcomes.

Transformative learning(107) involves the reconfiguration of ideas, knowledge and meaning stimulated by a process of critical reflection. Learners are empowered to identify and incorporate new learning as their own. The use of video recordings in the learning of communication skills is an example of these educational approaches. Video can result in reflection both in- and on-action, and through facilitated discussion after the event it can result in a transformative restructuring and the development of an action plan and new learning goals.(108–111)

Activity theory

Based on the work of Vygotsky and other Soviet psychologists(112,113) and Cole,(114) activity theory posits that conscious learning comes from activity. Activity denotes the forms of behaviour that are socially formed and conscious. Human activity is structured, dynamic and self-regulating, motivated by needs and objects. Activities create motor and mental actions directed by conscious goals. Actions themselves are implemented through operations, which are dependent on conditions in the (external and internal) system(115).

This seemingly complex interaction illustrates the underlying principle that learning, knowledge and activity are intrinsically interlinked and that learning is a socially mediated activity. Relationships between one activity system and another, for example, the simulated environment and the clinical setting might help us understand issues surrounding the transfer of skills and how clinical education might best be engineered. A crisis resource management or interprofessional exercise would find this educational approach most beneficial in a simulated setting. This would enable teams to rehearse their skills using hi-fidelity simulation and to transfer the skills into clinical practice.(116–118)

Models of expertise

In considering all the educational approaches above, it is also important to recognise the development of expertise and its impact on any simulated exercise. Expertise may be considered as the end point in a stepwise development of cognitive, psychomotor and affective skills. The Dreyfus brothers describe five levels of development of expertise from novice to expert,(119) and experiences in simulation should be modelled in accordance with the levels of expertise expected of the learner.

Feedback in Simulation

Feedback is an essential component in simulation – closing the learning loop. Feedback may be intrinsic or extrinsic. Intrinsic feedback, as described by Laurillard, refers to a conversational framework embedded within the teaching and learning experience.(120) Extrinsic feedback, by contrast, is usually available only after the event has taken place.

In an ideal world, learners should be able to compare their own performance with a standard, and be able to diagnose their own strengths and weaknesses. A simulated learning environment should permit such self-criticism, providing an atmosphere of trust and encouraging excellence. Most learners welcome the opportunity to discuss their strengths and areas for self-improvement, and in maximising the impact of learning from a simulation episode, extrinsic feedback is crucial. But when, how often and how well it is done is often disappointing.(121)

Who should give feedback?

In recent years, there has been a move towards the widespread use of multisource feedback, particularly as evidence of performance in the workplace.(122,123) Such a tool can also be useful in the simulated context where the event has involved a team.(124) Peer-group feedback can give learners a realistic perspective on standards of performance.

Simulators themselves can provide instant feedback by collecting data of events and interactions and from attached monitors. Video-recording a simulated learning event, whether a hi-fidelity scenario(109) or other simulated encounters,(125) may also provide the learner with an opportunity for later reflection,(126) although it may be no more superior for immediate feedback than for oral feedback alone.(111) Tutors and facilitators can provide feedback where the main focus is on striving for better professional practice, and trained simulated patients can also offer a unique perspective on the learning episode(127,128).

The purpose of feedback

Feedback ensures that learners are clear about the learning outcome expected, can have areas of performance clarified, are given time and space to make connections with what they already know and can generalise to what training might be required in the future.(129) Feedback also raises the learner's self-awareness. It can reinforce good practice and be corrective by encouraging modifications of behaviour. Feedback should be an integral component of the learning process and is analogous to the reflective thinking process needed for safe clinical practice.

The feedback process

Within any simulation event, there are four stages to the feedback process, although with practice they may be run together seamlessly.

1 Preparation for feedback: This is important and should be addressed prior to the simulation exercise. Learners can be asked to complete a questionnaire or to discuss in small groups the intended learning outcomes for the simulation exercise. This process helps to assess prior knowledge or similar experiences, to explore awareness of the learners' own competence and confidence, and to identify previous concerns or difficulties.

2 Coming out of role: During a simulation a learner takes on a health professional role caring for a 'patient' (simulator) in a situation of 'suspended disbelief'. Giving time to come out of role is important to allow the emotional responses of the learner to be addressed. This should not diminish the consequences of inappropriate action but helps promote conditions for deep learning. A learner has to acknowledge himself or herself as a student in learning, not a doctor or a healthcare professional responsible for the safety of the patient's life.(130) Concern for emotional impact must also be considered in relation to the experiences of simulated patients.(131–133)

3 Constructive feedback: Several models for constructive feedback exist which are relevant to learning from simulation. Most of these share a common goal of constructing what learning from performance has occurred. Examples include Pendleton's Rules(134) and the Cambridge–Calgary SETGO method,(135,136) both of which are widely used in consultation skills training; CORBS,(137) from the supervision literature; and GREAT,(138) a simple checklist developed specifically to debrief after simulator-based training.

4 Contemplation: In this final stage the facilitator encourages the student to link up what has happened in the simulator with prior relevant learning experiences and to think about transfer of learning to the workplace – to generalise their learning so it is accessible in different contexts. A subsequent post-encounter meeting can further support this process.

Feedback and its role in formative assessment and development is covered in more detail in Chapter 18.

Practical Approaches to Teaching, Learning and Assessment Using Simulation

To illustrate some of the theoretical concepts already highlighted in this chapter, this section explores the practical applications for simulation in the teaching and learning of technical and non-technical skills, and how the influence of the environment on practice can be analysed by recreating healthcare settings.

Teaching and learning a practical skill

Whether teaching components of a practical skill or learning more complex professional skills using simulation, knowledge is required to underpin practice. However, in medicine, as in other complex areas of professional work, it is not just necessary to recall facts, but it also necessary to be able to use knowledge.(139) Eraut categorises knowledge as propositional, procedural and personal; the latter two being gained only through experience and reflection, whether simulated or real practice.(140)

BOX 12.7 How to: Teach a technical, procedural or psychomotor skill(143)

- Demonstration of the skill in real time without discussing with the learners.
- Repeat the demonstration but with explanation of what is being done and why.
- A learner leads the tutor through another run of the demonstration.
- The learner performs the demonstration and then all learners practice.

BOX 12.8 How to: Teach a skill to a large group

S Set the foundation of prior learning, the importance of the skill and the context in which it will be learned and applied.

T Tutor demonstration in real time without commentary.

E Explanation with repeat demonstration.

P Practise under supervision with feedback from peer and tutor.

S Subsequent deliberate practice encouraged through self-directed learning and with peer assessment and feedback.

Gagne lists three phases in instructional design when contemplating the teaching of a technical skill.(141)

1 Early or cognitive phase – consciously developing a routine with cues from a facilitator.
2 Intermediate or associative phase – component parts become integrated.
3 Final or autonomous phase – skill becomes automatic, enabling other cognitive activities to be addressed.

Studies have shown that rest periods interspersed with periods of practice are more effective than continuous practice. A practical application of the above is found in the Advanced Trauma Life Support and Advanced Life Support courses, and this approach can be further adopted and adapted.(142) Joyce and Showers(143) stressed the importance of learning in context, modelling through real-time demonstration, repeat demonstration with explanation of actions, supervised practice and feedback to guide further development through further repeated practice. Their work also emphasised the importance of feedback and further coaching in ensuring effective implementation of new learning (*see* Box 12.7).

This standardised approach to skills teaching and learning is less easily transferable to a setting where there may be large cohorts of learners and smaller teaching faculties. However, it is possible to build on the model, as Joyce and Showers(143) also identified that while feedback and coaching were essential in skills training, they did not necessarily have to be done by the trainers or in the initial training session. Therefore, a modified approach may be adopted in which initial teaching is delivered to groups and learning is consolidated through deliberate practice and peer review (*see* Box 12.8).

Learning using patient scenarios

Planning and structuring are essential to developing successful patient-based scenarios, and here it is important to avoid the lure of the 'bells and whistles' of the technological capabilities of simulators. They are a means to an end. Patient scenarios can form a useful teaching aid in a variety of settings at all levels of simulation complexity. Salas *et al.* provide a simple but

BOX 12.9 Guide to effective simulation-based training(144)

- Understand the learner – the needs and the requirements.
- Embed measurements of performance both technical and non-technical for both individuals and teams.
- Ensure feedback is facilitated (e.g. video) and provided.
- Create scenarios based on learning outcomes.
- Guide the practice, including mistakes, and provide resources and support to seek improvement.
- Create synergy between content experts (clinicians) and process experts (educationalists).
- Evaluate the programme at all levels of the Kirkpatrick hierarchy.

effective blueprint for such an approach(144) (*see* Box 12.9).

In patient scenario teaching, particularly when using hi-fidelity simulators, the feedback is often referred to as the debrief. This has two elements: the clinical/technical aspects of the exercise and the non-technical professional skills. Useful frameworks have been validated to support non-technical skills debriefing, such as the Anaesthetic Non Technical Skills (ANTS) framework(145) and others.(146) Again, feedback to learners is absolutely essential,(147) and the stages of feedback described above should be followed.

Learning using different healthcare settings

Simulations representing the real healthcare environment are increasingly being used to develop and rehearse non-technical skills, such as prioritisation, decision making and situational awareness. Examples include simulated ward environments,(31,148) anaesthetic settings(149) and complete operating theatres.(117) In a simulated healthcare environment, significant events in practice can be recreated with errors and adverse events built in to test systems.(150)

Learning using team scenarios

There are several examples of where simulation has been used to explore the functioning of healthcare teams. In Basel, Switzerland, an operating theatre is used as a venue in which the whole team are presented with an emergency situation; video-recording facilitates analysis of team performance, leadership and follower roles, delegation of tasks, effective communication and feedback.(151) It also tests the safety procedures and organisational systems. This can lead to improved understanding of how teams can work better together and why errors arise.(152) At Imperial College, London, simulated operating theatres have also been used to explore the technical and non-technical differences between grades of surgeon.(153)

Other examples of simulated team scenarios are found in emergency medicine,(35) obstetrics,(94) the management of acutely ill patients,(154) advanced cardiac life support, trauma team training and neonatal resuscitation,(34) and many other disciplines.(155) Team and inter-professional simulation-based teaching and learning also occur in the undergraduate years, for example, in clinical skills,(156,157) communication skills,(158) resuscitation(158) and addressing patient safety issues,(118) although these bring challenges of their own.(160)

Assessment

The use of simulation in assessment usually focuses on the assessment of competence; therefore, the simulation needs to be as authentic as possible if the assessment is to offer a reasonable indication of whether a person is able to perform in the reality of practice. Miller's pyramid is often used as a model for the assessment of clinical competence, with four tiers representing 'knows', 'knows how', 'shows how' and 'does'.(161) Simulation sits at the top of the third level and is able to provide an environment for testing the 'shows how' of clinical ability. Formative assessment through debriefing and feedback should form an integral part of clinically oriented simulated assessment events. In more high-stakes summative assessment, the full range of simulators may be used, often in the format of an Objective Structured Clinical Examinations(162) or structured clinical skills assessment. In the classical format of this exam, candidates would typically rotate through a number of stations where they might encounter simulated patients, part-task simulators (e.g. venepuncture arm), simulated patient charts and results, resuscitation manikins, computer-based simulations and even whole-patient simulators, and will usually be tested on a range of psychomotor and communication skills. High levels of reliability and validity can be achieved in these exams,(163) where, interestingly, checklists and global scales show almost equal reliability.(164)

Hi-fidelity simulators offer the potential to examine higher levels of expertise among clinicians, testing knowledge, procedural and psychomotor skills, decision making, team working, communication and professional behaviour. Of key importance is that the testing process must be rigorously assessed itself for reliability and validity if the assessment is going to be used in a high-stakes stetting.(72,165,166) It should be noted that there is currently limited evidence to support the use of hi-fidelity simulators and complex clinical scenarios in high-stakes assessments.

The apex of Miller's pyramid – 'does' – can be assessed through simulation, but in the real practice environment, an example being incognito simulated patients who are trained to visit a practitioner in their practice and then score their performance.(167)

Transferability

Throughout this publication we have tried to highlight how simulations may be designed and delivered to most effectively promote transfer of learning to the workplace. These 'transferability factors' are summarised in Box 12.10. It should be noted that transferability is affected not only by the teaching regime, but also the characteristics of the individual learner.(168)

Limitations to Simulation

Simulation is not, and can never be, a replacement for authentic experiential learning in the real world of clinical practice. It can, however, prepare practitioners for the real world, providing a structure for deliberate practice analogous to the hours put in by a professional golfer on a golf range or a concert pianist working their way through books of technical studies.(169) Simulation is not a tool to replace other modes of learning, but a powerful adjunct, and at its most useful when fully integrated into the curriculum.(170) Simulation should not be viewed as limited to training but as enhancing all aspects of professional education, particularly in relation to clinical reasoning and professional judgement.

There is a question over the transferability of learning from the simulated to the clinical environment. Recently, there have been concerns expressed about a disparity between confidence and assessed competence of new graduates, and calls for the improved and systematic teaching of clinical skills.(171,172) However, it is still not clear how well these transfer into practice,(173) and it may be that simulation, while providing varying degrees of fidelity, does not attend to the noisy, messy and emotional reality of clinical practice. An approach exposing learners to this milieu may

- The role of the facilitator or tutor in a learning episode involving simulation is crucial in ensuring integration and transfer through a reflective action.
- Place the learning in context.
- Stage the simulation in a progressive and staged manner.
- A haptic component of a simulator in a simulated learning episode can add value to transfer of learning to context.
- The non-verbal skills of simulated patients, more than the content of their script, promote engagement with the learner. The resulting deep learning creates transferability potential.
- Recreation of the real clinical environment facilitates 'suspension of disbelief' and aids transfer of competence to performance.
- Structuring the learning to move from the specific to the general at the end of a learning session using simulation promotes transfer.
- Giving inexperienced learners specific relevant tasks in the workplace can reinforce learning in the simulated setting.
- Build a time into the learning session to encourage generalisability to the workplace.
- Feedback is crucial in enabling learners to generalise their learning for future practice.
- Ensure learning facilities using simulation are located close to or in the context of the workplace.
- Link the timing of the simulation to workplace experience.

have more relevance,(66,83) and it has also been suggested that close geographical location of workplace and simulated learning facilities where learners can more readily avail themselves of learning opportunities as their needs are identified is important. Training should be more aligned to fulfilling capability and less to time-limited competency end points.(174)

Planning of learning needs to support the development of skills through a process that stages acquisition linked to increasing authenticity.(101) It should be realised that learning in the simulated environment is not an end in itself. It is unrealistic to expect that one or two episodes of teaching and learning using simulation are sufficient to produce competence or proficiency. Learners still need to apply their learning in the real world, under supervision, and to receive feedback so that their skills base may become consolidated, refined and adaptable. In terms of unintended learning, there may be the danger of abnormal risk-taking behaviours being adopted by learners if their simulated experience, which is risk and harm free, is not tempered with the need for them to recognise their own limitations and to call for senior help in difficult circumstances.

Some learners may form a comfort zone within the simulated environment and might retreat to this in the face of a challenging clinical workplace – 'simulation-seeking behaviour'; these learners require encouragement and support to put the lessons from simulation into practice in the workplace, with suitable supervision and feedback, akin to Vygotsky's 'zone of proximal development'.(175)

The workplace may also be the source of contradictory practice and negative role modelling that causes dissonance for the learner, who needs to be prepared for this eventuality.

There is no doubt that there are significant costs associated with establishing simulation-based learning, whether this is in clinical skills facilities or simulation centres.(176) The costs relate not only to the technological aspects but also to the physical infrastructure, the personnel and the ongoing costs associated with a programme of this sort. This needs to be offset against the potential gain in terms of patient safety, potential reduced litigation and the satisfaction of a better-prepared healthcare workforce. However, it is important to ensure the most cost-effective approach is used for learning and to recognise that simulation may not always be appropriate.

The Future of Simulation

Simulation needs more supportive evidence, both in relation to its effectiveness and its efficiency in medical education (*see* Box 12.11). Simulation is resource intensive, both financially and in manpower costs,(176) and therefore has to justify its role both in terms of outcomes and deliverables. Despite an almost exponential boom in the simulation literature (*see* Figure 12.4), more robust studies are required that link educational theory with the demands of service, studies which demonstrate changes in workplace behaviour that impact on patient outcomes, occurring as a direct result of simulated interventions. More specifically, there is also a need for an explicit understanding of clinical thinking; rehearsal of decision-making processes through simulation may help to avoid errors and increase physician awareness,(192) but the most effective and efficient way of doing this has yet to be identified.

For the moment though, with an increasing professional and societal emphasis on patient safety, it looks like simulation is not only here to stay, but will become even bigger business over the next few years. Greater public accountability will require that doctors rehearse and practise their skills away from the bedside, consulting room or operating theatre before putting patients in the firing line. The challenge for simulation is to prove that it can make a difference.

BOX 12.11 Where's the evidence?

There is an increasing literature regarding the use of simulation in medical education (*see* Figure 12.4), but most studies have been at the lower levels of Kirkpatrick's evaluation hierarchy.(5) Some research has looked beyond learner satisfaction and has reported on impact on learning. For example, analysis of performance data from virtual reality simulators has shown that simulator training is associated with a reduction in performance time and enhanced proficiency(177) and, more importantly, that this gain transfers to the real world.(178)

Simulation is increasingly being used to investigate performance-shaping behaviours, such as fatigue(179) or the introduction of new equipment, techniques and facilities for trial and rehearsal prior to being implemented in the workplace.(180–184) The use of simulation may also improve cognitive ability, as suggested by Rogers *et al.* in a study of fourth-year medical students' thinking and application of skills for managing critically ill patients,(185) and similarly by Steadman *et al.*(186) There have also been reports of simulators used to teach basic sciences with the aim of bridging the theory–practice gap.(187,188) That said, there are also several studies that indicate simulation's lack of impact.(189–191)

In a recent systematic review,(170) Issenberg *et al.* identified that although much of the primary literature was weak, certain features of hi-fidelity simulation were consistently reported as facilitating learning. These were:

- providing feedback
- allowing repetitive practice
- integrating within curriculum
- providing a range of difficulties
- being adaptable; allowing multiple learning strategies
- providing a range of clinical scenarios
- providing a safe, educationally supportive learning environment
- active learning based on individualised needs
- defining outcomes
- ensuring simulator validity as a realistic recreation of complex clinical situations.

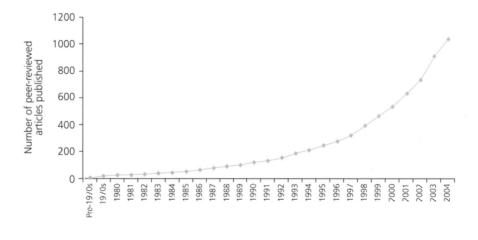

Figure 12.4 The growth in 'simulation' literature pre-1970s–2004.(193)

References

1 Leape LL (1994) Error in medicine. *Journal of the American Medical Association.* **272**: 1851–7.

2 Helmreich RL (2000) On error management: lessons from aviation. *British Medical Journal.* **320**: 781–5.

3 Reason J (2000) Human error: models and management. *British Medical Journal.* **320**: 768–70.

4 Burke CS, Salas E, Wilson-Donnelly K *et al.* (2004) How to turn a team of experts into an expert medical team: guidance from the aviation and military communities. *Quality & Safety in Health Care.* **13**(s1): i96–i104.

5 Kirkpatrick DL (1994) *Evaluating Training Programs: the four levels.* Berrett-Koehler Publishers, San Francisco, CA.

6 Bradley P (2006) History of simulation in medical education and possible future directions. *Medical Education.* **40**: 254–62.

7 Le Boursier du Coudray A (1759) *Abrégé de l'art des accouchements.* Vve Delaguette, Paris. Cited in: van Meurs WL (2006) Evolution of acute care simulation: a European perspective. *Medisch Journaal.* **35**: 116.

8 Tjomsland N and Baskett P (2002) Resuscitation greats: Armund S Laerdal. *Resuscitation.* **53**: 115–19.

9 Abrahamson S, Denson JS and Wolf RM (2004) Effectiveness of a simulator in training anesthesiology residents. *Quality & Safety in Health Care.* **13**: 395–7.

10 Good ML (2003) Patient simulation for training basic and advanced clinical skills. *Medical Education.* **37**(s1): 14–21.

11 Good ML and Gravenstein JS (1989) Anaesthesia simulators and training devices. *International Anesthesiology Clinics.* **27**: 161–6.

12 Gaba DM and DeAnda A (1988) A comprehensive anaesthesia simulation environment: re-creating the operating room for research and training. *Anaesthesiology.* **69**: 387–94.

13 Howard SK, Gaba DM, Fish KJ *et al.* (1992) Anesthesia crisis resource management training: teaching anesthesiologists to handle critical incidents. *Aviation, Space, and Environmental Medicine.* **63**: 763–70.

14 Gaba DM, Fish KJ and Howard SK (1994) *Crisis Management in Anesthesiology.* Churchill Livingstone, New York.

15 Flin R and Maran N (2004) Identifying and training non-technical skills for teams in acute medicine. *Quality & Safety in Health Care.* **13**(s1): i80–i84.

16 Glavin RJ and Maran NJ (2003) Integrating human factors into the medical curriculum. *Medical Education.* **37**(s1): 59–64.

17 Barrows HS (1993) An overview of the uses of standardized patients for teaching and evaluating clinical skills. *Academic Medicine.* **68**: 443–51.

18 Santen S, Hemphill RR, McDonald MF *et al.* (2004) Patients' willingness to allow residents to learn to practice medical procedures. *Academic Medicine.* **79**: 144–7.

19 Santen SA, Hemphill RR, Spanier CM *et al.* (2005) 'Sorry, it's my first time!' Will patients consent to medical students learning procedures? *Medical Education.* **39**: 365–9.

20 Sedlack RE and Kolars JC (2004) Computer simulator training enhances the competency of gastroenterology fellows at colonoscopy: results of a pilot study. *The American Journal of Gastroenterology.* **99**: 33–7.

21 Sedlack RE, Kolars JC and Alexander JA (2004) Computer simulation training enhances patient comfort during endoscopy. *Clinical Gastroenterology and Hepatology.* **2**: 348–52.

22 McManus I, Richards P and Winder B (1998) Clinical experience of UK medical students. *Lancet.* **351**: 802–3.

23 Hunt G and Wainwright P (eds) (1994) *Expanding the Role of the Nurse.* Blackwell Scientific Publications, Oxford.

24 Department of Health (2002) *Developing Key Roles for Nurses and Midwives: a guide for managers.* DoH, London.

25 Department of Health (2003) *The Chief Health Professions Officer's Ten Key Roles for Allied Health Professionals.* DoH, London.

26 Kohn LT, Corrigan JM and Donaldson MS (2000) *To Err is Human: building a safer health system.* National Academy Press, Washington, DC.

27 Department of Health (2000) *An Organisation with a Memory.* Stationery Office, London.

28 Blike G, Cravero J, Andeweg S *et al.* (2005) Standardized simulated events for provocative testing of medical care system rescue capabilities. In: *Advances in Patient Safety: from research to implementation*, pp. 193–207. Agency for Healthcare Research and Quality, Rockville, MD.

29 Maran NJ and Glavin RJ (2003) Low- to high-fidelity simulation – a continuum of medical education? *Medical Education.* **37**(s1): 22–8.

30 Donovan T, Hutchison T and Kelly A (2003) Using simulated patients in a multiprofessional communications skills programme: reflections from the programme facilitators. *European Journal of Cancer Care.* **12**: 123–8.

31 Ker J, Mole L and Bradley P (2003) Early introduction to interprofessional learning: a simulated ward environment. *Medical Education.* **37**: 248–55.

32 Macedonia CR, Gherman RB and Satin AJ (2003) Simulation laboratories for training in obstetrics and gynecology. *Obstetrics and Gynecology.* **102**: 388–92.

33 Beaubien JM and Baker DP (2004) The use of simulation for training teamwork skills in health care: how low can you go? *Quality & Safety in Health Care.* **13**(s1): i51–i56.

34 Ostergaard HT, Ostergaard D and Lippert A (2004) Implementation of team training in medical education in Denmark. *Quality & Safety in Health Care.* **13**(s1): i91–i95.

35 Shapiro MJ, Morey J, Small S *et al.* (2004) Simulation based teamwork training for emergency department staff: does it improve clinical team performance when added to an existing didactic teamwork curriculum? *Quality & Safety in Health Care.* **13**: 417–21.

36 Watterson L, Flanagan B, Donovan B *et al.* (2000) Anaesthetic simulators: training for the broader health-care profession. *Australia and New Zealand Journal of Surgery.* **70**: 735–7.

37 Shapiro MJ and Jay GD (2003) High reliability organizational change for hospitals: translating tenets for medical professionals. *Quality & Safety in Health Care.* **12**: 238–9.

38 Sexton J, Thomas E and Helmreich R (2000) Error, stress, and teamwork in medicine and aviation: cross sectional surveys. *British Medical Journal.* **320**: 745–9.

39 Leonard M, Graham S and Bonacum D (2004) The human factor: the critical importance of effective teamwork and communication in providing safe care. *Quality & Safety in Health Care.* **13**(s1): i85–i90.

40 Ulrich Ecke LK, Müller W, Ziegler R and Mann W (1998) Virtual reality: preparation and execution of sinus surgery. *Computer Aided Surgery.* **3**: 45–50.

41 Ladas SD, Malfertheiner P and Axon A (2002) An introductory course for training in endoscopy. *Digestive Diseases.* **20**: 242–5.

42 Letterie GS (2002) How virtual reality may enhance training in obstetrics and gynecology. *American Journal of Obstetrics & Gynecology.* **187**(s): s37–s40.

43 Reznek M, Harter P and Krummel T (2002) Virtual reality and simulation: training the future emergency physician. *Academic Emergency Medicine.* **9**: 78–87.

44 Adrales GL, Flanagan B, Donovan B *et al.* (2003) Evaluating minimally invasive surgery training using low-cost mechanical simulations. *Surgical Endoscopy.* **17**: 580–5.

45 Fichera A, Prachand V, Kives S *et al.* (2005) Physical reality simulation for training of laparoscopists in the 21st century. A multispecialty, multi-institutional study. *Journal of the Society of Laparoendoscopic Surgeons.* **9**: 125–9.

46 Aggarwal R, Grantcharov T, Moorthy K *et al.* (2006) A competency-based virtual reality training curriculum for the acquisition of laparoscopic psychomotor skill. *The American Journal of Surgery.* **191**: 128–33.

47 Education Committee of the General Medical Council (2002) *Tomorrow's Doctors: recommendations on undergraduate medical education.* General Medical Council, London.

48 Education Committee of the General Medical Council (2005) *The New Doctor: recommendations on general clinical training.* General Medical Council, London.

49 General Medical Council (2006) *Good Medical Practice.* GMC, London.

50 Accreditation Council for Graduate Medical Education (1999) *ACGME Outcome Project.* Accreditation Council for Graduate Medical Education, Chicago, IL.

51 Association of American Medical Colleges (1998) *Report I Learning Objectives for Medical Student Education: guidelines for medical schools.* Medical School Objectives Project, Washington, DC.

52 Frank JR (ed.) (2005) *The CanMEDS 2005 Physician Competency Framework. Better standards. Better physicians. Better care.* The Royal College of Physicians and Surgeons of Canada, Ottawa, ON.

53 UK Health Departments (2004) *Modernising Medical Careers – the next steps.* UK Health Departments, London.

54 Richards P and Gumpel M (1997) Save our service. *British Medical Journal.* **314**: 1756–8.

55 Rahman A (2005) Teaching students – whose job is it anyway? *British Medical Journal.* **330**: 153.

56 Richards T (1997) Disillusioned doctors. *British Medical Journal.* **314**: 1705.

57 Skinner DV, Camm AJ and Miles S (1985) Cardiopulmonary resuscitation skills of preregistration house officers. *British Medical Journal.* **290**: 1549–50.

58 Carter R, Aitchison M, Mufti GR *et al.* (1990) Catheterisation: your urethra in their hands. *British Medical Journal.* **301**: 905.

59 Feher M, Harris-St John K and Lant A (1992) Blood pressure measurement by junior hospital doctors – a gap in medical education? *Health Trends.* **24**(2): 59–61.

60 Taylor DM (1997) Undergraduate procedural skills training in Victoria: is it adequate? *Medical Journal of Australia.* **166**: 1–3.

61 Fox RA, Ingham Clark CL, Scotland AD *et al.* (2000) A study of pre-registration house officers' clinical skills. *Medical Education.* **34**: 1007–12.

62 Turner KJ and Brewster SF (2000) Rectal examination and urethral catheterization by medical students and house officers: taught but not used. *BJU International (formerly British Journal of Urology).* **86**: 422–6.

63 Goodfellow PB and Claydon P (2001) Students sitting medical finals – ready to be house officers? *Journal of the Royal Society of Medicine.* **94**: 516–20.

64 Boltri J, Hash R and Vogel R (2003) Are family practice residents able to interpret electrocardiograms? *Advances in Health Sciences Education.* **8**: 149–53.

65 Cartwright MS, Reynolds PS, Rodriguez ZM *et al.* (2005) Lumbar puncture experience among medical school graduates: the need for formal procedural skills training. *Medical Education.* **39**: 437.

66 Kneebone R, Nestel D, Yadollahi F *et al.* (2006) Assessing procedural skills in context: exploring the feasibility of an Integrated Procedural Performance Instrument (IPPI). *Medical Education.* **40**: 1105–14.

67 Ker JS, Dowie JS, Dowell A *et al.* (2005) Twelve tips for developing and maintaining a simulated patient bank. *Medical Teacher.* **27**: 4–9.

68 Ker J, Hesketh A, Anderson F *et al.* (2005) PRHO views on the usefulness of a pilot ward simulation exercise. *Hospital Medicine.* **66**: 168–70.

69 Morgan PJ and Cleave-Hogg D (2000) A Canadian simulation experience: faculty and student opinions of a performance evaluation study. *British Journal of Anaesthesiology.* **85**: 779–81.

70 Bradley P and Postlethwaite K (2003) Setting up a clinical skills learning facility. *Medical Education.* **37**(s1): 6–13.

71 McLaughlin SA, Doezema D and Sklar DP (2002) Human simulation in emergency medicine training: a model curriculum. *Academic Emergency Medicine.* **9**: 1310–18.

72 Devitt JH, Kurrek MM, Cohen MM *et al.* (2001) The validity of performance assessments using simulation. *Anesthesiology.* **95**: 36–42.

73 Forrest FC, Taylor MA, Postlethwaite K *et al.* (2002) Use of a high-fidelity simulator to develop testing of the technical performance of novice anaesthetists. *British Journal of Anaesthesiology.* **88**: 338–44.

74 Weller J, Wilson L and Robinson B (2003) Survey of change in practice following simulation-based training in crisis management. *Anaesthesia.* **58**: 471–3.

75 Meller G (1997) A typology of simulators for medical education. *Journal of Digital Imaging.* **10**(3, s1): 194–6.

76 Miller RB (1953) *Handbook on Training and Training Equipment Design.* Air Research and Development Command, United States Air Force, Dayton, OH.

77 Rehmann AJ, Mitman RD and Reynolds MC (1995) *A Handbook of Flight Simulation Fidelity Requirements for Human Factors Research.* Crew System Ergonomics Information Analysis Center, Wright-Patterson Airforce Base, Dayton, OH.

78 Farmer E, van Rooij J, Riemersma J *et al.* (1999) *Handbook of Simulator Based Training.* Ashgate, Aldershot.

79 Oser RL, Cannon-Bowers JA, Salas E *et al.* (1999) Enhancing human performance in technology-rich environments: guidelines for scenario-based training. In: Salas E (ed.) *Human/Technology Interaction in Complex Systems,* pp. 175–202. JAI Press Inc, Greenwich, CT.

80 Kneebone R (2003) Simulation in surgical training: educational issues and practical implications. *Medical Education.* **37**: 267–77.

81 Gordon MS, Ewy GA, Felner JM, *et al.* (1980) Teaching bedside cardiologic examination skills using 'Harvey', the cardiology patient simulator. *Medical Clinics of North America.* **64**: 305–13.

82 Takashina T, Shimizu M and Katayama H (1997) A new cardiology simulator. *Cardiology.* **88**: 408–13.

83 Kneebone R, Kidd J, Nestel D *et al.* (2002) An innovative model for teaching and learning clinical procedures. *Medical Education.* **36**: 628–34.

84 Pickard S, Baraitser P, Rymer J *et al.* (2003) Can gynaecology teaching associates provide high quality effective training for medical students in the United Kingdom? Comparative study. *British Medical Journal.* **327**: 1389–92.

85 Rochelson B, Baker DA, Mann WJ *et al.* (1985) Use of male and female professional patient teams in teaching physical examination of the genitalia. *Journal of Reproductive Medicine.* **30**: 864–6.

86 Wånggren K, Pettersson G, Csemiczky G *et al.* (2005) Teaching medical students gynaecological examination using professional patients – evaluation of students' skills and feelings. *Medical Teacher.* **27**: 130–5.

87 Dacre J, Nicol M, Holroyd D *et al.* (1996) The development of a clinical skills centre. *Journal of the Royal College of Physicians London.* **30**: 318–24.

88 du Boulay C and Medway C (1999) The clinical skills resource: a review of current practice. *Medical Education.* **33**: 185–91.

89 Bradley P and Bligh J (1999) One year's experience with a clinical skills resource centre. *Medical Education.* **33**: 114–20.

90 Gaba DM (2004) The future vision of simulation in health care. *Quality & Safety in Health Care.* **13**(s1): i2–i10.

91 Skinner B (1978) *Reflections on Behaviorism and Society.* Prentice-Hall, Englewood Cliffs, NJ.

92 Watson JB (1924) *Behaviorism.* Norton, New York.

93 Bandura A (2001) Social cognitive theory: an agentic perspective. *Annual Review of Psychology.* **52**: 1–26.

94 Thompson S, Neal S and Clark V (2004) Clinical risk management in obstetrics: eclampsia drills. *British Medical Journal.* **328**: 269–71.

95 Douglas JDM and Laird C (2004) Clinical fire drills and skill decay: can we develop an evidence base for policy and a language for training? *Medical Education.* **38**: 14–16.

96 McCarthy GJ and Reid DK (1981) *The Learning Theory of Piaget and Inhelder.* Brooks/Cole Pub Co., Monterey, CA.

97 Bruner J (1966) *Toward a Theory of Instruction.* Harvard University Press, Cambridge, MA.

98 Jarvis P, Holford J and Griffin C (2004) *The Theory and Practice of Learning (2e).* RoutledgeFalmer, London.

99 Lave J and Wegner E (1991) Situated learning: legitimate peripheral participation. Cambridge University Press, Cambridge.

100 Collins A, Brown JS and Newman SE (1986) *Cognitive Apprenticeship: teaching the craft of reading, writing, and mathematics.* BBN Labs Inc, Cambridge, MA.

101 Gott SP, Kane RS and Lesgold A (1995) *Tutoring Transfer of Technical Competence.* Armstrong Lab, Brooks AFB, TX.

102 Kolb D (1984) *Experiential Learning.* Prentice Hall, Englewood Cliffs, NJ.

103 Reeves S, Freeth D, McCrorie P *et al.* (2002) 'It teaches you what to expect in future': interprofessional learning on a training ward for medical, nursing, occupational therapy and physiotherapy students. *Medical Education.* **36**: 337–44.

104 Wahlstrom O, Sanden I and Hammar M (1997) Multiprofessional education in the medical curriculum. *Medical Education.* **31**: 425–9.

105 Schön D (1983) *The Reflective Practitioner.* Basic Books, New York.

106 Schön D (1987) *Educating the Reflective Practitioner.* Jossey-Bass, San Francisco, CA.

107 Mezirow J (1991) *Transformative Dimensions of Adult Learning.* Jossey-Bass, San Francisco, CA.

108 Seropian MA (2003) General concepts in full scale simulation: getting started. *Anesthesia and Analgesia.* **97**: 1695–705.

109 Byrne AJ, Sellen AJ, Jones JG *et al.* (2002) Effect of videotape feedback on anaesthetists' performance while managing simulated anaesthetic crises: a multi centre study. *Anaesthesia.* **57**: 176–9.

110 Roter DL, Larson S, Shinitzky H *et al.* (2004) Use of an innovative video feedback technique to enhance communication skills training. *Medical Education.* **38**: 145–57.

111 Savoldelli GL, Naik VN, Park J *et al.* (2006) Value of debriefing during simulated crisis management: oral versus video-assisted oral feedback. *Anesthesiology.* **105**: 279–85.

112 Bedny GZ, Seglin MH and Meister D (2000) Activity theory: history, research and application. *Theoretical Issues in Ergonomics Science.* **1**: 168–206.

113 Engeström Y (1999) Activity theory and individual and social transformation. In: Engeström Y, Miettinen R and Punamäki R (eds) *Perspectives on Activity Theory,* pp. 19–38. Cambridge University Press, Cambridge.

114 Brown K and Cole M (2001) Cultural historical activity theory and the expansion of opportunities for learning after school. In: Packer MJ and Tappan MB (eds) *Cultural and Critical Perspectives on Human Development,* pp. 225–238. SUNY Press, New York (http://lchc.ucsd.edu/People/MCole/browncole.html).

115 Engestrom Y (1987) *Learning by Expanding: an activity-theoretical approach to developmental research.* Orienta-Konsultit, Helsinki.

116 Small SD, Wuerz RC, Simon R *et al.* (1999) Demonstration of high-fidelity simulation team training for emergency medicine. *Academic Emergency Medicine.* **6**: 312–23.

117 Aggarwal R, Undre S, Moorthy K *et al.* (2004) The simulated operating theatre: comprehensive training for surgical teams. *Quality & Safety in Health Care.* **13**(suppl 1): i27–i32.

118 Kyrkjebø JM, Brattebø G and Smith-Strøm H (2006) Improving patient safety by using interprofessional simulation training in health professional education. *Journal of Interprofessional Care.* **20**: 507–16.

119 Dreyfus H and Dreyfus S (1986) *Mind Over Machine: the power of human intuition and expertise in the era of the computer.* Basil Blackwell, Oxford.

120 Laurillard D (1997) Learning formal representation through multimedia. In: Entwhistle NF (ed.) *The Experience of Learning,* pp. 172–83. Scottish Acdemic Press, Edinburgh.

121 Cowan G (ed.) (2001) *Assessment and Appraisal of Doctors in Training. Principles and practice.* Royal College of Physicians of London, Salisbury.

122 Lockyer J (2003) Multisource feedback in the assessment of physician competencies. *Journal of Continuing Education in the Health Professions.* **23**: 4–12.

123 Archer JC, Norcini J and Davies HA (2005) Use of SPRAT for peer review of paediatricians in training. *British Medical Journal.* **330**: 1251–3.

124 Beaubien J and Baker D (2003) Post-training feedback: the relative effectiveness of team- versus instructor-led debriefings. In: *47th Annual Meeting of the Human Factors and Ergonomics Society.* Human Factors and Ergonomics Society, Santa Monica, CA, 2003.

125 Fuller G and Smith P (2001) Rediscovering the wheel: teaching communication skills using video taped clinical consultations in specialist training. *Clinical Medicine.* **1**: 203–4.

126 Festa LM, Baliko B, Mangiafico T *et al.* (2000) Maximizing learning outcomes by videotaping nursing students' interactions with a standardized patient. *Journal of Psychosocial Nursing & Mental Health Services.* **38**: 37–44.

127 McGraw RC and O'Connor HM (1999) Standardized patients in the early acquisition of clinical skills. *Medical Education.* **33**: 572–8.

128 Howley L and Martindale J (2004) The efficacy of standardized patient feedback in clinical teaching: a mixed methods analysis. *Medical Education Online.* **9**.

129 Rogers J (2001) *Adults Learning (4e).* Open University Press, Maidenhead, p. 225.

130 Stafford F (2005) The significance of de-roling and debriefing in training medical students using simulation to train medical students. *Medical Education.* **39**: 1083–5.

131 Spencer J and Dales J (2006) Meeting the needs of simulated patients and caring for the person behind them? *Medical Education.* **40**: 3–5.

132 Bokken L, van Dalen J and Rethans J-J (2004) Performance-related stress symptoms in simulated patients. *Medical Education.* **38**: 1089–94.

133 Bokken L, van Dalen J and Rethans J-J (2006) The impact of simulation on people who act as simulated patients: a focus group study. *Medical Education.* **40**: 781–6.

134 Pendleton D, Schofield T, Tate P *et al.* (1984) *The Consultation: an approach to learning and teaching.* Oxford University Press, Oxford.

135 Silverman J, Draper J and Kurtz SM (1996) The Calgary–Cambridge approach to communication skills teaching 1: agenda-led outcome-based analysis of the consultation. *Education for General Practice.* **7**: 279–378.

136 Kurtz S, Silverman J and Draper J (1998) *Teaching and Learning Communication Skills in Medicine.* Radcliffe Medical Press, Oxford.

137 Hawkins P and Shohet R (2000) *Supervision in the Helping Professions: an individual, group and organizational approach (2e).* Open University Press, Milton Keynes.

138 Owen H and Follows V (2006) GREAT simulation debriefing. *Medical Education.* **40**: 488–9.

139 Bloom BS (1956) *Taxonomy of Educational Objectives: the classification of educational goals. Handbook I: Cognitive domain.* Longmans, New York.

140 Eraut M (1994) *Developing Professional Knowledge and Competence.* The Falmer Press, London.

141 Gagne RM (1985) *The Conditions of Learning and Theory of Instruction (4e).* Holt, Rinehart and Winston, New York.

142 Walker M (ed.) (1998) *Advanced Life Support Group, Pocket Guide to Teaching for Medical Instructors.* BMJ Books, London.

143 Joyce BR and Showers B (1980) Improving in service training: the messages of research. *Educational Leadership.* **37**: 379–85.

144 Salas E, Wilson KA, Burke CS *et al.* (2005) Using simulation-based training to improve patient safety: what does it take? *Journal on Quality and Patient Safety.* **37**: 363–71.

145 Fletcher G, Flin R, McGeorge P *et al.* (2003) Anaesthetists' non-technical skills (ANTS): evaluation of a behavioural marker system. *British Journal of Anaesthesiology.* **90**: 580–8.

146 Rudolph JW, Simon R, Dufresne RL, Raemer DB (2006) There's no such thing as "nonjudgmental" debriefing: A theory and method for debriefing with good judgment. *Simulation in Healthcare.* **1**: 49–55.

147 Gaba DM, Howard SK, Flanagan B *et al.* (1998) Assessment of clinical performance during simulated crises using both technical and behavioral ratings. *Anesthesiology.* **89**: 8–18.

148 Ker JS, Hesketh EA, Anderson F *et al.* (2006) Can a ward simulation exercise achieve the realism that reflects the complexity of everyday practice junior doctors encounter? *Medical Teacher.* **28**: 330–4.

149 Gaba DM and DeAnda A (1988) A comprehensive anesthesia simulation environment: re- creating the operating room for research and training. *Anesthesiology.* **69**: 387–94.

150 Crosskerry P (2003) The importance of cognitive errors in diagnosis and strategies to try and minimise them. *Academic Medicine.* **78**: 1–6.

151 Helmreich RL and Schaefer H (1994) Team performance in the operating room. In: Bogner M (ed.) *Human Error in Medicine,* pp. 225–53. Lawrence Erlbaum Associates, Hillsdale, NJ.

152 Helmreich RL and Davies JM (1996) Human factors in the operating room: interpersonal determinants of safety, efficiency, and morale. In: Aitkenhead AR (ed.) *Ballière's Clinical Anaesthesiology: safety and risk management in anaesthesia,* pp. 277–96. Ballière Tindall, London.

153 Moorthy K, Munz Y, Adams S *et al.* (2005) A human factors analysis of technical and team skills among surgical trainees during procedural simulations in a simulated operating theatre. *Annals of Surgery.* **242**: 631–9.

154 Smith GB, Osgood VM and Crane S (2002) ALERT(TM) – a multiprofessional training course in the care of the acutely ill adult patient. *Resuscitation.* **52**: 281–6.

155 Baker DP, Gustafson S, Beaubien JM *et al.* (2005) *Medical Team Training Programs in Health Care, in Advances in Patient Safety: from research to implementation.* Agency for Healthcare Research and Quality, Rockville, MD, pp. 253–67.

156 Freeth D and Nicol M (1998) Learning clinical skills: an interprofessional approach. *Nurse Education Today.* **18**: 455–61.

157 Tucker K, Wakefield A, Boggis C *et al.* (2003) Learning together: clinical skills teaching for medical and nursing students. *Medical Education.* **37**: 630–7.

158 Ross F and Southgate L (2000) Learning together in medical and nursing training: aspirations and activity. *Medical Education.* **34**: 739–43.

159 Pirrie A, Wilson V, Harden RM *et al.* (1998) AMEE Guide No. 12: Multiprofessional education: Part 2 – promoting cohesive practice in health care. *Medical Teacher.* **20**: 409–16.

160 Lorente M, Hogg G and Ker J (2006) The challenges of initiating a multiprofessional clinical skills project. *Journal of Interprofessional Care.* **20**: 290–301.

161 Miller GE (1990) The assessment of clinical skills/competence/performance. *Academic Medicine.* **65**(9 Suppl): S63–S67.

162 Harden R, Stevenson M, Downie WW *et al.* (1975) Assessment of clinical competence using objective structured examination. *British Medical Journal.* **1**: 447–51.

163 Newble D (2004) Techniques for measuring clinical competence: Objective Structured Clinical Examinations. *Medical Education.* **38**: 199–203.

164 Regehr G, MacRae H, Reznick RK *et al.* (1998) Comparing the psychometric properties of checklists and global rating scales for assessing performance on an OSCE-format examination. *Academic Medicine.* **73**: 993–7.

165 Byrne AJ and Greaves JD (2001) Assessment instruments used during anaesthetic simulation: review of published studies. *British Journal of Anaesthiology.* **86**: 445–50.

166 Devitt J, Kurrek MM, Cohen MM *et al.* (1998) Testing internal consistency and construct validity during evaluation of performance in a patient simulator. *Anesthesia and Analgesia.* **86**: 1160–4.

167 Rethans JJ, Drop R, Sturmans F *et al.* (1991) Assessment of the performance of general practitioners by the use of standardized (simulated) patients. *British Journal of General Practice.* **41**: 97–9.

168 Barnett SM and Ceci SJ (2002) When and where do we apply what we learn? A taxonomy for far transfer. *Psychological Bulletin.* **128**: 612–37.

169 Ericsson KA, Krampe RT and Tesch Roemer C (1993) The role of deliberate practice in the acquisition of expert performance. *Psychology Review.* **100**: 363–406.

170 Issenberg SB, McGaghie WC, Petrusa ER *et al.* (2005) Features and uses of high-fidelity medical simulations that lead to effective learning: a BEME systematic review. *Medical Teacher.* **27**: 10–28.

171 Barnsley L, Lyon PM, Ralston SJ *et al.* (2004) Clinical skills in junior medical officers: a comparison of self-reported confidence and observed competence. *Medical Education.* **38**: 358–67.

172 Evans DE, Wood DF and Roberts CM (2004) The effect of an extended hospital induction on perceived confidence and assessed clinical skills of newly qualified pre-registration house officers. *Medical Education.* **38**: 998–1001.

173 Silverman J and Wood DF (2004) New approaches to learning clinical skills. *Medical Education.* **38**: 1021–3.

174 Kneebone RL, Scott W, Darzi A *et al.* (2004) Simulation and clinical practice: strengthening the relationship. *Medical Education.* **38**: 1095–102.

175 Bockarie A (2002) The potential of Vygotsky's contributions to our understanding of cognitive apprenticeship as a process of development in sadult vocational and technical education. *Journal of Career and Technical Education.* **19**: 47–66.

176 Kurrek MM and Devitt JH (1997) The cost for construction and operation of a simulation centre. *Canadian Journal of Anaesthesia.* **44**: 1191–5.

177 Kneebone RL, Nestel D, Moorthy K *et al.* (2003) Learning the skills of flexible sigmoidoscopy – the wider perspective. *Medical Education.* **37**(s1): 50–8.

178 Grantcharov TP, Kristiansen VB, Bendix J *et al.* (2004) Randomized clinical trial of virtual reality simulation for laparoscopic skills training. *British Journal of Surgery.* **91**: 146–50.

179 Howard SK, Gaba DM, Smith BE *et al.* (2003) Simulation study of rested versus sleep-deprived anesthesiologists. *Anesthesiology.* **98**: 1345–55.

180 Kobayashi L, Shapiro MJ, Sucov A *et al.* (2006) Portable advanced medical simulation for new emergency department testing and orientation. *Academic Emergency Medicine.* **13**: 691–5.

181 Vadodaria BS, Gandhi SD and McIndoe AK (2004) Comparison of four different emergency airway access equipment sets on a human patient simulator. *Anaesthesia.* **59**: 73–9.

182 Sanders J, Haas RE, Geisler M *et al.* (1998) Using the human patient simulator to test the efficacy of an experimental emergency percutaneous transtracheal airway. *Military Medicine.* **163**: 544–51.

183 Lim TJ, Lim Y and Liu EHC (2005) Evaluation of ease of intubation with the GlideScope or Macintosh laryngoscope by anaesthetists in simulated easy and difficult laryngoscopy. *Anaesthesia.* **60**: 180–3.

184 Anderson K, Gambhir S, Glavin R *et al.* (2006) The use of an anaesthetic simulator to assess single-use laryngoscopy equipment. *International Journal for Quality in Health Care.* **18**: 17–22.

185 Rogers PL, Jacob H, Thomas EA *et al.* (2000) Medical students can learn the basic application, analytic, evaluative, and psychomotor skills of critical care medicine. *Critical Care Medicine.* **28**: 550–4.

186 Steadman RH, Coates WC, Huang YM *et al.* (2006) Simulation-based training is superior to problem-based learning for the acquisition of critical assessment and management skills. *Critical Care Medicine.* **34**: 151–7.

187 Morgan PJ, Cleave-Hogg D, Desousa S *et al.* (2006) Applying theory to practice in undergraduate education using high fidelity simulation. *Medical Teacher.* **28**: e10–e15.

188 Tan GM, Kti L, Suresh S *et al.* (2002) Teaching first-year medical students physiology: does the human patient simulator allow for more effective teaching? *Singapore Medical Journal.* **43**: 238–42.

189 Gordon J, Shaffer DW, Raemer DB *et al.* (2006) A randomized controlled trial of simulation-based teaching versus traditional instruction in medicine: a pilot study among clinical medical students. *Advances in Health Sciences Education.* **11**: 33–9.

190 Morgan PJ, Cleave-Hogg D, McIlroy J *et al.* (2002) Simulation technology: a comparison of experiential and visual learning for undergraduate medical students. *Anesthesiology.* **96**: 10–16.

191 Engum SA, Jeffries P and Fisher L (2003) Intravenous catheter training system: computer-based education versus traditional learning methods. *The American Journal of Surgery.* **186**: 67–74.

192 Eva KW and Norman GR (2005) Heuristics and biases; a biased perspective on clinical reasoning. *Medical Education.* **39**: 870–2.

193 Center for Medical Simulation, Simulation References. [Online] Available from: http://harvardmedsim.org/cms/simreferences.html [Accessed Feb 2nd 2007].

Patient involvement in medical education

John Spencer and Judy McKimm

KEY MESSAGES

- Patient involvement in medical education is embedded within a broader health services policy agenda.

- There is a growing literature on patient involvement but much of it is descriptive and lacks rigour.

- A wide variety of initiatives and settings has been described.

- A wide range of benefits has been shown for all stakeholders.

- There is a need for appropriate support, training and remuneration for all involved.

- 'Patients' include patients themselves, patient groups, and patient representatives and advocates.

- There is a need for further research, including an assessment of the strengths and weaknesses of different approaches, an evaluation of long-term impact and identification of factors that influence sustainability.

Introduction

My method (is to) lead my students by hand to the practice of medicine, taking them every day to see patients in the public hospital, that they may hear the patient's symptoms and see their physical findings. Then I question the students as to what they have noted in their patients and about their thoughts and perceptions regarding the causes of the illness and the principles of treatment. Sylvius (1614–1672)(1)

In the early 17th century Sylvius's teaching methods would have been unusual, and it would probably have been considered eccentric to involve patients in medical education to such a degree. Although the traditional apprenticeship approach – dating back at least to the time of Hippocrates – depended on contact with sick people, by the time medical education was formally established in the universities of Europe in the 13th century, the patient had all but 'disappeared'. It was not until after the Renaissance that some universities started to introduce bedside clinical experience. By the 18th century it was, in the words of one author, 'axiomatic' that students should supplement their book learning by spending time 'walking the wards',(2) although examination of patients as a component part of assessment did not appear until the following century. Clinical experience through patient contact gradually assumed its place at the centre of medical education such that by the turn of the 20th century, Sir William Osler's assertion that 'it is a safe rule to have no teaching without a patient for a text, and the best teaching is that taught by the patient himself'(3) had

become part of the rhetoric of a modern medical education.

The long-acknowledged, and crucial, role of the patient in clinical education has historically been a passive one, at worst, something imposed on a hapless hospital patient unable to say 'No' to a gaggle of students at the foot of the bed – think Sir Lancelot Spratt in the film *Doctor in the House*.(4) Even at best, the patient, although treated with courtesy, was more often than not just a medium – 'an interesting case' – through which the clinical teacher taught.

This chapter considers the importance of actively involving patients in the education of doctors and other health professionals, explores aspects of what is a growing literature on the subject, including evidence of benefits, describes models and approaches to involvement, discusses the problems and challenges, and identifies areas for further inquiry. Before doing that, however, it is important to consider some terminology.

Patients, Users and Consumers

Terminology in the area of patient involvement in medical education is a source of controversy and confusion, and the issues are complex. The language used generates strong emotions, affecting communication and collaboration between interested groups, and may even impair scholarly activity, such as searching and reviewing the literature.(5,6) Views vary greatly about which labels people prefer to have used to describe them and preferences may change over time.(6) For simplicity's sake we will mainly use the term 'patient' (and, where relevant, 'carer') throughout this chapter, because, for all its limitations, it is probably the most widely recognised term in medical education (*see* Box

Understanding Medical Education: Evidence, Theory and Practice.
Edited by T Swanwick. © 2010 Association for the Study of Medical Education.

BOX 13.1 Terminology

User or *service user* is commonly used in the UK, but in North America may be more associated with illicit drug use. However, 'user' does imply a degree of active participation.

Lay is also used frequently; it implies the person is not necessarily either sick or under active care. However, 'lay' defines a person essentially not by any positive attributes, but by what they are *not* (i.e. 'professional') and what they do not have (i.e. medical expertise).

Consumer, client or *customer* connote health as a commodity and healthcare as a market, thus a commercial relationship.

Survivor is a term mostly restricted to use in relation to cancer and mental health.

Patient is probably the most unambiguous term, although it implies that the person is sick and under active care; the term connotes passivity; and the care relationship is medicalised.

13.1). We use it to mean both people with health problems, whether or not they are currently receiving care, and healthy people, although we recognise that this may be contentious and will not acknowledge everyone's preference. We also recognise that 'on the ground' it is important to recognise the power of language.(5)

Context of Patient Involvement

Involving patients in the management and practice of healthcare has been an important aspect of UK government policy since the 1980s, developing through the 1990s to the point where it is now enshrined as the underlying principle of healthcare reform and modernisation in a 'patient-led National Health Service (NHS)', the aim being to make health services more responsive to the needs of the community. It is now a statutory requirement that 'patient and public involvement should be part of everyday practice in the NHS and must lead to action for improvement';(7) this inevitably encompasses involvement in the training and education of health professionals.(8,9) These trends are not confined to the UK.(10)

There is arguably a broader educational context, that of 'social accountability'. This has been defined by the World Health Organisation as:

the obligation [of medical schools] to direct their education, research and service activities towards addressing the priority health concerns of the community, region, and/or nation they have the mandate to serve.(11)

Social accountability has evolved as a major contemporary discourse embracing concepts such as 'social responsibility' (of doctors and other health professionals), 'the social contract' (between professions and society) and 'social responsiveness' (of institutions). At the same time, and influenced by much the same social and political forces, the concept of 'professionalism' has been revisited and redefined, with obvious implications for education.(12–14)

These developments have occurred in parallel with changes in public expectations of healthcare, changes often described as part of the move from paternalism to partnership. With the decline in an uncritical deference to the professions, rise of consumerism and greater understanding of what healthcare can achieve, many patients expect to have their concerns addressed and their requests heard, and to be fully informed about their condition, briefed about risks of treatment, involved in decisions about their care, and educated and supported to manage their own conditions.(15)

Aside from changes in patients' expectations, there is now a greater appreciation of the psychological and social consequences of ill health and healthcare treatments, and the need for new models to guide clinical practice, such as the 'bio-psycho-social model' and 'patient-centredness', which put the patient's perspective and priorities at the centre.(16,17) Increased knowledge about variation between patients in values, preferences and responses to illness and their effect on treatment outcomes has brought the healthcare professional's interaction with the patient to centre stage. At the same time, the technical complexity of medicine increases all the time, with greater choice of diagnostic tests and treatments, and more complicated procedures and interventions.

Such circumstances make working with patients even more demanding, for example, supporting patients to exercise choice in situations of uncertainty, enabling them to understand the various options available and the risks and dangers involved, and helping them appreciate restrictions on choice. Learning how to do all these things needs input from patients and challenges educators to seek the most appropriate ways of enabling students and trainees to learn, while respecting the rights and needs of patients.(18) We go on to explore some of the issues involved.

Scope of Patient Involvement

Most people would probably assume that when people talk about 'patient involvement in the curriculum' they mean direct involvement in teaching, learning and assessment; indeed these areas are the main focus of this chapter. Nonetheless, there is potential for people from the community to make a contribution to all aspects of the educational process. These include:
- student selection and admission
- curriculum development, design and content
- course management
- faculty development

- practice placements
- programme evaluation.

However, several recent major literature reviews highlight that patient involvement in the above areas is still relatively unusual in most educational institutions. A number of frameworks that can help us explore the potential scope of patient involvement in medical education exist. Here we describe three: Tew *et al.*'s 'ladder of patient involvement',(19) the 'Cambridge framework'(20) and a taxonomy of the active involvement of patients in healthcare professions education described by Towle *et al.*(6)

Ladder of patient involvement

Tew *et al.*(19) describe a 'ladder of involvement', which they propose can be used to monitor patients' levels of involvement within individual programmes and institutions. The tool was developed in the context of mental health education and training, but in theory should be applicable across the educational spectrum, whether undergraduate or postgraduate (*see* Box 13.2).

The Cambridge framework

Spencer *et al.* reviewed the patient's role in medical education and suggested a framework (the 'Cambridge framework') to facilitate discussion about involvement of patients in clinical education.(20) It is based on four sets of attributes of situations and environments in which patients, students and teachers interact, under the headings 'Who?', 'How?', 'Where' and 'What?'. The authors also provide a checklist against which patient involvement can be planned or evaluated.

Who?

This aspect of patient involvement reflects the individual background, culture, experience and expectations of each patient, his or her family and carers. Patients vary immensely in terms of the clinical problems with which they present, as well as their age, gender, ethnicity, sexual orientation, emotional and intellectual capacity, and socioeconomic status.(21)

How?

Students and trainees work in a wide range of settings (such as hospital wards, hospital and community ambulatory clinics, emergency departments) presenting different opportunities to work with patients. These depend on factors such as whether encounters are planned or opportunistic, pressures of time, available supervision and so on. The issues under this

---

BOX 13.2 Ladder of patient involvement(19)

Level	Description of involvement
1 No involvement	The curriculum is planned, delivered and managed with no consultation or involvement of service users or carers
2 Limited involvement	Outreach with local service user or carer groups. Service users/carers invited to 'tell their story' in a designated slot and/or be consulted about course planning or management, student selection, student assessment or programme evaluation. Payment offered but no opportunity to participate in shaping the course as a whole
3 Growing involvement	Service users/carers contribute regularly to at least two of the following: planning, delivery, student selection, assessment, management or evaluation. Payment at normal visiting lecturer rates. However, key decisions on matters such as curriculum content, learning outcomes or student selection made in forums in which service users/carers are not represented. Some support before and after sessions, but no consistent programme of training and supervision. No discrimination against service users and carers accessing programmes as students
4 Collaboration	Service users/carers involved as full team members in at least three of the following: planning, delivery, student selection, assessment, management or evaluation. Underpinned by a statement of values. Service users/carers contribute to key decisions on matters such as curriculum content. Facility for contributors to the programme to meet and regular provision of training, supervision and support. Positive steps to encourage service users and carers to access programmes as students
5 Partnership	Service users, carers and staff work together systematically and strategically across all areas, underpinned by an explicit statement of partnership values. All key decisions made jointly. Service users and carers involved in the assessment of practice learning. Adequately funded infrastructure to provide induction, support and training. Service users and carers employed as lecturers on secure contracts and/or contracts established between programmes and independent groups. Positive steps made to encourage service users and carers to join learning sessions even if not (yet) in a position to achieve qualifications

heading (*see* Box 13.3) may help teachers to consider and plan how patients may be involved, and to relate this to the intended learning outcomes and the setting. In fact, most of the issues apply to all patient encounters.

Where?

Recognising that healthcare and healthcare education take place in a wide range of locations and settings, and that context will inevitably influence the nature and quality of learning, questions addressed under this heading explore issues to do with place, safety, identity, power relationships and so on. The 'Where?' also includes whether it is a 'real or 'simulated environment', such as training wards and simulation centres, and the contrast between 'uniprofessional' or 'multiprofessional' settings to distinguish between clinical situations in which doctors alone are learning with patients and those in which a range of health and social care professionals are learning and working (Box 13.4).(21)

What?

This set of attributes deals essentially with 'content': the clinical problems presented, the specific skills and knowledge that may be learned, and underlying atti-

tudes and values. Consideration of these should help teachers realise the maximum potential of particular situations and assess the likely impact on both patients and learners in particular situations (Box 13.5).

Active patient involvement

As observed above, there are many different contexts in which students may encounter patients, although historically this has tended to be restricted to opportunistic contact with 'real' patients in the wards and clinics of a teaching hospital. In the past two to three decades, however, a number of other ways of providing patient contact have been developed or have evolved in response to changes in the way healthcare is organised, the changing characteristics of patients in hospital and increasing recognition of the need to protect patients from harm, including, most recently, the challenges of infection control. This has led to the use of new environments, notably 'the community', where patient encounters take place either in primary care or in people's homes. This inevitably changes the dynamics and power balance. The shift of clinical education into the community is a worldwide phenomenon, has been shown to be effective(22) and is now the norm in undergraduate programmes.

Towle *et al.*(6) propose a further classification with elements of both the Cambridge framework and 'Ladder of involvement', which they argue helps clarify the patient's role and makes communication of research findings easier to articulate, synthesise and compare. The taxonomy considers the wide variety of ways other than real patients in the workplace in which patients are encountered, describing a continuum of patient involvement grounded in five attributes at six levels (*see* Box 13.6).

Levels of Patient Involvement

In this section, we describe some of the issues that may arise for medical educators under each of the levels described in Box 13.6.

BOX 13.6 A taxonomy of patient involvement(6)

Degree to which the patient is actively involved in the learning encounter	Duration of contact with learner	Patient autonomy during the encounter	Training for the patient	Patient involvement in planning the encounter and curriculum	Institutional commitment to patient involvement in education
1 Paper-based or electronic case or scenario Patient is focus of a paper-based, electronic or web-based case or scenario	None	Not applicable	Not applicable	None	Low
2 Standardised/volunteer patient in clinical setting Patient encounter with student is scripted and serves as an example to illustrate or reinforce learning (e.g. teacher asks patient to provide student with history or student practices a clinical exam)	Encounter-based	None	None	None	Low
3 Patients share their experience with students within faculty-directed curriculum Patient is invited to share experience; faculty plan the encounter but patient determines personal comfort and level of participation	Encounter-based	None–low	Brief, simple	None	Low
4 Patient teacher(s) involved in teaching and/or evaluating students Patient is given preparation for specific teaching role, may actively question students and may be involved in giving feedback and evaluating their performance	Variable	Moderate	Structured, extensive	Low–moderate	Low–moderate
5 Patient teacher(s) as equal partners in student education, evaluation and curriculum development Patients are involved in many aspects of educational delivery, development and evaluation, beyond specific courses to the curriculum as a whole – a true partnership in which patients make meaningful and valued contributions to decision making	Moderate–extensive	High	Extensive	Moderate–extensive	Moderate
6 Patient(s) involved at the institutional level in addition to sustained involvement as patient teacher(s) in education, evaluation and curriculum development for students As (5) above but there also are institutional policies that ensure involvement in decision-making bodies within undergraduate, graduate and continuing health professional education	Extensive	High	Extensive	High	High

Note: In all instances patients are 'real' and assumed to be representing themselves

1 *Electronic or paper-based case or scenario*

Paper-based cases and scenarios have long been used to supplement real patient contact, with video-based and electronic cases increasing in use as the technology has developed. The use of virtual patients was first described in the early 1970s. A virtual patient has been defined as a:

specific type of computer program that simulates real-life clinical scenarios: learners emulate the roles of health care providers to obtain a history, conduct a physical examination, and make diagnostic and therapeutic decisions.(23)

A recent critical literature review concluded that the evidence base to inform their use was currently non-existent, at least in published form.(23) Within the definition there was wide variation, for example, in the degree of interactivity, amount of feedback provided and use in assessment. In terms of effectiveness, evidence suggests that virtual patient interventions are more likely than *no* intervention to improve learning, are better at promoting more technical knowledge-based aspects than interpersonal skills, and possibly more effective and better accepted as triggers in problem-based learning than paper cases. From both theoretical and empirical perspectives the most effective use for virtual patients is in the development of clinical reasoning, which requires exposure to multiple cases and their variations, and to reasoning modelled by experts.(24) However, there has been little helpful research into issues such as the most effective design, sequencing or balance within the curriculum. Consideration of the evidence-based principles that underpin simulation in general may be helpful (*see* Chapter 12).(25)

On a more holistic level, there have been increasing calls to adopt a narrative approach in all aspects of healthcare – clinical practice, therapy and research – and in the education of health professionals, with potential benefits claimed for all parties.(26,27) Guy Widdershoven, Professor of Ethics of Healthcare at Maastricht University, notes that 'we dream in narrative, daydream in narrative, remember, anticipate, hope, despair, believe, doubt, plan, revise, criticise, construct, gossip, learn, hate and love by narrative'.(26)

One kind of narrative account is what Aronson called the 'autopathography', more simply referred to as a 'patient's tale', or perhaps more cynically, the 'medical confessional'.(28) He identified nearly 300 such book-length tales, mostly written in the last 20 years, and analysed and classified some of their characteristics. Reading and reflecting on such stories may help health professionals, both in training and in practice, better understand and empathise with their patients, and 'teach them things they won't learn from textbooks',(28) indeed 'that cannot be arrived at by any other means'.(26)

There are many ways in which such resources may be used in an educational context. It is important though that intended aims and outcomes are congruent with overall curricular outcomes, and that teaching integrates with the rest of the course and meets other curricular requirements.(29) Powley and Higson suggest the following simple process for using written narratives in teaching(30):

- read
- discuss
- facilitate and analyse responses
- discuss applications.

Questions such as 'What is the story about?' and 'What effect did it have on me?' help learners focus the reading, apply it to different contexts and promote reflection. Grounding the exercise in reality reinforces relevance, which in turn helps motivate learners. Sufficient time must be allowed for reflection and discussion. In terms of choice of text, Aronson's own criteria for recommending a book are 'that it should provide a judicious balance between emotional expression and analytical discourse, and that it should have informed, and above all entertained me'. He suggests a 'top ten' in his article,(28) but there are many other sources of relevant advice and guidance (*see* Further reading section).

Another increasingly common source of such stories is the Internet. 'Google' any disease, common or rare, and a significant proportion of 'hits' will be personal accounts of the problem, as either patient or carer. Resources such as the 'Patient Voices' programme or Healthtalkonline (*see* Further reading section) are freely available. Others can be purchased or can be developed by teachers and learning technologists to suit specific purposes, although the cost, time and expertise required to do this should not be underestimated. Examples include interactive tutorials on various topics, such as epileptic seizure classification(31) or breaking bad news.(32)

Such resources can be included in face-to-face or e-learning tutorials or lectures (e.g. embedded in PowerPoint presentations), providing illustrative or trigger scenarios about different clinical conditions or situations. These are particularly helpful when it is inappropriate or difficult for learners to work with real patients, such as children and families, patients with rare conditions, terminally ill patients or patients with mental health problems. Learning technologies can also enable a more standardised approach to assessing clinical skills or knowledge. For example, the Royal College of Paediatrics and Child Health has developed an assessment of clinical skills using videos of very ill children; the Royal College of Ophthalmologists also uses video assessments in examinations, and personal digital assistants (a handheld or palmtop computer) have been used as an assessment tool.(29)

2 *Standardised or volunteer patient in a real clinical setting*

Learning from real patients in the clinical context has been the mainstay of clinical education, enabling students and trainees to consolidate and synthesise their learning from a range of sources. Indeed, 'bedside teaching' is the only setting in which the full panoply of technical and non-technical skills, attitudes and applied knowledge that constitute 'doctoring' are modelled by clinical teachers and can be learnt as an integrated whole.(33)

Ramani reminds us that 'the bedside is the perfect venue for unrehearsed and unexpected triangular interactions between teacher, trainees and patient ... physician teachers should be vigilant about grabbing teachable moments' during these encounters.(34) McKimm's clinical 'trialogue'(35) – a 'discussion between three groups with different principles, backgrounds and expectations'(36) that attends to the developing relationships between all three 'players', rather than consciously trying to think about teaching and clinical practice – is a useful model that may help teachers plan and work actively within these meetings with patients and learners.

Whenever and wherever clinical teaching occurs, however, real patients are usually the most vulnerable of the parties involved (i.e. teacher, learner, other professionals and patient). Notwithstanding, most patients find clinical teaching rewarding, often commenting that they feel students 'have to learn'. However, it should not be tacitly assumed that patients will engage in teaching; the patient's feelings should always be respected and they should know that whatever their decision, treatment and care will not be affected. If a facility is a teaching environment, patients must be informed that learners may be present and may be providing care. This allows the patient to prepare for the initial encounter and to raise any anxieties (*see* Ethical issues section). There are also potential educational benefits from briefing patients explicitly about a session's aims, what teacher and learners hope to get out of it, and what may be expected of the patient, for example, whether they will be asked to give feedback.(33) Patients need to be aware of the number and level of the learners who may be present and each person's role should be clarified and verbal or written agreement obtained and recorded.

3 *Patients share their experience with students within faculty-directed curriculum; and*

4 *Patient teacher(s) involved in teaching and/or evaluating students*

Selecting real patients for teaching in specified clinical areas is often opportunistic and based on availability. A more structured approach employing trained patients, that is, non-professional or patient educators who are simultaneously both patient and teacher, is being increasingly used within undergraduate and postgraduate training. Expert patients or patient educators can be drawn from many settings, even those where concerns might be expressed about the potential risk to patients, such as those who are terminally ill or have mental health problems.

The idea of the expert patient is also enshrined in the wider patient involvement agenda. The 'expert patient initiative was ... part of the government's commitment to place patients at the heart of healthcare which is ... part of the transformational focus of the clinical governance agenda'.(37) This initiative was primarily targeted at people with chronic conditions to help them 'become key decision makers in their own care'.(37) The expert patient initiative is supported by an educational programme for the patients themselves, and there is some evidence it has resulted in changes in confidence and self-efficacy in relation to self-management of symptoms (such as pain, tiredness, depression and breathlessness).(38) However, results of several well-powered randomised controlled trials looking at outcomes of such programmes in the UK failed to show any effect on use of healthcare; the authors of a review called for caution in rolling out the programme further without evaluation.(39)

There are a number of advantages in not involving patients who are primarily being treated in the clinical setting for clinical care in teaching. Patient educators have the benefits of being:

* motivated individuals with an interest in medical training
* 'real' (as opposed to simulated) with authentic clinical histories and possibly clinical signs
* able to give structured feedback from a patient's perspective, such as the pressure of the hands or the way in which a history was taken.(21)

One distinctive category of patient teacher is the gynaecology teaching associate. These are women trained to teach pelvic and breast examination, who are themselves examined. They are widely used in North America and Scandinavia, but interestingly are still a rarity in the UK. Such teaching can help free up clinical tutors as, once trained, they need little assistance in running sessions or participating in clinical assessments. They have been found to be acceptable and effective – in one comparative study students taught by associates had better skills in an end-of-attachment assessment than students who were not.(40) A call was made by the authors for wider use of associates to complement existing teaching programmes.

Well-managed patient involvement in clinical teaching can benefit both patients and learners. The challenge is to be sensitive to both patients' and learners' needs and to identify suitable patients who feel equipped to participate. Sometimes, however, it is neither possible nor appropriate to involve real patients in learning and this is where one needs to adopt alternative strategies.

5 *Patient teacher(s) as equal partners in student education, evaluation and curriculum development*

It is unusual in medical education to find this level of involvement, with some notable exceptions, but models have been developed particularly in mental health and social care education. Guidelines and recommendations derived through a variety of processes have been published,(5,19,41–44) and UK guidance about involving patients in health-related research highlights issues that may be relevant to professional education.(45) The British Medical Association has also published recommendations for medical education and training.(46)

6 *Patient(s) involved at the institutional level in addition to sustained involvement as patient teacher(s) in education, evaluation and curriculum development for students*

Involvement at this level is even rarer than Level 5. One of the best examples in the UK is the Universities/Users Teaching and Research Action Partnership (UNTRAP) based at Warwick University,(47) which is a partnership between Warwick and Coventry universities, users of health and social care services and their carers, and the NHS. Patients are involved at different levels, some in one-off events, others more heavily. The central philosophy of UNTRAP is that everyone will benefit if service users, carers, academics and professionals share their experience. Other institutional approaches have also been described.(19)

Benefits and Disadvantages

The thought of training doctors *without* patient contact would nowadays be considered absurd (although in some undergraduate medical education systems in mainland Europe it is still minimal); medical schools aspire to maximise it, clinical teachers and teaching administrators strive to deliver it, students demand as much as possible and patients seem only too willing to help. At the postgraduate level, with an increasing emphasis on in-service training, patient contact is a crucial element. A significant literature has accumulated [one of the most comprehensive bibliographies(6) identified nearly 300 relevant papers], providing corroboration for some of the theoretical benefits. Contact between patients and learners is generally very well received, with relatively few apparent adverse effects or disadvantages for the former, and even fewer for the latter. Patients intuitively recognise the contributions they can make to health professional's education, for example, by acting as 'experts' in and/or exemplars of their condition, showing and telling, aiding

the development of professional skills and attitudes, and boosting confidence.(48) Although the majority of studies report distinctive, largely positive outcomes for patients, one group, using a phenomenological approach, showed that involvement in clinical teaching for most patients was, in fact, characterised by its ordinariness.(49) A qualitative study of views of students and faculty concluded that there was strong support for patient involvement in teaching. The authors contended that patient contact creates a 'complex contextual learning environment', but there were concerns about the possible emotional and psychological impact on both patients *and* students of recounting painful and traumatic experiences, and 'professionalisation' of some patients through repeated telling of their stories. Interestingly, there was only muted support for the idea of extending patient involvement into non-teaching roles.(50)

Much of this literature, however, is descriptive, with 'low-level' evaluations (e.g. 'how was it for you?') often based on self-report. There is often insufficient information about the actual educational interventions and the research design used; interventions are often described in their early stages with few attempts at evaluating long-term impacts. Little research so far appears to have been informed by theory [exceptions include Rees *et al.*'s study that used socio-cultural theory(5)]. Finally, people have published in disparate outlets, which, along with problems posed by use of different terms, has bedevilled searching and synthesis of the literature.(6) Nevertheless, several comprehensive reviews have been published over the past few years (Boxes 13.7 and 13.8).(6,8,20,51–54)

Principles and Practice

In this section we explore general principles for involvement, focus on three important ethical issues and consider the challenge of representativeness.

General principles

As described above, a number of papers supporting and guiding patient involvement in medical education have been published, and these invariably also highlight barriers and challenges. From this growing literature we have distilled a set of principles to inform practice (*see* Box 13.9). We have not explored barriers and challenges in any further detail, but these are argued to include:

- value discordance
- power imbalances
- perceptions of intimidation (such as unfamiliar even hostile environments)
- a lack of consent, choice and confidentiality
- time constraints
- institutional inertia

BOX 13.7 Benefits of increased patient involvement

Based on theoretical considerations(20) and published evidence the main benefits to students are:

- motivation through relevance
- increased empathy
- development of professional skills and attitudes
- increased confidence
- social responsibility
- development of clinical reasoning
- new insights and understanding
- recognition of cultural diversity and lifestyle factors
- improved performance in examinations

For patients, the benefits appear to be:

- satisfaction at contributing to student learning
- improved relationships with professionals
- altruistic feelings, for example, giving something back to 'the system'
- being valued and increased self-esteem
- development of own skills
- catharsis
- increased knowledge about their own condition
- getting a better service from their clinicians, for example, 'a good going over'
- companionship and relief from social isolation

BOX 13.8 Disadvantages of increased patient involvement

Disadvantages to students

Few disadvantages are reported by students, but they include:

- embarrassment
- emotionally challenged in certain situations
- concern about representativeness of some patients

For patients, disadvantages are mainly in relation to:

- mental health problems and those in embarrassing situations (e.g. gynaecological problems)
- concerns about confidentiality and choice, previous poor experiences, large numbers of learners

There is little evidence of any significant adverse effects.

- inadequate resourcing
- lack of training, support and debriefing
- problems with language and communication.

Ethical issues

Ethical issues to be considered when involving patients in teaching can be summarised as the 'three Cs': consent, choice and confidentiality. The main message emerging from policy documents, good practice and

BOX 13.9 General principles for patient involvement

When considering involving patients and carers, the following issues should be addressed, *as appropriate to the proposed level of involvement.*

- Leadership – seek a 'champion', or, at very least, a dedicated clinical placement lead(46)
- Ensure institutional support and address underlying cultural issues
- Provide adequate resources
- Create a written strategy, including a statement of values
- Establish an infrastructure and appropriate policies (e.g. on payment, contracts, ethics)
- Provide safe and comfortable environments
- Offer training and support, for both patients and faculty in new ways of working
- Treat 'patients' as equals
- Pay attention to language and avoid technical jargon and terminology
- Develop mechanisms for responding to feedback
- Embrace change and be prepared to be challenged and think in new ways
- See involvement as a process, not a one-off event
- Seek opportunities for further development and to build capacity
- Work to ensure diversity is reflected and minority views represented

the literature is that simply assuming that patients will be involved in teaching and learning without making this explicit through formal systems, professional conversations and ethical practice is no longer enough.

Consent

A mindset shift needs to occur within the medical profession to enable informed partnership rather than informed consent (patient).(55)

This quote from the body that oversees postgraduate training in the UK highlights issues discussed earlier around the wider agenda of patient involvement. Medical law and ethics enshrine the principle of informed consent, which should guide routine involvement of patients, not just those encounters involving embarrassing situations or invasive procedures.(46) 'Arguments for not informing patients in advance seem to be based more on prejudice and on empirical evidence',(56) and providing information about learner involvement before the clinical encounter does not appear to adversely influence patients' decisions about participation. Perhaps not surprisingly, there is evidence that patients are more positive about involvement when consent is obtained.(57) Obtaining consent should be 'a continuous process that begins with the first contact the service has with the patient',(46) and all patients should be informed that students may be present and involved in care. It is important to recognise that the presence of a student will inevitably change the doctor–patient relationship and the dynamics of a consultation, although there is little if any evidence of significant negative effects on the quality of care.(58) An interesting argument has been made that there should be an expectation that all patients should be willing to contribute to medical education as a default stance, the *quid pro quo* being that all trainees should be required to demonstrate competence in the relevant task in simulation before being 'let loose'.(59)

Choice

Facilitating patient choice is challenging when students and trainees need to learn within the 'turbulent here and now of care delivery',(59) when there is little time to ensure that each encounter is set up as people would prefer. Promoting active choice about involvement shows basic respect but also acknowledges that the patient is an expert about the way his or her own condition affects them. It moves clinicians away from 'operating from within the safety of a powerful expert role and performing habitual and ritualized tasks that depersonalize the transaction of caring'.(60)

Informing patients and seeking consent should be done without the learner being present, then confirmed in the presence of learners.(43) Building in 'moment-to-moment' opportunities for patients to say 'No' is another way of empowering them and acknowledging their needs.(27) Patients should be informed about the level of experience and the identity of any doctor intending to carry out a procedure on them. Lack of personal power and space, and the more urgent need for treatment, mean that a different approach may need to be taken in hospital settings compared with primary care, where there is usually a more intimate relationship, more privacy and the patients have greater autonomy.(61)

Confidentiality

As in clinical practice in general, confidentiality in relation to patients involved in education has, in the past, been somewhat lax. This is clearly unacceptable in modern times, and institutions must develop strategies to ensure confidentiality is maintained. Some patients express concerns 'about students' access to their case notes and whether discussions about patients occurred after they had left the consulting room',(62) which raises questions about whether and how aspects of choice, consent and confidentiality should be raised with patients.

Practical steps that help to maintain confidentiality include:

- providing sufficient information to patients so they can assess and understand the boundaries of confidentiality

- reassuring the patient about the fact that students and trainees are bound by the same duty to respect confidentiality as are 'fully fledged' health professionals
- involving patients in discussions
- remembering that curtains around a bed or cubicle do not ensure silence or privacy
- finding private spaces to discuss intimate or distressing issues
- raising issues of confidentiality routinely with learners as part of preparation and debrief.

When patient information is being used in teaching, permission must be obtained for the use of images, sound recordings and extracts from case notes, particularly identifiable information. Patient information or body parts are not the property of organisations or clinicians unless formal consent has been obtained. Increasing use of electronic records is creating new challenges for ensuring confidentiality. In the UK in future, students will only have access using a smartcard.(63)

Medical ethics and law is complex and ever changing, and all clinicians have a responsibility to keep up to date and informed. Clinical teachers are key role models for their learners: keeping the 'three Cs' in mind ensures that these are seen as fundamental pillars of good medical practice, not as options. Embedding these principles in institutional practices and policies is an important step.(46)

Patient representation

It is easy to forget that the vast, ubiquitous population of people who might fall under the general heading of 'patient' is by no means homogeneous; indeed, diversity is the norm. 'Patients' do not think alike any more than professionals do, yet much of the literature on 'involvement' sidesteps this issue and, if only by an act of omission, seems to treat all users, carers, survivors, clients, patients, etc., as the same. Charlotte Williamson of Picker Institute, Europe, proposes three broad categories of 'patient' who might get involved.(64)

- 'Individual patients' can (obviously) describe their own experience but cannot necessarily speak for others, which raises questions about representativeness and begs the need for eliciting concerns from this group using survey methods.
- 'Patient group members' usually *do* know about the experiences of others like themselves, but may still have a narrow perspective. Consulting all relevant groups in locality is important.
- Finally 'patient representatives or advocates' usually have broader experience, perhaps of working with several groups, wider knowledge about issues at strategic and policy levels, and of 'the bigger picture'.

Ideally consultation with 'patients' should involve all three categories using appropriate methods. In Williamson's words:

The patient side of health care is complex but not mysterious. Consulting the 'right' patients can be feasible and rewarding.(64)

Simulated patients

Simulation is increasingly used at all levels of health professional education and training to complement both classroom and clinical learning. It cannot replace 'authentic experiential learning in the real world of clinical practice', but can ' … prepare practitioners for the real world, providing a structure for deliberate practice … clinical reasoning and professional judgement'.(26) Simulated, or 'standardised', patients were first introduced by Barrows and Abrahamson in the 1960s(65) and are now well established in the mainstream of health professional education. They were originally real patients trained to present standardised representations of their own problems;(65) nowadays, in the words of Barrow himself,(66) a simulated patient will generally be 'a well person trained to simulate a patient's illness', with or without a thespian background. The significant difference is that they usually portray a range of scenarios *outside* their own experience (Silverman J and Britten N, personal communication).

The advantages of using simulated patients include:
- authenticity
- opportunities for standardisation
- customisation
- convenience
- efficient use of time
- feedback.

It allows exploration and rehearsal of challenging situations such as breaking bad news or communicating about sensitive areas, and simulators can also teach, give feedback and contribute to assessment. Research has shown that people generally cannot easily distinguish between real patients and well-trained simulators.(67,68)

The use of simulated patients has been shown to be acceptable to learners and faculty, and effective, reliable and valid in both instruction and assessment. There is wide international experience of using simulated patients in most clinical specialties, although some mental health and paediatric problems as well as those of the very elderly can be difficult to simulate and may be under-represented, as may certain patient groups, for example, ethnic minorities.

There is a continuum between real patients and highly trained simulators, and the choice of which approach to use in a particular setting will be determined by a range of factors, including the nature of the phenomena to be simulated, intended aims and learning outcomes, local circumstances and available resources.(69) However, in the wider context of patient involvement and its aims, simulation's primary purpose is to enable skills development and rehearsal, *not* to ensure incorporation of the patient's voice (Silverman J and Britten N, personal communication).

The literature on the effects of simulation on simulated patients themselves is limited. There is evidence of potential harm in some situations (e.g. when portraying emotionally intense roles), but the general consensus is that benefits outweigh any disadvantages.(68) It is important to pay attention to recruitment (including exploring the person's reasons for wanting to get involved), training and support, and debriefing and de-roling.(66,68,70)

The use of simulation and simulated patients is discussed in detail in Chapter 12.

Areas for Further Research

In light of the variable quality of much of the research in this area, a large research agenda has been identified looking at a wide range of aspects. These include questions such as the following.
- What are the drivers of patient involvement?
- What are the strengths and weaknesses of different approaches, and how do these vary between professions and disciplines, and between countries and across cultures?
- What factors influence what works, and why?
- How do structural and organisational factors such as location, access and safety influence development of programmes?
- What factors influence patients' experiences of involvement?
- What are the key outcomes, short *and* long term, for all parties?
- What factors influence sustainability of programmes?

Conclusions

From an early stage of training, students and trainees need to actively engage with patients, carers and families so that they can learn to consolidate their learning and put learning from other contexts into practice in the real clinical environment. There are immense benefits not only for the learners, but also for patients, if involvement is appropriate and carried out professionally and sensitively. Many patients want to 'give something back' to those who care for them, and engaging in medical education at all levels is one of way of so doing.

Teachers and learners need to be aware when learning on 'real' patients is inappropriate. However, there are many alternatives available ranging from paper case scenarios to high-fidelity simulations. The greater emphasis on professionalism, including attending to legal and ethical issues, and the changing agendas relating to patient empowerment and social accountability mean that, for a host of reasons, educators need to pay close attention to seeking active, informed involvement in educational activities from patients and carers. This approach will help put the rhetoric of 'patients as partners' centrally into practice in the teaching and learning environment.

Acknowledgements

The original commission for this chapter, as one of the *Understanding Medical Education* series, was given to John Spencer, along with Janet Askham and Alison Chisholm of Picker Institute Europe. Unfortunately, early in the project, Alison took time out of work for personal reasons and, tragically, Janet died unexpectedly while in New Zealand; our condolences go to her family and friends. The project, unsurprisingly, stalled for a while, but as deadlines came and went, Judy McKimm came to the rescue.

References

1 Jolly B (1998) Historical and theoretical background. In: Jolly B and Rees L (eds) *Medical Education in the Millennium*, pp. 171–87. Oxford University Press, Oxford.
2 Rosner L (1997) The growth of medical education and the medical profession. In: Loudon I (ed.) *Western Medicine*, pp. 147–59. Oxford University Press, Oxford.
3 Osler W (1905) The hospital as a college. In: *Aequanimatus, and Other Addresses*. HK Lewis, London.
4 *Doctor in the House* (http://www.youtube.com/watch?v=oVWjAeAa52o; accessed August 2009).
5 Rees CE, Knight LV and Wilkinson CE (2007) User involvement is a sine qua non, almost, in medical education: learning with rather than just about health and social care service users. *Advances in Health Sciences Education*. 12(3): 359–90.
6 Towle A, Bainbridge L, William Godolphin W et al. (2010) Active patient involvement in the education of health professionals. *Medical Education*. 44: 64.
7 http://icn.csip.org.uk/_library/Creating_a_patient-led_NHS.pdf; accessed August 2009.
8 Morgan A and Jones D (2009) Perceptions of service user and carer involvement in healthcare education and impact on students' knowledge and practice: a literature review. *Medical Teacher*. 31: 82–95.
9 General Medical Council (2009) *Tomorrow's Doctors*. GMC, London.
10 Crawford MJ, Rutter D, Manley C et al. (2002) Systematic review of involving patients in the planning and development of health care. *British Medical Journal*. 325: 1263.
11 Woollard RF (2006) Caring for a common future: medical schools' social accountability. *Medical Education*. 40: 301–13.
12 Royal College of Physicians (2005) *Doctors in Society – medical professionalism in a changing world*. RCP, London.
13 Medical Professionalism Project (2002) Medical professionalism in the new millennium: a physicians' charter. *Lancet*. 359: 520–1.
14 Hilton S and Southgate L (2007) Professionalism in medical education. *Teacher and Teacher Education*. 23: 265–79.
15 Coulter A and Ellins J (2007) Effectiveness of strategies for informing, educating and involving patients. *British Medical Journal*. 335: 24–7.
16 Engel GL (1989) The need for a new medical model: a challenge for biomedicine. *Journal of Interprofessional Care*. 4: 37–53.
17 Stewart M, Brown JB, Weston WW et al. (2003) *Patient-Centred Medicine. Transforming the Clinical Method* (2e). Radcliffe Medical Press, Oxford.
18 Hasman A, Coulter A and Askham J (2006) *Education for Partnership*. Picker Institute, Oxford.
19 Tew J, Gell C and Foster S (2004) *Learning from Experience: involving service users and carers in mental health education and training*. Mental Health in Higher Education/NIMHE West Midlands/Trent WDC, York.
20 Spencer J, Blackmore D, Heard S et al. (2000) Patient-oriented learning: a review of the role of the patient in the education of medical students. *Medical Education*. 34: 851–7.
21 McKimm J (2008) *Involving Patients in Clinical Teaching*. London Deanery, London. (http://www.faculty.londondeanery.ac.uk/e-learning/involving-patients-in-clinical-teaching; accessed August 2009).
22 Spencer J (2002) What can undergraduate education offer general practice? In: Harrison J and van Zwanenberg T (eds) *GP Tomorrow* (2e), pp. 49–66. Radcliffe Medical Press, Oxford.
23 Cook DA and Triola MM (2009) Virtual patients: a critical literature review and proposed next steps. *Medical Education*. 43: 303–11.
24 Eva K (2005) What every teacher needs to know about clinical reasoning. *Medical Education*. 39: 98–106.
25 Issenberg SB, McGaghie WC, Petrusa ER et al. (2005) Features and uses of high-fidelity medical simulations that lead to effective learning: a BEME systematic review. *Medical Teacher*. 27: 10–28.
26 Greenhalgh T and Hurwitz B (1999) Why study narrative? *British Medical Journal*. 318: 48–50.
27 Engel JD, Zarconi J, Pethtel LL and Missimi SA (2008) *Narrative in Health Care. Healing patients, practitioners, profession, and community*. Radcliffe Publishing, Oxford.
28 Aronson JK (2000) Autopathography: the patient's tale. *British Medical Journal*. 321: 1599–602.
29 van Schoor AN, Navsa N, Meiring JH et al. (2006) Perspectives on the use of PDAs as assessment tools. *The Clinical Teacher*. 3: 170–4.
30 Powley E and Higson R (2005) *The Arts in Medical Education. A Practical Guide*. Radcliffe Publishing, Oxford.
31 Farrar M, Connolly AM, Lawson J et al. (2008) Teaching doctors how to diagnose paroxysmal events: a comparison of two educational methods. *Medical Education*. 42: 909–14.
32 Cleland J, Ford R, Hamilton NM et al. (2007) Breaking bad news: an interactive web-based e-learning package. *The Clinical Teacher*. 4: 94–9.
33 Spencer JA (2003) Teaching and learning in the clinical environment. *British Medical Journal*. 326: 591–4.
34 Ramani S (2003) Twelve tips to improve bedside teaching. *Medical Teacher*. 25: 112–15.
35 McKimm J (2008) The 'Trialogue': a new model and metaphor for understanding clinical teaching and learning and developing skills. Paper presented at the ASME Conference, Leicester, 10–12 September.
36 My Dictionary.com (http://www.mydictionary.com; accessed August 2009).
37 Hardy P (2009) *The Expert Patient Programme: a critical review*. MSc Lifelong learning, policy and research (http://www.

pilgrimprojects.co.uk/papers/epp_msc.pdf; accessed August 2009).

38 Squire S and Hill P (2006) The Expert Patients Programme. *Clinical Governance.* **11**: 17–21.

39 Griffiths C, Foster G, Ramsay J *et al.* (2007) How effective are expert patient (lay led) education programmes for chronic disease? *British Medical Journal.* **334**: 1254–6.

40 Pickard S, Baraitser P, Rymer J and Piper J (2006) Can gynaecology teaching associates provide high quality effective training for medical students in the UK? Comparative study. *British Medical Journal.* **327**: 1389–92.

41 Levin E (http://www.scie.org.uk/publications/guides/guide04/files/guide04.pdf; accessed August 2009)

42 http://depts.washington.edu/ccph/partnerships.html; accessed August 2009.

43 Howe A and Anderson J (2003) Involving patients in medical education. *British Medical Journal.* **327**: 326–8.

44 O'Keefe M and Jones A (2007) Promoting lay participation in medical school curriculum development: lay and faculty perceptions. *Medical Education.* **41**: 130–7.

45 http://www.invo.org.uk/pdfs/Briefing%20Note%20Final. dat.pdf; accessed August 2009.

46 British Medical Association (2008) *Role of the Patient in Medical Education.* (http://www.bma.org.uk/careers/medical_education/roleofthepatient.jsp; accessed August 2009).

47 http://www2.warwick.ac.uk/fac/cross_fac/healthatwarwick/untrap/; accessed August 2009.

48 Stacy R and Spencer J (1999) Patients as teachers: a qualitative study of patients' views on their role in a community-based undergraduate project. *Medical Education.* **33**: 688–94.

49 McLachlan E, King N, Wenger E and Dornan T (2009) *How does involvement in medical student education affect a patient's sense of identity?* Paper presented at the AMEE Conference, Malaga, Spain, September 2009.

50 Jha V, Quinton ND, Bekker HL and Roberts TE (2009) What educators and students really think about using patients as teachers in medical education: a qualitative study. *Medical Education.* **43**: 449–56.

51 Wykurz G and Kelly D (2002) Developing the role of patients as teachers: literature review. *British Medical Journal.* **325**: 818–21.

52 Repper J and Breeze J (2004) A review of the literature on user and carer involvement in the training and education of health professionals. (http://www.shef.ac.uk/content/1/c6/01/34/62/Finalreport.pdf; accessed August 2009).

53 Jha V, Quinton ND, Bekker HL and Roberts TE (2009) Strategies and interventions for the involvement of real patients in medical education: a systematic review. *Medical Education.* **43**: 10–20.

54 Moss B, Boath L, Buckley S and Colgan A (2009) The fount of all knowledge: training required to involve service users and carers in health and social care education and training. *Social Work Education.* **28**: 562–72.

55 Postgraduate Medical Education and Training Board (2008) *Training in Partnership: shaping the future of postgraduate medical education and training in the UK – the patient perspective, 2008.* PMETB, London. (http://www.gmc-uk.org/9_May_2008_ Patient_Perspective_Seminar_Report_pdf_30426823.pdf).

56 Westberg K, Lynøe N, Löfgren M and Sandlund M (2001) Getting informed consent from patients to take part in the clinical training of students: randomized control trial of two strategies. *British Medical Journal.* **323**: 488.

57 Haffling A and Håkansson A (2008) Patients consulting with students in general practice: survey of patient's satisfaction and their role in teaching. *Medical Teacher.* **30**: 622–9.

58 Price R, Spencer J and Walker J (2008) Does the presence of medical students affect quality in general practice consultations? *Medical Education.* **42**: 374–81.

59 Draper H, Parle J and Ross N (2008) Medical education and patients' responsibility. Back to the future? *Journal of Medical Ethics.* **34**: 116–19.

60 Hardy P and Stanton P (2007) Cultivating compassion: seeing patient voices. *British Medical Journal.* **335**: 184–7.

61 Benson J, Quince T, Hibble A *et al.* (2005) Impact on patients of expanded, general practice based, student teaching: observational and qualitative study. *British Medical Journal.* **331**: 89.

62 O'Flynn N, Spencer J and Jones R (1997) Consent and confidentiality in teaching general practice: survey of patients' views on presence of students. *British Medical Journal.* **315**: 1142.

63 http://www.connectingforhealth.nhs.uk/systemsandservices/rasmartcards/studentaccess; accessed August 2009.

64 Williamson C (2007) How do we find the right patients to consult? *Quality in Primary Care.* **15**: 195–9.

65 Barrows HS and Abrahamson S (1964) The programmed patient: a technique for appraising clinical performance in clinical neurology. *Journal of Medical Education.* **39**: 802–5.

66 Barrows HS (1993) An overview of the uses of standardized patients for teaching and evaluating clinical skills. *Academic Medicine.* **68**: 443–51.

67 Kurtz S, Silverman J and Draper J (2005) *Teaching and Learning Communication Skills in Medicine* (2e). Radcliffe Medical Press, Oxford.

68 Thistlethwaite J and Ridgway G (2006) *Making it Real. A Practical Guide to Experiential Learning.* Radcliffe Publishing, Oxford.

69 Collins JP and Harden RM (1998) Real patients, simulated patients and simulators in clinical examinations. AMEE guide no. 13. *Medical Teacher.* **20**: 508–21.

70 Spencer J and Dales J (2006) Meeting the needs of simulated patients and caring for person behind them. *Medical Education.* **40**: 3–5.

Further Reading

Association for Standardized Patient Educators (ASPE) (http://www.aspeducators.org). ASPE is the international organisation for professionals in the field of standardised patient methodology. It is based in the US and the web site provides good ideas around the use of simulated patients.

British Medical Association (2008) *Role of the Patient in Medical Education.* (http://www.bma.org.uk/careers/medical_education/roleofthepatient.jsp; accessed August 2009).

Farrell C, Towle A and Godolphin W (2006) *Where's the Patient's Voice in Health Professional Education?* University of British Columbia. Report of an international conference to explore the challenges of incorporating the patient's voice. (http://chd.ubc.ca/dhcc/sites/default/files/documents/PtsVoiceReport.pdf; accessed April 2010).

Healthtalkonline (http://www.healthtalkonline.org/ and http://www.youthhealthtalk.org/). The information on Healthtalkonline is based on qualitative research into patient experiences, led by experts at the University of Oxford. These personal stories of health and illness will enable patients, families and healthcare professionals to benefit from the experiences of others.

Patient Voices Programme Patient Voices Programme (http://
www.patientvoices.org.uk/). The Patient Voices programme
was founded in 2003, and aims to facilitate the telling and the
hearing of some of the unwritten and unspoken stories of ordinary people so that those who devise and implement strategy
in health and social care, as well as the professionals and clinicians directly involved in care, may carry out their duties in a
more informed and compassionate manner. It provides more
than 100 digital stories from patients, carers and health workers
on a range of topics.

Simulated Patients UK (http://www.simulatedpatients.co.uk).
This site provides a one-stop resource for users of simulated
patients throughout the UK.

Tew J, Gell C and Foster S (2004) *Learning from Experience: involv-
ing service users and carers in mental health education and training.*
Mental Health in Higher Education/NIMHE West Midlands/
Trent WDC, York.

UBC Division of Health Care Communication. Bibliography
(http://www.chd.ubc.ca/dhcc/node/67). This is possibly the
most comprehensive bibliography of relevant literature in the
public domain.

How to design a useful test: the principles of assessment

Lambert WT Schuwirth and Cees PM van der Vleuten

KEY MESSAGES

- Good assessment requires a variety of methods; no single method can test the whole of medical competence and performance.

- In a good assessment programme the total is more than the sum of the parts. To achieve this:

  - each instrument must be chosen on the basis of its strengths and weaknesses

  - all decisions are based on rational arguments and/or scientific underpinning

  - rational decisions are made about to how to combine results

  - the whole programme is part of a total quality management system.

- Modern assessment in medical education is more a matter of good educational design than psychometric measurement.

Introduction

Designing a system of assessment is not easy. Many different instruments have been described in the medical education literature, each with its own advantages and disadvantages. The volume of published research on assessment is huge, and research findings often contradict long-established practices based on tradition and intuition. Furthermore, the discipline has its own jargon and set of statistical concepts. In among all this, the responsibility regularly falls on medical teachers to set up fair assessment systems. The aim of this chapter is to explain the basic concepts behind assessment and thus help reduce this 'burden'. It is not a cookbook providing assessment 'recipes'; instead, we hope that after reading this publication the medical educator will be better equipped to make informed choices in matters of assessment.

What Is Assessment?

Although assessment is generally acknowledged to be fundamental to the educative process, there are many different constructions of the term, ranging from assessment as a certification procedure leading to a pass/fail decision, to assessment as an evaluative or feedback action in education. Here we will use 'any *purported* and *formal* action to obtain information about the competence and performance of a candidate' as our working definition of assessment.

Assessment is never undertaken without a specific purpose. This can be either summative or formative. Summative means that the assessment has been conducted for decision-making or certification purposes, such as deciding who is admitted, progresses or qualifies. Formative relates to the feedback function of assessment or, more precisely, how the assessment informs the students about their performance.

Some people argue that formative and summative assessment purposes should not be mixed in one assessment, but in educational settings we tend to advise otherwise. Pure summative assessment ('pass' or 'fail' only) does not help students to plan their study. If a student fails, they do not know what they need to work on in order to pass at the next attempt. On the other hand, pure formative assessment with no consequences at all is often not taken seriously.

How to Choose the Best Approaches to Assessment

A first step in setting up an assessment system is to choose the most appropriate methods. This is not an easy task. Over the past few decades, a wide variety of instruments have been developed and used in medical education, and often authors claim that their instrument is the best for all purposes. We may safely assume, however, that each method has its own strengths and weaknesses, and these must be weighed carefully against the desired purposes of the assessment. A testing authority whose purpose is licensing

Understanding Medical Education: Evidence, Theory and Practice.
Edited by T Swanwick. © 2010 Association for the Study of Medical Education.

may demand different strengths from the methods from, say, a medical school. Several criteria that can be used in this evaluative process have been described in the literature.(1) The most popular ones are as follows.

Reliability

The reliability of a method pertains mostly to the *reproducibility* of its results, that is, how often the same result is obtained. Let us illustrate this with three examples.

1 John scores 83% in a test. If John were given a different, but similar, test – a so-called parallel test – would he again score 83%?
2 John is the best-scoring student in his class. Harry comes next, Peter's score is slightly lower and Jim's score is the lowest. If this class of students were given a parallel test, would the rank ordering of scores be the same as in the first test?
3 In another test, John passes. He scores 83% and the cut-off score for the test was 50%. If John were given a parallel test would he pass again?

These examples illustrate three operational definitions of reliability. The first example is from a domain-referenced perspective. The test here aims to measure how much of a certain domain John knows. It may be intuitively clear that to be able to conclude that John's knowledge is *exactly* 83% you need a very fine – highly reliable – measurement. The second example – from a norm-referenced perspective – is somewhat less demanding. Here we are not interested in whether John's score was exactly 83%, but only whether his score was better than Harry's, Peter's and Jim's. The measurement can be slightly coarser. In the third case, demands on the measurement are even lower.

Now let us turn the concept around. If we have the test results of a class of students, depending on which of the three conclusions we want to draw, the test is more or less reliable. This is all very well in theory, but we do not have a parallel test, so how can we establish the parallel test score. A typical approach is to retrospectively divide the test into two halves randomly and treat them as parallel tests. Most of the well-known reliability tests in classical test theory, for example, Kuder–Richardson and Cronbach's alpha, build on this approach (*see* Box 14.1).

Why is it so hard to design a perfectly reliable test? The largest source of unreliability is sampling error. For pragmatic reasons, a test usually comprises a sample of questions from the whole domain of possible questions. But because items can differ in difficulty, and because different students find different items difficult – John does better on the myocardial infarction items and Harry does better on the arrhythmia items – sampling error arises. The same applies equally to other assessment modalities, such as the examiner's choice of question in oral or short essay examinations. So if sampling error is such a major issue, it follows

that brief assessments and assessments based on the observation of only one examiner are very likely to be unreliable.

There is one final issue to discuss in relation to reliability, namely the relationship between reliability and objectivity. A common misconception is that subjective assessment is always unreliable and objective assessments are always reliable.(2) The following two illustrations demonstrate that this is not necessarily the case. The first example is a one-item multiple-choice examination. This is a so-called objective test, but as it has only one item, it is not reliable. On the other hand, suppose we were to write 10 pieces of music ourselves and take, at random, 10 pieces written by Mozart, and submit them all to a panel of experts who have to assess the musical artistry of the composer. The panel would reach the decision that Mozart is the better composer. It would not matter if we took another sample of our own compositions or another sample of Mozart's compositions or even another sample of experts, the decision would still be the same. Musical artistry, however, is not 'objective'; it is highly subjective. Yet the decision of the panel is highly reproducible and thus reliable.

In conclusion, reliability is a matter of careful sampling. It relies on a sufficiently large sample through all possible sources of error, for example, items, examiners and test occasions. But reliability is not the whole story.

Validity

Validity is defined as the extent to which the competence that the assessment claims to measure is actually being measured. This is not always easy to demonstrate, and determining the validity of a particular test method is a matter of collecting evidence from different angles.

The first step is to define exactly for what purpose the method is valid. In the way that a thermometer is a valid instrument to measure temperature and only temperature (not weight, for example), an assessment method is valid only for a certain aspect of competence. Any claim by a test developer that their instrument is a valid instrument for medical competence is therefore to be regarded with suspicion. Validity has been defined in numerous different ways. For the purposes of this publication, we will classify the different varieties of validity into two categories.(3,4)

Content validity (often also referred to as *direct* validity)

An examination must be representative of the *whole* testable domain. An examination on cardiology should not be composed only of items on myocardial infarction. To ensure adequate coverage, a test is typically constructed according to a blueprint. The blueprint is a matrix in which the test maker determines how many items per subject or category are to be asked. A

BOX 14.1 Focus on: The measurement of reliability

Reliability is a central concept in test theory, as examiners and candidates want a test that gives a similar result on different occasions with different candidates. Test–retest analysis assesses the same candidate's performance in the same test on two separate occasions, whereas parallel testing assesses the same candidate using tests containing different questions that are thought to be equivalent. In each case, reliable tests should give very similar marks on both occasions. Mathematically, psychometricians *model* the responses of candidates in different ways, with three broad approaches.

Classical test theory (CTT)

This has been around for half a century or more. The main assumption is that a candidate has a true ability, or score, but because of measurement error, for whatever reason, the candidate does not obtain the exact same score even if an identical test is used on two occasions. The similarity of marks on the two occasions is used to calculate the reliability, which becomes higher as measurement error becomes lower. A similar approach can be used for comparing parallel tests.

CTT works best with multiple-choice tests where all candidates answer identical questions. Its major drawback is that reliability calculated from one group of candidates cannot be extrapolated easily to other groups. Apparent reliability of a test can be much inflated by including a few outstandingly bad candidates. CTT reliability is also very misleading as a description of the accuracy of a cutoff score (pass/fail boundary) in high-stakes examinations.

Generalisability theory (GT)

CTT does not work well with typical clinical examinations where not all candidates can see all patients or be seen by all examiners. There is therefore variability due to examiners (e.g. hawks and doves) and clinical scenarios, as well as case-specificity, with some candidates doing better with some types of case than others. GT generalises CTT to include such components. A measure equivalent

to reliability ('generalisability') can be calculated: in effect, how similar would a candidate's mark be with different examiners and different scenarios?

GT allows sophisticated calculations of the effects of different types of exam – 'what if' questions – such as, would the exam be more generalisable with more stations and fewer examiners per station? The untested, perhaps unrealistic, assumption is that examiners and candidates will behave in precisely the same way in such new situations. As with CTT, GT estimates of generalisability cannot be easily extrapolated to new situations.

Rasch modelling (RM) and item–response theory (IRT)

IRT is a more complex variant of Rasch modelling. RM starts with the assumption that every test item has a particular difficulty, with the probability of a candidate answering an item correctly depending on the item's difficulty and the ability of the candidate. Mathematical modelling then allows the item difficulties to be calculated, as well as candidate abilities. A new test comprised of previously used items from an item bank used in different combinations can have its reliability calculated before the test is used. The reliability can also be calculated for candidates of differing ability (e.g. fourth-year students rather than third-year). IRT is an extension of RM that not only calculates the difficulty of items, but also calculates discriminative value and chance-guessing rates.

IRT requires large data sets and is best used for large-scale examinations with a thousand-plus candidates. RM, however, is robust with small numbers. RM cannot handle clinical situations with different scenarios and examiners, but they can be handled with Facet theory. The major problem for RM and IRT is not the conceptual basis, which is rigorous, powerful and realistic, but the poor mathematical and statistical skills of most biomedical examiners.

Chris Mc Manus
University College London

subsidiary issue in content validity is the relevance of the items. Only relevant items contribute to the content validity of the examination.

Construct validity (often also referred to as *indirect* validity)

A construct is a personal psychological characteristic that cannot be observed directly but which is assumed to exist. A typical example is the notion of intelligence. We assume this construct to have certain characteristics: more intelligent people can learn faster, have superior memory skills and are better able to solve problems than less intelligent people. If we were to

design a new test to measure intelligence, we would hope that people who learn faster outperform people who learn more slowly, and demonstrating this would contribute to the validity of our new test. Applying this principle to tests for medical problem solving means that for a test to have good construct validity, it would be necessary for people who solve problems more expertly to outperform those who are less good problem solvers.

There are many other types of validity evidence: weak correlations between two tests that are supposed to measure different constructs; strong correlations between two tests that are assumed to measure the same construct; and so on. Although they are sometimes labelled as different forms of validity, in effect they all contribute to the evidence for the validity of a test for a specific construct.

The concept of validity has engendered a wide variety of view points. Some claim that only construct validity is worthwhile and dismiss content and face validity as just a collection of opinions.(5) Some take the usability of the test and the relationship between the test and its user as an important element of validity.(6) Others take a more holistic view, and we think that Messick strikes an intelligent balance in his unified definition of validity as 'the degree to which empirical evidence and theoretical rationales support the adequacy and appropriateness of inferences and actions based on test scores or other modes of assessment'.(7) 'Inferences' and 'actions' bring us neatly to considering the educational consequences of the test.

Educational impact

The saying 'Students don't do what you expect, students do what you inspect' epitomises the educational impact of assessment. Although there is not an abundance of empirical data in the medical educational literature, it is a commonly held belief that assessment has a major impact on students' learning behaviour.(8,9) Often the standard response of teachers is to chide students for this strategic approach to learning, but a more rational response is for the test maker to capitalise on this behaviour. It is normal human behaviour and it is not going to go away; indeed, we are all susceptible to these kinds of external motivator. More importantly, the driving influence of assessment is a powerful tool to ensure that students learn what, and how, teachers want them to learn. To maximise the effectiveness of this link, it is important to realise that assessment influences student learning in several ways: through its content, its format, the scheduling of examinations and the regulatory structure of the assessment programme.

The influence of *content* is obvious. Topics that come up repeatedly in the examinations will be perceived by students as the most important. When it comes to *format*, the literature gives different views. Some studies seem to indicate that students prepare differently for different formats, especially multiple-choice versus open-ended examinations.(10) Others indicate that this is only the perception of students, whereas in fact they prepare similarly.(11) As a rule of thumb, we advocate using a variety of formats in an assessment programme. This way, students will not become used to one type of preparation.

A typical problem of *scheduling* concerns annual examination periods. If several examinations are held during the same few weeks, students will not be able to prepare adequately for all of them. They will then have to select strategically the examinations for which they will prepare well and those for which they will not. From the faculty's point of view this is a waste of resources, as effort is put into constructing a high-quality examination that is not taken seriously. Better therefore to spread examinations, rather than to cluster them. The *assessment programme as a whole* defines academic success. The credit points attributed to each part, the way scores are combined, the minimum number of points needed to progress and so on all define how students will study or prepare for the examinations. Programmes with continuous assessment will promote continuous learning; pinpoint assessments will promote cramming behaviour. Because educational impact is such a major effect of assessment, it is often also seen as a part of validity, specifically termed 'consequential validity'.

Cost-effectiveness

This seems an easy and obvious issue, but the practice sometimes differs from the theory. For example, a prerequisite for a cost-effective assessment programme is an explicit description of its goals, both in terms of *what* is to be assessed and *how* it is to be assessed. Only then can an evaluation be conducted into whether the programme is optimally cost-effective. The most important factors hampering cost-efficiency are misconceptions based on tradition and intuition, poorly supportive infrastructure and lack of collaboration.

Typical examples of the first are interviews, oral examinations and open-ended questions. The literature on interviews for selection for medical schools converges on the conclusion that their predictive validity is unacceptably low.(12–14) Their use therefore constitutes a cost-ineffective assessment procedure. The same applies to many unstructured oral examinations.(15) Such orals have poor reliability and are often used to test simple factual knowledge, which can better be tested using more cost-effective methods. This is not to say that there is no place for oral examinations in an assessment programme, but they should be used only where they have an added value over other formats.(16) Similarly, there is an almost inextinguishable belief that open-ended questions test higher-order cognitive skills and multiple-choice questions do not. Again, the literature converges on the notion that in this matter the question format is quite unimportant, but the content of the question is.(17–19) Of course, in an assessment programme there may be indications to use open-ended questions, for example, if creativity or spontaneous generation of the answer is essential. In other cases there are more cost-effective alternatives.

Typical examples of poor infrastructure support are the lack of good item banking and the absence of a centralised management and administrative support for the logistics and administration of examinations. The consequences are that 'expensive' scientific staff members carry out work that could be done just as well – or even better – by administrative personnel.

The benefits of collaboration may perhaps be obvious. Many medical schools have comparable curricula with comparable end goals, and sharing test material would be a way to reduce costs, because it would mean not everybody has to reinvent the wheel.(20) This is not to say that collaboration is easy. Careful planning, commitment of all partners and some sort of pre-investment are all needed to make collaboration successful.

Acceptability

Setting up an assessment system cannot be done in a vacuum. A careful balance between what may be scientifically and educationally superior and what is acceptable to the stakeholders has to be struck. Even the best assessment method is useless if teachers and students will not subscribe to it. Some even go so far as to incorporate this issue into the argument for a test's validity.(6) This is not that strange a point of view because an instrument is valid only if it is used properly.

Popular Assessment Instruments

No single assessment instrument is perfect and no single instrument can test all aspects of medical competence and performance. Each instrument has its strengths and weaknesses. A good assessment programme should therefore include a combination of various methods, each selected for a specific purpose, and each with its indications and contraindications.(21,22) This section describes the major strengths and weaknesses of different groups of commonly used assessment methods, using the five criteria described above: reliability, validity, educational impact, cost-efficiency and acceptability.

Written assessment instruments

There are many different written assessment instruments currently in use. Some are case-based, some are context-free. Some use open-ended questions, some use multiple choice.

As a general rule, the amount of time it takes to answer a question has a negative impact on the reliability of the test. As you may recall, a test can only sample from the whole domain of possible items, and, as such, the sample must be large enough to be reliable. It follows then that the more items a test contains, the more reliable it is likely to be. This immediately places open-ended questions at a disadvantage because they require more answering time. So, essays are generally less reliable *per hour of testing time* than short-answer questions.

Where reliability is a fairly straightforward issue in written assessment, validity is much more complex. There are some popular beliefs about the validity of different types of question. For example, many people think that open-ended questions test higher-order cognitive skills and that multiple-choice questions can test only factual knowledge. This is a widespread misconception: the question *format* is quite unimportant with respect to validity, whereas the question *content* is very important.(17–19) So, *what* you ask is important, not how you record the answer. Of course, some contents do not fit certain formats. It is best not to ask items that require the spontaneous and creative generation of possibilities in multiple-choice format, while items requiring a selection from a finite list of realistic options are best not asked in an open-ended format.

Thus careful consideration of content is essential. A further and important distinction relates to context. Context-rich items contain a case description and questions that ask for (essential) decisions or an evaluation of the problem. Typical examples of these are extended-matching items or key-feature approach items.(23–25) Context-free items do not have a case description and simply ask for general knowledge. Context-rich approaches test application of knowledge and problem solving, but context-free items do not.(26) Both, however, can be equally important aspects to assess; one is not superior to the other.

The idea that open-ended questions test superior cognitive skills over multiple-choice questions is also widespread among students. Although this may not actually be true, it will still influence students' perception and their learning. Using a variety of methods sends a clear message to students that they have to master the subject matter irrespective of the assessment format.

Another aspect of educational impact is the influence that assessment has on test makers. If, for example, all tests have to be in multiple-choice format, examiners will construct items that fit this format, and questions requiring spontaneous generation of the answer will be under-represented. On the other hand, if all items are of the open-ended format, the examiner will be burdened with the high workload of correcting tests and will start asking simple questions that are easy to score, which also means that important aspects may be neglected.

The use of multiple-choice-based assessments is highly cost-effective. They may be slightly more difficult to produce, but the use of Optical Mark Reading scanners certainly makes them easier to score. This is a particularly relevant consideration in medical schools with a large number of students per year-class. Every pound, euro or dollar can be spent only once; therefore, money spent on unnecessarily expensive assessment methods cannot be spent on improving education. So, from the viewpoint of cost-efficiency, it is best to use open-ended questions only if more efficient formats will not suffice.

There might be a wealth of scientific literature proving that test format is unimportant, but sometimes beliefs may be so strong that stakeholders cannot be convinced. You will then hear arguments claiming that multiple-choice assessments are too easy, make students lazy and are not worthy of an academic environment, and that real life and real practice are not simply a question of selecting options from a list. Whether it is useful to try to fight such arguments is a political decision and will vary from institution to institution. However, if it proves impossible to overcome problems of acceptability at first, there may be good reasons to postpone the 'battle'. Your energy may be better spent on good teaching and good-enough assessment, and, more important, any test can be valid only if it is used correctly. For this, it has to be acceptable to all stakeholders.

Objective Structured Clinical Examinations and simulated patients

Objective Structured Clinical Examinations (OSCEs) and simulated patient (SP)-based examinations have become very popular for the assessment of (practical) skills.(27,28) Both are based on a series of structured cases that must be addressed by the candidate. In an OSCE, a candidate enters a series of different rooms or stations in sequence. In each room there is a specified assignment (e.g. perform a resuscitation or take the blood pressure), a simulated patient or dummy, and an examiner with a checklist or rating scale. The candidate has to complete the assignment and his or her performance is scored against the checklist or rating scale. After a fixed period of time, a signal is given and the candidate proceeds to the next station.

OSCEs and SP-based examinations were developed as an answer to the unstructured observations in practice. They are cleverly developed in that they address the inherent unreliability of observed practice in three ways. First, by adding structure to the observations, they become more reliable. Second, by keeping each of the observations short (the original OSCEs had five-minute stations), many different observations can be made per hour, thus enabling wider and more effective sampling. Third, by having the candidate move from station to station, such assessments also sample across different examiners. The 'hawks' will be compensated for by the 'doves', or better still all candidates will be examined by the same panel of examiners. The second of these issues – that of sampling across many cases – is the most important because the biggest threat to reliability is having too small a sample. The many reliability studies on OSCEs have demonstrated this over and over again. One of the practical implications is that it is better to have more stations with one examiner per station than fewer stations with two examiners per station. Despite the clever reliability approach, OSCEs still require a minimum average of two hours of testing per candidate to achieve an acceptable reliability for summative decisions.

With respect to validity, two issues are of overriding importance: the length of the stations and the use of checklists versus global rating scales. One might be inclined to think that longer stations, that is, longer than five minutes, may be more (content) valid but less reliable, but this is not necessarily the case. Longer cases contain more information than shorter ones, and there seems to be an optimum balance between the length and the number of cases in an OSCE. As a rule of thumb, it is best to adapt the length of the stations to the content of the case, so durations of stations may be designed to vary from 5 to 20 minutes.(29)

Checklists are detailed lists of behaviours, and they describe precisely the actions to be taken, for example, 'washes hands', 'puts left hand on the sternum of the patient'; whereas rating scales allow for more interpretation by the examiner, describing in broad terms only the skills to be performed, for example, 'explores patient's concerns', 'comes to the correct conclusions'. So should checklists or rating scales be used?

One would be inclined to think that as checklists are more structured they would be more reliable, but this is not always the case.(30) The choice of whether to use checklists or rating scales should be made mainly on the basis of the type of skill to be assessed. Technical skills, such as taking blood pressure or performing resuscitation, can easily be tested with checklists, whereas more complicated skills, such as short patient contacts, seem to be better tested with rating scales. Most medical schools use short stations with checklists for technical skills in the more junior year groups, and integrated longer stations with rating scales in the more senior years.

In general, OSCEs are taken very seriously by students and have a high impact on student learning behaviour. This provides both a risk and an opportunity. The risk comes with detailed checklists. Even if they are not handed out officially, a 'black market' in old checklists may develop, and memorising these may be a successful study strategy for students. Memorising rating scales is less useful. The use of rating scales in OSCEs induces a study behaviour that is aimed more at practising the skill, and an opportunity here is to allow some time – about two minutes – at the end of each station for specific feedback. When the OSCE is solely for certification purposes, this is not desirable. In such cases, optimising the reliability (and thus the sampling) is more essential. However, most OSCEs are held within the educational environment of medical schools and can provide a wonderful opportunity for learning.

Unfortunately, OSCEs are very expensive to conduct. They require extensive resources and good logistics. It is therefore important to use OSCEs effectively, and using an extensive part of the OSCE time to explore general knowledge is not efficient. This does not mean that no knowledge should be tested in an OSCE, but that the knowledge tested should be background knowledge and should have a direct relationship to the case.

OSCEs are widely accepted and popular throughout the world. The only threat to their acceptability is when OSCEs are used to test highly technical skills with very detailed checklists. They then tend to become monkey tricks and examiners may feel that their expertise is not being used or valued.

Oral examinations

Oral examinations come in various forms, ranging from the completely unstructured to the highly structured, case-based examination. The oral examination has tended to be discarded, being considered too unreliable and too expensive. But recently opinion on the oral has shifted in a more favourable direction,(16) and the prevailing view is that there is room for an oral examination in an assessment programme as long as it is used in the correct way and for the correct purpose.

This does imply, though, that to be acceptable, the oral examination must be constructed in such a way that it achieves sufficient reliability. For this, some structure – but not too much – is needed; a situation analogous to the OSCEs, where detailed checklists do not lead to higher reliabilities than rating scales. Reliability can be further enhanced by asking about a good variety of topics rather than homing in on only one. If multiple examiners are used, it is also better to 'nest' cases within examiners instead of using panels.(15)

There is a largely unsubstantiated view that orals are somehow more valid than written examinations. You may recall that in considering the validity of an assessment, the content is more important than the format. Often, the answers to oral questions require a good deal of (factual) knowledge, which can be assessed just as well by less expensive methods. If orals are to be used correctly, they have to be aimed at examining aspects that cannot be examined otherwise, such as hypothesis generation, explanations and the transfer of principles through various contexts. Another misapprehension is the perceived advantage that orals offer in following through on a certain topic – 'to see if they really understand it'. In such cases, the law of diminishing returns rules: the first question on a topic may prove a rich source of information about the candidate's competence, but the 10th question will add virtually nothing new.

Of course, just as with any type of examination, students will prepare strategically for the oral. In doing this they often try to get the lenient examiners or find out what the examiners' hobby horses are. It is therefore best to use a rotational approach in which students rotate from examiner to examiner, each of whom addresses a different, but predetermined, case or topic.

Despite the high costs of oral examinations, they are widely accepted in assessment programmes, apparently even by the students, since – astonishingly – they are not as often the subject of appeals and litigation as are written assessments.

Workplace-based assessment

Recent developments have placed the assessment in the authentic medical context once again. Where OSCEs were developed to test students in a simulated environment, instruments such as mini-CEX (Clinical Evaluation Exercise) and 360° feedback assess the candidate in their professional environment.(31,32)

Mini-CEX uses a generic form with rating scales, which an examiner uses to score a patient encounter. Items include history taking, physical examination, professionalism, clinical judgement, counselling, organisation and efficiency, and an overall impression. The competence of the candidate is assessed by a series of direct observations. Another workplace-based approach, 360° feedback, uses standard lists of rating scale items, which are sent to various parties. So, not only colleagues, but also nursing staff and patients, are sent a form and asked to give their rating on the items. Examples of items include:

- ability to diagnose patients
- ability to use evidence-based medicine approaches in practice
- verbal communication with colleagues.

At first sight, both of these methods may seem like a step back to the old in-training judgements, but this is not the case. The mini-CEX draws on the lessons learnt from the OSCEs about structure and sampling. Observations in practice, such as mini-CEX, can become reliable as long as the examiners have some criteria; a sufficient number (roughly 7 to 10) of different cases are observed; and there is more than one observer.(33,34) The added value is that what is being measured is more authentic than in a simulated environment. In many simulated assessments, certain symptoms cannot be simulated, but in real contexts these symptoms are present.

The 360° feedback method is not based on direct observations but on a judgement in retrospect. Normally, this is ill advised since such judgements tend to be very unreliable. But two aspects remedy this problem. First, many different people are asked, so a broad sample of observations is obtained. Second, judges are not asked for a global impression but to give a judgement about specific aspects of someone's strengths and weaknesses. In both cases judges need to be trained to use the instrument correctly.

Apart from being 'measurements' of competence or performance, these instruments are also intended to provide the candidate with extensive feedback. This is needed to influence learning behaviour. So rather than being measurement-only instruments, they are also educational tools aimed at improving the performance of candidates. Furthermore, the supervisor cannot complete them if he or she has not observed the candidate directly. So, in those educational environments where direct observation is not part of the educational culture, the use of these instruments may help to change the educational routine.

Using workplace-based instruments well does not have to be time-consuming, especially in those situations where frequent observation and feedback are already part of the teaching culture. However, it is important not to make the forms too long, as this will make such an approach less acceptable to users.

Portfolios

The word 'portfolio' is a container term used to describe all kinds of educational tools. From the assessment point of view there are two approaches that it may be useful to discuss here:

- portfolio as an instrument to measure the *reflective ability* of the candidate
- portfolio as an instrument to *collate assessment information* form various sources.

In both cases the portfolio contains an 'archive' and an 'analysis'. The analysis contains a self-assessment of strengths and weaknesses, learning goals and a learning plan.

The reflective portfolio focuses on self-assessment; it assesses the extent to which the self-assessment demonstrates a good reflective ability. The second portfolio approach collates all assessment information about the student. The analysis section is used to evaluate current performance and to plan future learning. This approach is best compared to a patient chart, in which information from various sources, such as laboratory data, imaging data, and results from history taking and physical examination, is collected, but it also contains a regular evaluation about the well-being of the patient and a plan for further diagnostic and therapeutic actions. So, the portfolio becomes not only an assessment but also an educational instrument.

It is difficult to say anything definitive about the reliability and validity of portfolios. Studies calculating reliability in the traditional psychometric way, using either generalisability theory or inter-rater agreement measures such as Cohen's Kappa, report moderate reliabilities at best.(35) Other authors suggest an organisational approach to rendering the portfolios dependable, using concepts from qualitative research methodologies, such as benchmarking, peer evaluation, member checking and stepwise replication.(36) In such cases, reliability cannot be expressed as a number but must be derived from the carefulness of the procedure.

The validity of the portfolio approach requires further study. It is apparent that conventional construct validity methods do not apply here, so other methodologies need to be developed. Moreover, since portfolios are used for so many purposes, content validity cannot easily be established.

It may also be obvious that portfolios are expensive. They are time-consuming not only to produce, but also to assess, especially if more than one judge has to assess each portfolio. It is tempting then to try to produce a simple scoring list or rubric to increase efficiency, but this only serves to trivialise the assessment. Training of assessors and using global criteria for judging the portfolio is a better approach, and it may be more efficient to set up a procedure in which multiple judges are used only if there is doubt about the result, with only a very limited number of judges used in all clear cases.(36)

Computers in assessment

There are many different ways in which computers can play a role in assessment. The most obvious is computerised administration. But there are other, and more important, roles for computers in assessment, and these are discussed briefly below.

Administrative support in assessment

Item banks can be very powerful in supporting quality control. Indeed, this aspect is often more important than their role in enabling the reuse of old items. Attempts to build a complete item bank from which items can be drawn at random often prove unsuccessful. There are two reasons for this. First, an examination is more than a randomly generated set of items, even if the individual items are of good quality. There is always an extra quality control step needed to ensure that the combination of items is good. A second reason is concerned with the nature of medicine and other health sciences. In these disciplines, things evolve quite rapidly, rendering items quickly outdated. Also, ideas about what constitutes a good item may evolve. Item banks are more useful in tracking an item in the quality control process. They also provide the opportunity to scan the domain coverage quickly, so that production of redundant items is prevented and under-represented subjects can be filled with specific new items.

There are many good commercial products available for item banking. For simple purposes it is also possible to use standard database software with self-produced scripts, shells or queries. Developing complete high-brow software systems is always more time consuming than one would expect. When an item bank system is needed, the best approach is to determine carefully the needs of the organisation, or the functional and operational specifications, and then determine which of the available software can meet these needs sufficiently.

Test analysis

In the quality control of tests, computers can be used to evaluate test results. The most well-known application is a standard item analysis with p-values, a-values, item–total or item–rest correlations and the calculation of reliabilities.

The p-value represents the proportion of students answering the question correctly. As such, it is an indication of how difficult this item was for this particular group of candidates. A p-value of 1.00 means that every candidate answered the item correctly, whereas a p-value of 0.00 means that nobody gave the correct answer.

The a-values indicate the proportion of candidates choosing each option in a multiple-choice question and, as such, is an indicator for the attractiveness of each distracter.

The item–total and item–rest correlations indicate the extent to which the item was answered correctly by the high achievers on the test and answered incorrectly by the low scorers on the test.

Standard statistical software such as SPSS often allows for such analyses, and such structured item analyses can be very valuable and may have a major impact on the quality of tests.

Computerised testing

There are many obvious advantages of computerised testing. Hand scoring is not needed; the results can be calculated immediately; and data files for further analysis are easily available. Also, there are no added costs for reproduction of test booklets and answer sheets. Audio and video clips are possible and can help to improve the content validity of the test.

But there are also downsides to computerised testing. First, open-ended questions are difficult to score automatically and may need hand scoring or at least verification of the computer scoring procedures. Although hand scoring of typed text may be easier than that of – sometimes illegible – handwriting, this still nullifies the advantages of immediate results and availability of data files. This may lead test developers to use multiple-choice-type questions exclusively.

Second, if there are many more candidates than there are computers available, equivalent test forms have to be developed. Although corralling of students is an option to prevent unwanted information exchanges, this is possible only to a limited extent. Producing extra equivalent tests is more expensive than reproduction costs.

Third, the necessity of a systems administrator for the computer network adds to the costs. Fourth, reading from a computer screen is more exhausting than reading from paper, which may limit the maximum test length. Finally, without sufficient back-up systems computer or network problems may disturb the test administration. Although with ongoing technology these problems are rare, and despite the fact that things can also go wrong with paper-and-pencil administration, problems are still more likely to occur with computerised testing. So, before deciding

to use computers to administer a test that could also be a pen-and-paper exercise, it is important to consider all the pros and cons very carefully.

Assessment possibilities unique to computer testing

There are some interesting and potential possibilities presented by computer-based assessment that are unique to the format and not merely logistical advantages. We discuss three of them here, namely real-time simulations, sequential testing and computer-adaptive testing.

Real-time simulations are useful to test the management of cases in which time is essential in real life, such as emergency medicine. As a formative tool it can also be helpful to demonstrate to the candidate how much time they took to solve the case and where a gain in efficiency could be made. For summative testing it tends to complicate things, as one cannot simply add up response time and proficiency. So, to come to a pass/fail decision, one has to find a valid way of combining these different qualities into one single score, and this is not easy.

Sequential testing is an approach that enables a more efficient use of time and resources in assessment. It basically comes down to administering a short screening test to all candidates. Based on the reliability of this test, a (95%) confidence interval can be calculated around the pass/fail score. For every candidate whose score is outside this interval, there is sufficient certainty ($p \leq 0.05$) to say that his or her score is either a pass or a fail. The remainder of the students must answer an additional set of questions. The scores of these are added to their scores in the first part of the test. In this way a longer test is presented only to those candidates where there is doubt about their passing or failing. Such an approach is feasible only if the scores and the confidence interval can be calculated quickly and an additional test is available on request.(37)

A further development is *computer-adaptive testing* (CAT). This approach is based on a so-called calibrated item bank – an item bank in which the precise difficulty of all items is known beforehand. For such a calibration, classical test theory (CTT) is often not sufficient. A more complicated statistical approach – item–response theory (IRT) – is used (See Box 14.1). Unlike CTT, the use of IRT allows the difficulty and discriminative power of items to be estimated regardless of the specific group of candidates. The computer selects an item of moderate difficulty for the candidate. When the candidate answers the item correctly, the computer selects a slightly more difficult item, and when the answer is incorrect, an easier item is selected. This process is repeated either until a specified number of items have been answered or until a certain level of preciseness of the test is reached.(38) In the former, the precision proficiency estimate varies across candidates (but in the majority of cases is better than a standard test); in the latter, the precision is fixed, but the number of items needed may vary from candidate to candidate (in the majority of cases this will be fewer than in a standard test). Although CAT is a wonderful concept, the statistical requirements for achieving a well-enough calibrated item bank are quite heavy, often requiring considerable pre-testing of all items.(38)

Combining Assessment Methods

It is currently generally accepted that to gain a complete picture of someone's competence and performance, one assessment instrument is not enough; a variety of well-chosen instruments is needed. How then should assessment methods be combined? Essentially, there are two approaches, one quantitative the other qualitative.

Quantitative methods
- Compensatory
- Partially compensatory
- Conjunctive

Qualitative methods
- Expert judgement
- Explicit procedures

In a quantitative combination, results are somehow translated into numerical values. These values are then combined in a compensatory, partially compensatory or conjunctive manner.

Compensatory means that the results of the tests are averaged and that the average needs to be above the pass/fail score, regardless of the scores on the individual tests. For example, averaging the two sets of marks 4/10 and 8/10, and 2/10 and 10/10, gives a result of 6 in both cases (which on a 10-point scale often means a pass). A model in which every test result contributes to a total score with a certain percentage, for example, test 1 accounts for 30% and test 2 for 20% and so on, is also a compensatory model. Compensatory models often result in high reliabilities for the final decision, as such decisions are made on the basis of many items within multiple tests held on different occasions, so sampling across many sources of error. The biggest downside is that compensatory models may induce a minimalist study strategy. Some students may have such high scores on previous tests that they tend not to take the later tests (and the related courses) seriously.

A *partially compensatory* model corrects for this. Here the scores can be averaged, but for each test there is an absolute minimum score, and if this is not reached the student has to repeat the test. This is a compromise in that the combined reliability is somewhat lower than in a completely compensatory model, but the negative educational impact is also diminished.

A (completely) *conjunctive* model requires that the student achieves a score above the pass/fail score in all the tests in order to gain an overall pass. Such an approach stimulates students to take all the individual tests (and courses) seriously and to study hard for all of them, but it is less reliable overall. In every test there is the possibility of a false negative result, that is, a student who fails who should in fact have passed. Such failure is then largely due to measurement error rather than incompetence. If each failure leads to a consequence (which is the case in conjunctive but not in compensatory models), the overall reliability is lower.

The results of some assessments are simply not quantitative in nature. So, it is not possible to add them up to form a total score. Although it is common practice to convert the results of qualitative assessments into numerical scores, we want to warn against this as a methodologically incorrect practice. This is perhaps best illustrated by an analogy to medical practice. You do not add your first impression of 'very sick patient' to a sodium level of 133 mmol/l – these two pieces of information need to be combined qualitatively. The same applies to different observations with results such as 'performed extremely well' and 'good bedside manner'. These cannot be combined in a quantitative way but need to be evaluated qualitatively. Such a combination requires – again similar to medical practice – expert judgement and careful procedures. Good examples of such approaches are the General Medical Council's practice performance procedures and some portfolio assessments.(36,39,40)

Standard Setting

Perhaps the most heavily debated issue in assessment is the issue of standard setting. It is the cut-off score that determines the consequences of the assessment, that is, who passes and who fails, and often quite small changes in cut-off scores represent substantial changes in the numbers of students who pass and fail. The holy grail is therefore the *true* cut-off score. Unfortunately, like its mythical counterpart, there is no such thing. The literature describes a wide variation of methods,(41) each of which has its own specific purposes, and a distinction is usually made between relative and absolute standards.

A relative standard implies that the performance of the group of candidates who are taking a test is used to determine the pass/fail score for that test. An example is the Wijnen method, in which the mean score of the group minus one standard deviation is the cut-off score. An absolute standard determines a prospectively defined minimum level of competence to be demonstrated. The most well-known example of this is the Angoff method.(42) The Angoff method entails the use of an expert panel in which each member judges each individual question and gives an estimate of the chance of a *borderline* student answering the item correctly. In some modifications there is a group discussion of the individual estimates to rule out misconceptions. The average estimate is calculated per item and then averaged across all items, thus providing a cut-off score. It can be seen that in the Wijnen method the group of candidates serve as their own reference group, and in the Angoff method a panel of experts serves as the reference group.

There is no one single best standard-setting method for all tests, but there is a most appropriate method for each individual test.

No matter which method of standard setting is used, it will always be arbitrary, as there will always be assumptions made about the required level. Relative methods are based on assumptions about the stability of the mean competence of large groups of students. Especially large year-classes of medical students appear to be very comparable across cohorts and universities in many, but not all, countries. Absolute methods are based on assumptions about the required level of competence, the teaching the candidates have had and the end goals of the curriculum. In every case, therefore, there must at least be an explicit rationale for the decisions about the standard-setting method. This is sometimes expressed in the aphorism 'standard setting may be arbitrary, it may never be frivolous'. Any standard set must be:

- explicable, through the rationales behind the decisions made
- defensible, to the extent that it can assure the stakeholders about its validity (An issue in this may be 'due diligence', that is, demonstrating that good effort was put into setting the standard.)
- stable, as it is not defensible that the standards vary from year to year.(43)

Future Directions

A section on future directions is always a dangerous one to write since so-called 'future developments' may, with hindsight, appear to have been flukes. Still, we would like to make some predictions.

The change from defining educational outcomes in constructs – such as knowledge, skills, attitudes and problem-solving skills – to actions, as described in Miller's pyramid (knows, knows how, shows how and does), and the further change from there into more or less complex tasks that require the timely availability of relevant knowledge, skills, attitudes and problem-solving ability, the so-called competencies, must have an influence on our way of thinking about assessment.

Also, the emergence of new assessment methods such as mini-CEX, 360° feedback and portfolio, in which the main goal is *not* to add up the individual items to give a total score, must have an influence on

our way of thinking about assessment. We see three main developments here.

1 Assessment will be less viewed as an external measurement of the results of the educational process but more as an integral part of the process. Currently, it is still fairly common to take students out of the authentic educational context to be tested on their competence. Assessments such as mini-CEX take the assessment back into the authentic educational context. Current approaches to assessing professional behaviour even acknowledge that it is impossible to evaluate this outside the authentic context. This leads, in our view, to a second development.

2 Assessment is no longer seen exclusively as a psychometric measurement problem, but more as an educational design problem. This implies that the purpose of assessment is not merely to determine whether a candidate is up to standard, but more how the information about the candidate's competence can best be used to tailor the teaching or the courses to individual needs. So, instead of striving for a standardised curriculum with standardised testing, it will entail a development to tailored assessment with flexible curricula. This may lead to a third development.

3 Standard psychometric approaches to issues such as fairness and defensibility of examinations will have to be expanded with other measures. For example, basic assumptions underlying the standard psychometric approach, such as stable and generic constructs, homogeneity of the universe (e.g. the total universe of possible items) and assumption of local independency of the observations, cannot always be met. Moreover, some modern instruments aim precisely at being locally dependent observations (mini-CEX, longitudinal testing), acknowledge the heterogeneity of the universe (360° feedback) and acknowledge the non-existence of traits in competence (portfolio). This does not make the issues of defensibility, fairness and carefulness go away but will require different – statistical – models. Our best guess at the moment would be that these are probabilistic and Bayesian in nature.(44)

Epilogue

Designing assessment programmes and selecting the best instruments for each purpose is not easy. To complicate matters further, medical education is a rapidly evolving discipline. This may lead one to despair of assessment science and argue that the truths of yesterday are obsolete and will be replaced with new ones. We would argue against this. Any evolving discipline questions truths critically and scientifically, and this is a strength rather than a weakness. In this respect, medical education does not differ from medicine – what was true when we were students often no longer holds true today. The purpose of this publication is to guide the reader through the field of assessment of medical competence and performance by providing background information and a few guidelines. The most important messages we have tried to convey are that in designing high-quality assessments, the most important foundations are rational decisions based on the best available evidence and careful quality control.

References

1 Van der Vleuten CPM (1996) The assessment of professional competence: developments, research and practical implications. *Advances in Health Science Education.* **1**(1): 41–67.

2 Van der Vleuten CPM, Norman GR and De Graaf E (1991) Pitfalls in the pursuit of objectivity: issues of reliability. *Medical Education.* **25**: 110–18.

3 Cronbach LJ (1983) What price simplicity? *Educational Measurement: Issues and Practice.* **2**(2): 11–12.

4 Ebel RL (1983) The practical validation of tests of ability. *Educational Measurement: Issues and Practice.* **2**(2): 7–10.

5 Downing SM and Haladyna TM (2004) Validity threats: overcoming interference with proposed interpretations of assessment data. *Medical Education.* **38**(3): 327–33.

6 Guba EG and Lincoln YS (2001) Guidelines and checklist for constructivist (aka fourth generation) evaluation (http://www.wmich.edu/evalctr/checklists; accessed 17 August 2004).

7 Messick S (1994) The interplay of evidence and consequences in the validation of performance assessments. *Educational Researcher.* **23**(2): 13–23.

8 Frederiksen N (1984) The real test bias: influences of testing on teaching and learning. *American Psychologist.* **39**(3): 193–202.

9 Newble DI and Jaeger K (1983) The effect of assessments and examinations on the learning of medical students. *Medical Education.* **17**: 165–71.

10 Stalenhoef-Halling BF, Van der Vleuten CPM, Jaspers TAM and Fiolet JBFM (1990) A new approach to assessing clinical problem-solving skills by written examination: conceptual basis and initial pilot test results. In: Bender W, Hiemstra RJ, Scherpbier A, Zwierstra RJ (eds) *Teaching and Assessing Clinical Competence. Proceedings of the Fourth Ottawa Conference*, pp. 552–7. Boekwerk Publications, Groningen, The Netherlands.

11 Hakstian RA (1971) The effects of type of examination anticipated on test preparation and performance. *Journal of Educational Research.* **64**(7): 319–24.

12 Eva K, Rosenfeld J, Reiter H and Norman G (2004) An admissions OSCE: the multiple mini-interview. *Medical Education.* **38**(3): 314–26.

13 McManus IC, Iqbal S, Chandrarajan A et al. (2005) Unhappiness and dissatisfaction in doctors cannot be predicted by selectors for medical school application forms: a prospective longitudinal study. *BMC Medical Education.* **5**(38). doi:10.1186/1472-6920-5-38.

14 Salvatori P (2001) Reliability and validity of admissions tools used to select students for the health professions. *Advances in Health Science Education.* **6**(2): 159–75.

15 Swanson DB (1987) A measurement framework for performance-based tests. In: Hart I and Harden R (eds) *Further Developments in Assessing Clinical Competence*, pp. 13–45. Can-Heal Publications, Montreal.

16 Wass V, Wakeford R, Neighbour R and Van der Vleuten C (2003) Achieving acceptable reliability in oral examinations: an analysis of the Royal College of General Practitioners membership examination's oral component. *Medical Education.* **37**: 126–31.

17 Maatsch J and Huang R (1986) An evaluation of the construct validity of four alternative theories of clinical competence. *Proceedings of the 25th Annual RIME Conference*, pp. 69–74. Association of American Medical Colleges, Chicago.

18 Norman GR, Smith EKM, Powles AC et al. (1987) Factors underlying performance on written tests of knowledge. *Medical Education.* **21**: 297–304.

19 Schuwirth LWT, Van der Vleuten CPM and Donkers HHLM (1996) A closer look at cueing effects in multiple-choice questions. *Medical Education.* **30**: 44–9.

20 Van der Vleuten CPM, Schuwirth LWT, Muijtjens AMM et al. (2004) Cross institutional collaboration in assessment: a case on progress testing. *Medical Teacher.* **26**(8): 719–25.

21 Schuwirth LWT, Southgate L, Page GG et al. (2002) When enough is enough: a conceptual basis for fair and defensible practice performance assessment. *Medical Education.* **36**: 925–30.

22 Van der Vleuten CPM and Schuwirth LWT (2005) Assessing professional competence: from methods to programmes. *Medical Education.* **39**(3): 309–17.

23 Bordage G (1987) An alternative approach to PMPs: the 'key-features' concept. In: Hart IR and Harden R (eds) *Further Developments in Assessing Clinical Competence, Proceedings of the Second Ottawa Conference*, pp. 59–75. Can-Heal Publications, Montreal.

24 Page G, Bordage G and Allen T (1995) Developing key-feature problems and examinations to assess clinical decision-making skills. *Academic Medicine.* **70**(3): 194–201.

25 Case SM and Swanson DB (1993) Extended-matching items: a practical alternative to free response questions. *Teaching and Learning in Medicine.* **5**(2): 107–15.

26 Schuwirth LWT, Verheggen MM, Van der Vleuten CPM et al. (2001) Do short cases elicit different thinking processes than factual knowledge questions do? *Medical Education.* **35**(4): 348–56.

27 Stillman P, Ruggill J, Rutala P and Sabers D (1980) Patient instructors as teachers and evaluators. *Journal of Medical Education.* **55**: 186–93.

28 Harden RM and Gleeson FA (1979) Assessment of clinical competence using an objective structured clinical examination (OSCE). *Medical Education.* **13**(1): 41–54.

29 Petrusa E (2002) Clinical performance assessments. In: Norman G, Van der Vleuten CPM and Newble DI (eds) *International Handbook of Research in Medical Education*, pp. 673–709. Kluwer, Dordrecht, Boston, MA, London.

30 Regehr G, MacRae H, Reznick R and Szalay D (1998) Comparing the psychometric properties of checklists and global rating scales for assessing performance on an OSCE-format examination. *Academic Medicine.* **73**(9): 993–7.

31 Norcini J, Blank LL, Arnold GK and Kimball HR (1995) The mini-CEX (Clinical Evaluation Exercise); a preliminary investigation. *Annals of Internal Medicine.* **123**(10): 795–9.

32 Garman AN, Tyler JL and Darnall JS (2004) Development and validation of a 360-degree-feedback instrument for healthcare administrators. *Journal of Health Care Management.* **49**(5): 307–21.

33 Williams M, Klamen D and McGaghie W (2003) Cognitive, social and environmental sources of bias in clinical performance ratings. *Teaching and Learning in Medicine.* **15**(4): 270–92.

34 Norcini JJ, Blank LL, Duffy FD and Fortna GS (2003) The mini-CEX: a method for assessing clinical skills. *Annals of Internal Medicine*. **138**(6): 476–81.

35 Roberts C (2002) Portfolio-based assessments in medical education; are they valid and reliable for summative purposes? *Medical Education*. **36**: 899–900.

36 Driessen E, Van der Vleuten CPM, Schuwirth LWT *et al.* (2005) The use of qualitative research criteria for portfolio assessment as an alternative to reliability evaluation: a case study. *Medical Education*. **39**(2): 214–20.

37 Smee S, Blackmore DE, Rothman AI *et al.* (1998) Pioneering a sequenced OSCE for the Medical Council of Canada: An administrative overview. In: Melnick D (Ed.) Evolving assessment: Protecting the human dimension. Proceedings of the 8th International Ottawa Conference on Medical Education and Assessment. Held July 12–15, 1998 Philadelphia (PA) USA. National Board of Medical Examiners, Philadelphia, USA.

38 Clauser BE and Schuwirth LWT (2002) The use of computers in assessment. In: Norman GR, Van der Vleuten CPM and Newble DI (eds) *International Handbook of Research in Medical Education*, pp. 757–92. Kluwer, Dordrecht, Boston, MA London.

39 Southgate L, Cox J, David T *et al.* (2001) The General Medical Council's Performance Procedures; peer review of performance in the workplace. *Medical Education*. **35**(1): 9–19.

40 Southgate L, Campbell M, Cox H *et al.* (2001) The General Medical Council's Performance Procedures; the development and implementation of tests of competence with examples from general practice. *Medical Education*. **35**(1): 20–8.

41 Cusimano MD (1996) Standard setting in medical education. *Academic Medicine*. **71**(s10): S112–20.

42 Angoff WH (1971) Scales, norms and equivalent scales. In: Thorndike RL (ed.) *Educational Measurement*, pp. 508–600. American Council on Education, Washington, DC.

43 Norcini J (2003) Setting standards on educational tests. *Medical Education*. **37**: 464–9.

44 Schuwirth LWT and Van der Vleuten CPM (2006) A plea for new psychometrical models in educational assessment. *Medical Education*. **40**(4): 269–300.

Written examinations

Brian Jolly

KEY MESSAGES

- Construct an assessment blueprint for the course or unit that is being assessed.
- Decide on the objectives or domains in the blueprint that need to be assessed with written formats. These would normally involve recall of information, recognition of patterns of presenting symptoms, clinical decision making, choice of investigations, analysis of data and synthesis of ideas, strategies and management.
- Decide whether a constructed response is necessary to assess the objective, or whether a selected response would do.
- Choose the appropriate format for each item of the blueprint.

- Collect all the items into their format groupings.
- Arrange a workshop to develop the required formats.
- Once the test is proofed and prepared, arrange a further workshop to set standards. Methods may vary depending on item type and the setting.
- Deliver the test.
- Prior to result determination thoroughly review the items using item analysis software. Make sure that key personnel know how to interpret the output.
- Determine the final scores of candidates and cut scores for the test with all the poorly performing items eliminated.

Introduction

Assessment has become accepted as a critical part of the educational and accreditation processes across the health professions. The senior guardians of those professions have traditionally set high standards and wished to find means of protecting them.(1) With the recent increased international concern for patient safety(2,3) the need for efficient, reliable and valid assessment has become even more important. This in turn has led to a search for an increased level of sophistication in testing, mostly targeted at the development of high-fidelity simulations and work-based assessment.(4,5) However, health professionals operate across a very broad spectrum of human activity, from listening and talking to patients, to intricate and physically demanding interventions. Knowledge and thinking play a crucial role in these activities and there is considerable evidence to suggest that knowledge, and its storage in clinically useful frameworks, are the most important attributes that divide the novice from the expert.(6,7)

One of the most useful ways of finding out what people know is to ask them a question. When such enquiries are written down or the person is required to give a written response, we are in the territory of

written assessment. This paper introduces the reader to the use of written assessment in medical and health professions' education and covers four key areas:

- the situation of assessment within a given curriculum
- different formats of written assessments
  - constructed response
  - selected response
  - combined constructed and selected response
- test item performance
- standard setting.

Assessment, particularly in medicine, historically involved oral activities: general discussion, case discussion, demonstration, answers at the bedside, etc. In this tradition, the long case was adopted by the newly established General Medical Council (UK) in 1858, as a means of assuring the competence of physician apprentices.(8) But with the post-Flexnerian (circa 1910) emphasis on scientific endeavour in medicine, the measurement of knowledge through reliable and explicit means became increasingly emphasised.(9) In general, psychometric perspectives on assessment have reflected the need for efficiency, reliability and validity, while the educational perspective has stressed the need for appropriate influences on learning of assessment processes.(10,11) In recent years these two heritages have converged considerably.

Research on assessment in medicine has been most productive in the past 20 years,(12) and I do not intend to summarise all of this research here. There are books available that summarise the area and will help the

Understanding Medical Education: Evidence, Theory and Practice.
Edited by T Swanwick. © 2010 Association for the Study of Medical Education.

interested reader.(13–15) I will try to provide a balanced overview of the field and consider the theoretical determinants of assessment in as much detail as is helpful.

Assessment in the Curriculum

Before designing any assessment event it is useful to think about the purpose of assessment. Although we use the term 'assessment' quite loosely, each assessment that a learner undertakes usually has, or is used to perform, a particular function, reflecting the complexity of professional training. Some of these functions include:

* measuring competence
* measuring performance
* diagnosing trainees' problems
* measuring improvement
* selecting individuals
* identifying effective learning/teaching
* self-evaluation
* showing effectiveness of curriculum
* measuring curriculum change.

Each of these purposes will have constraining influences on the content of the assessment, the strategy used and the techniques employed. For example, assessments used to certify competence need to be closely aligned to the core curriculum objectives (content validity), reliable and focused at pre-specified levels of competence. However, an assessment used to select trainees into a restricted-entry postgraduate training programme may be targeted at a level of excellence, and may need to contain specific elements that predict success in that programme.(16)

One process for assuring the content validity of assessment is called blueprinting.(17–19) Essentially, this needs to be done for the assessment regime or strategy for the whole course, *before* individual components are designed, because it is one way of ensuring that the content is appropriately assigned to those components. For example, there will be specific domains of activity that are better suited to some types of assessment and this will become apparent when a thorough blueprinting exercise, which reflects the complete assessment strategy, is conducted for the whole curriculum. Detailed descriptions of the rationale and technique of blueprinting can be found elsewhere.(17–19) Trying to design the written segments of an assessment process without adequate blueprinting of the whole assessment on the curriculum is likely to result in an imbalanced assessment.

Knowledge, Reasoning and Written Assessment

When the blueprinting is complete there will be a number of attributes of a qualified health professional that reflect the cognitive domain of human endeavour – understanding, recalling, recognising, reasoning, inferring, deducing and deciding. Such attributes can be assessed in a number of ways, and there is little doubt that an effective clinician needs to be able to do all these things with patients and colleagues in clinical situations. However, not only is it impractical to assess these attributes comprehensively or effectively in clinical situations, there is also some evidence that it leads to contamination of the measurement process by other factors – these factors are generally referred to as 'construct irrelevant variance'.(20) For example, oral examinations purportedly aimed at examining clinical reasoning can be reduced to the investigation of factual recall, frequently focus on minutiae or merely serve to reveal the examiners' 'cultural incompetence'.(21)

One way of avoiding these problems is to decontextualise the assessment. In the 20th century, this trend and the recognition that, psychometrically, a minimum number of questions on a topic is needed to give a reliable estimate of a person's knowledge, gave rise to a number of developments in assessment. These included the multiple-choice question (MCQ), in its various guises, and the short-answer question. However, over the past 20 years, researchers have rediscovered that context is a crucial element of thinking. Generally it has an important function in the formation of memory,(22) and in clinical reasoning in particular.(23) It has also been determined that expertise is significantly dependent on knowledge.(24) Moreover, the way that this knowledge is obtained and organised is much more important than its sheer volume. For clinicians, the usability of knowledge is critical, and depends on both the efficiency of learning, and where and how that learning has taken place.

In brief, clinical reasoning depends on integrated knowledge, preferably learnt or repeatedly accessed by the learner in complex clinical contexts, where appropriate scientific principles are articulated to address patient problems.(25) These findings mean that we now have new varieties of written assessments. In the newer MCQ formats, the extended-matching item and the script concordance test both typically establish a clinical context for the assessees' activities. And recent approaches to short-answer items now include the key features item. At the same time, previously endemic item types such as the multiple true/false question(26) have come under cogent criticism.

There is another dimension to written assessment that also needs to be considered: the nature of the response. This can be either a selected response or one constructed by the test taker. Although there has been some dispute over this, in general it is thought that constructed responses require candidates to operate at a higher level than selected responses, for example, recall and synthesis versus recognition and choice.

In the next section we look at each of the format types. There are exhaustive treatments of many of these available in the literature.(15) Here, I will abbreviate much of the extensive debate to help the newcomer make some practical decisions about assessment.

Formats of Written Assessment

Usefully, Epstein(27) has summarised a range of assessment techniques and their potential usage and I have adapted his summary for written assessment in the pages that follow (*see* Box 15.1). In doing so I have removed Epstein's suggestions about where each method might be best used, to allow more flexibility, based on the domains of activity or objectives that need to be assessed, the need to reflect the blueprint outcomes and the need to encompass local requirements for assessment of certain attributes. The test maker needs to think carefully about all these factors and make choices appropriately.

The various types of written assessment format are discussed in greater detail, subdivided into the following three categories:
- constructed response
- selected response
- combined selected and constructed response.

Constructed-response formats
Essays
An essay is:

> a test item which requires a response composed by the examinee, usually in the form of one or more sentences, of a nature that no single response or pattern of responses can be listed as correct, and the accuracy and quality of which can be judged subjectively only by one skilled or informed in the subject.(28)

On the face of it essays are one of the most effective ways of ascertaining how good a student is at constructing a complex response to a challenging question. The other approaches that might be used include oral examinations, projects and observation of discussion. However, many of these are subject to variability due to extraneous serendipitous factors. For example, in orals there is no 'product', so judgements about performance are made 'on the run', unless the examination is recorded and analysed later, and this would significantly increase the burden of administration.

Essays can be delivered in two contexts – 'unseen' or 'seen'. In the former, a question, or usually a suite of questions, is prepared and delivered *de novo* to students under examination conditions. In the latter, students are provided with a topic and given a time limit in which to address it. They may use any resources they can find. Occasionally questions may be given to students in advance, but the essay is written under examination conditions.

The attributes of the essay and issues in its construction, delivery and marking are far from straightforward. The key questions to consider when choosing any assessment are:
- What type of response is required?
- What cognitive processes are involved?
- How well do the response and the cognitive processes invoked map to the expectations of the assessor about student performance, and to the objectives of the curriculum?

Clearly, in the unseen examination, critical components of a successful essay will depend on memory (both short and long term). The essay's quality will also depend on the ability of the student to construct sentences of the appropriate length that are unambiguous and grammatically correct, and to organise their knowledge in a way that addresses the question. If these abilities are all critical elements of the curriculum or of the environment into which this examination might be the entry point (e.g. internship), then the essay may be a rational assessment. If they are only prerequisites and were assessed earlier, or if only knowledge and memory are important, another assessment method may be superior.

Constructing an essay question
- Decide on whether the essay is to be seen or unseen. For example, if most of the knowledge you require the student to have is basic, core and extensive, and must enable them to solve, manage and monitor a real clinical problem at some time in the future, and possess an in-depth knowledge of related or differential conditions, then an unseen essay would be most appropriate.
- Choose a problem or issue that can be addressed satisfactorily in the time allocated, or limit it in such a way as to make it answerable.
- Define the issue and describe the task clearly.
- Describe the structure that the answer should take and its scope.
- Avoid complex language in the question, such as double negatives, ambiguities and abbreviations.
- Use terms that cover the cognitive processes that you are expecting to be used in marshalling the answer. For example, compare, predict, prioritise, rather than examine, elucidate (*see* Box 15.2).
- Avoid questions where radically different answers will be acceptable. This is fine for a group discussion or debate, but it makes marking an essay difficult.
- For every question, construct a model answer or list the essential features expected.
- Trial-run the questions on a group who should know the answers.
- Make sure that *all* the defined essential features appear in the trial group's answers as a whole, although not necessarily in every member's answers.
- Proofread the paper three times, using a different reader each time.

BOX 15.1 Written assessment formats

Method	Domain and response mode	Design factors	Limitations	Strengths
Constructed-response format				
Essay				
The typical university essay, either seen or unseen, where the writer is required to describe, discuss and propose new perspectives on one or more issues. The answer may or may not be predetermined	Any situation where lengthy explanation or detail is required. Requires detailed synthesis of information; interpretation of literature; evaluation of management options. Context frequently provided by the candidate	Traditionally questions can vary from the blindingly obvious to the very obscure. Large number of dimensions to the constructed response. Getting questions right takes time. Model answers or protocols help marking. High marking workload	Can be usurped into provision of lists (e.g. of treatments) or a memory dump. Task may be misinterpreted. Long testing time per topic, so limited coverage possible. Reliability variable and susceptible to rater and candidate bias	Total flexibility in question setting. Can avoid cueing. Regarded as using higher order cognitive processes
Modified essay				
Specifically developed for medicine with track record in general practice. Highly structured case vignette followed by questions on any aspect. Focused on candidates' management of a case or cases. Answer(s) usually predetermined	Clinical management issues. Some cue identification and reasoning required to link, for example, signs and symptoms to investigations and management. Context provided by the question	Can move from one stage of clinical management to another easily, by using slightly different cases to address issues (e.g. patient management in one case, and ethics in a similar one). More efficient sampling of a wide area of knowledge possible	Needs careful design to avoid cueing. As a result can be patchy in sampling knowledge across cases	Can avoid cueing. Context is controllable by question setter. Can demand a wide range of cognitive processes. May be machine scoreable in the next 5–10 years
Short answer				
A short question that asks for a constructed specific answer, usually requiring one word, a short phrase or a line or two of text. Answers mostly predetermined	Recall of specific facts or statements about biomedical or clinical processes. Context provided by the question	Deceptively simple to construct. Can sample widely different domains of knowledge easily	Very wide variety of formats and little research on their use and psychometric properties. Can lead to cueing across items. Context provided by question	Scoring by machine becoming a reality. Can replace multiple-choice questions (MCQs) where recall is thought to be vital (e.g. decisions based on core knowledge and experience)
Extended short answer				
A question that asks for an extended answer, usually requiring a paragraph or two, which may address different aspects, or an extension, of the issue. Answers may be predetermined	Recall of related groups of concepts or relatively short explanations. Context provided by the question	Deceptively simple to construct. Can sample widely different domains of knowledge but in more depth than short answer	As above. Scoring more difficult as it depends on multiple attributes of answers involved in essay construction. Machine scoring not possible. Context provided by question. Recent research on analysis of answers can give more insight into level of functioning of candidate	Total flexibility in question setting

BOX 15.1 *Continued*

Method	Domain and response mode	Design factors	Limitations	Strengths
Selected response format				
MCQ – multiple true/false				
Typically a short statement or brief paragraph followed by several (3–6) options. Candidates are asked to identify which options are true and which ones are false in relation to the initial statement	Recognition of consonance between two facts, attributes or concepts. Can test recognition of clear-cut knowledge in many domains. Complex items requiring calculations or problem solving have been used	Requires all options to be absolutely true or false. Can test knowledge of contraindications through the 'false' option	Difficult to write. The number used in most assessments can lead to cross-cueing. Can involve silly or irrelevant options due to lack of absolute falsehoods. Getting statements into an absolute true/false mode sometimes requires convolutions such as double negatives. Extreme controversy over 'correction for guessing' as random choice of options results in 50% score. Rapidly waning in popularity	Can test range of knowledge in limited testing time. Machine scoreable. True/false requirement restricts applicability and engenders artificiality
Single best answer				
Typically a short statement or brief paragraph followed by several (3–6) options. Candidates are asked to identify the option that best fits with or is the best outcome for the initial statement	Recognition of consonance between two facts, attributes or concepts. Can reflect basic clinical decisions, basic science or hypothesis generation	Easier to write than true/false questions. Choosing one best answer is more salient to most areas of medicine	The number used in most assessments can lead to cross cueing. Need not involve a correction for guessing	Efficient sampling of knowledge. Allows more subtle distinctions than true/false types. Machine scoreable
Extended-matching question				
Typically a topic area (e.g. headache) followed by many (6–26) options homogenous to a clinical grouping (e.g. diagnosis). There is a linked question asking candidates to choose the most likely diagnosis. Then one or more paragraphs each comprising a clinical case vignette, including for example, headache presentation at various stages of progression, each of which may indicate different 'best' diagnoses	Recognition of consonance between (typically) clinical presentations and their underlying pathology, investigation and outcome; diagnoses, prognoses, tests, pharmacology, etc. Items appear to involve basic clinical reasoning. Students report fidelity to 'real' medicine	Relatively easy to generate first drafts. Salient to most areas of medicine that depend on a clinical context	Not easy to write in some areas of medicine, especially non-clinical ones, for example, epidemiology. Some argue that the 'extended' list of options is not as useful as first thought – many options are redundant	Seems to be more reliable than single best answer and true/false questions due to increased difficulty. No corrections for guessing needed. Good discriminators at higher levels of ability

Script concordance

Typically a case vignette followed by an additional sign or symptom and a question that asks whether a specific diagnosis would be more or less likely if such an attribute were present in the case, for example, given a description of a 67-year-old man with chest pain, if pain radiating down the left arm were present would the likelihood of myocardial infarction be 'strongly increased', … , 'strongly decreased'	Recognition of relationship between, and agreement with an expert group on, attributes of case presentations that are predictive of diagnoses, prognoses, findings on investigation, etc. Appears to involve basic clinical reasoning and personal probabilities	New type of item, limited experience available of construction. Scoring generated by expert group. May have more than one answer that scores marks. Appears to discriminate effectively between experts and non-experts in some specialties	Probably limited to diagnostic and prognostic decisions	More research needed, but does show high construct validity for clinical experience. Writing protocols and rules still in development

Combined constructed-and selected response format

Key features

Usually a short case vignette followed by between one and three questions that investigate the candidate's knowledge of the main aspects of the case. Answers may be constructed or selected, usually requiring words or short phrases.	Answers that attempt to focus *only* on the critical aspects of clinical cases, for example, key decisions and the factors underpinning those. Developed to counter arguments that short answers led to isolated recall of facts and trivialisation. Context provided by the question	Strict rules for design, done usually by a small team. Items may involve some *selected* responses as well as *constructed* ones. Can explore a wide variety of cases. Can match response mode to attributes of the context, for example, selecting the most important features in clinical investigation results. Shares some properties of modified essay questions	Scoring and standard setting can be complex. For example, although single-word answers are common, there may be several answers to one question, each differentially weighted. There may be totally inappropriate or dangerous answers given by test takers. Can be challenging to avoid cueing between different parts of the item	Partial scoring by machine is now becoming a reality. Can replace MCQ-style questions where recall is thought to be important (e.g. decisions based on core knowledge and experience). Has embedded quickly into assessment technology in medicine

When it comes to marking, each essay should
ideally be scored by a pair of assessors working
independently. If that is not possible, the same marker
should score the same question for all candidates. This
minimises extraneous variance stemming from the different ways each examiner marks different questions.
To help with the quality control of marking, all examiners of a particular question should preferably see all,
or at least the complete range, of answers to that question. Scores for a question should be the mean of all
the examiners marking that question.

Although assessor training is helpful, a model
answer is better than attempts at calibration. In fact, a
series of model answers specifically written to be at the
boundaries between two grades is a very useful way
of enabling accurate classification. For example, in an
A–E grade system, model answers should be at A/B
and B/C boundaries. This enables most essays to be
rated using two anchor points, since most will fall
between the boundaries. A model answer is also useful
when there is a common core of content that needs to
be covered in the essay. Where students each write an
individual assignment on a pre-assigned or selected
topic it may not be possible to have a model answer
(there would have to be as many models as there are
questions/students). In this case a process-based
framework can be used (*see* Box 15.3). Papers should
be marked anonymously.

A procedure needs to be in place to address wide
marking variations within one question.

Assessors are commonly urged to use the complete
scoring range and avoid centralising tendencies.
However, health profession students tend to be very
high achievers, so it is not uncommon to have skewed
distributions on tests. If high scores seem warranted
they should be given.

There are constraints on the essay. Many clinical
teachers do not regard them as relevant, but others
suggest that they give training in marshalling arguments and practice in writing. However, the practice
that essays give may be that of 'bad' writing – rushed,
unedited, poorly planned (because of time constraints)
and incompletely organised.(29) Many authors like to

let the issues sit in their minds for some time before
launching into print (like the author of this chapter),
but that is not possible in an examination essay and
may be difficult even in a seen paper.

An essay question does not necessarily assess higher
order cognitive skills. It often merely assesses recall,
dressed up as something more profound. This happens
in two ways, caused either by the students or the
teacher. Students can memorise vast tracts. Asking students how they went about answering the questions
in a debriefing session will assist you in deciding how
your essays performed. However, beware of the bright
student who unwittingly uses memory and reports
that he or she is 'thinking'. If you design an essay question meant to assess higher order processing but then

arrange the scoring framework in a way that allots marks to recall, or biases towards recall processes, you are not assessing higher order cognition.

Finally, the major disadvantage of the traditional essay is that it samples a small area in-depth and this restricts inferences that you can make about a person's competence in those specific areas.

Where's the evidence for essays?

There is a great deal of evidence about the impact of construct irrelevant variance on essay and other qualitative assessments; however, little of this comes from tertiary sector medical and health sciences. Experiments that change the quality of writing but not the content show moderate influences of style or construction factors on assessments of language and writing but not for other content areas such as science and mathematics.(30) In addition:

> Content scores do not seem to be appreciably affected by writing style when the scoring is done by teachers who have been trained by scoring professionals. Ratings in reading, social studies, science, and mathematics should be unaffected by writing style, and the results indicate that the scorers were reasonably successful at assessing the content of these responses without meaningful confounding with writing style.(30)

In a study on law essays, agreement among law professors on how they graded a single typical essay was 0.58 (intra-class correlation).(31) However, although the basis for this agreement was not investigated, and it was not clear in the paper whether these essays were marked anonymously, assessors' marks were higher for longer answers and for those written by brighter students. Notably the measures of length of essay and intellectual ability were unrelated. However, a combination of these two factors yielded a very high correlation with the assessors' grades. In other words, longer essays were marked higher even if written by the poorer students, and long essays by more able students attracted even higher marks. Markers who had no law training generally assigned the same grades to the papers as did the law professors. It appeared, therefore, that both professors and lay markers could and did identify and reward those papers that presented a persuasive 'common sense' answer to the question.

A more refined study showed that the amount that a student wrote on major issues, the use of jargon, the use of transitional phrases and quality handwriting all had significant positive correlations with grade, and grammatical and construction errors both had significant negative ones.(32) Two further predictors of success were 'strength of argument for conclusions reached' and 'tendency to argue both sides of an issue'. In further studies, quality of handwriting has been confirmed to be a factor.(33) However, on the whole, handwritten essays tend to score higher than computer-generated ones.(34)

An experimental study of structuring the essay question in medicine showed that the reliability of the structured questions was higher, due to the reduced variance between examiners in this format, and the better agreement between scores on individual questions in the structured format.(35)

Modified essay questions

A modified essay question (MEQ) consists of a brief scenario or clinical vignette followed by one or more short but searching questions. Test takers are required to construct answers, usually of a paragraph or two. Each question is designed to test a wide range of issues and the ability to think rationally and laterally. They have been used extensively in general practice specialty assessment. By way of illustration and with acknowledgement to the UK Royal College of General Practitioners membership examination, here are two examples.

- Daisy Boyd, aged 68 years, arrives late for her routine appointment smelling of urine. How would you manage this situation?

This question could contain issues as diverse as the management of incontinence to the management of time and the doctor's own feelings.

- Mike Hornby, aged 44 years, is in the terminal phase of motor neurone disease. He says 'Will you help me when the time comes?' What factors influence your response?

Such a question could raise clinical, ethical, legal, referral and personal issues. It may require further qualification to limit the range of answers to the areas you want, or the length of response to a scoreable one.

The MEQ was first developed in Australia and the UK to overcome the major restrictions of sampling and scoring pertaining to the traditional essay and to the now largely disused 'patient management problem' (PMP). The PMP had some potentially useful attributes; the technique required the candidate to fully explore a case from initial diagnosis to management and follow-up, through a series of largely selected responses. However, it was dogged by psychometric inadequacies.(36) The MEQ allows exploration of different aspects of a case using mostly constructed responses. Initially, whole cases were followed through, but the impact of cueing in this format is high and, in general, the principle now is to explore candidate's knowledge of cases and management through a wider sampling of content. There is a broad literature on MEQs(37,38) and they are ideally suited to computer administration and response collection, but not yet to computerised marking.

The major difficulty with MEQs involves the same issues that apply to essays: there is variability between markers on most constructed-response types of question,(39,40) and score weighting can be problematic. Increasing the number of markers and number of questions can ameliorate the problem but is frequently impractical.(40) Also, because cueing is so difficult to eradicate in an MEQ, many assessment developers limit the scope of each clinical problem to just one or two issues, so that dealing with a whole case across a time frame (one of the original arguments for using MEQs) becomes impossible. This can be circumvented by computer presentation of the segments of the MEQ.

Constructing a modified essay question

Decide first on the type of objectives that you wish to assess – diagnosis, decision making, patient or self-management. In the example essay questions, the designer was looking for affective and professional components of the encounters as well as cognitive ones. With some examinees this requirement may need signposting more clearly.

Decide how far it is possible to delve down into the specific case without risking cueing and avoid vaguely worded questions. To illustrate these points, here is an (deliberately flawed) example.

- Mrs Brown, a 38-year-old primary school teacher, complains of fatigue and tachycardia. She has been admitted to the general medical unit on which you work, for further investigation.
  Q1 What are the three most likely diagnoses?
  Q2 List five specific questions that would help you distinguish between these possibilities.
- A routine blood test reveals microcytic hypochromic anaemia with a haemoglobin level of 9.8 g/dl.
  Q3 List two typical signs you would look for when you examine the patient.
  Q4 Did this information affect your first diagnosis? If yes, how (explain briefly)?

In this example, computer delivery or physical removal of the answers to Q1 and Q2 would be required before giving the information about anaemia and asking candidates Q3 and Q4 in order to avoid both backward and forward cueing. Q1 and Q2 test broad knowledge of such clinical presentations and initial diagnostic strategy. They require understanding of the clinical significance of the scenario. Q3 tests linkage between data from investigation (that may not have been initially considered by the test taker) and subsequent questioning. Q4 is vague and open to misinterpretation – which one of Q1's 'three most likely diagnoses' does Q4 refer to? Is the test taker supposed to assume certain positive or negative outcomes from their examination of signs in Q3? What does 'information' mean in Q4? What does 'affect' mean? What is the designer's rationale for asking Q3 after the delivery of the information about the blood test? Would this information be better after Q3?

Where's the evidence for modified essay questions?

There were some psychometric studies done on the MEQ in the 1980s. These showed that reliabilities ranged between 0.43 and 0.90 (Alpha) for a 60-item test depending on the content area.(41) However, a recent study suggested that over 50% of MEQ items in a general test for undergraduates in medicine and surgery tested nothing more than factual recall.(42) This contrasts with the rationale for MEQs that emphasises their ability to reflect analysis, interpretation and clinical decision making.

Short-answer questions

Many educators use short-answer questions (SAQs) in some form. Frequently they are used as a means of gauging students' factual knowledge or understanding, for example, in lectures and ward rounds. In the verbal form they tend to be quite short, asking for one word or a few alternative answers, within a specific context, as in the following example.

- What is the most common feature of diabetic retinopathy we are likely to see in this patient?

The other major use of SAQs is in assessments. Various forms exist requiring the test taker to complete the sentence or supply a missing line (Cloze test), give short descriptive or analytical answers, or annotate diagrams. Such questions can demand a wide range of responses, from one or several words to a paragraph or more than a page. The different forms of SAQ provide for great versatility in usage, but make classification difficult. An individual question can be used to assess a specific objective, and unlike multiple-choice questions, SAQs have the advantage of requiring students to construct an answer rather than choosing (or guessing) from provided options, so avoiding cueing (at least when SAQs are used sparingly).

SAQs are easier to mark than essay questions and usually involve a structured marking sheet that indicates all possible answers, and ones that should or should not get credit. Marking sheets should also indicate whether spelling needs to be perfect or which common misspellings are acceptable. One-word answers are computer scoreable. But anything longer than a few words usually requires a marker.

Items should be marked with assessors blind to the identity of candidates and different markers allocated to different questions or sets of questions, In this way, examiner bias is diluted for each candidate. Some assessors report that having the marking done at one time in a large room with all examiners able to talk to each other as unexpected responses are discovered is beneficial to efficient and equitable scoring. Test designers need to be prepared to accept answers not on the scoresheet, some of which may or may not have been predicted. There will need to be a system for referring these to the test convenor or committee – do *not* allow discretion at the marker level, some markers may be unable to make this judgement.

Marking poses the major difficulties with this form of assessment although there is variability between markers on most constructed-response types of question.(39,40) Increasing the number of markers and number of questions can ameliorate the problem but is frequently impractical.(40) Many educators allege that SAQs reduce the likelihood that students will look for the relations between objectives or sections of the subject while studying, and that complex issues cannot always be satisfactorily addressed in short answers. However, there is little empirical evidence for these assertions.

Constructing a short-answer question

- Identify the specific learning objectives the item will cover. These are generally in the area of factual recall, comprehension, application or analysis. Higher levels such as evaluation or synthesis will probably require a longer test format, such as a modified essay.
- Choose the most appropriate SAQ format for the objective – a Cloze or completion item, an open one-word or phrase answer, a series of answers or a question that requires a short paragraph.
- State the item concisely in clear, unambiguous simple language. A good SAQ tests factual knowledge or capacity to analyse and clinically interpret a scenario. Introducing an element of the test taker's ability to make sense of the question introduces construct irrelevant variance into the assessment.
- Look at the draft item from a number of different perspectives – mentally try out adequate and inadequate responses. Ideally an item aimed at one fact should have just one answer, and one aimed at alternatives (e.g. differential diagnoses) should have as many as are appropriate. However, what you may think of as a clear, straightforward question may frequently be answered in multiple ways, depending on how the reader reads it.
- It is good practice to give the test taker an indication of the length of answer required.
- Indicate how many marks are available for the question.
- Some research suggests that items asking for positive perspectives (e.g. knowing the best method, describing good practice or identifying the most relevant facts) have greater educational significance (e.g. in terms of capacity to measure objectives) than knowing the poorest method, unsatisfactory practice or the least relevant issues. However, clinical science sometimes depends on the capacity to rule out rare or unlikely occurrences, so research done in general educational settings may not always apply in the health context. If you have to word an item negatively it is advisable to use some form of emphasis for the negative words (e.g. 'what is *not* an appropriate management option in this situation?'), using italics, bold type or underlining to stress this for the test taker.
- Try to avoid grammatical cues to the answer or providing answer spaces that are equal or proportional to the lengths of the required responses.
- Where a numerical answer has to be supplied, for example, from a calculation based on clinical data, indicate both:
  - the degree of precision expected *and*
  - that the appropriate units must be indicated.

Where's the evidence for short-answer questions?
There is very little research on SAQs, particularly in medicine. However, there is some evidence from secondary education that constructed-response SAQs measure exactly the same thing as MCQ items, as long as the stems are the same.(43) In other words, the cognitive task set to the test taker is more important than the response format. However, once the task diverges, even in the same content domain, the correlation between the two forms falls off. Also, SAQs are more reliably scored than essays,(44) largely because the pitfalls of scoring lengthy answers are avoided, and because SAQs can sample more widely in a given time. In addition, using SAQs may reduce the reported differences between men and women, and black and white racial groups on propensity to omit items in MCQ tests.(45,46) In medicine, SAQs have been used successfully as a reliable alternative to MCQ items in a progress test in the Netherlands.(47) One study showed that SAQ tests could produce better retention of information over time, as long as the delayed test was a short-answer test. There was no difference between groups if the test was an MCQ test.(48)

Selected-response formats
Multiple-choice questions – multiple true/false
Multiple-choice testing was once seen as an enduring solution to the reliable and valid measurement of knowledge in 'knowledge-rich' or knowledge-dependent environments such as medicine, bioscience and engineering. Invented in 1914 by Frederick Kelly, head of a training school in Kansas, US, by 1926 the multiple-choice test had become the right of passage for entering post-secondary education in the US. The MCQ was developed into several forms. One of these is the multiple true/false item (called an 'X-type' item in North America), which has become a significant feature of assessment of knowledge in medicine and many other professions over the past 50 years.

In essence, an MCQ is a question that proffers several answers from which the correct one or ones must be chosen. In multiple true/false types, a set of options, usually between four and six, is given, of which each can be either true or false. The candidate is required to indicate which is correct for each option. An example is shown in Box 15.4.

Over the past few years the multiple true/false item has received a good deal of critical attention. Many examining bodies (e.g. the National Board in the US) have given up using it altogether. The main reasons have been elucidated with a good deal of empirical evidence.(26) In brief, Case and Swanson state that:

BOX 15.4 Example of a multiple true/false item

Stem	Option	
The following present as chronic (>3 months) airspace disease on a chest radiograph	(a) Streptococcal pneumonia	T/F
	(b) Adult respiratory syndrome	T/F
	(c) Pulmonary oedema	T/F
	(d) Asbestosis	T/F

BOX 15.5 Example of a single-best-answer item

Stem	Option
A 65-year-old man has difficulty rising from a seated position and straightening his trunk, but he has no difficulty flexing his leg. Which of the following muscles is most likely to have been injured?	(a) Gluteus maximus*
	(b) Gluteus minimus
	(c) Hamstrings
	(d) Iliopsoas
	(e) Obturator internus

- the distinction between 'true' and 'false' is not always clear and it is not uncommon for subsequent reviewers to alter the answer key
- reviewers rewrite or discard true/false items far more frequently than items written in other formats
- some ambiguities can be clarified, but others cannot
- to avoid ambiguity, item writers are pushed towards assessing recall of an isolated fact
- application of knowledge, integration, synthesis and judgement questions can better be assessed by alternative formats such as single-best-answer questions.

It is also the case that using true/false restricts the choice of answers, as discussed in the National Board of Medical Examiners (NBME) guide,(26) to a subset that can best be classified as completely true all of the time or completely false all of the time. For this reason I strongly recommend not using this type of item and for any further information the reader is referred to other sources.(49)

Multiple-choice questions – single best answer

In single-best-answer questions a stem question asks the test taker to choose the one best answer, typically from a set of four to five options. An example, taken from the NBME's item writing manual(26) is given in Box 15.5.

MCQ items are usually scored optically or directly by computer. There are standard programs for marking and analysing test data straight from a scanner. The answer 'key' – a line of data containing the correct option for each item – is used in this process and should be double- or even triple-checked before use. The most common reason for problems at the marking or item analysis stage is a key that contains wrong answers. This may be because the answer has been wrongly transcribed from the item writer's design or (and this is not as rare as it should be) because they have not provided the best answer.

Most MCQs are scored 1 or 0 for correct or incorrect answers, respectively. Weighting is not necessary for best-answer items; it has very little impact on rankings of students and can reduce reliability. A so-called 'correction for guessing' need not be used.(50)

How to construct a single-best-answer question

Writing multiple-choice items involves following a series of basic rules, and a sensible approach to item construction is to have item-writing workshops that force item writers to work in small groups and then have their items immediately reviewed by a larger group. During the workshops the basic rules are as follows and should be applied as a test to each of the items that you construct. Each item should pass *all* the rules.

- Focus on an important (non-trivial) concept, typically a common or potentially serious clinical problem. Avoid trivial, 'tricky' or overly complex questions.
- Focus on how knowledge is applied to a clinical situation, not on recognising an isolated fact or association between concept and exemplar.
- The stem must state a clear question, and it should be possible to arrive at an answer with the options covered. To determine if the question is clearly focused, cover up the options and read the stem to make sure it is lucid and that other item designers can supply an answer dependent only on reading the stem (the cover test).
- All distractors and the correct answer should be homogeneous, that is, they should fall into the same category. For example, in an anatomy question all answers should be the same type of structure – bones, vessels, nerves, etc. In a clinical item they should all be diagnoses, tests, treatments, prognoses, and so on.
- All distractors should be salient and plausible. Order the options in numeric or alphabetical order.
- Try to write questions of moderate difficulty – if any of the item constructors has a problem with the item it is probably too difficult. Make sure the correct answer has a sufficiently different degree of correctness when compared with the distractors across all the conditions identified in the stem.
- Avoid technical item flaws – all items and options should be grammatically consistent, logically compatible and of the same (relative) length as the correct answer.

- Writing questions of the form 'Which of the following is correct?', followed by a set of brief, possibly unrelated postulates, one of which is correct, is *not* advisable. It is basically a true/false item masquerading as a one best answer. Furthermore, it is a good way of ensuring that the questions focus on trivia. These questions will not be directed at course objectives in a coherent fashion and will contain multiple heterogeneous options.

Where's the evidence for multiple-choice questions?

There is far too much research on MCQs to summarise in this chapter. The interested reader should look at recent evidence-based guidelines by Wood,(15) Downing(51) and Haladyna(49) for comprehensive treatments of many issues. One interesting fact to emerge is that the appropriate number of options to use in a one-best-answer item is more likely to be two or three than four or five. There is long-standing theoretical and empirical evidence to support this position.(52) However, this effect is generated when distractors are not performing adequately. In an item where the four or five distractors operate effectively, the item tends to have increased reliability. There is also contradictory evidence that extended-matching question (EMQ) distractors, usually a naturally occurring fairly large set of 10–15 (see below), may operate more effectively than three or four pre-selected ones.(26,53) We would hope that the processes that students use to answer one-best-answer MCQ items are at least analytical and at best reasoning rich. However, evidence suggests that 'the problem with multiple-choice items is not that they are mere exercises in recognition, but that we are unable to predict the processes that will be evoked'.(54)

Extended-matching questions

EMQs were developed in the early 1990s.(26) However, the kernel of the idea was developed by Sue Case in her PhD thesis as early as 1983.(55) She and David Swanson are credited with most of the development work on this format while at the NBME. An EMQ is a selected-response item in which the item stem has been extended, usually, to a short clinical vignette or scenario and the choices have been extended to include all potentially acceptable ones for the clinical problem or issue that is being addressed by the item. This format was originally targeted towards the application of clinical knowledge to diagnostic and management problems, but has been extended to other areas, such as basic science. For example, in Box 15.6 there are 20 options pertaining to the theme of diagnosis of abdominal pain. The options are followed by one or more clinical vignettes. The options are all causes of abdominal pain. It is usual in such items to attempt to make all the questions and options homogenous in this way, so other issues concerning abdominal pain, such as initial management or investigations,

---

BOX 15.6 Extended-matching question example

Area: Abdominal pain – diagnosis

Options

A Abdominal aneurysm	K Kidney stone
B Appendicitis	L Mesenteric adenitis
C Bowel obstruction	M Mesenteric artery thrombosis
D Cholecystitis	N Ovarian cyst – ruptured
E Colon cancer	O Pancreatitis
F Constipation	P Pelvic inflammatory disease
G Diverticulitis	Q Peptic ulcer disease
H Ectopic pregnancy – ruptured	R Perforated peptic ulcer
I Endometriosis	S Pyelonephritis
J Hernia	T Torsion

Lead in: For each patient with abdominal pain described below, select the most likely diagnosis.

Scenario/Stem: A 25-year-old woman has sudden onset of persistent right lower abdominal pain that is increasing in severity. She has nausea without vomiting. She had a normal bowel movement just before onset of pain. Examination shows exquisite deep tenderness to palpation in right lower abdomen with guarding but no rebound; bowel sounds are present. Pelvic examination shows a 7cm, exquisitely tender right-sided mass. Hematocrit is 32%. Leukocyte count is $18\,000/mm^3$. Serum amylase activity is within normal limits. Test of the stool for occult blood is negative.

Answer:

Next stem in the domain (diagnosis of abdominal pain) would appear here.

(courtesy of the NBME(49))

---

are not included. An item should focus on a specific area of clinical cognitive activity that pertains to a specific phase of the clinical process – in this case, diagnosis.

EMQs are usually scored 1 for a correct response and 0 for an incorrect one. It is sometimes possible to have more than one best answer, for example, when two (or more) diagnoses are equally likely, given the information in the vignette. However, the scoring of these requires more attention during the scanning process, as for optical scoring, one pass of the score sheet is necessary for each correct answer keyed. Unless it is clinically important to be able to recognise both potential diagnoses from the same vignette, such multiple responses are probably best avoided (e.g. by removing one of the options from the list).

Investigations of the reliability and construct validity of EMQs suggest that they have good measurement properties, and correlate well with other measures of recall, recognition and cognitive functioning.(56) They seem to be easier to write than true/false or other types of one-best-answer items, because in that style of item the convolutions that writers go through to reduce the item set to a smaller number where each is true or false, or there is clearly one best answer, are not needed.(57) Clinicians from some disciplines (e.g. public health, epidemiology, statistics) have suggested that EMQs are difficult to write for these content domains, but recent articles suggest they have been adopted or are being developed in some of these hitherto unexplored areas [e.g. psychiatry(58)].

How to construct an extended-matching question

It is best to write these items first by considering the area or domain of the assessment blueprint for which items need to be written (e.g. abdominal pain in our example). A general question is then posed, followed by all the possible answers to that question (e.g. What are the causes of abdominal pain in adults?). After these have been identified, scenarios that pertain to one or more of the answers are constructed. Ideally, create items (particularly the stems/scenarios) in pairs of writers at workshops of about 8–12 people in total (4–6 pairs), with review every two hours or so in a larger group. This is an effective, and in most examiners' experience, an enjoyable way of generating items. The stages are as follows.

- *Identify the domain or subject for the set.* The domain is an area of cognitive activity, for example, diagnosis, management planning. The subject can be a presenting complaint in a body system or systems (e.g. abdominal pain, so that diagnosis is the focus of the item), or a pre-diagnosed condition (e.g. community-acquired pneumonia, so that management is the focus of the item). Sometimes it might be appropriate to move directly from a non-diagnosed presenting complaint (e.g. abdominal pain) to an investigative option (e.g. ultrasound) or management plan (e.g. restricted diet). However, the more cognitive steps involved in moving between the presenting complaint and the focus of the item (e.g. asking about management), the less will be known about why an examinee might have answered the item wrongly. For example, the examinee might have thought a patient with ulcerative colitis had appendicitis and ordered surgical intervention.
- *Write the lead-in for the set.* The lead-in indicates the relationship between the stems and options. It must be a clear question for examinees. It is an essential component of an extended-matching set. Sometimes two lead-ins can be written at the same time, for example, one based on diagnosis and one on indications for investigations or management. Subsequent scenarios can be used, usually with only

minor modification, with either lead-in. In summary, the lead-in should consist of a single, clearly formulated task so that the examinee could, if necessary, create an answer without looking at the options.

- *Prepare the list of options.* The list of options should be single words or very short phrases. This list is best developed in a whole-group format. It will be generated in a fairly random order, but the options should be rearranged in alphabetical order for the final item presentation. For example, the initial list for Box 15.6 should contain all the likely causes of abdominal pain as options. Sometimes there are specific causes that occur only or predominantly in a particular subset of the population, for example, in women (e.g. ectopic pregnancy), in men (testicular torsion), in the elderly (dementia). Such options can sometimes become 'zebras',(26) which stand out as so obviously applying to one subgroup of patients that their inclusion is ill-advised. In Box 15.6 there are some such options, but there are also sufficient important differential diagnoses in the list to warrant their inclusion for the given scenario.
- *Write the stems.* The stems (items) within a set should be similar in structure. Most often, patient vignettes are appropriate. The scenario should contain all the information that one would normally expect to be available from any conscious patient: the presenting problem, the history (including duration of signs and symptoms), the physical findings and then the results of any immediate diagnostic tests carried out. Sometimes, for a complex case, further data pertaining to development of symptoms over several days might also be given, for example, initial management and subsequent clinical changes. Scenarios can include a smaller set of information, but it is unwise to exclude the information that would normally be collected by or available to the test taker in the real clinical context at the time they were seeing this patient. Specifying this information in a standardised order makes shorter reading time and hence allows more items to be delivered in a given time.
- *Review the items.* Make sure there is only one 'best' answer for each question. Having two right answers is possible but entails more marking effort than it is usually worth. Also make sure that there are at least four reasonable distractors for each item to minimise guessing effects. Evaluate the extent to which the lead-in clearly formulated the task. See if the other examiners can create an answer without looking at the options. Satisfying this 'cover-the-options' rule is an important feature of a good question because, if the examinee cannot do that, it means the question is too vague, is not appropriately targeted to the skills the examination is testing or exhibits some other flaw of test writing. As a final check, review the items (without the correct answer indicated) across other pairs in the writing group. If

the pair has difficulty determining the correct answer, modify the option list or the item to eliminate the ambiguity.

Where's the evidence for extended-matching questions?

There is evidence that MCQs, of which the EMQ type seems to be the most suited to clinical tasks, can involve substantially more than recognition of knowledge learnt by rote memorisation.(54) As mentioned previously, Skakun *et al.* suggest that 'the problem with multiple-choice items is not that they are mere exercises in recognition but rather that we are unable to predict the processes that will be evoked'.(54) They nevertheless suggest that unfocused items or those with negatively worded stems, as sometimes of necessity occur in the typical true/false or best of five types, do not appear to provoke problem-solving skills and forward reasoning. While the evidence for the link between item type and cognitive response is being developed, they suggest concentrating on items that are low-fidelity simulations of clinical situations with examinee tasks that are relevant for them (e.g. diagnosis and management). EMQs are ideally suited to this role. EMQs also substantially reduce the likelihood of obtaining a correct answer by chance alone. Although this area is fraught with controversy, and not all of the options provided for any one EMQ stem will be active for that item, modelling suggests that EMQs with between 7 and 12 active distractors will provide good insulation against the need to be concerned about the so-called 'guessing' factor in multiple choice tests.(59) The use of a smaller number of options reduces time spent on each item by candidates and therefore increases the number of items that can be used in a set time.(60) Swanson *et al.* advise: 'From a practical perspective, we are still encouraging … item writers to use the EMQ format with large numbers of options because of the efficiencies this approach affords in item preparation. However, pending the results of future research, we plan to begin advising (examiners) to reduce the number of options included on option lists in order to make more efficient use of testing time.'(60)

Script concordance items

Over the past 15 years interest has developed in constructing a multiple-choice test that can reflect clinicians' capacity to weigh evidence in a clinical encounter. This work has its foundations in a clearer understanding of how clinicians approach the diagnostic task and how this information is remembered.(61,62)

Memory for clinically important information is developed in stages. As a student, possibly because of the preclinical/clinical divide in most educational programmes, biomedical knowledge dominates. Additional insight into clinical problems develops as students gain more experience with patients and elaborate their knowledge into explanatory frameworks and linkages between symptoms, causes, basic mechanisms and management. With more experience of patients, these frameworks depend less on biomedical detail and more on 'illness scripts' that involve applied (functional) knowledge and relate to both common (easy) and uncommon (more difficult) patient presentations. Eventually these illness scripts are used by their owners to promote rapid recognition of patterns of patient presentation and reconcile these with previous presentations. However, when a challenging presentation occurs, expert clinicians muster their existing knowledge and strive to activate biomedical principles and knowledge (albeit usually tied to specific patient or contextual exemplars), but these occasions occur less frequently as expertise develops.(63) Previously, attempts to create tests that reflect this process through patient management problems and modified essay questions have foundered, primarily because clinicians disagree about these issues and this, coupled with the variety of constructed responses that such items can generate from the test takers, results in great difficulty in scoring them. Moreover, in a typical MCQ item when the test makers cannot agree on the best answer, either before or after it has been used, the item is usually removed from the test.

However, a group in Canada have devoted a considerable amount of effort to the task of developing an item format that overcomes these problems – this is the script concordance item (SCI).

The SCI is a selected-response item that depends on respondents choosing how well pieces of information contribute to a diagnostic or management strategy for a particular clinical problem. As described above, the script is the internal rubric experts use to classify data and generate or choose a hypothesis quickly. In the SCI, concordance is the congruence of the takers' script with elements of rubrics deemed by 'experts' to be most plausible. The items estimate the relative likelihood of diagnoses given a certain piece of clinical or biomedical information. The test items ask for choices to be made based on the subjective clinical probabilities of the test takers. However, they are scored in such a way that takes into account the degree of similarity (concordance) between the illness scripts of the test takers and the test makers. An example is shown in Box 15.7.

The marking scheme is based on the performance of an expert group. There are various ways to derive the marks. In one method, a consensus is reached between the experts on the best answer for each item. In others, each response attracts a mark that is proportional to the frequency of its choice by the expert group. Recommendations for exactly how this is done vary according to source. Some authors suggest awarding one mark for the experts' modal answer and then giving marks for alternatives based on the frequency ratios for the other answers. For example, if a group of 20 experts opted 12, 6 and 2 for the options +2, +1 and

BOX 15.7 Script concordance item example

A 25-year-old male patient is admitted to the emergency room after a fall from a motorcycle with a direct impact to the pubis. Vital signs are normal. The X-ray reveals a fracture of the pelvis with a disjunction of the pubic symphysis.(64)

If you were thinking of	And then you find	This hypothesis can be rated: (circle best response)
Urethral rupture	Urethral bleeding	−2 −1 0 +1 +2
Retroperitoneal bladder rupture	Bladder distension	−2 −1 0 +1 +2
Urethral rupture	Perineal haematoma	−2 −1 0 +1 +2

Where:

−2 = the hypothesis is almost eliminated
−1 = the hypothesis becomes less probable
 0 = the information has no effect on the hypothesis
+1 = the hypothesis has become more probable
+2 = the hypothesis is very likely to be correct

(courtesy of Charlin *et al.*(62))

0 in any one item, these options would be awarded 1, 0.5 and 0.167 marks, respectively, and the others zero marks. Other sources suggest awarding marks on a percentage distribution basis, so this would work out at 0.6, 0.3 and 0.1 per option for the three 'correct' options.

Another interesting feature of the marking scheme is that it can have more than one reference panel, depending on the context in which the item is to be used, for example, in a metro or rural environment, a general practice, the emergency department or medical ward. This is because the probabilities of some decisions or hypotheses may change depending on the context.

A test made up of SCIs is therefore a very flexible one, and one capable of rewarding partial or incomplete knowledge to some extent. Data so far suggest that a test composed of SCIs is very efficient; good reliability can be achieved with relatively small numbers of items.(65)

The way that SCIs are constructed clearly has implications for how best to use them. They are a specialised item suitable for investigating test takers' ability to formulate and progress specific diagnostic and management decisions.

How to construct a script concordance item

An SCI is created in a similar fashion to an EMQ, except that the specific diagnostic decision is the key

to the choice of vignette, rather than a list of potential diagnoses, and hence there may be less data in an SCI than an EMQ. There are two stages.

- A vignette is created containing data that presents a challenging clinical situation. This is usually text, but other information such as blood analysis (or the X-ray from the item in Box 15.7), can be given, depending on the clinical decisions that are being investigated. Not all the data needed are provided because these can be revealed as part of the item – the one or more (in this item three) hypotheses–information links in Box 15.7. Each of these clinically relevant pieces of information might help the clinician refine, improve, confirm or eliminate the clinical decisions or hypotheses made about what is happening. The response required from the test taker is to appraise the effect of each piece of new information on their hypothesis.

- Responses are pre-prepared using a five-point scale running from −2 (the hypothesis or decision is almost eliminated) to +2 (the hypothesis or decision is very likely to be correct). To get the best out of the item, and to sample knowledge broadly, there should be no links (cues) between the different provided responses. Once designed, a group of experienced clinicians complete the SCIs and their answers are collated. These answers are then used to decide on the marking scheme for scoring items.

Although it would seem relatively easy to design such items, Charlin and van der Vleuten(64) warn that the expert group writing the items must be familiar with the tool and be able to choose cases that are complex enough to fit with the level of training being assessed. Also the item is designed to assess decision making that is grounded in evidence, as opposed to received wisdom, so there must be enough data available on the clinical solution to the case, and the links provided in the case must be widely known by experts in the area.

Where's the evidence for script-concordance items?

There is not much evidence yet about how SCIs perform from a reliability and validity perspective. However, good construct validity has been shown in a number of studies. SCIs discriminate between different levels of surgical expertise and have also been used in pharmacy education.(66,67) SCIs are in many ways still in the development stage, and a number of important questions about their use still remains, for example, how many points on the scale are the most useful?(65)

Combined constructed- and selected-response formats

Key features items

A key features item (KFI) is an SAQ that can use both selected and constructed responses. The defining characteristic of a KFI is that it is aimed at assessing whether the test taker can recognise, deduce or infer the most important features of a clinical problem and, if required, subsequently choose the most salient, urgent and effective management strategies for that clinical problem.(68)

Readers may think that it could be reasonably assumed that all SAQs would possess these properties. Unfortunately, in the 1970s and 1980s this was not the case.(69) Curricula and assessments were frequently designed from discipline or specialty perspectives, with each concentrating on unusual or esoteric aspects of their craft to discriminate between the truly well-grounded student and the rest. This led to a culture in which trivia, rare morbidity, atypical presentations and specialty-specific issues dominated short-answer tests. It was also believed that decision-making skill was generic, so many short-answer tests focused on one or two problems, with the 'short' answers practically exhausting the available knowledge about that problem.(70)

Two researchers, Georges Bordage and Gordon Page, coined the term 'key feature' after a critique of and further research on the nature and assessment of clinical decision-making skills.(69) Their central concept was that 'in any clinical case, there are a few unique, essential elements in decision making which, alone or in combination, are the critical steps in the successful resolution of the clinical problem'.(68) With funding from the Medical Council of Canada their concept led to the creation of a new format for assessing decision-making skills. Furthermore, by testing only critical steps, candidates were tested on both important objectives and a much larger number of clinical problems than was the case with previous formats.

The 'key features' tested by such questions are (a) the ability to synthesise presenting complaints for recognition of an important and life-threatening condition; and (b) the ability to identify essential areas to investigate in the history to confirm or rule out this hypothesis. A typical key features item with the scoring key is shown in Box 15.8. Questions 1 and 2 directly address each of these key features. Each challenges the candidate to apply their knowledge in making clinical decisions. In this item there is a constructed response for Question 1, with only one answer required, and a selection of six options only from a list of 28 for Question 2. Usually both Question 1 and Question 2 answers would be written by the test taker on an optical scoring sheet. There would be space for free text to Question 1 and buttons or ovals to fill in for Question 2.

KFIs require a scoring rubric that reflects the importance of the various key elements of the case. It helps to test out the scoring rubric with colleagues and a few 'dummy' test takers. Higher weighted scores for more important answers should be encouraged. In Box 15.8, the diagnosis was awarded one mark and the elements

of the history a total of six marks. The scoring key shows that only seven of the 28 options would be considered appropriate, so the candidate must select six of these to score maximum marks. The question also weights aspects of the history more highly than obtaining the correct diagnosis. This may be because in this situation knowing the best questions to ask would probably result in a change of diagnostic preference if an inappropriate answer was initially given to Question 1.

There are very few question formats that truly assess clinical decision making, but KFIs can make this claim. Certainly the foundation work done on the validity and reliability of the format(71) would suggest that KFIs robustly measure these facets of competence, and test takers seem to like their salience to clinical practice. However, KFIs are difficult to construct well, and although scoring seems simple, some questions can be very difficult to weight appropriately. Standard setting with KFIs can also be complex, as although both the modified Angoff and Ebel methods have been used, some assessors report that they do not work very well for this format. This is because the items are generally multidimensional and can include many aspects of a case, some of which are interdependent. Making decisions about how borderline test takers would respond to such items is challenging.

How to write a key features item

- Select a clinical problem from the assessment blueprint in which analysis of the context, identification of clinical conditions and synthesis of the diagnosis and/or management (clinical decisions) are required objectives.
- Think of several real instances of the case in everyday practice and consider what the essential (necessary and sufficient) steps are to resolve this problem. This will allow you to focus solely on the critical decisions for each case. Make an effort to distinguish between decisions or steps that are appropriate, but not critical, and those that are vital.
- Any of the typical cognitive processes used or actions planned can be tested in KFIs – the scope depends on the objectives being tested and the case presentation. For example, framing initial hypotheses, looking for particular clinical findings, choosing tests, management options or specific drugs are all possible.
- Select one of the real cases for development into a problem scenario and related questions. The attributes of the case can be written according to the same rules as for EMQ items, that is age, sex, setting of the encounter. When you have written the scenario, use the key features to frame the questions for the case. Usually only two or three questions are possible without invoking prompting or cueing. The more questions that are asked about a particular case the more opportunities arise for cueing. For

---

BOX 15.8 Key features item example

Paul Young, a 56-year-old male, consults you in your surgery because of pain in his left leg that began two days ago and has been getting progressively worse. He states his leg is tender below the knee and swollen around the ankle. He has never had similar problems. His other leg is fine.

Question 1

What is your principal working diagnosis? List, in note form only, your single (1) diagnosis.

Answer 1 ....

Question 2

To establish your diagnosis, what elements of his history would you particularly want to elicit? Choose up to six (6) from the following list.

1 Activity at onset of symptoms	15 Palpitations
2 Alcohol intake	16 Paraesthesia
3 Allergies	17 Paroxysmal nocturnal dyspnoea
4 Angina pectoris	18 Polydipsia
5 Anti-inflammatory therapy	19 Previous back problems
6 Cigarette smoking	20 Previous knee problems
7 Colour of stools	21 Previous neoplasia
8 Cough	22 Previous urinary tract infection
9 Headache	23 Recent dental procedure
10 Haematemesis	24 Recent immobilisation
11 Impotence	25 Recent sore throat
12 Intermittent claudication	26 Recent surgery
13 Low back pain	27 Wounds on foot
14 Nocturia	28 Wounds on hand

Answer 2

1)   2)   3)   4)   5)   6)

Scoring key

Question 1

Deep venous thrombosis must be the differential diagnosis (score 1)

(Total requested = 1 Total accepted = 1 Total score = 1) More than 1 answer scores zero.

Question 2

Any six (6) of the following items are required:

>   Activity at onset of symptoms

>   Cigarette smoking

>   Previous knee problems

>   Previous neoplasia

>   Recent immobilisation

>   Recent surgery

>   Wounds on foot

Each scores 1

(Total requested = 6 Total accepted = 6 Total possible score = 6) More than 6 answers scores zero.

(courtesy of the Royal Australian College of General Practitioners)

---

example, to ask about management, further information may need to be given about test results that will strongly imply the diagnosis, so asking about differential diagnosis, history and investigations, management and follow-up all in the same item becomes difficult (the same issue arises in MCQs).

- Select the response format – write-in (constructed) or option choice (selected). This needs to be done carefully. The guiding principle is that if the key feature entails a cognitive process that is or should be generated by the professional (e.g. recognition of a myocardial infarction and decision on immediate action) then the response should be write-in. The number of required answers must be stated. This is to inhibit 'blunderbussing' – the tendency of test takers to write down everything they can think of in the hope that the correct one(s) are included in their responses. Exceeding the number required should be penalised. Write-in items need to be marked, whereas options can be electronically scored.

Where's the evidence for key features items?

KFIs have been used for both summative and formative assessment in a number of different contexts.(72,73) The reliability of the KFI paper (26 items) of the Royal Australian College of General Practitioners increased from 0.64 in 1999 to around 0.83 currently.(72) KFIs were rated adequate on average as tests of clinical decision-making skills by approximately 90% candidates in the 2004 Fellowship examination. Colo-rectal surgeons (n = 256) found them useful as a means of self-assessment, and nine KFIs were almost as reliable as 50 MCQs (0.95 versus 0.97 respectively).(74)

Item Analysis

After items have been used in a test, we want to know how well each item has performed. There are two parts to this: first, did the item cover its own cognitive territory appropriately; and second, how did it do in relation to its contribution to the test as a whole. In essence, we want to know the following.

- Did the item do its job in capturing the understanding of an individual on that particular element of the content of the test? This would include identifying any problems with its construction that led to misinterpretation by test takers. For selected-response items, distractors might have been included that did not work effectively or were too close to the correct response to allow even good candidates to make an appropriate choice.
- Did the item have demonstrable relationships with the content of other items on the test and with the content of the test as a whole? This would include looking at inter-item correlation, item–test correlation, relationships with other parts of an assessment regime, for example, other assessments of the same domain, and other assessments in different domains, such as procedural skills.

These questions can be answered in a number of ways. One way to approach the problem would be to read every item on the test again carefully, alongside the answers generated. Of course, most items will have been read many times already, and after reading hundreds of items, test designers will have become immune to the potential inadequacies of the items. Another way is to use basic item analysis. However, all item analysis data must be interpreted with extreme caution and with reference to the overall purpose of the test. Rules of thumb about deleting or modifying items (e.g. based on poor discrimination indexes for items) should probably be avoided.

Many programs are available to process item data, and most operate in similar ways. The core of item analysis is to look at a set of parameters for each item that describe its performance as an item, its relationship to the test as a whole and its contribution to the performance of the current cohort on that test. In a selected-response test such parameters include:

- the difficulty of the item – how many takers got the item correct?
- which of the options were chosen most frequently?
- which options were chosen by high, medium and low performers on the test as a whole?
- how did success on each item correlate with performance on the test as a whole?
- what were the inter-item correlations? (This might be particularly important for SAQ and key features questions.)

This section demonstrates how to use a typical set of item analysis data to make inferences about these questions. The particular one shown here is from the IDEAL Consortium item analysis software, but many others provide analogous output. Consider the item in Box 15.9, which is question 87 of a 100-item MCQ test on emergency care that has been administered to third-year medical students.

A cohort of 148 students answered this item as part of a test on emergency management. The item was

---

BOX 15.9 Sample item (question 87) for analysis

In Melbourne, Australia, a man collapses in the presence of a single healthcare worker who, after careful assessment of the patient and while waiting for the paramedic team, decides to deliver cardiopulmonary resuscitation (CPR).

Choose the most appropriate ratio for breaths:compressions with which the health worker should commence CPR.

A	1:30
B	2:30
C	2:15
D	3:15
E	3:30

The correct answer (Australian Resuscitation Council Guidelines) is B.

chosen because it was thought that students needed to be aware of the repeated changes to guidelines over the years and that recognition of the correct guideline was a vital decision. Some previously recommended ratios were included as distractors.

The output from the programme for this item is shown in Box 15.10. Box 15.10 shows a number of item parameters in the top row, then below this row it can be read as a table comparing the proportions of whole cohort (Total) and tertile groups (High, Mid and Low) that selected each of the options in the test. The final three rows describe parameters of the various groups that selected the different distractors.

Returning to the areas we need to investigate:

• Did the item do its job in capturing the understanding of an individual on that particular element of the content of the test?

Well, the item was completed by all test takers. The values for INV, the number of examinees not providing a valid response to this item, and for OMIT, the number of examinees omitting this item, were zero. Furthermore, the number of examinees not finishing the test from this item onwards (NF) was also zero. Takers did not get 'stuck' answering this item and not have time to finish as a result. As this item was number 87 of 100, we can probably conclude that all candidates finished the test and we already know that all did this item. Most test takers got it right, 90% in fact – expressed in the table as a difficulty index (the proportion of candidates who got the item right or DIF = 0.90). In some data analysis packages the difficulty index is often more appropriately called the facility index. This number also appears in the box for the proportion of the Total test takers who identified B as the correct answer – 0.90 in column B. So if this item covers core knowledge, the indications are that this was achieved in the majority of candidates.

How did the item work? Well, as we have seen, there were very few takers who got the item wrong, only 15 of 148, or 0.10 as a proportion. The proportions choosing each of the distractors varied between 0.03 and 0.01 (see the other proportions in the Total row of

the table). Because of the low numbers choosing distractors it is not possible to say with confidence that any one of the distractors was more or less attractive than the others. The Test score mean % is the mean score on the total test of those candidates giving the indicated response to this item. Variation in this row would indicate that perhaps there was one, or more, distractors that was attractive to a high- or low-scoring group. If a particular distractor was chosen by a group that collectively did well on the test overall, there may have been some teaching that impacted on this issue for those students. This may have been the case for the 5% of the cohort choosing C, the old guideline, who collectively scored 79% on this test. However, the very small numbers involved would make this interpretation risky.

• Did the item have demonstrable relationships with the content of other items on the test and with the content of the test as a whole?

This would include looking at inter-item correlation, and looking at item–test correlation. RPB is the point biserial correlation between item 87 and the score on the whole test, including the present item. Point biserial correlations are used to determine the covariation of a continuous variable (the total score on the test) with one that has a truly dichotomous distribution (in this case item 87). The point biserial is mathematically equivalent to a Pearson correlation coefficient in which one variable has only two values. The RPB for this item is almost zero. If the purpose of this test were to make discriminations between individual test takers, there would be a case for excluding this item, because it does not separate good from less good candidates. However, the focus of this item is to assess a core piece of knowledge that everyone should know – which is, in fact, what the item analysis shows the item does.

CRPB is the corrected point biserial. In this calculation the present item is removed from the test total while the correlation is calculated. This is done because in some test situations the inclusion of the analysed item (item 87) in the test total can inflate this value and introduce additional covariation. This problem is more

---

BOX 15.10 Item analysis data for question 87

DIF = 0.90, RPB = −0.039, CRPB = −0.075 (95% CON = −0.298, 0.157), RBIS = −0.068, CRBIS = −0.130, IRI = −0.012

Group	N	INV	NF	OMIT	A	B*	C	D	E
Total	148	0	0	0	0.03	0.90	0.01	0.03	0.03
High	38	0			0.05	0.84	0.05	0.05	0.00
Mid	64	0			0.00	0.97	0.00	0.00	0.03
Low	46	0			0.04	0.87	0.00	0.04	0.04
Test score mean %					68	68	79	69	67
Discriminating power (DP)					0.01	−0.03	0.05	0.01	−0.04
Standard error of DP					0.07	0.11	0.05	0.07	0.05

troublesome when SAQs are being analysed. Typically each short answer has a weight greater than one mark and so variation in the item can make a large difference to the total score and hence to differences between the corrected and uncorrected versions of the statistic, with the uncorrected score being somewhat inflated (more positive). Even in the data for item 87, we can see considerable variation between the RPB and the CRPB.

RBIS and CRBIS are the 'non-point' versions of the previously discussed correlations. Strictly speaking, the biserial coefficient is used where the dichotomous variable in fact has an underlying continuity and has been separated or recoded into a dichotomous one. The RBIS and CRBIS are always larger than their respective 'point' values, and may give an inflated value for variables where the continuity does not in fact exist.

IRI is the item's overall reliability index, which is virtually zero. However, whether it is retained in future tests depends on the purpose of the test. As discussed above, if the test is designed to be a test of competence in decisions around emergency medicine, then excluding all the items on which students scored highly might defeat the objective of the test. If the test has some selective purpose, for example, identifying students who might be competing for an elective in emergency medicine in later years, then excluding item 87 might be appropriate.

In summary, the item is correctly answered by almost all the cohort, has little discriminating power as a predictor of total test score and appears to reflect the possibility that the previous CPR guideline (option C) was being used by a few individuals, while the majority were aware of the new recommendation to use 2:30 in single bystander CPR.

Item analysis is a relatively quick way to identify problems with items, especially when such problems reside with their distractors. It is surprising how often items are identified as having distractors that are chosen by a significant proportion of students and then issues are discovered with the validity of the

'correct' option or with ambiguous wording of the question.

It is crucial that one or more of the group of academics/clinicians who designed the items understand how to interpret item analysis software, and that they appreciate the need to tailor decisions about items to the purpose of the test. Indiscriminate use of the item parameters as a criterion for exclusion is highly undesirable; even though this may appear more 'objective' it will introduce more problems than it solves

In Box 15.11, we have another item in the test, item 46, and in Box 15.12, the item analysis data for that item. See if you agree with my interpretation.

In brief, this shows that there is competition in the cohort's mind as to which is the correct answer, with sport and alcohol being the two main contenders, and hereditary a minor one. The item is not worded particularly well, as the options do not all follow grammatically from the stem. This may introduce some bias in the option choices. It is also double negatively worded. It might have been better to ask: 'Which of the following is *not* a predisposing factor for osteoarthritis?'

The difficulty is 0.50, that is, only half the cohort answered the item correctly. As it happens, items with difficulties within the 0.45–0.55 range are usually the most discriminating (this is a mathematical function),

---

BOX 15.11 Sample item (question 46) for analysis

Predisposing factors for osteoarthritis include all of the following *except*:

A   Sport

B   Alcohol abuse*

C   Occupation

D   Obesity

E   Hereditary

*The correct answer is B – alcohol abuse.

BOX 15.12 Item analysis data for question 46

DIF = 0.50, RPB = −0.438, CRPB = 0.378 (95% CON = 0.164, 0.559), RBIS = 0.549, CRBIS = 0.474, IRI = 0.219

Group	N	INV	NF	OMIT	A	B*	C	D	E
Total	148	0	0	0	0.23	0.50	0.07	0.08	0.12
High	38	0			0.11	0.68	0.05	0.05	0.11
Mid	64	0			0.12	0.63	0.06	0.09	0.09
Low	46	0			0.48	0.17	0.09	0.09	0.17
Test score mean %					64	72	66	65	67
Discriminating power (DP)					−0.37	0.51	−0.03	−0.03	−0.07
Standard error of DP					0.14	0.15	0.08	0.08	0.11

although of course they can be negatively discriminating (this is rare in well-chosen content, and is usually the result of an error in keying the correct answer). Here the discrimination is good, nearly half (0.48) of the third tertile chose 'A' as the correct answer, but roughly a tenth (0.11) of the top tertile did too. Perhaps this is because sport is featured so strongly in health promotional literature that some students believe it has few side effects. Although the item is discriminating, and has good item–test correlations in both corrected and uncorrected versions, one might argue that in an emergency setting this knowledge might be less relevant; perhaps it would be more appropriate in a musculoskeletal clinic or in general practice assessment. The overall item reliability is good – a test of 100 similar items would provide a highly discriminating test, although with a pass mark of around 50%, and may not be defensible from a blueprinting perspective. If all such items were of 50% difficulty, it would be difficult to argue that the knowledge they contained was 'core'.

Standard Setting for Written Assessments

In the previous section we noted that the purpose of the test is a fundamental consideration in how to interpret item analysis data. We noted that our main example item was answered correctly by 90% of the cohort. So what should be an appropriate pass score for the test that this item comes from? The mean score on the test was 69% and the standard deviation was 5.7, the highest score was 91% and the lowest 52%, so even the one student scoring three standard deviations below the mean obtained more than 50%.

There has been much recent interest in trying to define standards for written tests, because 'standards are always arbitrary but should not be capricious', a quote often attributed to Ronald Berk, but which is borrowed from the US legal system for appeals.(41) There seems nothing quite as arbitrary in a test of high-quality health professionals as a pass mark of 50% – is this doctor half full or half empty of the knowledge needed to perform in practice?

Consequently, effort has gone into describing what the appropriate level of performance on any test should be. Clearly this might vary from test to test and year to year, as knowledge changes, items have different inherent difficulty and expectations change. There is no room here to discuss standard setting in great detail, but there are very good, practically focused, treatments elsewhere.(42) However, there are some important principles.

- Production of all written high-stakes tests should entail effort to set *a priori* standards. This is perfectly possible in both 'objective' and other types of written items, such as SAQs.
- Usually, these standards should be based on careful consideration of test content and its appropriateness to meet course/professional requirements by a group of judges familiar with the cohort, the curriculum, the content and the context.
- Standard-setting methods that best fit the purpose of a test should be chosen. Setting a minimum standard of competence may be a different purpose to selecting students to enter an advanced course, or certifying to a specialty. Giving feedback to students is a different purpose to accrediting them to lead the advanced life support team.
- Norm referencing is unacceptable for written items used in competency licensing tests. These tests are focused on candidates' safety to practise, among other things. A clear and defensible standard needs to be identified.
- Usually, for written assessments, the minimum acceptable standard should be decided before the test. In this setting (high-stakes examinations and patient safety concerns), variation in test, and hence item, difficulty is a critical issue. Standards should be set for each test, item by item, using item-focused methods such as Angoff, modified Angoff or Ebel.(75,76)
- The final choice of method will be governed by the available resources and the consequences of misclassifying examinees as having passed or failed.
- In general, setting standards for selected-response single-best-answer questions is less complex than setting standards for script concordance and, particularly, for key features items. This is because, especially in the latter, decisions in one part of a key feature may have impact on responses to other parts, and each may also be weighted quite differently. This problem is still being grappled with.(72)
- The most robust methods [e.g. Angoff(75)] are invariably also the most time-consuming, but frequently result in excellent insights into test construction flaws because each item or response is carefully examined.

Summary

Written assessment is the most commonly used form of testing in tertiary and professional education. Huge amounts of research have been carried out on multiple-choice item formats and essay assessments. There are many variations of these methods used for assessment in the health professions. Newer formats, such as key features and script concordance items, are still very much in development.

Here I have presented the basic principles behind the most commonly used ones. While there are many other topics that could be discussed in relation to item design, such as standard setting, blueprinting, principles of scoring and weighting, these are addressed by other papers in this series.

Assessments of the types we have discussed here usually happen at the end of a term or year. However, they require a significant amount of time to prepare well, as each item needs to be written, reviewed, verified against the blueprint and compiled into the whole test. Then the test needs to be reviewed to check for cross-cueing or repetition between items, and optical score sheets prepared to reflect the different categories of responses in the test (e.g. for key features items) and then printed for the assessment. This can require between two and five months for a complex and/or comprehensive assessment.

Faculty development is a key component of improvements in assessment strategies. Some written assessments are deceptively simple when given a cursory glance, but their quality is dependent on expertise in the discipline, as an educationalist and in item writing. Good items also require detailed preparation and extensive trialling and analysis of items.

Finally, it is clear that there are different uses for different items. It is unlikely that a good assessment of cognitive skills in health disciplines can be undertaken with 'an MCQ'. It will require a carefully chosen group of items, matched to the curriculum, using an array of different response modes to reflect the complexity of healthcare in the 21st century.

Acknowledgements

I would like to thank Madeleine Gayler (our office administrative assistant, now a medical student in Western Australia) and Pamela Collum for extensive work on formatting the document and the references.

References

1 Dauphinee D (2002) Licensure and certification. In: Norman G, van der Vleuten C and Newble D (eds) *International Handbook of Research on Medical Education*, vol. 2, pp. 835–82. Kluwer, Dordrecht.
2 Smith J (2004) *The Shipman Inquiry Fifth Report. Safeguarding Patients: lessons from the past – proposals for the future*. HMSO, London (http://www.the-shipman-inquiry.org.uk/fifthreport.asp; accessed 1 January 2009).
3 Walton M, Shaw TJ, Barnet S and Ross J (2006) Developing a national patient safety education framework for Australia. *Quality and Safety in Health Care*. 15: 437–42.
4 Scalese RJ, Obeso VT and Issenberg SB (2008) Simulation technology for skills training and competency assessment in medical education. *Journal of General Internal Medicine*. 23(s1): 46–9.
5 Norcini JJ (2003) ABC of learning and teaching in medicine: work based assessment. *British Medical Journal*. 326: 753–5.
6 Glaser R (1984) Education and thinking: the role of knowledge. *American Psychologist*. 39: 93–104 (http://edr.

sagepub.com/cgi/external_ref?access_num=10.1037/0003-066X.39.2.93&link_type=DOI).
7 Boshuizen HPA and Schmidt HG (1992) On the role of biomedical knowledge in clinical reasoning by experts, intermediates and novices. *Cognitive Science*. 16: 153–84.
8 Newble DJ (1991) The observed long case in clinical assessment. *Medical Education*. 25: 369–73.
9 Hubbard JP and Clemens WV (1961) *Multiple-Choice Examinations in Medicine*. Lea & Febiger, Philadelphia, PA.
10 Newble DI and Swanson DB (1988) Psychometric characteristics of the objective structured clinical examination. *Medical Education*. 22: 325–34.
11 Newble DI and Jaeger K (1983) The effect of assessments and examinations on the learning of medical students. *Medical Education*. 17: 165–71.
12 Norman G (2002) Research in medical education: three decades of progress. *British Medical Journal*. 324: 1560–2.
13 Newble DI, Jolly BC and Wakeford RE (eds) (1994) *Certification and Recertification in Medicine: issues in the assessment of clinical competence*. Cambridge University Press, Cambridge.
14 Norman G, van der Vleuten C and Newble D (eds) (2002) *International Handbook of Research on Medical Education*, vol. 2. Kluwer, Dordrecht.
15 Wood R (1991) *Assessment and Testing*. Cambridge University Press, Cambridge.
16 Newble DI and Cannon R (2001) *A Handbook for Medical Teachers* (4e). Springer, New York, p. 126.
17 Dauphinee D (1994) The content of certifying examinations. In: Newble DI, Jolly BC and Wakeford RE (eds) *Certification and Recertification in Medicine: issues in the assessment of clinical competence*, pp. 92–104. Cambridge University Press, Cambridge.
18 Hamdy H (2006) Blueprinting for the assessment of health care professionals. *Clinical Teacher*. 3: 175–9.
19 Kane MT (1992) The assessment of professional competence. *Evaluation and the Health Professions*. 15: 163–82.
20 Downing SM (2002) Threats to the validity of locally developed multiple-choice tests in medical education: construct irrelevant variance and construct underrepresentation. *Advances in Health Sciences Education*. 7: 235–41.
21 Roberts C, Sarangi S, Southgate L *et al.* (2000) Oral examinations – equal opportunities, ethnicity, and fairness in the MRCGP. *British Medical Journal*. 320: 370–5.
22 Hobus PP, Schmidt HG, Boshuizen HP and Patel VL (1987) Contextual factors in the activation of first diagnostic hypotheses: expert–novice differences. *Medical Education*. 21: 471–6.
23 Bowen JL (2006) Educational strategies to promote clinical diagnostic reasoning. *New England Journal of Medicine*. 355: 2217–25.
24 Mylopoulos M and Regehr G (2007) Cognitive metaphors of expertise and knowledge: prospects and limitations for medical education. *Medical Education*. 41: 1159–65.
25 Croskerry P and Norman G (2008) Overconfidence in clinical decision making. *American Journal of Medicine*. 121: 24–9.
26 Case S and Swanson D (1998) *Item Writing Manual* (3e). National Board of Medical Examiners, Philadelphia, PA (http://www.nbme.org/publications/item-writing-manual-download.html; accessed 1 January 2009).
27 Epstein R (2007) Assessment in medical education. *New England Journal of Medicine*. 356: 387–96.
28 Stalnaker JM (1951) The essay type of examination. In: Lindquist EF (ed.) *Educational Measurement*, pp. 495–530. George Banta, Menasha, WI.

29 Ebel RL and Frisbie DA (1986) *Essentials of Educational Measurement* (4e). Prentice Hall, Englewood Cliffs, NJ.

30 Schafer WD, Gagné P and Lissitz RW (2005) Resistance to confounding style and content in scoring constructed-response items. *Educational Measures: Issues and Practice*. 24: 22–8.

31 Klein SP and Hart FM (1968) Chance and systematic factors affecting essay grades. *Journal of Educational Measurement*. 5: 197–206.

32 Linn RL, Klein SP and Hart FM (1972) The nature and correlates of law school essay grades. *Educational and Psychological Measurement*. 32: 267–79.

33 Markham LR (1976) Influences of handwriting quality on teacher evaluation of written work. *American Educational Research Journal*. 13: 277–83.

34 Powers D, Fowles M, Farnum M and Ramsey P (1994) Will they think less of my handwritten essay if others word process theirs? Effects on essay scores of intermingling handwritten and word-processed essays. *Journal of Educational Measurement*. 31: 220–33.

35 Verma M, Chatwal J and Singh T (1997) Reliability of essay type questions – effect of structuring. *Assessment in Education: Principles, Policy & Practice*. 4: 265–70.

36 Grosse ME and Wright BD (1988) Psychometric characteristics of scores on a patient-management problem test. *Educational and Psychological Measurement*. 48: 297–305.

37 Lim E, Hian C, Seet H *et al.* (2007) Computer-based testing of the modified essay question: the Singapore experience. *Medical Teacher*. 9: e261–8.

38 Feletti GI (1980) Reliability and validity studies on modified essay questions. *Journal of Medical Education*. 55: 933–41.

39 Smith B, Sinclair H, Simpson J *et al.* (2002) What is the role of double marking? Evidence from an undergraduate medical course. *Education for Primary Care*. 13: 497–503.

40 Cannings R, Hawthorne K, Hood K and Houston H (2005) Putting double marking to the test: a framework to assess if it is worth the trouble. *Medical Education*. 39: 299–308.

41 Cizek GJ (ed.) (2001) *Setting Performance Standards. Concepts, Methods and Perspectives*. Erlbaum, Mahwah, NJ.

42 Norcini JJ (2003) Setting standards on educational tests. *Medical Education*. 37: 464–9.

43 Rodriquez MC (2003) Construct equivalence of multiple-choice and constructed-response items: a random effects synthesis of correlations. *Journal of Educational Measurement*. 40: 163–84.

44 Grant DL (1957) Studies in the reliability of the short-answer essay examination. *Journal of Educational Research*. 51: 109.

45 Matters G and Paul C (2003) Psychological predictors of the propensity to omit short-response items on a high-stakes achievement test. *Educational and Psychological Measurement*. 63: 239–56.

46 Edwards BD and Arthur Jr W (2007) An examination of factors contributing to a reduction in subgroup differences on a constructed-response paper-and-pencil test of scholastic achievement. *Journal of Applied Psychology*. 92: 794–801.

47 Rademakers J, Ten Cate THJ and Bar PR (2005) Progress testing with short answer questions. *Medical Teacher*. 27: 578–82

48 Gay LR (1980) The comparative effects of multiple-choice versus short-answer tests on retention. *Journal of Educational Measurement*. 17: 45–50.

49 Haladyna TM (2004) *Developing and Validating Multiple Choice Items*. Lawrence Erlbaum, Mahwah, NJ.

50 Downing SM (2003) Guessing on selected-response examinations. *Medical Education*. 37: 670–1.

51 Downing SM (2002) Assessment of knowledge in written test forms. In: Norman G, van der Vleuten C and Newble D (eds) *International Handbook of Research on Medical Education*, vol. 2, pp. 647–72. Kluwer, Dordrecht.

52 Haladyna TM and Downing SM (1993) How many options is enough for a multiple-choice test item? *Educational and Psychological Measurement*. 53: 999–1009.

53 Case SM, Swanson DB and Ripkey DR (1994) Comparison of items in five-option and extended-matching format for assessment of diagnostic skills. *Academic Medicine*. 69(s): S1–3.

54 Skakun E, Maguire T and Cook D (1994) Strategy choices in multiple choice items. *Academic Medicine*. 69(s): S7–9.

55 Case SM (1983) The development and evaluation of a new instrument to assess medical problem solving. *Dissertation Abstracts International*. 44: 1764.

56 Bhakta B, Tennant A, Horton M *et al.* (2005) Using item response theory to explore the psychometric properties of extended matching questions examination in undergraduate medical education. *BioMed Central Medical Education*. 5: 9.

57 McCoubrie P (2004) Improving the fairness of multiple-choice questions: a literature review. *Medical Teacher*. 8: 709–12.

58 George S (2003) Extended matching items (EMIs): solving the conundrum. *Psychiatric Bulletin of the Royal College of Psychiatrists*. 27: 230–2.

59 Zimmerman DW and Williams RHA (2003) New look at the influence of guessing on the reliability of multiple-choice tests. *Applied Psychological Measurement*. 27: 357–71.

60 Swanson DW, Holtzman KZ, Clauser BE and Sawhill AJ (2005) Psychometric characteristics and response times for one-best-answer questions in relation to number and source of options. *Academic Medicine*. 80(s): S93–6.

61 Charlin B, Brailovsky C, Leduc C and Blouin D (1998) The diagnosis script questionnaire: a new tool to assess a specific dimension of clinical competence. *Advances in Health Sciences Education*. 3: 51–8.

62 Charlin B, Brailovsky C, Roy L *et al.* (2000) The script concordance test: a tool to assess the reflective clinician. *Teaching and Learning in Medicine*. 12: 189–95.

63 Schmidt H, Norman G and Boshuizen H (1990) A cognitive perspective on medical expertise: theory and implications. *Academic Medicine*. 65: 611–21.

64 Charlin B and van der Vleuten C (2004) Standardised assessment of clinical reasoning in contexts of uncertainty: the script concordance approach. *Evaluation and the Health Professions*. 27: 304–19.

65 Gagnon R, Charlin B, Roy L *et al.* (2006) The cognitive validity of the script concordance test: a processing time study. *Teaching and Learning in Medicine*. 18: 22–7.

66 Sibert L, Darmoni SJ, Dahamna B *et al.* (2006) On line clinical reasoning assessment with script concordance test in urology: results of a French pilot study. *BMC Medical Education*. 6: 45.

67 Meterissian S, Zabolotny B, Gagnon R and Charlin B (2007) Is the script concordance test a valid instrument for assessment of intraoperative decision-making skills? *American Journal of Surgery*. 193: 248–51.

68 Farmer EA and Page G (2005) A practical guide to assessing clinical decision-making skills using the key features approach. *Medical Education*. 39: 1188–94.

69 Norman G, Bordage G, Curry L *et al.* (1985) Review of recent innovations in assessment. In: Wakeford R (ed.) *Directions in Clinical Assessment*. Report of the Cambridge Conference on the Assessment of Clinical Competence, pp. 8–27. Office of the

Regius Professor of Physic, Cambridge University School of Clinical Medicine, Addenbrookes Hospital, Cambridge.

70 McGuire CH, Solomon LM and Bashook PG (1976) *Construction and Use of Written Simulations*. Psychological Corporation of Harcourt Brace Jovanovich, New York.

71 Page G and Bordage G (1995) The Medical Council of Canada's key features project: a more valid written examination of clinical decision-making skills. *Academic Medicine*. 70: 104–10.

72 Farmer EA and Hinchy J (2005) Assessing clinical decision making skills in general practice: the key features approach. *Australian Family Physician*. 34: 1059–61.

73 Fischer M, Kopp V, Holzer M *et al.* (2005) A modified electronic key feature examination for undergraduate medical students: validation threats and opportunities. *Medical Teacher*. 27: 450–5.

74 Trudel JL, Bordage G and Downing SM (2008) Reliability and validity of key feature cases for the self-assessment of colon and rectal surgeons. *Annals of Surgery*. 248: 252–8.

75 Cizek GJ (1996) Standard setting guidelines. *Educational Measurement: Issues and Practice*. 15: 13–21.

76 Ebel RL (1972) *Essentials of Educational Measurement* (2e). Prentice Hall, Englewood Cliffs, NJ.

Further Reading

Case S and Swanson D (1998) *Item Writing Manual* (3e). National Board of Medical Examiners, Philadelphia, PA (http://www.nbme.org/publications/item-writing-manual-download.html; accessed 1 January 2009).

Ebel RL and Frisbie DA (1986) *Essentials of Educational Measurement* (4e). Prentice Hall, Englewood Cliffs, NJ.

Newble DI, Jolly BC and Wakeford RE (eds) (1994) *Certification and Recertification in Medicine: issues in the assessment of clinical competence*. Cambridge University Press, Cambridge.

Norman G, van der Vleuten C and Newble D (eds) (2002) *International Handbook of Research on Medical Education*, vol. 2. Kluwer, Dordrecht.

Wood R (1991) *Assessment and Testing*. Cambridge University Press, Cambridge.

Workplace assessment

John J Norcini

KEY MESSAGES

- Assessment in the setting of clinical training is not well developed, but methods based on observation of routine encounters offer a rich and feasible alternative.

- A framework for assessment based on observation includes two dimensions: the grounds on which judgements are made (single encounter or routine performance) and the nature of the judgements themselves (occurrence, quality or suitability).

- Tools such as the mini-CEX, DOPS, CbD and mini-PAT offer valid assessment.

- Faculty development is a key to the successful use of the methods.

- The opportunity for educational feedback as part of these methods is as important as their contribution to the assessment process.

- A series of challenges remains, including reliability, equivalence, stakes, relationships, the need for other forms of assessment and feasibility.

Introduction

Assessment in the context of medical education has changed dramatically over the past 50 years.(1) From near exclusive reliance on the essay question and the clinical viva, assessment methods have proliferated, particularly those appropriate to use in the setting of undergraduate medical education. These newer methods cover more of the competencies of a doctor, and there is much better understanding of how to deploy them to produce scores that are valid and reliable.

Assessment in the setting of clinical training, particularly postgraduate training, is not as well developed as assessment in the undergraduate arena. The curriculum in most clinical training settings is less structured, and the trainees often have more responsibility. Consequently, assessment needs to pose a broader range of patient problems and include more complex and acute care, multi-system disease and procedural skill. Moreover, the focus is more often on the assessment of integrated skills rather than on specific aspects of competence. Compared with practising doctors, trainees in clinical settings are not yet completely responsible for patients, and they have not differentiated within specialty. As a result, assessment needs to focus on the potential to practise, not actual practice, so assessments of work products are likely to be less useful.(2) Moreover, the results of an assessment programme need to support the educational enterprise.

It is difficult to develop high-quality written or performance-based assessments locally, especially in the context of postgraduate training. There are small numbers of trainees and staff; resources are fragmented across the specialties; and assessment expertise is rare. There is also a need to address sophisticated content and skills, which are difficult to simulate at the level of advanced trainees.

Despite these challenges, there are two aspects of training in a clinical setting that offer significant advantages for assessment. First, there are routine interactions among members of the healthcare team and between trainees and patients, so the clinical material that can serve as the basis for assessment is readily available. Second, there are skilled clinician-educators in the setting who, with some training, can act as judges. Consequently, assessment methods that are based on observation of routine encounters are most feasible in the setting of clinical training. In addition, the use of these methods supports the educational process because they offer the opportunity for formative feedback and the development of a plan for remediation when it is needed.

In 1990, Miller proposed a structure, in the form of a pyramid, for categorising methods of assessment.(3) Knowledge (knows) is at the lowest level of the pyramid followed by competence (knows how), performance (shows how) and action (does) (*see* Figure 16.1). Assessments based on observation in the setting of work are representative of the top two levels of the pyramid. Miller distinguished between these two levels depending on whether trainees were in an artificial testing situation (i.e. they were aware that they were being assessed). Underlying this distinction is the reasonable but unproven assumption that the assessment methods that come closest to capturing a doctor's

Understanding Medical Education: Evidence, Theory and Practice.
Edited by T Swanwick. © 2010 Association for the Study of Medical Education.

Figure 16.1 Miller's pyramid for assessing clinical competence.

unobserved, routine functioning will yield the most valid results. Of course, capturing authentic performance has problems as well since the clinical context poses a number of threats to validity (e.g. differences between doctors in case mix and the severity of illness of their patients).(2)

A Framework for Assessment Based on Observation

Assessors have been asked to make a number of different kinds of judgement based on their observations. For the purpose of this chapter, a two-dimensional framework will be used to describe these judgements.(4,5) The first dimension relates to the grounds on which the judgements are made – a single encounter or routine performance. The second dimension relates to the nature of the judgement – whether it is occurrence, quality or suitability.

Grounds for judgement
Single encounter
In this instance, the assessors base their judgements on observation of a single event. For example, a faculty member might observe the trainee in interaction with a particular patient, patient record or procedure and then provide an evaluation of it. The traditional clinical viva illustrates this. A trainee examines and interviews a patient, draws conclusions and then presents all of this to one or more assessors. Judgements about the trainee are made on the basis of that one event.

The advantage of basing judgements on single events is the reassurance that the assessor has actually observed the performance and is focused on reaching a conclusion about it. Theoretically, this reduces the biasing effects of previous contact and clarifies what is to be evaluated. The disadvantage is that the performance of doctors is case or task specific.(6) This means that performance on one event does not predict with high accuracy performance on another. Therefore, several different events need to be sampled to obtain a generalisable estimate of performance (Box 16.1).

Routine performance
In this instance, the assessors base their judgements on observations they have made over a period of time. This is one of the most common types of assessment, and most training programmes in the US and UK ask faculty members to periodically complete rating forms that attest to the competence of their trainees.

The major advantage of this basis for judgement is that it should include observations of the trainee on a number of different occasions. In this way, it reduces, to some degree, the problems of case specificity of performance. However, assessors sometimes offer evaluations of aspects of performance they do not observe. For example, Pulito *et al.* found that faculty members primarily observe cognitive skills and professionalism and have little basis for assessing other aspects of competence.(7) Moreover, Silber *et al.* found that faculty members tend to assess competence along the two dimensions of medical knowledge and interpersonal skills and do not make distinctions among other aspects of competence.(8)

Nature of the judgement

Based on their observations of single encounters or routine performance, the nature of judgements assessors have been asked to make falls into three categories:

- occurrence – whether particular behaviours were demonstrated
- quality – the goodness of the performance
- fitness or suitability – whether the performance was good enough for a particular purpose.

Occurrence

Assessors are sometimes asked to indicate whether they have observed a particular behaviour, and they are often given a checklist on which to note the occurrence. For instance, Martin *et al.* developed procedure-specific checklists containing 22–32 task steps.(9) They were applied by assessors to their observation of procedures done by trainees. Each time one of the steps on the checklist was completed, the assessor noted it, and after the procedure, the marks were tallied.

Simply noting the occurrence of behaviours is often viewed as objective, leaving less to the judgement of the observer. It structures the task of the assessor and ensures that it is more focused and consistent over observations and assessors. If they are clinician-educators, however, simply asking the assessor to note the occurrence of particular behaviours does not make best use of their ability to discriminate among performances.

Quality

More often, assessors are asked to make a judgement about the quality of the performance they observe. They typically record these judgements on a rating scale. For example, in the study by Martin *et al.*, observers were also asked to complete a seven-item global rating form that captured the quality of the trainees' procedural skills on a five-point scale.(9) The same form was used for all procedures, and after the examination the ratings were tallied.

In the Martin *et al.* study, the global assessments of quality were strongly correlated with the checklists, which simply noted the occurrence of aspects of performance.(9) This is not an unusual finding, and it suggests that they are capturing the same aspects of competence.(10) However, the global ratings tend to be a bit more valid. For instance, in the Martin *et al.*

study, they discriminated among levels of training, while the checklists did not.

Fitness

In some instances, assessors are asked to determine whether a performance is satisfactory or fit for purpose. For example, in the Martin *et al.* study, the assessors were also asked to make a pass–fail judgement.(9) In essence, this required them to make two judgements in sequence. They needed to first establish the quality of a performance, and then they had to decide whether it was good enough for a particular purpose. In the Martin *et al.* study, pass–fail results were not correlated with other measures (e.g. year of training) because so many of the participants passed.(9)

The simultaneous decision making underlying a single judgement about fitness is very efficient in academic settings where it is important to identify individuals for advancement and remediation. However, it combines two somewhat unreliable judgements into one and renders the meaning of the results unclear to a degree. For example, a failing judgement can be rendered because the performance was poor or the assessor had high standards. Since it is not possible to disentangle these, it is best to ask for judgements about quality and fitness separately, as they did in the study by Martin *et al.*

Common Methods

A number of different methods of assessment based on observation have been used in the setting of clinical training. The four assessment methods recommended as part of the Foundation Programme in the UK serve as a good example of these:

- mini-clinical evaluation exercise (mini-CEX)
- direct observation of procedural skills (DOPS)
- case-based discussion (CbD)
- multi-source feedback (MSF).(13)

In addition, the programme requires that trainees complete an educational portfolio. These methods will be the focus of this section.

The Foundation Programme is a two-year period of postgraduate training, which acts as a bridge between undergraduate and specialist/general practice training.(13) It is composed of placements in a variety of healthcare settings, which provide experiences in primary care and the specialties. Learning objectives have been developed for each stage of training, and the assessment procedures are focused on the demonstration of clinical competencies.

Mini-CEX

In the mini-CEX, a faculty member observes a trainee interact with a patient in a clinical setting.(13,14) The trainee engages in a clinical activity (e.g. taking a focused history and performing relevant aspects of the physical examination) and afterwards summarises the encounter (e.g. provides a diagnosis and/or treatment plan). The faculty member scores the performance and then provides educational feedback. The encounters are intended to take about 15 minutes, and trainees are expected to be evaluated several times and by different faculty members.

The method was originally devised for use in internal medicine postgraduate training programmes in the US. Individual faculty members were responsible for deciding when trainees were to be assessed and for identifying appropriate patients. Ratings were gathered on a nine-point scale, where 1–3 was unsatisfactory, 4–6 was satisfactory and 7–9 was superior. The dimensions of performance observed and evaluated were interviewing skill, physical examination, professionalism, clinical judgement, counselling, organisation and efficiency and overall competence. Not every encounter permitted assessment of all of these dimensions. Depending on the purpose of the assessment, the ratings were aggregated across dimensions and encounters for each trainee.(13,14)

Given its structure, the ground for judgements underpinning the mini-CEX is always the single encounter. Depending on how it has been deployed, however, the nature of the judgements has varied depending on the purpose of the assessment. For instance, in the US, assessors were asked to judge both the quality (ranking from 1 to 9) of the performance and its fitness (unsatisfactory versus satisfactory-superior) for a first-year postgraduate trainee.

In the US, the mini-CEX has been used in a number of different inpatient, outpatient and emergency department settings. In these settings, the mini-CEX has been applied to a broad range of patient problems. For example, in a study by Norcini *et al.*, the presenting complaints included abdominal pain, chest pain, cough, dizziness, fever, headache, low back pain, shortness of breath and weight gain. Common internal medicine problems, such as arthritis, asthma, chronic obstructive pulmonary disorder, congestive heart failure (CHF), coronary artery disease, diabetes and hypertension, formed the basis for assessment, as well as other common problems, such as seizure, substance abuse, depression, dementia and rash. The mini-CEX was also applied to trainees using patients with multiple problems, such as CHF, hypertension and diabetes, and with acute problems such as sepsis and myocardial infarction.(12)

The mini-CEX is analogous to a classroom test for the clinical setting. It is intended to identify the few trainees whose performance is wholly unsatisfactory and to provide the remainder with an opportunity for ongoing assessment and formative feedback. It is also designed to ensure that the clinical skills of trainees have been observed and evaluated by faculty members. Unfortunately, this occurs far too rarely in the context of many busy clinical placements.(15)

The mini-CEX is not intended for use in a high-stakes examination setting, nor should it be used to compare or rank trainees across different programmes.

There is growing literature suggesting that the mini-CEX has the expected relationships with other assessments of competence. In the undergraduate setting, Kogan *et al.* found that mini-CEX scores had modest correlations with examination scores, inpatient clerkship ratings, outpatient clerkship ratings and final course grades.(16) In a postgraduate setting, During *et al.* found correlations between the individual components of the mini-CEX and the corresponding monthly evaluations by faculty members, as well as the results of an in-training examination.(17) In a study by Boulet *et al.*, videotapes of standardised patient (SP)–student encounters were evaluated by faculty using the mini-CEX form.(18) The SP checklists predicted faculty global ratings, and SP ratings of doctor–patient communication correlated with faculty ratings of communications. Finally, Holmboe *et al.* scripted videotapes of trainees whose performance was unsatisfactory, satisfactory or superior. Using the mini-CEX form, faculty successfully discriminated among the three levels of performance.(19)

Since its initial development, the mini-CEX has been modified for use in a number of different settings. The original forms have been translated into several different languages. The competencies assessed have been tailored to particular needs (e.g. the Professionalism Mini-Evaluation Exercise) and to a variety of undergraduate and postgraduate disciplines and clinical settings.(20–22) The rating scales have been modified as well, with changes in both the number of points on the scale and the definitions of those points. All of these modifications are appropriate, and they ensure the relevance of the method to the setting in which it is being used.

The assessment portion of the Foundation Programme provides an example in which the mini-CEX has been appropriately modified to make it more relevant to a particular setting.(13) Trainees are assessed four to six times throughout the year with different faculty members for each encounter. Both the assessor and the patient are selected by the trainee, but the assessor must agree that the encounter is appropriate. Assessors include consultants, experienced specialist registrars, staff grade and associate specialists and general practitioners. There is a list of core problems as part of the curriculum, and trainees are expected to sample from them. The immediate feedback given after the encounter includes strengths, weaknesses and an action plan for further effort.

Figure 16.2 shows a typical assessment form. It has been anglicised, and a six-point rating scale is being used. The descriptors require the assessors to judge both the quality of the trainee's performance and whether it meets expectations for completion of the year of training.

Please refer to www.hcat.nhs.uk for guidance on this form and details of expected competencies for F1

Mini-Clinical Evaluation Exercise (CEX) - F1 Version

Please complete the questions using a cross: ☒   Please use black ink and CAPITAL LETTERS

Doctor's Surname

Forename

GMC Number: **GMC NUMBER MUST BE COMPLETED**

Clinical setting:
A&E	OPD	In-patient	Acute Admission	GP Surgery
☐	☐	☐	☐	☐

Clinical problem category:
Airway/ Breathing	CVS/ Circulation	Gastro	Neuro	Pain	Psych/ Behav	Other
☐	☐	☐	☐	☐	☐	

New or FU:
New	FU	Focus of clinical encounter:	History	Diagnosis	Management	Explanation
☐	☐		☐	☐	☐	☐

Number of times patient seen before by trainee:
0	1-4	5-9	>10	Complexity of case:	Low	Average	High
☐	☐	☐	☐		☐	☐	☐

Assessor's position:
Consultant	GP	SpR	SASG	SHO	Other
☐	☐	☐	☐	☐	

Number of previous mini-CEXs observed by assessor with <u>any</u> trainee:
0	1	2	3	4	5-9	>9
☐	☐	☐	☐	☐	☐	☐

Please grade the following areas using the scale below:	Below expectations for F1 completion		Borderline for F1 completion	Meets expectations for F1 completion	Above expectations for F1 completion		U/C*
1. History Taking	☐	☐	☐	☐	☐	☐	☐
2. Physical Examination Skills	☐	☐	☐	☐	☐	☐	☐
3. Communication Skills	☐	☐	☐	☐	☐	☐	☐
4. Clinical Judgement	☐	☐	☐	☐	☐	☐	☐
5. Professionalism	☐	☐	☐	☐	☐	☐	☐
6. Organisation/Efficiency	☐	☐	☐	☐	☐	☐	☐
7. Overall clinical care	☐	☐	☐	☐	☐	☐	☐

*U/C Please mark this if you have not observed the behaviour and therefore feel unable to comment.

Anything especially good?   **Suggestions for development**

Agreed action:

Have you had training in the use of this assessment tool?:   ☐ Face-to-Face   ☐ HaveReadGuidelines   ☐ Web/CDrom

Assessor's Signature:

Date (mm/yy):
M M   /   Y Y

Time taken for observation: (in minutes)

Time taken for feedback: (in minutes)

Assessor's Surname

Assessor's registration number:

<u>Please note</u>: Failure of return of all completed forms to your administrator is a probity issue
Acknowledgements: Adapted with permission from American Board of Internal Medicine

Figure 16.2 Typical mini-CEX assessment form.

DOPS

DOPS is a variation on the mini-CEX, which was originally designed by the Royal College of Physicians to assess and provide feedback on procedural skills.(23) Just as with the mini-CEX, trainees are observed with real patients, but in DOPS they are conducting procedures. After the encounter, the faculty member rates the trainee's performance and provides educational feedback. The encounters are necessarily brief (usually less than 15 minutes, with 5 minutes for feedback), and trainees are expected to be evaluated several times and by different faculty members.

Trainees must select from an approved list that contains many of the procedures used routinely in practice.(13) For example, it includes various injections, intubation, electrocardiogram, nasogastric tube insertion, venepuncture, cannulation and arterial blood sampling. Trainees are assessed on their understanding of indications, anatomy, technique, aseptic technique, proper analgesia, communication and other important aspects of procedural skill. They are also asked how often they have performed the procedure.

Trainees are to be assessed six times throughout the year with different procedures and faculty members for each encounter.(13) As with all the tools used as part of this programme, the timing, procedure and assessor are selected by the trainees, but the assessor must agree that the procedure is appropriate. Like the mini-CEX, assessors include consultants, experienced specialist registrars, staff grade and associate specialists and general practitioners. However, nurses and other appropriate allied health professionals can also act as assessors. The immediate feedback given after the encounter includes areas of strengths and suggestions for development.

Since it is a variation, studies indicating the validity of the mini-CEX apply to DOPS as well. In addition, there is considerable research showing that global ratings of procedural skills can produce valid results.(24) For example, Goff *et al.* demonstrated that in an objective structured assessment of technical skills, judgements of occurrence, quality and fitness by two assessors were able to distinguish among levels of training.(25) Similarly, a study of actual performance by Winckel *et al.* found that both checklists and global ratings distinguished among levels of training for 41 operations (*see* Box 16.2).(26)

CbD

CbD is a variation on chart-stimulated recall (CSR) developed by Maatsch for use by the American Board of Emergency Medicine.(27) In the Foundation Programme, the trainee must select two case records from patients they have seen recently and in which they have made entries.(13) The assessor selects one of the two cases and explores one aspect of it with the trainee. For example, they might choose to focus on which investigations the trainee ordered or on the

ethical issues raised by a particular patient. In all instances, the assessor is interested in understanding the reasoning behind the trainee's choices.

CbD is designed to stimulate trainees to discuss why they acted as they did. It offers the opportunity for assessment of the application of knowledge, decision making and ethical issues. The primary purpose is not to assess medical record keeping, but since it is used as the basis for discussion, it allows evaluation of this aspect of performance. CbD uses single encounters as the grounds for measurement, and assessors are asked to make judgements about both the quality of the clinical assessment, investigation and referrals, treatment, professionalism, medical record keeping and overall clinical care and about whether they meet or exceed expectations (i.e. fitness). The assessment form is shown in Figure 16.3.

As with other methods used in the Foundation Programme, each encounter is intended to take 15 minutes, followed by 5 minutes of feedback, and there should be four to six encounters during the year.(13) Assessors include consultants, experienced specialist registrars, staff grade and associate specialists and general practitioners. There is a list of core problems as part of the curriculum, and trainees are expected to sample from them. The feedback given after the encounter should include strengths, suggestions for development and an action plan that outlines a response to these suggestions.

The original work on the validity of the CSR was done in conjunction with the certification and recertification programmes of the American Board of Emergency Medicine.(27) When given to a sample of practising doctors, CSR score distributions and pass–fail results were consistent with those for initial

Please refer to curriculum at www.mmc.nhs.uk for details of expected competencies for F1 and F2

Case-based Discussion (CbD) – F2 Version

Please complete the questions using a cross: ☒   Please use black ink and CAPITAL LETTERS

Doctor's   Surname

Forename

GMC Number: **GMC NUMBER MUST BE COMPLETED**

Clinical setting: A&E ☐   OPD ☐   In-patient ☐   Acute Admission ☐   GP Surgery ☐

Clinical problem category: Pain ☐   Airway/Breathing ☐   CVS/Circulation ☐   Psych/Behav ☐   Neuro ☐   Gastro ☐   Other

Focus of clinical encounter: Medical Record Keeping ☐   Clinical Assessment ☐   Management ☐   Professionalism ☐

Complexity of case: Low ☐   Average ☐   High ☐   Assessor's position: Consultant ☐   SpR ☐   GP ☐

Please grade the following areas using the scale below:	Below expectations for F2 completion		Borderline for F2 completion	Meets expectations for F2 completion	Above expectations for F2 completion		U/C*
	1	2	3	4	5	6	
1 Medical record keeping	☐	☐	☐	☐	☐	☐	☐
2 Clinical assessment	☐	☐	☐	☐	☐	☐	☐
3 Investigation and referrals	☐	☐	☐	☐	☐	☐	☐
4 Treatment	☐	☐	☐	☐	☐	☐	☐
5 Follow-up and future planning	☐	☐	☐	☐	☐	☐	☐
6 Professionalism	☐	☐	☐	☐	☐	☐	☐
7 Overall clinical judgement	☐	☐	☐	☐	☐	☐	☐

*U/C Please mark this if you have not observed the behaviour and therefore feel unable to comment.

Anything especially good?   **Suggestions for development**

Agreed action:

	Not at all								Highly
Trainee satisfaction with CbD	1 ☐	2 ☐	3 ☐	4 ☐	5 ☐	6 ☐	7 ☐	8 ☐	9 ☐	10 ☐
Assessor satisfaction with CbD	1 ☐	2 ☐	3 ☐	4 ☐	5 ☐	6 ☐	7 ☐	8 ☐	9 ☐	10 ☐

What training have you had in the use of this assessment tool?:   ☐ Have Read Guidelines   ☐ Face-to-Face   ☐ Web/CD rom

Time taken for discussion: (in minutes)

Assessor's Signature: Date: ☐☐ / ☐☐ / ☐☐

Time taken for feedback: (in minutes)

Assessor's Surname

Assessor's GMC Number   **Please note:** Failure of return of all completed forms to your administrator is a probity issue

2466400642

Figure 16.3 Typical CbD assessment form.

certification. They were also correlated with scores from a variety of other methods, including an oral examination and an audit of practice records. Of all the methods used, CSR was considered most valid by practising doctors.

In a later study, Norman *et al.* applied several different assessment methods to a group of doctors, who were referred because of practice problems, and a group of volunteers.(28) CSR was correlated with an SP examination (0.74) and an oral examination (0.51) given to these same groups. In addition, CSR was able to distinguish the 'referred' from the volunteer group.

Finally, Solomon *et al.* gave CSR to a group of doctors eligible for recertification.(29) It was correlated with an oral exam (0.49), and when it was combined with the oral exam, CSR had correlations with written and oral exams administered 10 years earlier (0.45, 0.37).

Mini-PAT

Making judgements about the performance of peers has formed the basis of the referral process in medicine and other professions for centuries.(30) In recent years, these judgements have been collected in a systematic fashion and aggregated to provide an assessment of performance. There are several variations on the process, and (at the time of writing) two are used as part of the Foundation Programme.(13) This chapter focuses on the mini-PAT.

Trainees nominate eight assessors who are consultants, experienced specialist registrars, staff grade and associate specialists, general practitioners, nurses or allied health personnel. Each is sent a questionnaire, which, after completion, is returned to a central location for processing. This ensures that the trainee does not know the views of their assessors. The trainee self-assesses and submits the questionnaire for processing as well. Figure 16.4 shows the questionnaire that is being used. It contains 16 questions addressing the categories of
- good clinical care
- maintaining good medical practice
- teaching and training – appraising and assessing
- relationships with patients
- working with colleagues
- an overall assessment.

Unlike the other methods in the Foundation Programme, the judgements underpinning the mini-PAT are grounded in routine performance. As with the other methods, however, assessors are asked to make judgements about both quality and fitness.

The questionnaires are collated electronically in a central location, and feedback is prepared for the trainee. It is presented in graphical form, which depicts self-ratings, the mean ratings of the assessors and the national mean ratings. All comments are included verbatim, but they are anonymous. The trainee and their educational supervisor review the results together and agree on strengths, areas for development and an action plan. This entire process is repeated twice every year.

Peer assessment programmes of this type have been used at a number of different institutions. For 30 years, medical students in the obstetrics/gynecology and internal medicine clerkships at the University of Missouri-Kansas have been asked to evaluate the professionalism of their peers.(31) The programme has evolved over the years, but recently most of the negative reports about professional behaviours received by the promotions committee emanated from peers.(32)

Similarly, the University of Florida uses a peer assessment system to identify those medical students whose professionalism is outstanding.(33) The information is included in the Dean's letter of recommendation for postgraduate training, and there are reports that it has enabled some students to acquire a more desirable post.(32)

There is a growing body of evidence supporting the validity of peer assessments. A study of certification in the US by Ramsey *et al.* compared certified internists and non-certified internists who were 5–10 years past certification or training.(34) Several assessments were collected, and the certified doctors had higher peer ratings, even though their peers did not know their certification status. The results were also correlated with written examination performance.

In a follow-up study, Ramsey *et al.* focused only on practising internists who were 5–15 years past certification.(35) Two lists of peers were solicited, one from the participants and one from their medical supervisors. In addition, the questions on the assessment form were divided into two scales, one for cognitive/technical skills and one for professionalism. The source of the peers (participant versus medical supervisor) did not affect the ratings. Further, a written examination had a statistically significant correlation with the cognitive/technical scale but not the professionalism scale.

The mini-PAT is a shortened form of the Sheffield Peer Review Assessment Tool, which was studied with paediatricians.(36) Results of that work indicate that it was feasible, produced scores with reasonable reliability and was not significantly influenced by extraneous factors, such as occupation of assessor, length of working relationship and the clinical setting in which the relationship took place. Moreover, it was able to distinguish between doctors of different grades.

Portfolios

A portfolio is simply a collection of information (methods for the purposes of this chapter) that is intended to demonstrate achievement. However, there are many variations on this simple theme. Portfolios

Please refer to curriculum at www.mmc.nhs.uk for details of expected competencies for F1 and F2

mini-PAT (Peer Assessment Tool) - F1 Version

Please complete the questions using a cross: ☒   Please use black ink and CAPITAL LETTERS

Doctor's   Surname

Forename

GMC Number:

How do you rate this Doctor in their:	Below expectations for F1 completion	Borderline for F1 completion	Meets expectations for F1 completion	Above expectations for F1 completion		U/C*
	1	2	3	4	5	6	
Good Clinical Care							
1 Ability to diagnose patient problems	☐	☐	☐	☐	☐	☐	☐
2 Ability to formulate appropriate management plans	☐	☐	☐	☐	☐	☐	☐
3 Awareness of their own limitations	☐	☐	☐	☐	☐	☐	☐
4 Ability to respond to psychosocial aspects of illness	☐	☐	☐	☐	☐	☐	☐
5 Appropriate utilisation of resources e.g. ordering investigations	☐	☐	☐	☐	☐	☐	☐
Maintaining good medical practice							
6 Ability to manage time effectively / prioritise	☐	☐	☐	☐	☐	☐	☐
7 Technical skills (appropriate to current practice)	☐	☐	☐	☐	☐	☐	☐
Teaching and Training, Appraising and Assessing							
8 Willingness and effectiveness when teaching/training colleagues	☐	☐	☐	☐	☐	☐	☐
Relationship with Patients							
9 Communication with patients	☐	☐	☐	☐	☐	☐	☐
10 Communication with carers and/or family	☐	☐	☐	☐	☐	☐	☐
11 Respect for patients and their right to confidentiality	☐	☐	☐	☐	☐	☐	☐
Working with colleagues							
12 Verbal communication with colleagues	☐	☐	☐	☐	☐	☐	☐
13 Written communication with colleagues	☐	☐	☐	☐	☐	☐	☐
14 Ability to recognise and value the contribution of others	☐	☐	☐	☐	☐	☐	☐
15 Accessibility/Reliability	☐	☐	☐	☐	☐	☐	☐
16 Overall, how do you rate this doctor compared to a doctor ready to complete F1 training?	☐	☐	☐	☐	☐	☐	☐

Do you have any concerns about this doctor's probity or health?   ☐ Yes   ☐ No
If yes please state your concerns:

*U/C Please mark this if you have not observed the behaviour and therefore feel unable to comment.   6927534062

Figure 16.4 The mini-PAT questionnaire.

can include a number of different types of information, both single encounter and routine performance. For example, they can contain a summary of educational experiences (e.g. a procedure log or participation in continuing medical education), reflection on those experiences, research papers, critical incidents, mini-CEX results or scores on a written examination. In some instances, the content of the portfolio is left wholly to the trainee, while in others they must all include exactly the same information. Typically, the portfolio is reviewed by assessors, who are asked to make judgements about it.

There is a portfolio as part of the Foundation Programme, and it has five sections.(13) In the first section, trainees need to include a plan for the development of their portfolio. The second section contains the completed and signed forms that mark their progress through each placement. The third section is voluntary and is designed to encourage reflection on workplace experiences and self-appraisal. The fourth section documents that all of the assessments described above have been completed. The final section is a signoff, which officially documents that all the requirements of the Foundation year have been satisfactorily completed (i.e. the nature of the judgement is occurrence or whether the first four sections of the portfolio are complete).

Because portfolios used for different purposes might contain different forms of assessment, it is not reasonable to extrapolate the validity of one portfolio from another. However, it is sensible to extrapolate the validity of the portfolio from the validity of the contents (i.e. mini-CEX, DOPS, CbD, mini-PAT), and in the case of the Foundation Programme there is good evidence in this respect.

Regardless of the particular application, the use of portfolios in assessment requires that one or more experts make judgements about their contents. Applying the framework presented above, these judgements can be made about occurrence (e.g. whether a trainee has had the required number of mini-CEX encounters), quality (e.g. whether the mini-CEX results indicated good performance) and fitness (e.g. whether the mini-CEX results indicated satisfactory completion of a year of training). There are several factors that will contribute to the quality of these judgements, and they are similar to those for all assessments based on observation.

First, the purpose of the portfolio must be clear (e.g. it is intended for summative use). Second, it is important to be specific about what each portfolio must contain and to have as much commonality across them as possible; this enhances the ability to make comparisons both among trainees and against standards. Third, the portfolios should be based on as many independent assessments of performance as is feasible. This is equivalent to having a number of different encounters in the mini-CEX or DOPS. Fourth, several examiners should be involved in making judgements about each portfolio; this reduces the effects of examiners who differ significantly in stringency. Portfolio-based learning and assessment is covered in more detail in Chapter 7 of this book.

Influence on Learning

The workplace offers a rich environment for assessment, and the observational methods described above can be of considerable use in this regard. It is perhaps more important, however, that several of them offer the opportunity for formative assessment and feedback at the same time. Unfortunately, there are data suggesting that a sizeable majority of postgraduate trainees are never observed in a patient encounter.(15) Not only do the methods described above require that observation, but in addition to summative assessment, the observations are intended to serve as a basis for formative assessment and educational feedback (see Chapter 18).

Holmboe *et al.* have developed an excellent programme for providing feedback, which has been incorporated into the Foundation Programme.(43) At the completion of the assessment process, the observers need to provide an evaluation of the trainees' strengths and weaknesses while enabling them to react to these. Faculty members then need to encourage self-assessment and develop action plans that will enable the trainees to address any deficiencies. These components are documented on the mini-CEX, DOPS and CbD forms used as part of the Foundation Programme. Feedback between the educational supervisor and trainee is also an important part of the mini-PAT.

Faculty Development

Faculty development is one key to the success of workplace assessment based on observation. Holmboe *et al.* have developed an excellent workshop, which has applicability to a variety of observational methods.(44) It consists of three major pieces. First, there is training in behavioural observation, including knowing what to look for, preparing the trainee and patient and minimising intrusiveness and interference. Second, there is performance dimension training, in which faculty members decide on the dimensions of performance that are important. Finally, there is frame of reference training, where faculty members practise to improve their accuracy and discrimination and reduce differences in stringency.

The workshop consists of didactic mini-lectures, small group and videotape evaluation exercises and practice with standardised trainees and patients. A randomised control trial of this model showed that faculty members who underwent training thought it was excellent, felt more comfortable performing direct observation and were more stringent than the control group faculty members.

In addition to the focus on assessment, faculty development efforts should also be provided for the provision of educational feedback. This goes well beyond the methods presented here, but given the few times trainees are actually observed in their work, workplace-based assessment offers an opportunity that should not be missed.

Challenges for Workplace-based Assessment

For the methods described above, as well as others that are based on observation, there is a series of challenges to the assessment process. Among them are reliability, equivalence, stakes, relationships, the need for other forms of assessment and feasibility.(30)

Reliability

If the same trainee were examined on different occasions with different patients by different assessors, we would want their results to be the same. This is called reliability or reproducibility. In the observation of clinical performance, three major factors affect reliability: the number of encounters observed (both single encounters and routine performance), the number of assessors and the aspects of performance being evaluated.(45)

Seminal work by Elstein *et al.* in the mid-1970s indicated that doctors' performances were case specific; performance on one case only weakly predicted performance on others.(6) This finding has been replicated several times. Consequently, it is important to observe trainees with a number of different patients before having confidence in the results of their assessment. All of the methods used in the Foundation Programme require multiple encounters with patients.

Likewise, there is research showing that experienced assessors, even when observing exactly the same encounter, differ in their opinions about its difficulty and quality.(46) More importantly, they interact with each encounter along the lines of their own strengths, weaknesses and experiences. Consequently, it is important to include assessments from different faculty members to achieve reliable results. Again, all of the methods used in the Foundation Programme require multiple observers and a different assessor for each different encounter.

Finally, there is research indicating that more reliable results are obtained when assessors are asked to judge a number of aspects of a performance rather than making a single overall judgement about it.(35) At the same time, asking for too many judgements does little to improve reliability and adversely affects feasibility. The exact number will, of course, vary with the characteristics of the performance and the nature

of the judgements being made (more for quality and fitness, less for occurrence), but generally 5–10 questions should be sufficient.

Some factors, such as the exact wording of the questions and the number of points on the scale, have only a very modest influence on reliability. But because these things are obvious and easy to change, some users spend considerable effort on them. Assuming that reasonable care has been taken, this effort would better be spent recruiting and training assessors or observing additional encounters.

Equivalence

An important issue in the use of observational methods is whether the assessments of trainees are equivalent to one another. In most of the methods described above, different patients or their records serve as the basis for assessment, and these may differ in complexity. Likewise, different faculty members and different peers act as assessors for the trainees, and they are not equally stringent. In portfolios that do not have strict requirements for what is included, there is considerable variability in the basis for assessment. As a consequence, it is not clear whether trainee differences are due to their ability or to the difficulty of the encounters and assessors that trainees face.

This is less of a problem within each training programme, where presumably the assessors and clinical settings are similar. It is also less troublesome when the stakes are lower and there is an emphasis on feedback and formative assessment. However, the observational assessments of the type described above do not yield comparable scores at the regional or national level because faculties can differ appreciably, as do the clinical settings for training. Using a common problem list, involving a number of assessors for each trainee and providing good faculty development will lessen the impact of these problems, but they remain significant.

Stakes

Although it has not been studied extensively, there is some evidence to indicate that assessments based on observation are influenced by what is at stake. Certainly, authors have found that when used for an important purpose (e.g. promotion, continued certification), grades tend to be very high and very few trainees are considered unsatisfactory.(47–49) Although it is possible that doctors in these studies are well above average, it is more likely that peers and faculty members are reluctant to provide negative assessments when the stakes are moderate or high.

There is no way to avoid this problem completely, but there are some things that will lessen its effect. The use of external examiners reduces the amount of prior information available and lessens the assessors' personal stake in the trainee. For both external assessors and internal assessors, faculty development is important and has been shown to increase the stringency of the grades they provide.(43) For peer assessment, anonymity is crucial. Where appropriate, it is also helpful to restrict the nature of the judgements to occurrence or quality rather than fitness. The latter requires a high-stakes decision, and these are often better made using other faculty members and other methods.(50)

Relationships

The relationship between trainees and their observers can adversely affect the validity of the assessments. In the Foundation Programme, these effects might be exacerbated by the fact that trainees choose their assessors.(13) In addition, when assessors are faculty members, their role as educator is in conflict with their role as evaluator. Likewise, the relationships between the trainee and the peers who complete the questionnaires are varied and might influence the results.

Although there is no way to avoid the effects of relationships, there are some steps that might decrease their influence. Where feasible, using external assessors reduces some of the concerns. Similarly, ensuring anonymity in the context of peer assessment is important. It may also be useful if the assessor selects the trainee, the patients and the peers rather than having them chosen by the trainee. However, the effect of self-selection of assessors versus selection by others did not make a difference when studied by Ramsey *et al.*(35)

The need for other forms of assessment

Observation in the workplace constitutes a powerful tool for assessment and feedback. However, it does not serve all purposes, and other forms of assessment are better suited to some functions. For example, differences in assessors and clinical material make it unwise to compare trainees regionally or nationally. Consequently, assessment based on observation in the workplace should not be the sole basis on which to rank trainees and select them for additional educational experiences. Likewise, this form of assessment alone is not suitable for making high-stakes end-of-training decisions such as those for certification in the US. In both instances, assessment based on observation in the workplace needs to be supplemented with a national programme that includes tests of knowledge and clinical skill.

In addition to national ranking and achievement testing, observation in the workplace is best suited to an assessment of integrated skills in the context of patient care. Where problem trainees are identified, this form of assessment is neither ideal nor efficient in determining relative areas of strength and weakness. For diagnostic purposes, it is best to follow with assessments of medical knowledge and clinical skill.

Feasibility

There are significant resource constraints in the workplace setting, and the methods described here were designed to be as efficient as possible given this context. Nonetheless, there remain serious challenges to carrying out this form of assessment. Clearly, the centralisation of functions, such as collecting and reporting data for the mini-PAT, significantly enhances the feasibility of the method. Likewise, a national programme of faculty development is useful.

Despite these efficiencies, local administration strategies are still needed. In the case of the Foundation Programme, trainees are given responsibility for ensuring that the assessments are completed.(13) This is effective but creates challenges based on the assessor–trainee relationship. In the US, the assessors have chosen the trainee and patient, but enlisting the cooperation of busy clinician-educators is difficult. This is an area that requires more attention to ensure the validity and feasibility of the methods.

Summary

Assessment in the setting of clinical training, particularly postgraduate training, is not as well developed as assessment in the undergraduate arena. Over the past decade, several methods based on the observation of routine trainee–patient encounters and interactions with colleagues have been proposed. The Foundation Programme in the UK has assembled the best of these methods and applied them in the setting of postgraduate training.

The mini-CEX, DOPS and CbD are based on the observation of a single performance with a patient or a medical record, while the mini-PAT captures routine performance. In all instances, judgements about the quality and fitness of the performance(s) are made by assessor(s), and there is considerable research supporting the validity of these methods.

The opportunity for educational feedback as part of these methods is as important as their contribution to the assessment process. At the completion of each assessment, the observers need to provide an evaluation of the trainees' strengths and weaknesses while enabling them to react to these. Faculty members then need to encourage self-assessment and develop action plans, which will enable the trainees to address any deficiencies. In a sense, the methods bring together summative and formative assessment and create a teaching moment that skilled faculty members can grasp.

A portfolio is a collection of a variety of different assessments and experiences. Because of the variability in their contents, it is not reasonable to generalise from studies of the validity of one portfolio to another. However, in the case of the Foundation Programme, it is possible to extrapolate the validity of the portfolio from the validity of the contents (i.e. mini-CEX, DOPS, CbD, mini-PAT).

Faculty development is a key to the successful use of these methods. A model workshop would consist of training in behavioural observation, performance dimension training and frame of reference training, along with considerable practice. Periodic but shorter versions of the workshop are needed to maintain faculty involvement and proficiency. In addition, the provision of educational feedback should be an important part of the overall faculty development effort.

Finally, a series of challenges remains, including reliability, equivalence, stakes, relationships, the need for other forms of assessment and feasibility. Given the nature of the methods, some (e.g. equivalence) will be very difficult to surmount. Consequently, it will be important to deploy these methods appropriately and to ensure that they are only one piece of a larger assessment programme.

Acknowledgements

The Foundation Programme assessment examples are reproduced here with grateful acknowledgement to the North American Board of Internal Medicine (mini-CEX), the Federation of Royal Colleges of Physicians (DOPS), the American Board of Emergency Medicine (CBD) and the University of Sheffield (mini-PAT). Further information can be found at http://www.mmc.nhs.uk/.

References

1 Norman GR (2002) Research in medical education: three decades of progress. *British Medical Journal.* **324**: 1560–2.

2 Norcini JJ (2005) Current perspectives in assessment: the assessment of performance at work. *Medical Education.* **39**: 880–9.

3 Miller GE (1990) The assessment of clinical skills/competence/performance. *Academic Medicine.* **65**(9): s63–7.

4 Norcini JJ (2003) Peer assessment of competence. *Medical Education.* **37**: 539–43.

5 Norcini JJ (2006) Faculty observations of student professional behaviour. In: Stern D (ed.) *Measuring Professionalism,* pp. 147–58. Oxford University Press, Oxford.

6 Elstein AS, Shulman LS and Sprafka SA (1978) *Medical Problem-solving: an analysis of clinical reasoning.* Harvard University Press, Cambridge, MA.

7 Pulito AR, Donnelly MB, Plymale M and Mentzer Jr RM (2006) What do faculty observe of medical students' clinical performance? *Teaching and Learning in Medicine.* **18**(2): 99–104.

8 Silber CG, Nasca TJ, Paskin DL et al. (2004) Do global rating forms enable program directors to assess the ACGME competencies? *Academic Medicine.* **79**(6): 549–56.

9 Martin JA, Regehr G, Reznick R et al. (1997) Objective structured assessment of technical skill (OSATS) for surgical residents. *British Journal of Surgery.* **84**(2): 273–8.

10 Norcini JJ and Boulet JR (2003) Methodological issues in the use of standardized patients for assessment. *Teaching and Learning in Medicine.* **15**(4): 293–7.

11 Brennan RL (2001) *Generalizability Theory.* Springer-Verlag, New York.

12 Norcini JJ, Blank LL, Duffy FD and Fortna G (2003) The mini-CEX: a method for assessing clinical skills. *Annals of Internal Medicine.* **138**: 476–81.

13 National Health Service. Modernising Medical Careers: Foundation Programmes (http://www.mmc.nhs.uk/pages/foundation; accessed 28 September 2006).

14 Norcini JJ, Blank LL, Arnold GK and Kimball HR (1995) The mini-CEX (clinical evaluation exercise): a preliminary investigation. *Annals of Internal Medicine.* **123**: 795–9.

15 Day SC, Grosso LG, Norcini JJ et al. (1990) Residents' perceptions of evaluation procedures used by their training program. *Journal of General Internal Medicine.* **5**: 421–6.

16 Kogan JR, Bellini LM and Shea JA (2003) Feasibility, reliability, and validity of the mini-clinical evaluation exercise (mCEX) in a medicine core clerkship. *Academic Medicine.* **78**(s10): S33–5.

17 Durning SJ, Cation LJ, Markert RJ and Pangaor LN (2002) Assessing the reliability and validity of the mini-clinical evaluation exercise for internal medicine residency training. *Academic Medicine.* **77**(9): 900–4.

18 Boulet JR, McKinley DW, Norcini JJ and Whelan GP (2002) Assessing the comparability of standardized patient and physician evaluations of clinical skills. *Advances in Health Sciences Education.* **7**: 85–97.

19 Holmboe ES, Huot S, Chung J et al. Construct validity of the miniClinical Evaluation Exercise (miniCEX). *Academic Medicine.* **78**: 826–30.

20 Cruess R, McIlroy JH, Cruess S et al. (2006) The professionalism mini-evaluation exercise: a preliminary investigation. *Academic Medicine.* **81**(s10): S74–8.

21 Hatala R, Ainslie M, Kassen BO et al. (2006) Assessing the mini-clinical evaluation exercise in comparison to a national specialty examination. *Medical Education.* **40**(10): 950–6.

22 Kogan JR and Hauer KE (2006) Brief report: use of the mini-clinical evaluation exercise in internal medicine core clerkships. *Journal of General Internal Medicine.* **21**(5): 501–2.

23 Wragg A, Wade W, Fuller G et al. (2003) Assessing the performance of specialist registrars. *Clinical Medicine.* **3**(2): 131–4.

24 Larson JL, Williams RG, Ketchum J et al. (2005) Feasibility, reliability and validity of an operative performance rating system for evaluating surgery residents. *Surgery.* **138**(4): 640–7.

25 Goff BA, Nielsen PE, Lentz GM et al. (2002) Surgical skills assessment: a blinded examination of obstetrics and gynecology residents. *American Journal of Obstetrics and Gynecology.* **186**(4): 613–17.

26 Winckel CP, Reznick RK, Cohen R and Taylor B (1994) Reliability and construct validity of a structured technical skills assessment form. *American Journal of Surgery.* **167**(4): 423–7.

27 Maatsch JL, Huang R, Downing S and Barker B (1983) *Predictive validity of medical specialty examinations.* Final report for Grant HS 02038-04, National Center of Health Services Research. Office of Medical Education and Research and development, Michigan State University, East Lansing, MI.

28 Norman GR, Davis D, Painvin A et al. (1989) Comprehensive assessment of clinical competence of family/general physicians using multiple measures. In: *Proceedings of the Annual Conference on Research in Medical Education,* pp. 75–9. Association of American Medical Colleges, Washington, DC.

29 Solomon DJ, Reinhart MA, Bridgham RG et al. (1990) An assessment of an oral examination format for evaluating clinical competence in emergency medicine. *Academic Medicine.* **65**(s9): S43–4.

30 Norcini JJ (2003) Peer assessment of competence. *Medical Education*. **37**: 539–43.

31 Arnold L, Willoughby L, Calkins V and Eberhart G (1981) Use of peer evaluation in the assessment of medical students. *Medical Education*. **56**: 35–42.

32 Arnold L and Stern D (2006) Content and context of peer assessment. In: Stern D (ed.) *Measuring Professionalism*, pp. 175–94. Oxford University Press, Oxford.

33 Small PA, Stevens B and Duerson MC (1993) Issues in medical education: basic problems and potential solutions. *Academic Medicine*. **68**: S89–98.

34 Ramsey PG, Carline JD, Inui TS *et al*. (1989) Predictive validity of certification by the American Board of Internal Medicine. *Annals of Internal Medicine*. **110**(9): 719–26.

35 Ramsey PG, Wenrich MD, Carline JD *et al*. (1993) Use of peer ratings to evaluate physician performance. *Journal of the American Medical Association*. **269**: 1655–60.

36 Archer JC, Norcini JJ and Davies HA (2005) Peer review of paediatricians in training using SPRAT. *British Medical Journal*. **330**: 1251–3.

37 Martin JA, Reznick RK, Rothman A *et al*. (1996) Who should rate candidates in an objective structured clinical examination? *Academic Medicine*. **71**(2): 170–5.

38 Hodges B, McNaughton N, Regehr G *et al*. (2002) The challenge of creating new OSCE measures to capture the characteristics of expertise. *Medical Education*. **36**(8): 742–8.

39 Hodges B, Regehr G, McNaughton N *et al*. (1999) OSCE checklists do not capture increasing levels of expertise. *Academic Medicine*. **74**(10): 1129–34.

40 Rothman AI, Blackmore D, Dauphinee WD and Reznick R (1997) The use of global ratings in OSCE station scores. *Advances in Health Sciences Education*. **1**: 215–19.

41 Regehr G, MacRae H, Reznick RK and Szalay D (1998) Comparing the psychometric properties of checklists and global rating scales for assessing performance on an OSCE-format examination. *Academic Medicine*. **73**(9): 993–7.

42 Regehr G, Freeman R, Robb A *et al*. (1999) OSCE performance evaluations made by standardized patients: comparing checklist and global rating scores. *Academic Medicine*. **74**(s10): S135–7.

43 Holmboe ES, Yepes M, Williams F and Huot SJ (2004) Feedback and the mini clinical evaluation exercise. *Journal of General Internal Medicine*. **19**(5 Pt 2): 558–61.

44 Holmboe ES, Hawkins RE and Huot SJ (2004) Effects of training in direct observation of medical residents' clinical competence: a randomized trial. *Annals of Internal Medicine*. **140**(11): 874–81.

45 Norcini JJ (2001) The validity of long cases. *Medical Education*. **35**: 735–6.

46 Noel GL, Herbers JE, Caplow MP *et al*. (1992) How well do internal medicine faculty members evaluate the clinical skills of residents? *Annals of Internal Medicine*. **117**: 757–65.

47 Hay JA (1995) Tutorial reports and ratings. *Evaluation Methods: a resource handbook*. McMaster University, Hamilton, Ontario.

48 Ramsey PG, Carline JD, Blank LL and Wenrich MD (1996) Feasibility of hospital-based use of peer ratings to evaluate the performance of practicing physicians. *Academic Medicine*. **71**: 364–70.

49 Hall W, Violato C, Lewkonia R *et al*. (1999) Assessment of physician performance in Alberta: the physician achievement review. *Canadian Medical Association Journal*. **161**: 52–7.

50 Norcini JJ (2005) Standard setting. In: Dent JA and Harden RM (eds) *A Practical Guide for Medical Teachers*, pp. 293–301. Elsevier Churchill Livingston, Edinburgh.

Structured assessments of clinical competence

Katharine AM Boursicot, Trudie E Roberts and William P Burdick

KEY MESSAGES

- Objective Structure Clinical Examinations (OCSEs) have become widespread in the assessment of clinical competence.

- OSCEs should be blueprinted to the learning outcomes of the course and curriculum.

- Training of simulated patients and examiners is essential for high levels of consistency.

- Developing high-quality OSCE stations takes time and effort.

- Authenticity is important in enhancing the validity of the test.

- OSCEs are often complex and costly to run, but they are a fair and reliable method of assessing clinical skills.

- Future developments of OSCEs are likely to be in the area of acute medical simulations, which are difficult to test by other means.

Introduction

The reliable and valid assessment of clinical competence has become an increasingly important area of concern in medical education. Various stakeholders, with legitimate interests in the clinical competence of graduates from medical schools and of postgraduate trainees, are requiring evidence that assessments are discriminating between the sufficiently and insufficiently competent at all levels of medical training and education.

While clinical competence is based on a thorough base of specialist medical knowledge,(1) the term *clinical competence* also encompasses other professional practice elements such as history taking and clinical examination skills, skills in practical procedures, doctor–patient communication, problem-solving ability and management skills, relationships with colleagues and ethical behaviour.(2–4)

As it cannot be assessed by written tests, the assessment of clinical competence has historically involved the direct observation of candidates by professional colleagues. With the development of work-based learning methods to assess clinical performance in a more authentic and naturalistic way there is the potential for confusion over terminology. For the purposes of this chapter we will consider assessments of clinical competence to be measures of what doctors can do in controlled representations of professional practice. We will restrict the use of performance assessment to

measurements of what doctors do in their professional practice.(5) In other words, we shall consider competency-based assessments to be those assessments undertaken outside the 'real' clinical environment and performance-based assessment to be those administered within the natural clinical setting.

A variety of formats for assessing clinical competence has been developed over the years and in this extended chapter we review the more 'classic' long- and short-case formats, and also describe newer formats such as the Objective Structure Clinical Examination (OSCE) and Objective Structured Long Case Examination Record (OSLER). We discuss the stages of planning and implementing OSCEs and offer practical advice on blueprinting, station development, examiner training, simulated/standardised patient training, organisational issues and standard setting. We do not discuss workplace-based assessment instruments as these are covered comprehensively in Chapter 16.

The Long Case

In the traditional long case, candidates spend one hour with a patient, during which they are expected to take a full formal history and perform a complete examination. The candidate is not observed. On completion of this task the candidate is questioned for 20–30 minutes about the case, usually by a pair of examiners, and is occasionally taken back to the patient to demonstrate clinical signs.

Holistic appraisal of the examinee's ability to interact, assess and manage a real patient is a laudable goal of the long case. However, in recent years there has

Understanding Medical Education: Evidence, Theory and Practice.
Edited by T Swanwick. © 2010 Association for the Study of Medical Education.

been much criticism of this approach, related to issues of reliability pertaining to examiner, examinee and patient factors.(6) The lack of measurement consistency caused by examiner bias and variations in examiner stringency is a major argument against the long case. Reliability is further compromised when there is little prior agreement between pairs of examiners as to what constitutes acceptable competence. Unstructured questioning and global marking without anchor statements compounds the problem. Reliability in the long case encounter is also diminished by variability in degree and details of information disclosure by the patient, as well as variability in patients' demeanour, comfort and health. Furthermore, some patients' illnesses may be straightforward, whereas others may be extremely complex. Examinees' clinical skills also vary significantly across tasks (i.e. task or case specificity),(7) so that assessing examinees on one patient may not provide generalisable estimates of a candidate's overall ability.(6,8,9)

While validity of the inferences from a long case examination is one of the strengths of the genre, inferring examinees' true clinical skills in the time-constrained environment of actual clinical practice from a one-hour long case encounter is also debatable. Additionally, given the evidence of the importance of history taking in achieving a diagnosis,(10) and the need for students to demonstrate good patient communication skills, the omission of direct observation in this process is surprising.

Objective Structured Long Case Examination Record

In an effort to address these shortcomings, while at the same time attempting to retain the concept of seeing a 'new' patient in a holistic way, the OSLER was developed by Gleeson in the 1990s.(11)

The OSLER has 10 key features:

- it is a 10-item structured record
- it has a structured approach – there is a prior agreement on what is to be examined
- all candidates are assessed on identical items
- construct validity is recognised and assessed
- history process and product are assessed
- communication skill assessment is emphasised
- case difficulty is identified by the examiner
- it can be used for both criterion- and norm-referenced assessments
- a descriptive mark profile is available where marks are used
- it is a practical assessment with no need for extra time over the ordinary long case.

The OSLER also consists of 10 items, which include four on history, three on physical examination, and three on management and clinical acumen. For any individual item, examiners decide on their overall

grade and mark for the candidate and then discuss this with their co-examiner and agree on a joint grade. This is done for each item and also for the overall grade and final agreed mark. The recommended time allocation for the OSLER examination is 30 minutes.(12)

There is evidence that the OSLER is more reliable than the standard 'long case'.(13) Most recently it has been shown that assessments using structured long cases can be highly reliable (predicted Cronbach's alpha of 0.84),(14) but this did require 10 separate cases and 20 examiners and thus raises issues of practicality.

Short Cases

In addition to the long case described above, students also classically undertook a series of (usually three to six) short cases. In these cases they were taken to a number of patients with widely differing conditions and asked to examine individual systems or areas and give differential diagnoses of their findings, or to demonstrate abnormal clinical signs or produce spot diagnoses. Although in some ways similar to an OSCE in that they provide a wider range of cases on which the examiner is able to base his or her opinion of the student's ability, there are important differences. Different students rarely saw the same set of patients, often cases differed greatly in their complexity and the same two assessors examined the student at each case. These cases were not meant to examine communication skills but instead concentrated on clinical examination skills, with communication with the patients as merely incidental. The examination was not structured and the examiners were free to ask any questions they wanted. Like the long case there was no attempt to standardise the expected level of performance. For all these reasons OSCEs have superseded this type of assessment.

Objective Structured Clinical Examinations

The remainder of this chapter relates to the OSCE, an assessment format in which the candidates rotate sequentially around a series of structured cases located in 'stations', at each of which specific tasks have to be performed. The tasks usually involve a clinical skill, such as history taking, examination of a patient or a practical skill. The marking scheme for each station is structured and determined in advance. There is a time limit for each station, after which the candidates have to move on to the next task.

The basic structure of an OSCE may be varied in the timing for each station, the use of a checklist or rating scale for scoring, the use of a clinician or standardised patient as examiner and the use of real patients or manikins, but the fundamental principle is that every candidate has to complete the same assignments in the same amount of time and is marked according to a structured marking schedule.

The terminology associated with the OSCE format can vary – in the undergraduate area they are more consistently referred to as OSCEs, but in the postgraduate setting a variety of terminology exists. For example, in the UK, the Royal College of Physicians' membership clinical examination is called the Practical Assessment of Clinical Examination Skills (PACES), while the Royal College of General Practitioners' membership examination is called the Clinical Skills Assessment (CSA).

Rationale

The use of OSCEs in the quantitative assessment of competence has become widespread in the field of undergraduate and postgraduate medical education(15–19) since they were originally described,(20) mainly due to the improved reliability of this assessment format. This has resulted in a fairer test of candidates' clinical abilities, since the score has become less dependent on who is examining the candidate and which patient is selected for the encounter. The criteria used to evaluate any assessment method are well described(21) and summarised in Chapter 12. We will examine these criteria – reliability, validity, educational impact, cost-efficiency and acceptability – in some detail, as they relate to OSCE design.

Reliability

Essentially, the OSCE was developed to address the inherent unreliability of classical long and short cases. OSCEs are more reliable than unstructured observations in four main ways.

- Structured marking schedules allow for more consistent scoring by examiners according to predetermined criteria, hence reliability is improved.
- Candidates have to perform a number of different tasks across clinical, practical and communication skill domains – this wider sampling across different cases and skills results in a more reliable picture of a candidate's overall competence. The more stations or cases each candidate has to complete, the more generalisable the test is.
- The reliability of the global test score increases with increasing number and increasing homogeneity of stations or cases. Reliability of sub-scores must be carefully reviewed before reporting.
- As the candidates move through all the stations, each is examined by a number of different examiners, so multiple independent observations are collated. Individual examiner bias is thus attenuated.

It is worth bearing in mind that sampling across different cases makes the most important contribution to reliability; the more stations in an OSCE, the more reliable it will be. However, increasing the number of stations has to be balanced with the practicability of an OSCE exercise. Practically, to enhance reliability it is better to have more stations with one examiner per station than fewer stations with two examiners per station.(22,23)

Validity

Validity assessment asks the question 'What is the degree to which evidence supports the inference(s) made from the test results?' Each separate inference or conclusion from a test may require different supporting evidence. Note that it is the inferences that are validated, not the test itself.(24,25)

Inferences about ability to apply clinical knowledge to bedside data gathering and reasoning, and to effectively use interpersonal skills, are most relevant to the OSCE model. Inferences about knowledge, rather than clinically relevant application of knowledge, or clinical and practical skills, are less well supported by this method.(26)

Types of validity evidence include *content validity* and *construct validity*. Content validity (sometimes referred to as *direct validity*) of an OSCE is determined by how well the sampling of skills matches the learning objectives of the course or degree for which that OSCE is designed.(26,27) The sampling should be representative of the whole testable domain for that examination purpose. The best way to ensure an adequate spread of sampling is to use a *blueprint* method, which we will describe later in the chapter.

Construct validity (sometimes referred to as *indirect validity*) of an OSCE would be the implication that those who performed better at this test had better clinical skills than those who did not perform as well. In an OSCE testing situation, we can only make inferences about a candidate's clinical skills in actual practice, as the OSCE is an artificial situation.

To enhance the validity of inferences from an OSCE, the length of any station should be best fitted to the task to achieve the best authenticity possible. Thus, for example, a station in which blood pressure measurement is tested would authentically be achieved in five minutes, whereas taking a history of chest pain or examining the neurological status of a patient's legs would be more authentically achievable in 10 minutes.(28)

Educational impact

The impact on students' learning resulting from a testing process is sometimes referred to as *consequential validity*. The design of an assessment system can reinforce or augment learning, or undermine learning(29,30): it is a well-recognised phenomenon that students focus on their assessments rather than the learning objectives of the course. Explicit, clear learning objectives allied with clinical skills assessment content and format can be a very effective way of encouraging students to learn the desired clinical competencies. Objectives that include action verbs like 'demonstrate' or 'perform', which are then linked to OSCEs that measure ability to demonstrate or perform certain skills, will encourage students to practise these skills. By contrast, an assessment system that measures students' ability to answer multiple-choice questions about clinical skills will encourage students to focus on knowledge acquisition. Neither approach is wrong – they simply demonstrate that assessment drives education and that assessment methods need to be thoughtfully applied. There is a danger in using detailed checklists as this may encourage students to memorise the steps in a checklist rather than learn and practise the skill. Rating scale marking schedules encourage students to learn and practise skills more holistically.

OSCEs may be used for formative or summative assessment. When teaching and improvement are a major goal of an OSCE, time should be built into the schedule at the end of each station to allow the examiner to give feedback to the student on their performance, providing a very powerful opportunity for student learning. For summative certification examinations, expected competencies should be clearly communicated to the candidates so they have the opportunity to learn the skills prior to taking such examinations.

Cost-efficiency

OSCEs can be very complex to organise. They require meticulous and detailed forward planning, and engagement of considerable numbers of examiners, real patients, simulated patients, and administrative and technical staff to prepare the circuits and station materials and manage the examination. It is therefore most cost-effective to use OSCEs to test clinical competencies and not knowledge, which can be tested more efficiently in a different examination format. Effective implementation of OSCEs requires thoughtful deployment of resources, with attention to production of examination material, timing of sittings, suitability of facilities, catering, and collating and processing of results. Other critical logistics include examiner and standardised patient recruitment and training. This is possible even in resource-limited environments.(31)

Acceptability

The increased reliability of the OSCE format over other formats of clinical testing and its perceived fairness by candidates has helped to engender the widespread acceptability of OSCEs among test takers and testing bodies.

Since Harden's original description in 1979,(20) the use of OSCEs has become widespread in the undergraduate level of testing of clinical competence,(17,18,32,33) as well as increasingly in postgraduate assessment.(16–19,34–39) More recently, OSCEs have been used to replace traditional interviews in recruitment processes in both undergraduate and postgraduate settings.(40,41) For example, for recruitment to general practice training schemes in the UK, candidates go through an OSCE format of scenarios in assessment centres where different exercises are assessed by trained assessors, who observe various job-related competencies, including communication skills, team involvement and problem-solving ability.

In North America, clinical skills assessment has been accepted on a massive scale. In 1992, the Medical Council of Canada (MCC) added a standardised patient component to its national licensing examination because of the perception that important competencies expected of licensed physicians were not being assessed.(40) Since inception, approximately 2500 candidates per year have been tested at multiple sites at fixed periods of time during the year throughout Canada. The MCC clinical skills examination uses physicians at each station to score the encounter.

In the US, the Educational Commission for Foreign Medical Graduates (ECFMG) instituted a performance-based examination in 1998 to assess bedside data gathering, clinical reasoning, interpersonal skills and spoken English communication skills of foreign medical graduates seeking to enter residency training programmes. From 1998 to 2004, when it was incorporated into the United States Medical Licensing Examination (USMLE), there were 43642 administrations, including 37930 first-time takers, making it the largest high-stakes clinical skills examination in the world at the time.(42) A single test centre was used until 2001, when examinees were randomised to two centres.

The 11 scored encounters had a standardised format, with each requiring the candidate to elicit a medical history, perform a physical examination, communicate in spoken English with a patient in a clinical setting and generate a written record of the encounter. In each station, the candidate encountered a unique standardised patient – a lay person recruited and trained to give a realistic portrayal of a patient with a standardised medical and psychosocial history, and standardised findings on physical examination. Each case had a case-specific checklist containing the elements of medical history and physical examination considered pertinent to that particular case. Simulated patients were trained to recognise appropriate queries and/or physical examination manoeuvres, including acceptable equivalents or variants, and to document each checklist item achieved by the candidate. Simulated patients also evaluated each candidate's interpersonal skills and spoken English proficiency. After each encounter, the candidate generated a patient note on which the pertinent positive and negative elements of history and physical examination were recorded, a differential diagnosis constructed and a diagnostic work-up plan proposed. Performance was evaluated by averaging scores across all encounters and determining the mean for the integrated clinical encounter (data gathering combined with the patient note score) and communication (interpersonal skills and spoken English). Generalisability coefficients for the two conjunctively scored components of CSA were approximately 0.70–0.90.(43)

In 2004, the USMLE adopted the ECFMG clinical skills assessment model and began testing all US medical graduates in addition to foreign medical graduates seeking ECFMG certification.(44) The two-centre model of the ECFMG examination was expanded to five centres, with additional computer and standardised patient training infrastructure added to ensure comparability across all centres.

The USMLE Step 2 (Clinical Skills) uses 12 standardised patient encounters, each 15 minutes in length followed by 10 minutes to write a patient note. As in the ECFMG CSA examination, standardised patients document the items asked in the history and performed in the physical examination to specified criteria, and evaluate interpersonal skills and spoken English skills, while physician raters score the patient note. Approximately 35 000 administrations take place each year.

OSCE Design

We turn now to the elements of good OSCE design, which are summarised in Box 17.1.

Blueprinting

For any particular OSCE, the content, that is, clinical tasks chosen for the stations, should map onto the learning objectives of the course and the candidates' level of learning. It is only reasonable to test candidates on what they have been taught.(27)

To map the assessment to the learning objectives, the categories of skill to be tested should be mapped on one axis and the elements of the course being tested should be mapped on the other. Usually in OSCEs,

the skills domains are categorised into clinical examination skills, practical skills and communication skills, which can be further subgrouped into history-taking skills and other doctor–patient/colleague interactions. The subject content of the OSCE will be determined to a certain extent by how the elements of the course are categorised, that is, by subject discipline or systems.

Blueprinting is a powerful tool that helps to focus the OSCE designers on the exact nature of what they wish to test and relate this to the teaching. Once this blueprint or framework for an OSCE is agreed, the individual stations can be planned and classified according to this blueprint. This ensures adequate sampling across subject area and skill, in terms of numbers of stations covering each skill and the spread over the subjects/systems of the course being tested.

The feasibility of testing a particular task also needs to be considered. Real patients with clinical signs can be used to test clinical examination skills, while simulated patients are best for testing communication skills. Simulated patients can also simulate a number of clinical signs (e.g. loss of visual field, localised abdominal pain). Healthy volunteers can be used when testing the technical process of a clinical examination. There are many manikins on the market for testing invasive practical skills, for example, intravenous cannulation, urethral catheterisation and arterial blood gas sampling.

It is essential to use a blueprint to plan the content of an OSCE as this helps to ensure that different domains of skill are tested equitably and that the balance of subject areas tested is fairly decided. An example is provided in Box 17.2.

Station development

It is important to write out station specifications well in advance of the examination date so the stations can be reviewed and trialled prior to the actual assessment. Sometimes stations that seem like a good idea at the time of writing may turn out to be unfeasible in practice. When writing a station specification, the following sections should be considered.

- *Construct:* a statement of what that station is supposedly testing, for example, this station tests the candidate's ability to examine the peripheral vascular system.
- *Clear instructions for the candidate:* to inform the candidate exactly what task they should perform in that station.
- *Clear instructions for the examiners:* including a copy of the candidate instructions, to assist the examiner at that station to understand his or her role and conduct the station properly.
- *List of equipment required.*
- *Personnel requirements:* whether the station requires a real patient or a simulated patient and the

---

BOX 17.1 Elements of Objective Structure Clinical Examination design

Blueprinting: ensuring the test content maps across the learning objectives of the course.

Station development and piloting: writing stations that function well.

Examiner training: engaging examiners, ensuring consistency of marking contributes to reliability.

Simulated patient training: consistent performance ensures each candidate is presented with the same challenge.

Organisation: making detailed plans well in advance. *Be prepared!*

BOX 17.2 Example of a system-based blueprint

	History	Explanation	Examination	Procedures
Cardiovascular	Chest pain	Discharge drugs	Cardiac	BP
Respiratory	Haemoptysis		Respiratory	Peak flow
Gastrointestinal	Abdominal pain	Gastroscopy	Abdominal	PR
Reproductive	Amenorrhoea	Abnormal smear	Cervical smear	
Nervous	Headache		Eyes	Ophthalmoscopy
Musculoskeletal	Backache		Hip	
Generic	Pre-op assessment	Consent for post-mortem		IV cannulation

details of such individuals (e.g. age, gender, ethnicity).

- *Simulated patient scenario:* if the station requires a particular role to be played.
- *Marking schedule:* this should include the important aspects of the skill being tested, a marking scheme for each item and how long the station should last. The marking schedule may be either a checklist or a rating scale as there is good evidence that despite the apparent objectivity of structured checklists, global rating scales have been shown to be equally as realible (*see* Box 16.2). Items can be grouped into the broad categories of process skills, content skills and clinical management skills.

Process skills

For clinical examination stations with a real patient or simulated patient, these could include introduction and orientation, rapport, professional manner and communicating with the patient appropriately during examination.

For history-taking stations, these could include introduction and orientation, listening skills, questioning skills, demonstration of empathy and appropriate closure.

For explanation stations, these could include introduction and orientation, rapport, establishing what the patient knows/understands, demonstration of empathy, appropriate organisation of explanation, checking the patient's understanding and using clear language, avoiding jargon.

Content skills

Appropriate technical steps or aspects of the task or skill being tested.

Clinical management skills

It may be appropriate to ask the candidate some set questions in relation to the specific case.

Figures 17.1 and 17.2 provide examples illustrating the checklist and rating scale marking schedules, respectively.

Piloting

Ideally, stations should be piloted before they are used in examinations to ensure that all stations are functional in terms of the following.

- *Timing:* can the candidates realistically perform the task in the time allotted?
- *Difficulty:* how difficult is the station?
- *Equipment:* is all the equipment required available and on the list?
- *Is an additional helper required* to assist the examiner, for example, catheterisation, suturing stations?
- *Candidate instructions:* do the instructions tell the candidate exactly what the task is?
- *Examiner instructions:* do the instructions tell the examiner how to conduct the station? Does the examiner know what the candidate has been told to do?
- *Real patient specifications:* are the medical conditions specified?
- *Simulated patient scenario:* is the age/gender/ethnicity specified? Is there enough information for the simulated patient to learn and play the part effectively?
- *Construct validity:* is the station testing what it is meant to test? Does the marking schedule reflect the elements of the task appropriately?

Simulated patient training

For consistent performances, particularly in communication skills stations, it is best to use well-trained simulated patients. Depending on location, it may be possible to organise a database of actors who assist in the teaching as well as assessment of communication skills. It is desirable to have people across a range of ages and ethnicities as well as a balanced gender mix. Training and monitoring simulated patients is essential to ensure consistent performance – a significant factor in the reliability of the examination. The simulated patients should be sent their scenarios in advance and then asked to go through their roles with other simulated patients playing the same role, while being supervised by a communication skills teacher

THIS IS A 10-MINUTE STATION	Good	Adequate	Not done/ Inadequate
1 Introduction and orientation (name and role, explains purpose of examination, confirms patient's agreement)	[ ]	[ ]	[ ]
2 Rapport (shows interest, respect and concern, appropriate body language)	[ ]	[ ]	[ ]
3 Appropriately exposes the patient and positions them at 45 degrees		[ ]	[ ]
4 Looks at hands, commenting on peripheral stigmata (i.e. cyanosis, clubbing, splinter haemorrhages)		[ ]	[ ]
5 Checks the radial pulse, commenting on the rate and rhythm		[ ]	[ ]
6 Asks for patient's blood pressure **Examiner please give correct BP**		[ ]	[ ]
7 Looks for central stigmata of cardiovascular disease (i.e. anaemia, central cyanosis, hyperlipidaemia)		[ ]	[ ]
8 Examines the JVP correctly (positions the patient's chin and neck; assesses the waveform in the correct area) and comments on findings		[ ]	[ ]
9 Palpates the carotid or brachial pulses, commenting on the character		[ ]	[ ]
Inspects and palpates the praecordium:			
10 Localises the apex beat, commenting on the position		[ ]	[ ]
11 Examines for RVH		[ ]	[ ]
12 Auscultates in all four cardiac areas		[ ]	[ ]
13 Moves patient to left side and sits patient forward in expiration	[ ]	[ ]	[ ]
14 Comments on heart sounds and times heart sounds against central pulse	[ ]	[ ]	[ ]
15 Comments on any murmurs		[ ]	[ ]
16 Listens to the lung bases		[ ]	[ ]
17 Candidate attempts to assess peripheral pulses **Examiner please stop candidate**		[ ]	[ ]
18 Checks for ankle/sacral oedema		[ ]	[ ]
19 Presents a brief summary and conclusions	[ ]	[ ]	[ ]
20 Communicates with patient appropriately during examination (explains what they are doing, gains patient's cooperation)	[ ]	[ ]	[ ]
21 Examines patient in a professional manner (gentle, watches for pain, maintains dignity and privacy)	[ ]	[ ]	[ ]
22 Closure (thanks patient, leaves patient comfortable)	[ ]	[ ]	[ ]
23 Candidate cleans hands after examination		[ ]	[ ]

Figure 17.1 Example checklist mark sheet for cardiovascular examination.

	Clear fail	Borderline fail	Borderline pass	Clear pass	Excellent
1 **Physical examination:** inspection, pulses, JVP, carotids, palpation of precordium, auscultation of valve areas	□	□	□	□	□
2 **Identification and interpretation of physical signs:** identifies and interprets signs correctly; makes reasonable diagnosis	□	□	□	□	□
3 **Management:** suggests appropriate investigations, treatment and follow-up	□	□	□	□	□

Figure 17.2 Example rating scale mark sheet for cardiovascular examination.

and/or a clinician, to develop the role to a suitable standard.

Examiner training

OSCEs require large numbers of examiners. This can be a strength, as candidates are observed and scored by clinicians, but it is also one of the potential weaknesses of OCSEs, as inconsistency between examiners will reduce the fairness and reliability of an OSCE.

Considerable resources should be devoted to examiner training. In our own institutions we offer structured half-day training sessions. The programme for these events is interactive and very much acknowledges the inherent expertise that experienced clinicians bring to the assessment process. These training sessions cover:

BOX 17.3 Focus on: Simulated patients as assessors

Scoring standardised patient examinations can be done by third-party observers (usually physicians) or by the standardised patients themselves. Physician examiners enhance the validity of the assessment because they can apply holistic judgements and integrate subdomains of sequence, logic and other factors that may be difficult for a non-professional completing a binary checklist to capture. Boulet *et al.*,(45) however, demonstrated that holistic judgements from physician examiners are similar to aggregate scores from trained standardised patients, at least in assessing a general, entry-level physician. Physician evaluator models using holistic scoring models may have greater utility in capturing higher levels of expertise – something that checklist models may not be able to do. Any examiner, whether simulated patient or physician, must be thoroughly trained and then monitored to ensure consistent use of the score scale, since variability diminishes reliability.(46)

Ratings of interpersonal and communication skills provide a unique challenge in determining who is best able to provide the ratings. Although the assessment of doctor–patient communication skills can be accomplished by a physician or other observers, and can be done 'live' or via video-taped reviews, it is unclear whether someone watching the interplay between a doctor and a patient can adequately measure the complex, multidimensional nature of the communication. Many aspects of this communication, especially those that are non-verbal, are best assessed by the patient or the person trained to be the patient.(44)

Spoken English is another domain that might be better scored by non-physicians. The generalisability coefficient of this component of the Educational Commission for Foreign Medical Graduates Clinical Skills Assessment (CSA), scored by standardised patients, was 0.94.(47)

From a logistical and cost perspective, the examinee volume for the CSA and now the United States Medical Licensing Examination Step 2 (CS) (approximately 35 000 per year) makes it effectively impossible to entertain using physician examiners. Cost analysis also needs to account for training time and quality assurance for standardised patients or physician raters as well as the different nature of the training needed by each group. It may also be harder to standardise a large number of highly educated, typically independently thinking physicians across five test centres in a year-round testing model.

Currently in the UK, at both the undergraduate and postgraduate levels, examiners are clinicians or other healthcare professionals. It would probably need a considerable shift in cultural acceptance to move to standardised patients as the sole assessors of clinical competence. The prospect of a national large-scale assessment on the back of recent proposals for revalidation and recertification may give cause for reconsideration.

- principles of OSCEs
- role of examiners (i.e. to assess not to teach, conduct vivas, adhere to marking schedules and respect the role of the simulated patient)
- marking video-recorded OSCE stations, after which we go through the marking with the clinicians and get them to think through their mark allocation
- marking 'live stations' with group members playing the candidate, the assessor and the simulated patient. This demonstrates how stressful this assessment is for the candidate and how difficult it can be to play the part of a good simulated patient
- standard-setting procedure used. This can be crucial when using a student-centred approach, and all the examiners are integral to the standard-setting process. The more the assessors understand their vital role in this process the more likely they are to do it in a satisfactory way. The use of non-clinicians in assessment is discussed in Box 17.3.

Working with real patients

Patients do not always give the same history each time they are asked to repeat it; they can become tired or unwell and they may develop new signs and symptoms to the ones you were told about; they may even lose old clinical findings. However, they can be a most valuable resource and need to be treated as such. Using 'real' patients in OSCEs adds greatly to the validity of the assessment. Ideally, patients should be used to assess the detection of common chronic clinical signs. For each clinical sign assessed you will need several patients and even the most stoical patient should not be expected to be examined by more than 10 students in the course of a day. Ideally, patients should be swapped in and out of the station to allow them to have sufficient rest time.

Practical considerations

The smooth running of OSCEs is highly dependent on the detail of the practical arrangements made in advance and it is worth putting some effort into this to ensure a tolerable day of examinations. There are many aspects to consider.

Prior to the OSCE
Suitable venue

Depending on the number of stations and candidates, more than one circuit may need to be conducted simultaneously. There are advantages (less noise, more privacy for patients) to conducting each station in a separate room (e.g. in an outpatient department), but larger halls divided up with soundproofed partitions can also be suitable. Venues may need to be booked well in advance of examination dates. Appropriate adjacent rooms to the OSCE circuits are required for the gathering of the students, where they can be registered and briefed prior to the examination. Rooms may be required for patients to rest in between each examination. A floor plan of the stations and rests is an invaluable aid to planning.

Recruitment of examiners

Busy clinicians and other teachers will need advance notice to enable them to attend and play the vital role of assessors in each station. It is helpful to send out a grid of dates and times so people can tick the sessions they wish to attend. This is best done by central coordination.

Recruitment of simulated patients

Once the OSCE has been blueprinted, the simulated patients required should be listed and actors contacted to engage them for the dates of the exam.

Running order of the stations

Stations should be numbered to avoid confusion over mark sheets, equipment and people involved. Rest stations should be provided: usually one rest per 40 minutes in a circuit is suitable. If many candidates are sitting the OSCE, running multiple circuits of the same stations enables more candidates to be examined at any one time.

Using stations of different lengths

It is best to group stations of the same length together and run these circuits separately. If there are 5-, 10- and 15-minute stations, then the candidates should be asked to attend on three separate occasions to undertake each circuit. Mixing stations of different timings in one circuit is possible, but can lead to confusion.

A list of all the equipment required

Detailed by station, this is vital for the preparations to be successful. Arrange to go round the circuit the day before the OSCE and check that all the equipment is correctly set up.

Production and processing of mark sheets

Calculate the numbers required for each station and allow extra for spoilage. Allow time for proofreading. If there are a large number of candidates it may be worth looking into using sheets that can be processed by electronically scanning after the OSCE. Alternatively, marking by hand will require the organisation of people to mark and ensure that results are entered correctly.

Liaison with clinical skills centre staff

Close cooperation with clinical skills centre technical and teaching staff is vital in the planning. It is useful

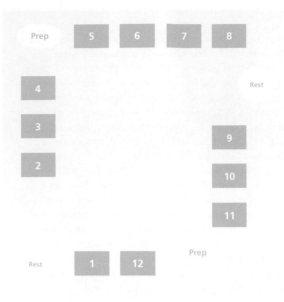

Figure 17.3 Example of a floor plan for an Objective Structure Clinical Examination in a large room.

to draw up a circuit plan to indicate the layout required and for the numbering of the stations to be agreed (*see* Figure 17.3).

On the day of the OSCE

Signs

It is very helpful to have signs indicating the rooms for the students, the patients and the examination, so that people unfamiliar with the venue can find their way easily. All the stations should be numbered on large signs to help candidates follow the circuit successfully.

Timing

An electronic timing programme is the ideal, but a reliable stopwatch and loud manual bell is an acceptable alternative. It is important to ensure that all candidates and examiners can hear the bells so the candidates move onto the next station promptly.

Helpers/marshals

A vital part of the smooth running of OSCEs depends on having a small army of helpers to direct the candidates, examiners, simulated patients and patients to ensure everyone is in the right place at the right time. This should include looking after the welfare of all the people involved on the day.

Catering

Examining, acting, being examined and helping at OSCEs can be tiring and sometimes stressful work. The very least one can do is provide refreshments for all participants – water for the candidates at rest stations, drinks for all other staff and lunch for those who spend the whole day assisting or being examined.

Briefing
It is helpful to gather all candidates in a room where they can be registered and briefed about the practical arrangements for the day. Examiners, even if they have attended a training session, should be reminded about how to score the mark sheets and conduct the stations appropriately, and also to switch off their mobile phones.

After the OSCE
Collection of mark sheets
Collection should be organised meticulously, as missing sheets can be very prejudicial to a candidate's overall score. It is also helpful to check the sheets for completeness of scoring and to ask examiners to check they have completed the sheets before leaving.

Care of patients/simulated patients
A system to ensure that patients have transport to take them home is always appreciated. Arrangements to ensure the simulated patients are paid are also welcome and encourage future participation.

Thank-you letters
Patients, examiners and helpers are much more likely to take part again if they receive acknowledgement of their contribution to the examination process.

Standard setting
Standard setting or establishing the pass mark is critical for determining who passes and who fails any particular assessment of clinical competence. The standard or pass mark indicates the minimum score that every candidate has to reach to pass the OSCE. While it is difficult to quantify a concept as complex as clinical competence, the reality is that examinations such as OSCEs are used to discriminate between those who have sufficient clinical skills and those who do not, for a particular level or purpose.

The fundamental principle underlying all standard-setting methods is to reach a consensus on professional values and standards.(48) There are many standard-setting methods described in the literature,(49–52) but all the traditional ones were developed for multiple-choice questions. It is debatable whether it is appropriate for these methods to be used for complex performance-based examinations such as OSCEs.

Norcini, in his comprehensive review of standard setting,(48) suggests that the Fixed Percentage and Hofstee methods can be applied to OSCEs directly, while Angoff's method can be used in a modified version. The issue for examination setters is whether they are prepared to use either relative methods (Fixed Percentage) or compromise methods (Hofstee) rather

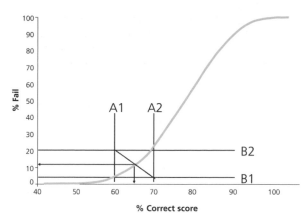

Figure 17.4 Hofstee method of standard setting.

than absolute or criterion-referenced methods (such as Angoff and the Borderline Group methods).

Fixed percentage method
This relative method essentially fixes the percentage of candidates who will pass the examination, usually by discussion among judges on a panel. This method is independent of test content and the clinical competence of the candidates as the standards will vary from one sitting to another, depending on the ability of the group of candidates taking the test. It is best suited when there is a requirement for determining a proportion of the best or worst candidates.

Hofstee method
This is a compromise between relative and absolute standard-setting methods. The judges have to set their minimum (A1) and maximum (A2) acceptable pass marks and their minimum (B1) and maximum (B2) acceptable rates of failing candidates (*see* Figure 17.4). A diagonal line is drawn across the rectangle formed by these four lines and the point at which it intersects with the cumulative performance data of the candidates determines the pass mark. In this example, the pass mark would be 65%. As this method has elements of relative standard setting, it is not the method of choice for high-stakes examinations.

Angoff's method
This criterion-referenced method has been described extensively in the literature(48,52,53) and can be used in two different ways for OSCEs.

Classical Angoff method
The judgements from all the judges on the standard-setting panel are collected for every item on a checklist for every station in the OSCE. The usual process of discussion, iteration and summating the judgements is carried out for every station, yielding a pass mark for each station. This can be a very time-consuming process.

Modified Angoff method

The judgements of all members of the standard-setting panel are made at the level of each station, rather than each checklist item. The usual discussion and summation of judgements is carried out to yield a pass mark for each station.

Borderline group method

In the past 15 years, a method of standard setting has been developed specifically for performance-based examinations such as OSCEs, where a clinician-examiner is present to observe and score the candidates.(54–56) In this method, the examiner at each station completes the checklist scoring as usual but is also asked to allocate a 'global' score, based on his or her overall judgement of how well he or she thinks each candidate has performed at that station.

The global rating scale can be:
- a three-point scale: pass – borderline – fail
- a six-point scale: outstanding – clear pass – borderline pass – borderline fail – poor – inadequate.

Other variants are also possible.

For each station, the scores of all candidates rated as 'borderline' (if using the three-point scale) or all the 'borderline passes' and 'borderline fails' (if using the six-point scale) are extracted and averaged to obtain a pass mark. In this way, a pass mark is generated for each station.

This standard-setting method is very efficient in terms of using the clinician-examiners to set the pass mark and not having to convene a separate panel of judges. It is highly credible, as it utilises the expertise of the examiners in making judgements about professional standards, and collates the judgements over a large number of examiners. It does require some expertise in processing the data, and is more reliable if the examiners are trained,(56) but overall, it has become regarded as the 'gold standard' method of standard setting for OSCEs.(57)

Conclusions

Assessment of clinical competence is a crucial part of the basis on which decisions are made about the ability of clinicians and doctors in training. But any method of assessing clinical skills should be considered in the context of a wider programme of assessment, which should include the assessment of knowledge, clinical examination skills, practical procedure skills, doctor–patient communication, problem-solving ability, management skills and relationships with colleagues, as well as professional attitudes and behaviour.

One of the most important aspects of assessing clinical skills is the range of sampling across a candidate's skill base; this has to be taken into account when designing any assessment. OSCEs can assess clinical, communication and practical skills but are still situated in the context of an examination setting. To assess doctors in the context of their professional practice requires the use of different formats in the workplace.

As workplace-based assessment becomes more widespread, the focus of testing in OSCEs may be directed towards earlier stages of clinical skill acquisition and technical proficiency. Another development might be that OSCEs become more specialised, possibly focusing on acute clinical scenarios, which would be difficult to assess reliably *in vivo*. Complex high-fidelity teamworking scenarios are being developed in some areas and may become more appropriate as interprofessional training in the postgraduate arena becomes more common.

Acknowledgement

Some of the material used in this section has previously been published in an article by one of the authors in *The Clinical Teacher*,(58) and is reproduced here with permission.

References

1 Miller G (1990) The assessment of clinical skills/competence/performance. *Academic Medicine*. **65**(s9): S63–7.
2 General Medical Council (2003) *Tomorrow's Doctors*. London, GMC.
3 General Medical Council (2001) *Good Medical Practice*. London, GMC.
4 Frank JR, Jabbour M and Tugwell P (1996) Skills for the new millennium: report of the Societal Needs Working Group, CanMEDS 2000 Project. *Annals of the Royal College of Physicians and Surgeons of Canada*. **29**: 206–16.
5 Rethans JJ, Norcini JJ, Baron-Maldonado M *et al*. (2002) The relationship between competence and performance: implications for assessing practice performance. *Medical Education*. **36**: 901–9.
6 Norcini JJ (2001) The validity of long cases. *Medical Education*. **35**: 720–1.
7 Swanson DB, Norman GR and Linn RL (1995) Performance based assessment: lessons learned from health professions. *Education Research*. **24**(5): 5–11.
8 Norcini JJ (2002) The death of the long case? *British Medical Journal*. **324**: 408–9.
9 Norcini JJ (2001) Does observation add to the validity of the long case? [letter]. *Medical Education*. **35**: 1131–3.
10 Hampton JR, Harrison MJG, Mitchell JRA *et al*. (1975) Relative contributions of history taking, physical examination and laboratory investigations to diagnosis and management of medical outpatients. *British Medical Journal*. **2**: 486–9.
11 Gleeson FA (1997) Assessment of clinical competence using the objective structured long examination record (OSLER). *Medical Teacher*. **19**: 7–14.
12 Gleeson FA (1994) The effects of immediate feedback on clinical skills using the OSLER. *Proceedings of the Sixth Ottawa Conference in Medical Education*, pp. 412–15.

13 van Thiel J, Kraan HF and van der Vleuten CPM (1991) Reliability and feasibility of measuring medical interviewing skills. The revised Maastricht history and advice checklist. *Medical Education.* **25**: 224–9.

14 Wass V, Jones R and van der Vleuten CPM (2001) Standardized or real patients to test clinical competence? The long case revisited. *Medical Education.* **35**: 321–5.

15 Reznick RK, Blackmore D, Cohen R *et al.* (1993) An objective structured clinical examination for the licentiate of the Medical Council of Canada: from research to reality. *Academic Medicine.* **68**(s10): S4–6.

16 Sloan DA, Donnelly MB, Schwartz RW and Strodel WE (1995) The Objective Structured Clinical Examination. The new gold standard for evaluating postgraduate clinical performance. *Annals of Surgery.* **222**: 735–42.

17 Cohen R, Reznick RK, Taylor BR *et al.* (1990) Reliability and validity of the objective structured clinical examination in assessing surgical residents. *American Journal of Surgery.* **160**: 302–5.

18 Davis MH (2003) OSCE: the Dundee experience. *Medical Teacher.* **25**: 255–61.

19 Newble D (2004) Techniques for measuring clinical competence: objective structured clinical examinations. *Medical Education.* **38**: 199–203.

20 Harden RM and Gleeson FA (1979) Assessment of clinical competence using an Objective Structured Clinical Examination (OSCE). *Medical Education.* **13**: 41–54.

21 van der Vleuten CPM (1996) The assessment of professional competence: developments, research and practical implications. *Advances in Health Science Education.* **1**: 41–67.

22 Swanson DB (1987) A measurement framework for performance-based tests. In: Harvey I and Harden RM (eds) *Further Developments in Assessing Clinical Competence*, pp. 13–45. Can-Heal, Montreal.

23 van der Vleuten CPM and Swanson DB (1990) Assessment of clinical skills with standardized patients: state of the art. *Teaching and Learning in Medicine.* **2**: 58–76.

24 Messick S (1994) The interplay of evidence and consequences in the validation of performance assessments. *Educational Researcher.* **23**(2): 13–23.

25 Downing SM and Haladyna TM (2004) Validity threats: overcoming interference with proposed interpretations of assessment data. *Medical Education.* **38**: 327–33.

26 Downing SM (2003) Validity: on the meaningful interpretation of assessment data. *Medical Education.* **37**: 830–7.

27 Biggs J (1999) *Teaching for Quality Learning at University.* Open University Press and Society for Research into Higher Education, Buckingham.

28 Petrusa E (2002) Clinical performance assessments. In: Norman GR, van der Vleuten CPM and Newble DI (eds) *International Handbook of Research in Medical Education*, pp. 673–709. Kluwer, Dordrecht, Boston and London.

29 Kaufman DM (2003) ABC of learning and teaching in medicine: applying educational theory in practice. *British Medical Journal.* **326**: 213–16.

30 Newble DI and Jaeger K (1983) The effect of assessments and examinations on the learning of medical students. *Medical Education.* **17**: 165–71.

31 Vargas AL, Boulet JR, Errichetti AM, van Zanten M and Lopez MJ (2007) Developing performance-based medical school assessment programs in resource-limited environments. *Medical Teacher.* **29**(2–3): 192–8.

32 Adamo G (2003) Simulated and standardized patients in OSCEs: achievements and challenges 1992–2003. *Medical Teacher.* **25**: 262–70.

33 Newble DI (2004) Techniques for measuring clinical competence: objective structured clinical examinations. *Medical Education.* **38**: 199–203.

34 Townsend AH, McIlvenny S, Miller CJ and Dunn EV (2001) The use of an Objective Structured Clinical Examination (OSCE) for formative and summative assessment in a general practice clinical attachment and its relationship to final medical school examination performance. *Medical Education.* **35**: 841–6.

35 Hodges B (2003) Validity and the OSCE. *Medical Teacher.* **25**: 250–4.

36 Hodges B, Turnbull J, Cohen R *et al.* (1996) Evaluating communication skills in the OSCE format: reliability and generalizability. *Medical Education.* **30**: 38–43.

37 Mavis BE and Henry RC (2002) Between a rock and a hard place: finding a place for the OSCE in medical education. *Medical Education.* **36**: 408–9.

38 Reznick RK, Blackmore D, Dauphinee WD *et al.* (1996) Large-scale high-stakes testing with an OSCE: report from the Medical Council of Canada. *Academic Medicine.* **71**(s1): S19–S21.

39 Rymer AT (2001) The new MRCOG Objective Structured Clinical Examination – the examiners' evaluation. *Journal of Obstetrics and Gynaecology.* **21**: 103–6.

40 Eva KW, Rosenfeld J, Reiter HI and Norman GR (2004) An admissions OSCE: the multiple mini-interview. *Medical Education.* **38**: 314–26.

41 Lane P (2005) Recruitment into training for general practice – the winds of change or a breath of fresh air? *British Medical Journal Career Focus.* **331**: 153.

42 Whelan GP, Boulet JR, McKinley DW *et al.* (2005) Scoring standardized patient examinations: lessons learned from the development and administration of the ECFMG Clinical Skills Assessment (CSA). *Medical Teacher.* **27**: 200–6.

43 Boulet JR, Ben David MF, Ziv A *et al.* (1998) High-stakes examinations: what do we know about measurement?: using standardized patients to assess the interpersonal skills of physicians. *Academic Medicine.* **73**(10): S94–6.

44 Whelan GP, McKinley DW, Boulet JR *et al.* (2001) Validation of the doctor–patient communication component of the Educational Commission for Foreign Medical Graduates Clinical Skills Assessment. *Medical Education.* **35**: 757–61.

45 Boulet JR, McKinley DW, Norcini JJ and Whelan GP (2002) Assessing the comparability of standardized patient and physician evaluations of clinical skills. *Advances in Health Sciences Education, Theory and Practice.* **7**: 85–97.

46 Noel GL, Herbers JE Jr, Caplow MP *et al.* (1992) How well do internal medicine faculty members evaluate the clinical skills of residents? *Annals of Internal Medicine.* **117**: 757–65.

47 Boulet JR, van Zanten M, McKinley DW and Gary NE (2001) Evaluating the spoken English proficiency of graduates of foreign medical schools. *Medical Education.* **35**: 767–73.

48 Norcini JJ (2003) Setting standards on educational tests. *Medical Education.* **37**: 464–9.

49 Norcini JJ and Shea JA (1997) The credibility and comparability of standards. *Applied Measurement in Education.* **10**: 39–59.

50 Livingstone SA and Zeiky MJ (1982) *Passing Scores: a manual for setting standards of performance on educational and occupational tests.* Educational Testing Service, Princeton, NJ.

51 Zeiky MJ (2001) So much has changed. How the setting of cutscores has evolved since the 1980s. In: Cizek GJ (ed.) *Setting Performance Standards: concepts, methods, and perspectives*, pp. 19–52. Lawrence Erlbaum Associates, Mahwah, NJ.

52 Cizek GJ (2001) *Setting Performance Standards: concepts, methods, and perspectives*. Lawrence Erlbaum Associates, Mahwah, NJ.

53 Angoff WH (1971) Scales, norms and equivalent scores. In: Thorndike RL (ed.) *Educational Measurement*, pp. 508–600. American Council on Education, Washington, DC.

54 Cohen R, Rothman AI, Poldre P and Ross J (1991) Validity and generalizability of global ratings in an objective structured clinical examination. *Academic Medicine.* **66**: 545–8.

55 Dauphinee WD, Blackmore DE, Smee SM *et al.* (1997) Using the judgements of physician examiners in setting standards for a national multicentre high stakes OSCE. *Advances in Health Science Education.* **2**: 201–11.

56 Hodges B (2003) Analytic global OSCE ratings are sensitive to level of training. *Medical Education.* **37**: 1012–16.

57 Smee SM and Blackmore DE (2001 Setting standards for an objective structured clinical examination: the borderline group method gains ground on Angoff. *Medical Education.* **35**: 1009–10.

58 Boursicot K and Roberts T (2005) How to set up an OSCE. *The Clinical Teacher.* **2**: 16–20.

Formative assessment

Diana F Wood

KEY MESSAGES

- Formative assessment promotes desirable educational outcomes, including learner self-regulation and the development of lifelong learning skills.

- Students with a high level of self-regulation are more effective learners, showing increased resourcefulness, persistence and success.

- A well-designed programme of formative assessment linked to overall curriculum aims and the teaching and learning goals of individual modules enhances the learning experience for students.

- Effective feedback is central to the process of formative assessment.

- Teachers in medical education identify the development of constructive feedback skills as the most important aspect of their professional development.

- Formative assessment linked to curriculum design should be an essential component of medical education at all levels.

Introduction

Assessment forms a major element of any teaching and learning programme and should be recognised as integral to the whole educational enterprise, not just delivered as an 'add-on' at the end of a course. Traditionally, in medical education, assessment is used to demonstrate that information has been transmitted in some way from the teacher to the learners, the latter memorising notes diligently and reproducing them as necessary in formal examinations requiring factual recall.

One of the most obvious developments in medical education over the past 20 years or so has been a greater understanding of assessment and the way it can be used to enhance both students' learning and the overall quality of the educational experience. At its most pragmatic level, this reflects our recognition that 'assessment drives the curriculum'.[1] Students learn what is needed to pass examinations and use weighting of assessments as a means to rank the importance of various parts of the syllabus. If assessments are developed independently and added on to the teaching programme to test 'what students have learned' (usually by factual recall), then well-meaning attempts to foster deep learning and understanding of a subject will founder.

Furthermore, students expect to be assessed and tend to use grading systems that compare them with their peers as a means of evaluating the amount of work required of them to perform well in the course.[2] This in itself has provided a challenge to many medical educators faced with introducing minimum-competency 'pass–fail' assessments in which students are not ranked against their peers but against pre-set, minimal-competency guidelines.

The key is to align assessment with the educational desires of the faculty and the aims of curriculum planners. In a well-designed curriculum, faculty are aware of their educational goals from the outset and build in the design and timing of assessments to ensure that these goals are addressed by the teaching programme.

This paper predominantly relates to the use of formative assessment in undergraduate medical education. However, the principles described are derived from a variety of sources, including the general educational literature, and can be extrapolated to all levels of medical education. In many cases, formative assessment methods described here can be directly transferred to the postgraduate arena with correction only for the level of the learners in relation to the educational goals.

The paper considers the following areas:
- definitions of formative and summative assessment
- teacher and learner perspectives on formative assessment and the research evidence underpinning them
- the role of feedback in formative assessment, including examples from experiential learning settings in communication skills teaching
- how formative assessment may be used within a curriculum
- examples of formative assessment in different teaching and learning environments.

Understanding Medical Education: Evidence, Theory and Practice.
Edited by T Swanwick. © 2010 Association for the Study of Medical Education.

BOX 18.1 Some functions of assessment

Assessment may be used to:

• Measure student learning	Against a pre-set criteria
• Grade students	Against a standard
	Against a comparative group
• Summarise achievement	For the student
	For the faculty
	For other interested bodies (university, potential employer, etc)
• Indicate readiness to progress	
• Provide feedback	On learning
	On why a mark was given to teaching staff
• Diagnose specific misunderstandings	
• Motivate students to learn	
• Focus and direct student learning	
• Help students learn more effectively	
• Inform the teaching programme	Review what students do not know or understand
	Review teaching and learning methods
• Promote staff development	Ensure that faculty are aware of the curriculum goals and understand how assessment forms part of the programme
• Contribute to education quality assurance	

Assessment is a complex construct, and recognition of its various purposes will help ensure that an individual educational programme achieves its multiple goals (*see* Box 18.1).

Assessment has classically been divided into two categories: *formative* and *summative*. In essence, formative assessment provides feedback to learners about their progress, whereas summative assessment measures the achievement of learning goals at the end of a course or programme of study. In undergraduate medical education, summative assessments are used at various points in the course to determine progression, to signify the need for remediation in one or more areas and ultimately for graduation, allowing registration with national medical certification bodies and progression into postgraduate and continuing medical education. In general, little feedback is provided to students from summative assessments except in the case of failure. However, the general principles attached to the development of formative assessments also apply – it is essential that summative and high-stakes assessments test appropriate curricular content using methodologies compatible with the teaching programme of the individual institution.

In recent years, particularly in postgraduate medical education, the distinction between formative and summative assessment has become blurred, with essentially formative workplace-based assessments being collated and used for summative purposes. This trend has presumably been driven by a desire to reconnect assessment with learning. Workplace-based assess-

ment is covered in more detail in Chapter 16. Much of the literature related to formative assessment derives from studies in secondary schools and in general higher education. However, a focus on the development of learner self-regulation and lifelong learning means that the general principles described below can be related to medical education at all levels.

Characteristics of Formative Assessment

Formative assessment describes any assessment that is designed specifically to provide feedback. It has been defined as follows:

> … encompassing all those activities undertaken by teachers, and/or by their students, which provide information to be used as feedback to modify the teaching and learning activities in which they are engaged.(3)

Formative assessment should be an active process in which the evidence from assessment is used to adapt teaching to meet student needs.(4) Some of the characteristics of formative assessment are shown in Box 18.2. Feedback is central to effective formative assessment. In general, formative assessment should be ongoing, frequent, non-judgemental and carried out in informal settings. For students, the availability of a regular, dynamic interaction with their tutors helps them engage with the learning process, acting as a motivator and encouraging deep learning and understanding. Furthermore, it offers them the opportunity

General	Informal
	Ongoing and frequent
	Dynamic
	Non-judgemental
	Part of the overall teaching and learning process
Effects on students	Allows detailed feedback
	Promotes self-directed learning
	Raises self-esteem
	Engages students in the learning process
	Encourages deep learning and understanding
	Motivates learning
	Identifies insecurities
	Offers help with specific remediation
Effects on staff	Allows detailed feedback
	Promotes self-directed learning by the students
	Fosters interactive teaching and learning methods
	Encourages varied and challenging teaching methods
	Identifies students in difficulty early in the curriculum
	Develops teaching skills
	Evaluation feeds into curriculum development

to identify their learning difficulties in a safe environment and to take up remedial assistance if appropriate.

For teachers, formative assessment encourages the development of skills associated with the promotion of self-directed learning in the student. Teachers are motivated by better understanding of their students' needs and by helping them become more self-regulated in their learning. Review of the teaching and assessment programme feeds into curriculum development and forms part of ongoing curriculum evaluation.

Overall, consideration of the effects of formative assessment on students and teachers suggests that it should be a positive experience for both groups. Students are encouraged to engage in active learning and teachers to develop skills with which to provide a challenging educational experience in a supportive environment.

Formative assessment can play a major role in the acquisition of lifelong learning skills by helping students self-regulate their learning activities. A well-designed series of formative assessments can make a major contribution to the educational impact of an overall assessment programme, a characteristic that is

as important as the reliability and validity of the individual assessments themselves.(5) Thus, in the ideal situation, formative assessment is a two-way process between learner and teacher, placing the student at the centre of the activity.

In reality, assessment is usually seen as the province of teachers, most of whom regard feedback primarily as a means of transmitting information to students. Often, little thought is given to how feedback information received during formative assessment is processed by students. In this respect, assessment has not kept pace with other developments in teaching and learning in higher education, where the emphasis has shifted towards a dialogue between teacher and student, fostering self-direction and motivation to learn. An assessment process that focuses solely on the teacher's role overlooks the need to help students gain the skills of self-regulation necessary for lifelong learning and ignores the way in which feedback interacts with students' motivation and beliefs. To understand how formative assessment can be most effective, it is therefore necessary to consider the process from the point of view of both teacher and students.

Teacher Perspectives

A simple description of a formative assessment process from the teacher's perspective could be as follows:
1 Review the student's work.
2 Evaluate the work against a reference framework that reflects the pre-set learning objectives and the level expected of students at a particular stage in the course.
3 Make a judgement on the work and provide verbal or written feedback to the student on that judgement.

The apparent simplicity of these steps is misleading, mainly because it disguises the expertise of individual teachers and their differing levels of skill and experience, particularly in giving feedback. Such 'teacher factors' were reviewed by Sadler in 1998,(6) in which he identifies six important characteristics that highly competent teachers bring to the assessment process. These characteristics are summarised in Box 18.3.

Highly competent teachers are not only knowledgeable but also bring a positive attitude to teaching, with their ability to empathise with their students and desire to see them improve. Such teachers are reflective about their own skills and show concern for the integrity of the judgements they make. They demonstrate skill in constructing assessments using a variety of methodologies and are aware of assessment criteria and the standards expected of students at different levels within the curriculum. They learn from their experience in assessment and develop expertise in giving constructive feedback.

BOX 18.3 Characteristics of highly competent teachers that affect the quality of formative assessment

Characteristic	Effect on formative assessment
Knowledge	Greater knowledge base and understanding of the subject matter than the students
Attitude to teaching	Empathy with students, ability to communicate educational goals, desire to help students improve, concern for the integrity of their own judgements
Skill in constructing assessments	Use of varied assessment tools to develop different skills in students
Knowledge of assessment criteria and appropriate standards	Awareness of standards and appropriate expectations of students' performance at a certain level within the curriculum based on learning outcomes and previous experience of student achievement
Evaluative skills	Ability to make qualitative judgements informed by experience as assessors
Expertise in giving feedback	Identification of strengths and weaknesses, evaluative comments in relation to criteria, suggestions for alternative learning methods, examples of different ways to achieve the goals

Adapted from Sadler.(6)

Clearly, in any given faculty, the level of expertise will vary between teachers. The importance of the skills of individual teachers in formative assessment reinforces the requirement for assessment to be designed as part of an institutional educational programme, particularly in relation to staff development and appraisal.

Student Perspectives

From the student perspective, formative assessment should be a means to improve performance and aid development as self-directed and motivated learners. The term 'self-regulation' is used to describe the way in which students monitor their learning behaviour by setting and achieving goals, managing resources and adapting to external feedback. In doing so, students generate their own internal feedback, helping them evaluate their progress towards goals and to adapt their learning processes in the face of obstacles or changes in motivation. Self-regulated learners are aware of their own knowledge, beliefs and cognitive skills, and they use these to interpret external feedback effectively.(7)

Nicol and Macfarlane-Dick recently reviewed the literature relating to formative assessment and self-regulated learning, elaborating the student's role in developing internal feedback mechanisms and modelling the relationship between internal and external feedback (Figure 18.1).(8) This model is useful as it

Adapted from Nicol and Macfarlane-Dick. (8)

Figure 18.1 A model of self-regulated learning illustrating the relationship between external factors and internal self-regulation in the student.

illustrates the way in which a task set by the teacher acts as a trigger for internal regulatory processes within the student, drawing on prior knowledge and motivation to learn. The process generates a set of internal outcomes, such as increased understanding or changes in motivational state, in addition to the external outcomes reflected in a piece of work submitted for assessment. External and internal outcomes are linked by external feedback requiring the student to engage actively with such input. Evidence from the literature suggests that students with a higher level of self-regulation are more effective learners, showing increased resourcefulness, persistence and success.

This student-centred approach to formative assessment described in the general educational literature is consistent with the constructivist approach to learning widely adopted in medical education through formal problem-based learning and other forms of problem-orientated learning and assessment.(9) Translation of constructivist theories into practice places the relationship between teacher and student and the effective use of feedback at the centre of the educational endeavour.(10)

Feedback

Feedback provides the route by which assessment becomes a tool for teaching and learning, and it is central to the concept of formative assessment. Feedback following assessment encourages student and teacher to work together to improve the student's understanding of a subject. The teacher shows that they are interested in the student's opinions, seeks clarification where appropriate and, where necessary, encourages the student to approach a topic in a different way. Feedback provided in a non-judgemental and open fashion allows the student to feel more confident to discuss their difficulties and plan better approaches to learning where necessary.

It has been recognised for many years and across all educational sectors that effective feedback is positively correlated with student achievement,(11) although it is also clear from early studies that the quality of feedback is vital. Poor-quality feedback may have no effect or may even be detrimental.(3)

Effective feedback
Feedback can be defined as a way in which learners become aware of the gap between their current level of knowledge or skill and the desired goal. It provides guidance towards reaching the goal, but effective feedback is achieved only when the student takes action to narrow the gap.(12,13) This implies not only that the educational goals are clearly described but also that students are able and empowered to take the necessary action to achieve them. This in turn means that effective feedback is a collaboration between teachers and learners rather than just a function of teaching *per se*.

Nicol and Macfarlane-Dick propose seven principles of good feedback that can facilitate the development of self-regulation (*see* Box 18.4).(8) These emphasise the need for learner and teacher to work together towards learner self-regulation. They clarify the teach-

---

BOX 18.4 Good feedback practice

- Helps clarify what good performance is
- Facilitates the development of self-assessment (reflection) in learning
- Delivers high-quality information to students about their learning
- Encourages teacher and peer dialogue around learning
- Encourages positive motivational beliefs and self-esteem
- Provides opportunities to close the gap between current and desired performance
- Provides information to teachers that can be used to help shape teaching

Adapted from Nicol and Macfarlane-Dick.(8)

---

er's role in providing information to the student about their performance and also, crucially, about what is expected of them and how to recognise the gap between current and expected attainment. These principles raise a number of issues pertinent to undergraduate medical education that can be considered under the heading 'Education for feedback'.

Education for feedback
On entry into medical school, students are generally very well motivated and academically capable, having achieved high standards in national school exit examinations, prior higher degrees and/or medical school selection examinations. Despite this, some students fail, contributing to internal demotivation and a cycle of further failure. Paradoxically, for the small number of students who underachieve in medical school, the learning habits developed to produce high-level performance in pre-medical school examinations may be the reason for their failure at the undergraduate level.(14) In particular, students who have learnt previously in a didactic teaching environment and become successful at memorising facts may be challenged by small group learning, problem solving, dealing with 'grey areas' of knowledge and scoping vast amounts of information to contain their learning goals within reasonable limits.

A programme of formative assessment and feedback introduced early in a course can go a long way towards preventing the onset of the cycle of failure and demotivation in these students. A well-designed formative assessment programme will ensure that students are aware of their goals and the ways in which these might be achieved. However, it is incumbent on the faculty to explain this process to the students at the beginning of the course. Individual and group feedback can be difficult for students and, if handled badly, can be detrimental to their progress. Educating students about formative assessment and feedback is essential to ensure maximum gain from the process. This in itself requires planning and thought – it is unlikely that a single lecture at the start of a course will be effective. Integrating the educational process with early feedback sessions and modelling good feedback within a learning group is more likely to be educationally valuable.(15)

Much of the research into feedback in medical education comes from the field of teaching communication skills, and these principles have been carried forward into other experiential and reflective learning environments. In the following section, two well-known approaches to feedback developed in the field of communication skills teaching are compared to provide examples of how effective feedback can be used in practical teaching situations.

Feedback in experiential learning settings: experience from communication skills teaching

Experiential learning in one-to-one or small group settings forms the basis of communication skills teaching programmes, usually in the form of observed simulated consultations. Students learn through frequent practice accompanied by feedback and reflection. This type of teaching can be particularly challenging for students who may feel exposed when required to perform difficult communication tasks in front of their tutors and peers. It places demands on teachers, who need to be aware of the dynamics within a learning group and who need to be trained and capable of handling students' responses and reactions. In these situations, feedback should not only be constructive but is best delivered within a framework that is known and accepted by both teachers and students.

The most widely used set of guidelines for providing feedback during teaching about consultation skills was described by Pendleton *et al*. in 1984(16) and has become known as 'Pendleton's Rules'. The stimulus for developing these guidelines was primarily the observation that feedback in medical education is traditionally negative, pointing out students' errors while failing to draw attention to their strengths and successes.

Application of this type of feedback to the experiential learning settings being introduced in communication skills teaching was more destructive than constructive, leading students to develop negativity about the whole teaching process and resent the use of role play and other observational teaching methods. In experiential learning it is clearly important that students should feel that they are in a safe environment. Actions must be confidential to the teacher and the learning group, and students should be supported in identifying their own strengths and weaknesses and helped in addressing areas of concern.

Pendleton's Rules stress the need for safety in the learning environment by emphasising the need to discuss the learners' strengths before commenting on their weaknesses, and to make recommendations rather than criticise. Furthermore, in each part of the process, the learner makes the first comments – this self-evaluation not only encourages them to develop skills of reflection but also enables the teacher to assess these skills and address any difficulties students may have in self-reflection.

Pendleton's rules applied to a small group learning session following a simulated consultation model can be summarised as follows from the teacher's point of view:
- clarify any issues of fact
- ask the learner to comment on what went well and why
- ask the group to discuss what went well and why, and add comments
- ask the learner to comment on what went less well and how it could be done differently
- discuss what could be done differently and how with the whole group.

There are a number of advantages to this approach to feedback. From the student's point of view, it provides a consistent framework in a safe environment – the student knows what to expect at the end of an observed consultation. The emphasis on self-assessment helps the student become more reflective about learning. The 'rules' force the student to think about positive aspects of their performance and to become aware of their individual strengths in communication. The requirement for positive comments by the student, the teacher and the group means that no student receives only negative feedback, and any adverse comments must be presented in a constructive way as recommendations for change. The overall effect is that the feedback experience should enhance motivation to learn and encourage the development of self-regulation. Finally, from the teacher's point of view, it provides a simple structure within which much can be achieved – this is particularly important for relatively inexperienced teachers.

There are, however, a number of disadvantages to Pendleton's Rules, mainly related to their enforcement of a strict order for the way in which feedback is given. By ensuring that each student receives positive feedback at the beginning of the process, the individual student's own agenda may be overlooked – students themselves feel that within the time available during a teaching session, there is little opportunity for the constructive criticism they desire. Interestingly, this may reflect much-needed change in the culture of teaching and learning in medical schools over recent years, and the improved methods used by teachers for experiential learning activities. Increasingly, students expect their opinions to be sought by the faculty, and the culture of persistently negative feedback prevalent at the time of the development of Pendleton's Rules is disappearing. Students appreciate the opportunity to reflect on their successes but are anxious to receive advice on how they might improve their performance.

The agenda-led outcome-based analysis (ALOBA) of the consultation, described by Silverman *et al.* in 1996,(17) provides an alternative mechanism for giving feedback in small group and one-to-one experiential learning situations. The ALOBA approach is built around the students' own agenda, allowing them to identify their individual problems in the context of their own and the patient's desired outcomes for a consultation. It provides opportunities for a group to give feedback, thus encouraging the development of feedback skills in all the learners in a small group setting. Finally, it allows the teacher to introduce a wider discussion of theoretical concepts and research evidence. The principles of the ALOBA method are shown in Box 18.5.

For a teacher using the ALOBA method, the task can be divided into three sections:
- organising the feedback
- group feedback

- ensuring that feedback leads to greater understanding.

Following a real or simulated consultation, the feedback process is organised in terms of the learner's agenda, requiring them to identify the problems they have encountered and the help they would like from the group. The student should first identify what outcomes they wished to achieve from the consultation and, with the rest of the group, should consider the patient's agenda in terms of outcomes (this part of the process may include the opinions of simulated or trained patients where present). The learner can then be asked to comment on the process, and the whole group is asked to join in the problem-solving process, identifying the issues, feeding them back to the learner and generating solutions.

In the second part of the process, specific feedback is invited from all members of the group. It is the teacher's responsibility to ensure that feedback is balanced, non-judgemental and descriptive in nature and that the group offers suggestions and alternatives rather than prescriptive comments. This is a particular

---

BOX 18.5 Agenda-led, outcomes-based analysis of the consultation (ALOBA)

Task for the teacher	Reason
Organise the feedback	
Identify the learner's agenda	Helps the learner to express their views on the consultation and describe what help they would like from the group
Discuss the outcomes that both learner and patient were trying to achieve	The learner starts to recognise the importance of their own desired outcomes and those of the patient
Allow the learner to comment first	Encourages self-assessment and reflection
Involve the whole group in problem solving	All students become more analytical of the consultation and reflect on how they might perform in the same situation
Group feedback	
Invite feedback from all members of the group	Helps all students develop feedback skills, including making specific non-judgemental comments
Ensure balanced feedback	Allows all students to support the learner by considering both what went well and what was less successful
Suggest alternatives rather than make prescriptive comments	The learner can consider alternative approaches and how they might work
Be supportive, act as a role model	All students can observe the use of constructive feedback
Ensure that feedback leads to greater understanding	
Rehearse suggestions	Allows the learner time to try out alternatives and for group comment on the effects
Use the consultation as learning material	All group members can contribute to the session and can learn as much as the learner under observation
Develop a wider discussion	Allows the introduction of concepts and research evidence to the group
Structure, summarise and record	Provides structure for the teaching allowing maximum learning benefits for the students; record the learning to inform future sessions

Adapted from Silverman *et al.*(17)

opportunity for the teacher to be seen as a role model, providing constructive criticism in a supportive environment.

In the final part of the process, the teacher has more freedom to optimise the learning opportunities of the session. Thus, the learner may be given time to rehearse suggestions made by the group, allowing other group members to see the effects of their suggestions. The teacher may take the opportunity to widen the discussion, introducing aspects of their own experience or drawing on the research evidence for a particular aspect of the consultation. Finally, the teacher should summarise the session, providing structure and offering suggestions for further learning within an appropriate conceptual framework. Recording the learning that has occurred in a session is another useful activity that can form the foundation of future sessions.

The advantages of the ALOBA method for providing feedback are, paradoxically, that having placed the individual student and their own agenda at the centre of each learning experience, the session becomes of more value to all the students involved. By offering the opportunity for students to consider the problems inherent in a consultation and engage in problem solving, all participants are more involved in the learning process. Whereas Pendleton's method may result

in the learner becoming the passive recipient of feedback from all the other participants, the ALOBA technique ensures that everyone is equally engaged in the process. From the teacher's point of view, the ALOBA method also provides an opportunity to introduce some of the concepts underlying good communication skills, providing a theoretical structure for the students to understand their learning. However, the ALOBA method does require more-experienced teachers and may be daunting for the less skilful.

Other methods for giving feedback in experiential learning have been described,(18–20) all of which contain aspects of the models described above.

Helpful and unhelpful feedback

Feedback is central to the process of formative assessment. Constructive feedback can enhance the learning experience and develop learner self-regulation; destructive feedback can have profoundly negative effects on learning. For many teachers in medical education, the development of constructive feedback skills is seen as the most important aspect of their professional development.(21) The principles of constructive feedback for experiential learning situations have been described elsewhere(22–24) and are summarised in Box 18.6. In essence, helpful feedback is specific, non-

---

BOX 18.6 How to: Give helpful feedback in experiential learning

Unhelpful feedback	Reason	Helpful feedback	Reason
'Your body language wasn't very good at the start'	Judgemental	'At the beginning you were looking at the computer screen records and not at the patient as she started to tell her story'	Descriptive, detailed, behavioural
'You weren't very empathetic'	Non-specific	'You didn't acknowledge the problems she has dealing with her husband's illness'	Identifies specific problem
'You're very abrupt'	Personality issue	'You interrupted a lot, for example…' (give specific points in consultation)	Behavioural, specific
'I think it would be better if you did it this way'	Advice	'Have you thought about trying it like this?'	Generating alternatives
'I don't think you heard everything with your hearing problem'	Hearing problem not resolvable in this situation	'You have always discussed your hearing problems with us. Was there any point at which you thought it was affecting the consultation?'	Supportive, possibly can be changed by altering the environment
'You didn't notice how upset she was'	Judgemental	'At one point she was looking down and appeared quite upset. You quickly continued by asking her direct questions about her medication and she never returned to the problem of what was upsetting her. Did you notice that?'	Descriptive, non-judgemental, specific
'It was really good'	Non-specific	'At the start you asked an open question and then allowed her to tell her story. You left silences so that she continued in her own words'	Positive, specific, descriptive

Level	Descriptor
1 Prestructural	Use of irrelevant information or no meaningful response
2 Unistructural	Answer focuses on one relevant aspect only
3 Multistructural	Answer focuses on several relevant features, but they are not coordinated
4 Relational	The several parts are integrated into a coherent whole: details are linked to conclusions; meaning is understood
5 Extended abstract	Answer generalises the structure beyond the information given: higher-order principles are used to bring in a new and broader set of issues

From Biggs and Collins.(25)

judgemental, behavioural and descriptive, and is provided within a supportive educational environment close to the time of the learning experience.

Similar criteria can be applied to feedback given in other formative assessments. For example, when marking written pieces of work, simply giving a grade or making a comment such as 'Good work' is less helpful to the learner than a description of why the work is good and offering suggestions for other issues that might have been included or arguments that might have been presented. A number of systems for classifying students' responses have been described, of which the most well known is the structure of the observed learning outcome (SOLO) taxonomy(25) (*see* Box 18.7). The levels described in this scheme are not content specific and can be applied to students' work at any stage in a curriculum, assuming the teacher is aware of the aims of the module and the level of attainment expected. Student work that scores in levels 4 and 5 shows evidence of categorising and structuring knowledge, characteristics associated with deep learning. Feedback offered to the students within this (or a similar) framework is more helpful to their learning than simple judgemental statements.

Finally, it is useful to check with the students that they have understood the feedback they have been given and that their interpretation of the feedback is correct. The students' perception of feedback they have received may vary greatly from that of the teacher

who gave the feedback,(26) and only by checking can these discrepancies be addressed.

Formative Assessment in the Curriculum

A programme of formative assessment with effective feedback can be used to develop self-regulation in learners, leading to better outcomes in terms of their learning and overall success. Formative assessment should be considered as part of a teaching institution's assessment strategy alongside summative assessments. The following section reviews the way in which a programme of formative assessment can be designed within a curriculum and considers some examples of different types of formative assessment used in medical education.

Formative assessment and module design

A programme of formative assessment should be built into the design of a teaching module that has explicit learning outcomes (which can be assessed). The module design should show clearly how evaluation of teaching, learning and assessment will be performed, allowing development of the teaching programme in the future. A number of schemata for module design incorporating assessment, feedback and evaluation have been described, such as the one shown in Figure 18.2.

This basic pattern of module design is appropriate for all types of learning in medical education, including classroom-based activities and experiential learning.(27) The example given in Figure 18.2 is based around threshold criteria (pass–fail assessments) but can be adapted to include grading, where appropriate. The model takes into account not only the aims of the teaching module but also the level of attainment

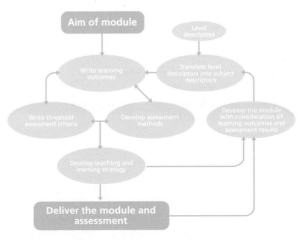

Adapted from Moon. (27)

Figure 18.2 Curriculum module development and review.

expected at the particular point in the curriculum. Module designers can therefore translate the level descriptors into learning outcomes and hence threshold assessment criteria. At that point the assessment methods are designed alongside the teaching and learning strategy for the module. Having delivered the module and performed the assessment as designed, evaluation of the module includes the teaching methods and the appropriateness of the learning outcomes and assessments used.

Using this format for curriculum design, assessment forms an integral part of the teaching programme and can easily be blueprinted against curriculum content and teaching methodologies. Linking the assessment programme explicitly to the design and evaluation of the module should ensure that evaluation of the assessment process itself is not overlooked.(28)

Examples of formative assessment in undergraduate medical education

Recognition of the value of formative assessment as a means of enhancing teaching and learning in medical education has led to an increase in its use in undergraduate programmes. The ability of formative assessment to identify students with difficulties and to offer remedial teaching is an important feature of the widening use of formal formative assessment. The principles of good formative assessment can be applied to all areas of assessment in medical education, including

- knowledge testing
- testing competence – practical, communication and clinical skills
- experiential learning settings – hospital clinical placements, general practice, community placements
- portfolios.

Often the most appropriate formative assessment includes elements of different learning activities (for example, an Objective Structure Clinical Examination plus written work), allowing the faculty to give a rounded assessment of student performance and provide help in specific areas. This section focuses on examples of formative assessment in three areas of undergraduate medical education:

- hospital clinical placements
- teaching consultation skills in general practice
- assessment of portfolios and reflective writing.

Hospital clinical placements

Much of the teaching and learning in medical schools occurs in the context of hospital clinical placements (clerkships). One of the most well-recognised and disheartening aspects of traditional medical education programmes was the ability of students to pass through a clinical teaching programme and only be identified as having problems when they failed a summative assessment or even their final examinations (often not to the surprise of teaching staff). Formative assessment can identify struggling students earlier in the course and, coupled with appropriate identification of the learning difficulties and additional teaching, can result in improved student performance.(14)

Most medical schools expect students on clinical placements to receive feedback on their performance, usually in the form of a grade, which is regarded as highly subjective by the students. It is less common to have a formative assessment process in which the 'firm grades' form part of the overall assessment. In my own medical school, we have established a major formative assessment at the end of the first stage in the clinical programme, supplemented by additional teaching tailored to students' needs. Other schools have made similar changes to their assessment programmes with improved student performance.(14,29)

However, the format of the assessment programme is crucial – the introduction of an in training assessment (ITA) consisting of a range of assessment formats to an internal medicine clerkship was not found to increase the number of supervisions or the quality of feedback received by the students.(30) The ITA was complex, requiring the student to undertake a number of supervised encounters or presentations related to 13 core competencies and was accompanied by feedback. The commitment of the senior clinicians to such a programme needs to be very high as it is ongoing and time-consuming. Asking too much of busy clinicians by way of formative assessment and feedback may be counterproductive. It may still prove to be more valuable to organise centralised assessment formats assessing competence, which can be used in either formative or summative ways, and to ask for workplace-based assessment only where it is absolutely vital in the assessment of performance.

Consultation skills in general practice

General practice placements often provide particularly good environments for formative assessment with appropriate feedback. In general, students are attached to a practice in small numbers and may be given the opportunity to see patients on their own or in observed consultations. A wide range of assessment methods for postgraduate trainees in general practice have been described, including observed consultations, review of video-taped consultations, multi-rater assessment and evaluation by peers and patients. General practitioner teachers are therefore skilled in assessment and feedback, and many of these methods can be extended to the undergraduate curriculum. Work reported from the Department of General Practice in Leicester suggests that postgraduate assessment methods can be transferred successfully with high levels of reliability, validity and educational impact.(31)

Portfolios

Much has been written about the use of portfolios in medical education, and there remains a debate about what the term actually means and what should be contained in a medical student's learning portfolio. To some, it is a repository for assessment grades, written pieces of work and lecture notes. Others have tried to harness the potential of portfolio learning to encourage students to develop reflective practice and adult learning skills.(32,33) Online learning portfolios have the potential to enhance the progression towards adult learning.(34)

Portfolios lend themselves to use in formative assessment as they can be the centre of discussion at student progress meetings. Inclusion of a variety of assessments within a portfolio is helpful if they have been marked according to appropriate criteria and with effective feedback given as part of the overall formative assessment process. The attraction of the portfolio as a means of assessment is strong – the collection of a series of pieces of work or assessments of competencies together with self-reflective pieces and evidence of professional development is a unique addition to the assessment opportunities open to medical educators. Portfolios are now increasingly used in formative assessment, and recent work suggests that it may be possible to combine this with a summative element.(35,36)

Conclusion

Formative assessment is a valuable part of the assessment programme in medical education. A well-designed programme of formative assessment linked to overall curriculum aims and the teaching and learning goals of individual modules enhances the learning experience for students and promotes desirable educational outcomes, including learner self-regulation and the development of lifelong learning skills.

References

1 Newble DI and Jaeger K (1983) The effect of assessments and examinations on the learning of medical students. *Medical Education.* **17**: 165–71.

2 Rust C (2002) The impact of assessment on student learning: how can research literature practically help to inform the development of departmental assessment strategies? *Active Learning in Higher Education.* **3**: 128–44.

3 Black P and William D (1998) Assessment and classroom learning. *Assessment in Education.* **5**: 7–74.

4 Black P and William D (1998) Inside the black box: raising standards through classroom assessment. PhiDeltaKappa International (http://www.pdkintl.org/kappan/kbla9810.htm).

5 van der Vleuten C (1996) The assessment of professional competence: developments, research and practical implications. *Advances in Health Science Education.* **1**: 41–67.

6 Sadler DR (1998) Formative assessment: revisiting the territory. *Assessment in Education.* **5**: 77–84.

7 Butler DL and Winne PH (1995) Feedback and self-regulated learning: a theoretical synthesis. *Review of Educational Research.* **65**: 245–81.

8 Nicol DJ and Macfarlane-Dick D (2006) Formative assessment and self-regulated learning: a model and seven principles of good feedback practice. *Studies in Higher Education.* **31**: 199–218.

9 Schuwirth LWT and van der Vleuten CPM (2004) Changing education, changing assessment, changing research? *Medical Education.* **38**: 805–12.

10 Rushton A (2005) Formative assessment: a key to deep learning? *Medical Teacher.* **27**: 509–13.

11 Hattie JA (1987) Identifying the salient factors of a model of student learning: a synthesis of meta-analyses. *International Journal of Educational Research.* **11**: 187–212.

12 Ramaprasad A (1983) On the definition of feedback. *Behavioural Science.* **28**: 4–13.

13 Sadler DR (1989) Formative assessment and the design of instructional systems. *Instructional Science.* **18**: 119–44.

14 Sayer M, Chaput de Saintonge M, Evans D and Wood D (2002) Support for students with academic difficulties. *Medical Education.* **36**: 643–50.

15 Henderson P, Ferguson-Smith AC and Johnson MH (2005) Developing essential professional skills: a framework for teaching and learning about feedback. *BMC Medical Education.* **5**: 11 (http://www.biomedcentral.com/1472-6920/5/11).

16 Pendleton D, Schofield T, Tate P and Havelock P (1984) *The Consultation: an approach to learning and teaching.* Oxford University Press, Oxford.

17 Silverman JD, Draper J and Kurtz SM (1996) The Calgary–Cambridge approach to communication skills teaching. 1. Agenda-led outcome-based analysis of the consultation. *Education in General Practice.* **7**: 288–99.

18 Neher JO, Gordon K, Meyer B and Stevens N (1992) A five-step 'microskills' model of clinical teaching. *Journal of the American Board of Family Practice.* **5**: 419–24.

19 Brukner HA, Altkorn DL, Cook S et al. (1999) Giving effective feedback to medical students: a workshop for faculty and house staff. *Medical Teacher.* **21**: 161–5.

20 Wall D (2004) Giving feedback effectively. In: Mohanna K, Wall D and Chambers R (eds) *Teaching Made Easy: a manual for health professionals.* Radcliffe Medical Press, Oxford.

21 Hewson MG and Little ML (1998) Giving feedback in medical education: verification of recommended techniques. *Journal of General Internal Medicine.* **13**: 111–16.

22 Ende J (1983) Feedback in clinical medical education. *Journal of the American Medical Association.* **250**: 777–81.

23 Kurtz S, Silverman J and Draper J (2005) *Teaching and Learning Communication Skills in Medicine.* Radcliffe Publishing, Oxford, pp. 123–9.

24 Roy Chowdhury R and Kalu G (2004) Learning to give feedback in medical education. *The Obstetrician and Gynaecologist.* **6**: 243–7.

25 Biggs JB and Collis KF (1982) *Evaluating the Quality of Learning: the SOLO taxonomy.* Academic Press, New York.

26 Sender Liberman A, Liberman M et al. (2005) Surgery residents and attending surgeons have different perceptions of feedback. *Medical Teacher.* **27**: 470–2.

27 Moon JA (2004) *A Handbook of Reflective and Experiential Learning*. Routledge Falmer, London, pp. 149–57.

28 Fowell SL, Southgate LJ and Bligh JG (1999) Evaluating assessment: the missing link? *Medical Education*. **33**: 276–81.

29 Denison AR, Currie AE, Laing MR and Heys SD (2006) Good for them or good for us? The role of academic guidance interviews. *Medical Education*. **40**: 1188–91.

30 Daelmans HEM, Hoogenboom RJI, Scherpbier AJJA *et al.* (2005) Effects of an in-training assessment programme on supervision of and feedback on competencies in an undergraduate internal medicine clerkship. *Medical Teacher*. **27**: 158–63.

31 McKinley RK, Fraser RC, van der Vleuten C and Hastings A (2000) Formative assessment of the consultation performance of medical students in the setting of general practice using a modified version of the Leicester Assessment Package. *Medical Education*. **34**: 573–9.

32 Snadden D (1999) Portfolios – attempting to measure the unmeasurable? *Medical Education*. **33**: 478–9.

33 Hays RB (2004) Reflecting on learning portfolios. *Medical Education*. **38**: 800–4.

34 Benson J, Chaudhry A, Lillicrap M *et al.* (2006) From directed learning to self-directed learning via a student portfolio: initial student experience. *Presented at the 12th International Ottawa Conference on Clinical Competence, New York, 2006. Abstract number OM1-2*, p. 110.

35 Friedman Ben David M, Davis MH *et al.* (2001) AMEE Medical Education Guide 24. Portfolios as a method of student assessment. *Medical Teacher*. **23**: 535–51.

36 Driessen E, van der Vleuten C, Schuwirth L *et al.* (2005) The use of qualitative research criteria for portfolio assessment as an alternative to reliability evaluation: a case study. *Medical Education*. **39**: 214–20.

Self-regulated learning in medical education

Casey B White and Larry D Gruppen

KEY MESSAGES

- Self-regulated learning is vital for continuing professional development.

- There is little evidence to suggest that medical schools and postgraduate institutions are successfully helping students become effective self-regulated learners.

- Researchers in medical education have most often studied self-regulated learning in the narrower context of self-assessment.

- Self-regulated learning involves four steps: planning, learning, assessment and adjustment.

- Self-regulated learning skills can be learnt – and therefore taught.

Introduction

The need for physicians to engage in effective self-regulated learning (SRL) is well documented and pressing, given the links between continuing medical education and the quality of healthcare.(1,2) However, there is little published evidence that medical schools and postgraduate institutions are successfully helping students become effective self-regulated learners. This is in spite of formal goals for 'lifelong learning' prevalent among medical schools and residency programmes, and the availability of research findings to guide efforts to integrate SRL into education and training programmes.

Since the 1980s, educators and psychologists outside medicine have conducted extensive research into SRL. Characteristics and habits of identified self-regulated learners have been compiled and explored, and specific strategies have been identified and tested. Psychological dimensions, task conditions, attributes and processes have been categorised under constructs bounded by the scientific questions of why, how, what and where learners engage in SRL. Models have been presented characterising the complex and intersecting networks that underlie SRL and that include personality, cognition and development. Outcomes of this research provide evidence that SRL comprises a set of skills that *can* be learnt.

Undergraduate and graduate medical programmes have yet to grapple with this concept in a systematic and uniform way. Difficulty in doing so has been attributed in part to different interpretations among teachers and students,(3) and also the inconsistency with which medical educators define and study SRL. In a 2005 review of the medical education literature reporting on SRL, Ainoda *et al.* found that only five out of 63 articles (8%) identified actually defined SRL, and those definitions were not consistent with one another.(4)

In medical education, among the studies conducted on self-assessment and self-regulation, agreement on and evidence of a systematic, feedback-driven programme of SRL appears to be highly variable.(5–7) In fact, researchers in medical education have most often studied SRL in the narrower context of self-assessment, based on the notion that self-assessment is the first step in a two-step process: (a) self-assessment of knowledge and skills, followed by (b) self-regulated education to address areas of concern or weakness.(8) Yet there is evidence that physicians have limited ability to self-assess their strengths and weaknesses,(9) and that those physicians who are the least skilled are also the most confident and the weakest self-assessors.(10) This is perhaps why we have focused our research efforts on self-assessment and its accuracy – if one cannot self-assess accurately, one cannot focus self-education where it is most needed. While this is in fact correct, our limited success in predicting factors that are key to effective self-assessment then leave us nowhere in terms of helping learners become effective self-assessors. Perhaps the problem in achieving this very important outcome lies in our perception of SRL and self-assessment.

Educational psychologists view SRL as a complex cycle comprising intermingling elements such as

Understanding Medical Education: Evidence, Theory and Practice.
Edited by T Swanwick. © 2010 Association for the Study of Medical Education.

psychological characteristics (e.g. self-efficacy, motivation, beliefs and learning style), personal choices (effort expended, learning strategies), judgements (self-assessment, attributions) and personal actions (e.g. goal setting, adjustment). They recommend a systematic integration of SRL into educational programmes, with monitoring and feedback to assure effective skills are acquired.

This chapter is meant to assure medical educators that SRL *can* be taught and that educators play a pivotal role in helping learners to develop SRL skills.(11) It provides theoretical and practical information about a broader and more complex cycle of SRL, and proposes a model for integrating SRL into medical education. The model, adapted from research in educational psychology, reflects four steps that comprise the cycle of SRL (planning, learning, feedback/assessment and adjustment), and the underlying elements within each. Adoption of a consistent, evidence-based model within and across the continuum of medical education (i.e. undergraduate to postgraduate) and across programmes (i.e. around the country or around the world) will help us explore the effectiveness of this approach in helping learners set personal goals, consider how what they bring to their learning as unique individuals influences their learning, monitor (i.e. self-assess) their learning and make adjustments to assure that they meet their goals. Such a model can also help medical educators meet their own goals of training physicians who are prepared for self-regulated, life-long learning.

A Model for Self-Regulated Learning

Medical educators are understandably eager to help students and physicians become capable of effective SRL. However, even medical programmes with clear expectations and requirements for their learners to engage in SRL do not necessarily have programmes in place to monitor the quality or effectiveness of SRL strategies used by students.(12)

Zimmerman reported that learners can be described as self-regulating to the extent that they are 'metacognitively, motivationally, and behaviourally active participants in their own learning process'.(13) Much of the research focused specifically on SRL has been grounded in elementary or middle school educational contexts, with some studies at more advanced educational levels. However, this work can be adapted and used as a framework for integrating SRL into medical education. The framework in Figure 19.1 adapts this research and models SRL as a cycle of four phases: planning, learning, feedback and adjustment.

Educators can contemplate different contexts (lecture hall, classroom, clinic, hospital) for applying elements of the model. Although it is important for learners to understand that ultimately the principles

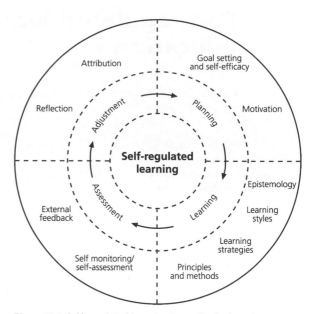

Figure 19.1 Self-regulated learning in medical education.

must apply across learning contexts, the elements can be introduced at earlier stages and then reinforced at later stages. In the next section of this chapter, each phase and element of the model is explicated, followed by an example of how the model may be applied (Box 19.1).

Planning

To self-regulate effectively, learners must set personal goals. Goals guide the decisions we make related to learning (e.g. value, strategies) and they are the specific measure against which we self-assess learning and performance. Motivation is a goal-guided process through which individuals instigate and sustain activities directly linked to goal achievement.(14) In the cycle of SRL, achievement of learning goals influences self-efficacy, which in turn reinforces motivation. (Box 19.2).

Goal setting and self-efficacy

Goal setting is the establishment of specific standards of performance or resulting outcomes. The motivational benefits of goals are dependent not just on goal setting, but on learner commitment to achieving them.(15)

Personal and social-environmental factors influence goal choice and goal commitment. Personal factors include skill level, previous performance, beliefs about goal value and attribution of performance. However, self-efficacy is the most important influence on personal goal setting.(15) Self-efficacy is an individual's belief in his or her ability to achieve specific goals.(16) A strong, positive sense of self-efficacy is critical to setting and achieving challenging yet attainable goals, which translate into personal successes that support setting more difficult goals.

Social-environmental factors include group norms (higher norms lead to higher personal goals), group and peer goals, and role modelling by peers. Feedback from others is an essential influence, especially when it comprises positive self-efficacy information that emphasises challenge, mastery, self-improvement and achieved progress towards goal (Box 19.2).(15)

Motivation

It is useful to distinguish between intrinsic motivation, doing something because it is inherently interesting and enjoyable, and extrinsic motivation, doing something to obtain an outcome separate from the activity. Although intrinsic motivation results in high-quality learning, educators cannot depend on all learners to be intrinsically motivated across all learning tasks.

Self-Determination Theory emphasises that learners who are intrinsically motivated embrace learning as a valued activity in and of itself, regardless of rewards or outcomes.(17) Although this would seem to be an ideal orientation to learning, frankly, many of the tasks learners need to engage in to reach their learning goals are not inherently enjoyable.

Categories of extrinsic motivation range from the learner feeling the task(s) is controlled by external forces that produce rewards or punishments, to the learner feeling some sense of control over the task(s).

Within this extrinsic framework, learner attitudes can range from resentment or disinterest to willingness.

The least autonomous form of extrinsic motivation is *external regulation*, in which individuals perform to satisfy an external demand or to reap an external reward. Next is *introjection*, in which individuals still feel external control, but perform to maintain self-esteem or a feeling of self-value. *Identification* is a more autonomous form of motivation in which an individual finds personal importance in an action and internalises it as a means to a broader personal goal. The most autonomous form of extrinsic motivation is *integration*, in which individuals internalise reasons for an action and assimilate them totally into themselves. Although identification and integration share important qualities with intrinsic motivation, these are still extrinsic motivation because individuals are motivated to achieve a goal that they see as separate from their behaviour.

Although all learners bring some level of motivation to their learning,(18) educators can create environments that support development of intrinsic motivation and autonomy. Such environments offer optimal challenges, interpersonal involvement in learning, acknowledgement of feelings, opportunities to make choices about learning, and also opportunities for learners to evaluate their own and others' learning.(19)

Medical students and junior doctors are certainly, at least generally, viewed as highly motivated learners. While this might be true within the boundaries and 'safety' of a formal educational programme, autonomy will be key to lifelong learning and intrinsic motivation is key to autonomy. Also, extrinsically motivated learners who no longer have a strong reward system or direct oversight/feedback might not be effective self-regulated learners. If our goal is to help students and trainees become self-regulated learners who will pursue excellence throughout their professional careers, research relevant to motivation needs to become a greater focus in medical education (Box 19.3).

Learning

Learning can be defined as 'a persisting change in performance or performance potential that results from experience and interaction with the world'.(21) Individuals perceive and interact with the environment in personal and unique ways based on characteristics such as intelligence, personality, beliefs, experiences and culture. Because of this, there is no single idea, principle, paradigm or belief that defines how individuals learn most effectively. Furthermore, educators should be aware of how their own and their learners' beliefs about learning influence learning, as well as the presence of learning styles and their potential to influence the effectiveness of learning.

BOX 19.2 Focus on: Factors that influence goal choice and commitment(16)

Personal factors

Previous performance	Individuals are most likely to attempt goals with which they have had previous success
Skill level	It is unlikely that individuals will attempt to achieve goals that are far beyond their level to achieve
Value	An individual's personal beliefs about the importance or value in achieving a specific goal
Attributions	Attributing failure to unstable (controllable) causes such as low effort can lead to setting higher goals on subsequent tasks
Self-efficacy*	There is a positive correlation between high self-efficacy (personal belief that a goal is achievable) and strong commitment to goals

Social-environmental factors

Normative environment	Higher group norms encourage individuals to set higher personal goals
Group and peers	A peer or group can exert pressure in support of a group goal that encourages group members (or partner)
Role modelling	Positive role modelling of goal setting by others encourages individuals to set higher personal goals
Feedback*	Feedback that stresses challenge, mastery, self-improvement and achievement towards goal has the most positive effect

*Key factor.

BOX 19.3 Self-regulated learning in practice: Planning

At the first meeting of the longitudinal case (LC) small groups, early in the first year, students are introduced to the format of the cases and the nature of the problems/questions, as well as the expectations for their performance and participation. Personal responsibility for ensuring self-learning (with guidance and resources as needed/requested) and peer learning is emphasised to foster and support appropriate motivation for learning.

At this first meeting, students are asked to set personal learning goals for the LCs. Goals should address all domains, not just knowledge, and they should be articulated at an appropriate level (Bloom's Taxonomy(20) is used as a guide). Students discuss their goals with their facilitator (briefly) in an early small group. They may adjust their goals/learning outcomes and re-submit them at any time, and they are encouraged to do so at the start of each term (if detailed, these can also serve as a learning plan for the next stage of the cycle).

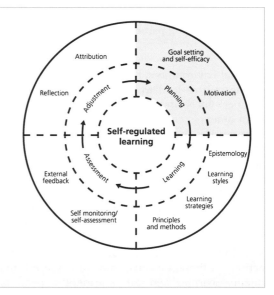

Epistemology

Personal epistemology is an individual's beliefs about knowledge and knowing. There is growing interest in how epistemology influences knowledge acquisition cognition (i.e. thinking and reasoning), and decisions educators and learners make about learning.

Research provides evidence that individuals traverse through a patterned sequence of development in their beliefs about knowledge and knowing, becoming more complex as they advance through college.(22) One schema proposes four distinct catego- ries and transition stages along a continuum ranging from a simplistic belief that knowledge exists as a fixed entity to be transmitted from knower to learner, to a more complex belief that knowledge is fluid, changing and contextual, and must be individually discovered (*see* Figure 19.2). This journey tends to be reinitiated when new areas of knowledge are first addressed.

In their progress towards self-regulation, learners should be aware of their own beliefs and how they influence their efforts to reach their academic goals.

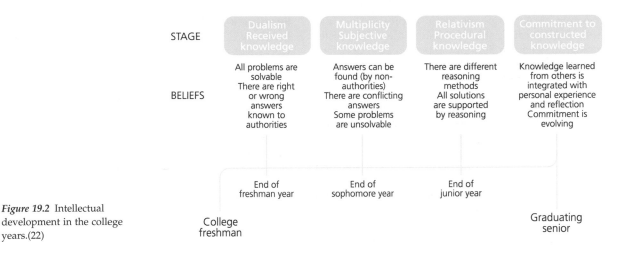

STAGE

| Dualism Received knowledge | Multiplicity Subjective knowledge | Relativism Procedural knowledge | Commitment to constructed knowledge |

BELIEFS

All problems are solvable
There are right or wrong answers known to authorities

Answers can be found (by non-authorities)
There are conflicting answers
Some problems are unsolvable

There are different reasoning methods
All solutions are supported by reasoning

Knowledge learned from others is integrated with personal experience and reflection
Commitment is evolving

End of freshman year   End of sophomore year   End of junior year

College freshman   Graduating senior

Figure 19.2 Intellectual development in the college years.(22)

Using a number of methods, educators can help learners understand where they are along the epistemological (i.e. developmental) continuum and how they can move forward.

Most college students have advanced beyond viewing knowledge as concrete and static; they are moving towards seeing it as dynamic and changing, and see themselves as active constructors of their own knowledge. Autonomous learning, including accurate and effective self-assessment, requires the ability to look at one's self objectively, something that is only possible at the higher levels of the developmental continuum.(23)

Given this evidence, it makes sense for medical students and trainees to be challenged to learn and practise these skills in increasingly complex contexts, if only because physicians use self-assessment skills in complex contexts in their professional lives. Based on evidence of strong correlations between epistemological beliefs and cognitive strategies that students use for learning, both educators and learners should have a solid understanding of their own beliefs about the acquisition of knowledge and how these can influence decisions related to teaching and to learning.

Learning styles

Learning styles can be thought of as innate characteristics possessed by learners that underlie and influence their learning, as opposed to learning strategies, which are the techniques learners choose. Although there is skepticism about the validity of learning styles as a construct, researchers continue to propose and categorise individual styles; one example of many is Kolb's 'cycle of experiential learning'.(24)

It is important for teachers and learners to recognise that individuals can and do have different preferences for learning, just as they have different personalities. Knowledge about how they learn most effectively can help learners strategise and choose techniques as they approach their learning, and also help them assess more effectively their progress towards learning goals.

Both learning styles and learning strategies are critical to effective SRL because of their key and personal connections to achieving learning outcomes or goals.

Learning strategies

Learning strategies are key to self-regulation because they are one area in which learners, in formal educational programmes, can exercise direct control or autonomy. Making decisions about strategies is a dynamic process that requires attention to different learning elements: individual learner needs (e.g. high aptitude for particular content versus low aptitude); styles (e.g. visual learner versus auditory); contexts (e.g. studying biochemistry versus studying the cardiac examination); and other factors such as environment and time of day.(25)

The effectiveness of strategies will also change as learners advance or change contexts in a particular discipline or domain. A strategy for learning the very basics of the cardiac examination (e.g. how to place a stethoscope) will not be effective for more advanced skills (e.g. detecting/recognising a cardiac abnormality). Learners need to be attentive to this and to self-monitoring outcomes that indicate the success or failure of specific strategies in helping them to achieve learning goals.

Finally, learners can encounter problems choosing and deploying the most appropriate strategies. They might not effectively match strategies with study/learning conditions, they might not be proficient in strategies they choose, or they might even lack the motivation necessary to employ certain strategies.(26) Such problems can be mitigated with effective monitoring and formative feedback.(27)

Principles and methods

Connecting principles with methods is key to building a bridge of understanding between teachers and learners. As epistemological beliefs evolve, that is, as learners begin to see they have a personal role in their acquisition of knowledge and see knowledge as more dynamic, problem-solving skills improve. This suggests that educators should consider their own epistemological beliefs in light of the pedagogical decisions they make based on those beliefs, and how those decisions affect the beliefs, knowledge acquisition and cognitive development of their learners.

It is important for educators to articulate specific principles underlying expectations and approaches if they are to help individuals become autonomous, self-regulating learners; it is equally important that learners understand these principles so they are prepared to meet these expectations. For example, in a course or programme one underlying principle might be to help individuals become self-directed learners. This should be stated explicitly and learners should be given specific information about what is expected of them. For instance, as self-directed learners 'in training' they will be expected to set their own goals, use experts and resources to help them achieve their goals, be willing to take responsibility for their own learning and productivity, be able to manage their own time and projects, and assess themselves and their peers.(28)

Teachers can conceptualise, construct and model specific learning activities that encourage ongoing cognitive growth and acquisition of increasingly complex reasoning skills. Approaches that foster development and provide logical opportunities for self-regulation include pedagogies with progressively increased emphasis on learners' participation and responsibility for their own and their peers' learning. Active learning methods such as collaboration and opportunities for learners to discuss and analyse ill-structured problems and controversial issues help foster the advanced cognitive skills that are inherent in higher levels of development (Box 19.4).(29,30)

Feedback and assessment

Feedback is a key component of SRL.(27) In a perfect world, self-regulated learners generate criteria against which to monitor their progress as they create their own goals for achievement. They then systematically monitor and interpret their progress against goals and adjust as needed. However, their interpretation of their progress might vary in accuracy because learners hold differing beliefs about learning and about their own self-efficacy, and they might also have knowledge or learning deficits of which they are not aware (i.e. 'you don't know what you don't know'). Thus, it is critical that learners receive timely, targeted and systematic feedback to help improve learning and to help them develop skills for effective self-monitoring and SRL.

Internal monitoring/self-assessment

Educational psychologists study the impact of feedback on the self-monitoring process as a means of exploring links between self-monitoring and self-regulated learning.(31) Engaging in SRL activities improves academic performance within formal educational structures where it is fostered and where feedback is part of the SRL cycle.(32,33) In fact, SRL and feedback are inextricably linked in school, where learners begin to understand and practise and then ultimately master SRL. Formative assessment includes both feedback and self-monitoring. The goal of many instructional systems is to facilitate the transition from feedback to self-monitoring.(34)

Internal monitoring is a conscious, pivotal element of learning that guides SRL. Learners identify goals, choose strategies and apply those strategies to a task(s) that yields a specific (learning) product or outcome.

BOX 19.4 Self-regulated learning in practice: Learning

Expectations for student performance are presented and discussed in the first meeting. There is not an explicit assessment of learning styles or strategies; rather, students choose their own strategies for personal learning, and they are given the control and autonomy to choose the methods by which they will teach in the longitudinal cases.

Questions/problems related to the cases are presented in a provocative manner to challenge students to grapple with complex and uncomfortable issues, to help them develop appropriate problem-solving skills, to encourage introspection and reflection, and to foster integration of personal experiences into new learning. The processes and heuristics students use to tackle these problems – thinking through potential and alternate solutions, applying values, and considering and weighing evidence and opinions – provide essential information about developmental level and cognitive and professional characteristics. Peers and facilitator provide feedback.

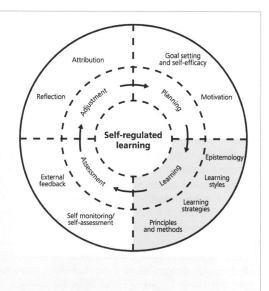

Self-monitoring during this process produces internal feedback (self-assessment) that compares the evolving state of the task to the goal. This provides the basis for further action(s) on the part of the learner, such as adjustment of strategies or even adjustment of goals.

Research on self-monitoring suggests that most learners do not inherently possess optimal skills.(35) When left to regulate on their own, learners will often monitor their progress incorrectly (e.g. believing they have mastered what they intended to) and terminate learning activities before achieving goals. Reasons for this vary, and some are linked with learners' choice of learning strategies. If the strategy chosen is not linked effectively with what the learner needs to accomplish in the task at hand, the same faulty thinking that led to that choice might contribute to incorrectly judging progress towards goals.(31) Also, during self-monitoring, learners might misperceive cues (specific criteria representing their progress) and thus misperceive progress, or they might be overwhelmed by cognitive demands that skew internal feedback on progress.

Studies of self-assessment across undergraduate and postgraduate medical education have tended to focus on assessment of outcomes, rather than internal formative feedback that guides learning and sharpens self-regulated learning actions. Many of these studies ask medical students or trainees to estimate their performance in a small group setting, an examination or essay, or a clinical performance (e.g. Objective Structured Clinical Examination station with a standardised patient), treating self-assessment as a separate and distinct entity. These studies focus on learner accuracy, usually as a comparison of a self-estimated performance measured against an 'actual' performance as scored or judged by an expert.

The medical education literature on self-assessment (*see* Box 19.5) reports at least one finding that is similar to the educational psychology literature on self-monitoring: while some learners are accurate self-assessors, many or even most are not.(36–38) Self-assessment accuracy is task- and context-specific (as are SRL strategies), but when the context changes, the better self-assessors remain better than the poorer self-assessors.(39) Attempts to identify characteristics of good self-assessors (i.e. reasons why some learners are more accurate than others) have provided limited useful information.(40)

There are those who blame the lack of enlightening findings on the methodologies used for the various studies on medical student self-assessment.(41) While this might certainly be true, another basic problem might be how medical education perceives and conceptualises the role of self-assessment. Educators believe self-assessment is a critical element in the process or cycle of SRL.(42,43) However, few medical educators or medical education programmes focus on the process of self-monitoring to achieve personal

> ### BOX 19.5 Where's the evidence: Self-assessment(41)
>
> There is a lack of published research to answer the important questions:
>
> - Does self-assessment help identify learning needs?
> - Does self-assessment bring about change in learner activity or clinical practice?
>
> Most research focuses on the accuracy of self-assessment.
>
> Some studies have looked at the impact of gender. The evidence is inconclusive, although a very large study ($n = 1152$) indicates men overestimate their ability more than women do.
>
> Poor performers tend to overestimate their ability while competent individuals are more likely to be accurate.
>
> Students are more accurate at self-assessing practice skills than knowledge.
>
> Feedback in the form of video, benchmarking and instruction can improve self-assessment accuracy.
>
> Research on self-assessment has been fraught with methodological problems.
>
> There is need for further research in this area to examine the impact of self-assessment.
>
> With thanks to Jan Illing at the University of Newcastle.

and external learning outcomes, or on how formative feedback can influence both performance and self-monitoring of performance. Rather, medical education is focused on the outcome of self-assessment – whether students self-assess their grade/score accurately. This means our assessment systems are focused more on providing summative information than formative feedback, and without formative feedback, attempts to integrate self-regulation are likely to have only limited success.

External formative feedback

Formative feedback occurs when teachers provide information to learners designed to enable them to learn better, improve performance, and enhance their self-reflective and self-monitoring processes. Effective formative feedback focuses learners' attention on their progress towards achieving goals, provides specific information that helps them to recognise and close gaps, and integrates review, reflection and self-assessment components. In its purest form, formative feedback does not involve scoring or grading.

Educators can serve as guides as learners develop their goals and choose learning strategies, but learners must self-monitor their own progress; faculty can then provide formative feedback that confirms or rectifies internal feedback. Both roles must be integrated into the curriculum and into expectations for learners and faculty.

Longitudinal case (LC) facilitators are exposed to relevant developmental theory.(22,23) The continuum of how individuals believe knowledge is constructed and stored provides a foundation for observing and assessing learner development and for providing feedback to learners that is focused on helping them advance developmentally.

Students are advised that one of the intended outcomes is advancing their cognition, skills and attitudes along a continuum that leads ultimately to autonomy, or 'self-authorship',(23) which are hallmark characteristics of higher order development. Students receive feedback in the context of development – where they appear to be along a continuum, how they are progressing in general, and methods and strategies they can use that foster development specifically.

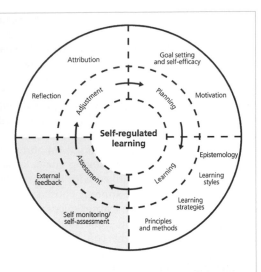

Effective self-assessment requires advanced cognitive and personal development. The LCs are designed to foster, support and measure medical student development in specific cognitive skills and attitudinal domains. At the end of each session, the group engages in peer assessment guided by the faculty facilitator. At the end of each term, each student completes the identical assessment instrument that the faculty facilitator completes for each student; the faculty facilitator meets individually with each student in the group to discuss both assessments.

Unfortunately, we know that the paucity of formative feedback in medical education is a critical issue and stems from two major causes: infrequent faculty observation of trainees/students; and discomfort among preceptors in giving feedback. Both lead to general and non-specific feedback (student to preceptor: 'How am I doing?'; preceptor to student: 'Fine') that fails to give students sufficiently specific information to reflect on their performance in the context of progress towards goals, and to adjust personal goals, strategies or techniques.

Problems with sufficient time to give formative feedback are exacerbated by regulations restricting the number of hours juniors can work; such legislation has influenced the availability of preceptors to provide feedback to learners in many clinical disciplines.(44) Experienced educators have proposed teaching models such as the 'One-minute Preceptor' that incorporate timely formative feedback.(45,46) Another model is the Clinical Encounter Card, which incorporates specific, timely feedback to students. At one institution medical students used the feedback to improve their performance and were encouraged by faculty using the cards to develop their own learning objectives on the rotation.(47)

Faculty development workshops designed to help preceptors sharpen feedback skills and improve comfort levels with giving feedback have been well received.(48) At the very least, specific guidelines for what constitutes formative feedback can help improve the timing and quality of formative feedback, which in turn provides learners with the information they need

to reflect on their performance and make necessary adjustments. Formative feedback is covered in more detail in Chapter 18 (Box 19.6).

Adjustment

Self-regulated learners must synthesise self- and externally generated feedback related to progress towards learning goals and take action such as adjustments to goals or strategies. Reflection (as a foundation for synthesis) and attribution (as a foundation for action) are central issues to consider in this part of the cycle.

Affect plays a key role in this phase. Preceptors are cautioned to keep their own personal feelings separate from the feedback they provide to learners. However, learners are bound to have feelings related to what they hear about their performance. In the process of reflection, learners can acknowledge their feelings and then learn to put them to productive use. Positive feedback and successful progress can boost feelings of self-efficacy and motivation and thus begin another round through the cycle. Negative feedback can diminish self-efficacy and motivation, especially if learners let their emotions interfere with understanding where and how they can adjust. Placing the blame for disappointing or frustrating performance on poor choices of goals (perhaps too ambitious) or strategies (perhaps not aligned well with goals) will help learners make the changes they need to make and to continue effectively through the SRL cycle. Placing the blame on self (not smart enough) or others (the resident did not like me) can get learners 'stuck' in the cycle and unable to move forward. Insufficient feedback leaves learners with insufficient information to move forward as well.

It is important for learners to acknowledge feelings (particularly where learning is focused on attitudes), but it is just as important for them to have a sense of control over their learning – a sense that if efforts are not entirely successful, they can adjust as needed and achieve success.

Reflection

Reflection is an advanced cognitive skill that requires individuals to examine new information/material, weigh its validity and relevance, and draw conclusions that they either incorporate into existing cognitive structures, or construct new structures with links to existing ones.(49) Reflection, an essential element of learning, is just as essential for developing SRL competency in learners.(50) In the context of SRL, reflection encourages individuals to consider themselves as learners with personal goals, beliefs and styles, to evaluate the processes or strategies they have chosen, and then to weigh the level of success these have contributed towards achievement of goals. Reflection provides important information as learners approach learning in the future (i.e. continue once again through the cycle).

Schön conceptualised the reflective practitioner, who possesses certain tacit expertise that is revealed through skilful performance.(51) Reflection-*on*-action is a process individuals use to ponder their performance after a task has been completed, reflecting on what worked well and what would they have done differently. Reflection-*in*-action is a process individuals use as they are working on a task and encounter situations in which their knowledge-in-action does not work in some new or changed context; in this circumstance reflection allows the learner to adjust an activity or task 'on the fly', that is, while it is ongoing.

Reflection-in-action can also be conceptualised as reflection-in-learning, where reflection during the learning process is encouraged and enhanced by self-monitoring and external, formative feedback. Guidance or feedback on the reflection process might be in order because some learners do not naturally engage in reflection and others can become more productive in their reflective activities.

Educators can employ different methods to help learners become comfortable with reflection, such as portfolios or writing in journals. As development advances, reflection can also be integrated as a key step in solving complex or ill-structured problems.

Attribution

Learners make causal attributions about whether specific performances are the result of ability or effort extended. Poor performance attributed to insufficient ability can discourage efforts to improve, while poor performance attributed to learning strategies can encourage efforts to experiment with different strategies in order to improve.(25)

Attribution theory provides a useful contemporary framework for thinking about specific factors to which learners attribute their academic successes or failures.(52) There are three types of explanation that individuals tend to make about success or failure.

- The cause of success or failure might be *internal* or *external* (factors within us or factors within the environment).
- The cause of success or failure might be *stable* or *unstable* (stable if we believe the outcome will be the same if we perform the same behaviour again, unstable if we believe the outcome might be different).
- The cause of success or failure might be *controllable* or *uncontrollable* (we can alter controllable factors if we wish, we cannot easily alter uncontrollable factors).

Learners will be most successful at achieving learning goals and outcomes when they attribute poor academic performance to internal, unstable factors over which they have control (i.e. effort). However, a key assumption of attribution theory is that learners will want to attribute academic success or failure in ways that maintain a positive self-image. Thus, when they achieve intended outcomes learners will tend to attribute success to their own effort or ability, but when they do *not* achieve intended outcomes they will tend to attribute failure to poor teaching or bad luck – factors over which they have no control. The ideal attribution for academic success is ability plus effort, and in practical terms effort can be defined as devoting effective learning time and strategies to academic tasks.

Learners who engage in the strategic, step-by-step learning that characterises SRL will tend to attribute success or failure on learning tasks to the presence or absence of sufficient strategic approaches, and they will blame failed efforts on their approaches rather than on their innate ability or on others. They can adjust their approaches to assure better outcomes, that is, they are in control of this process and thus they are in control of the outcomes.(53)

Outcomes of successfully employed SRL include learners' positive feelings about their accomplishments and the responsibility and self-control they engaged to accomplish what they did, which cyclically provides motivation to progress to the next step of learning (Box 19.7).(54)

Conclusion

This chapter has described a model for SRL that was synthesised from existing theory and evidence, most of which was undertaken and reported by educational psychologists. Scholars and educators involved in this research believe that effective SRL habits can be learnt,

BOX 19.7 Self-regulated learning in practice: adjustment

Given the nature of the psychosocial issues in the longitudinal cases and the presence of attitudinal intended learning outcomes, students are provided with opportunities for reflection about issues. These opportunities for practising reflection are meant to prepare them for reflection on personal issues such as beliefs, goals and performance.

Students are provided with a variety of resources, but they are free to make decisions about strategies they use to study and methods they use to learn and to help their classmates learn. With that freedom comes responsibility for assuring that learning is occurring and progress is made towards goals or learning outcomes. If progress is slower than expected or off-target, reflection about what might be wrong and how to adjust is encouraged.

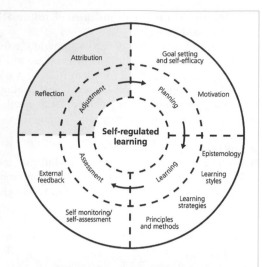

Each (end-of-term) assessment period, facilitators submit their assessments of students and then review and discuss with each student faculty assessment, self-assessment, and progress towards course and personal goals. Because the assessment instrument is scaled on distal learning outcomes, proximal goals are encouraged. In their one-on-one meetings with students (formal meeting times are scheduled twice each year), facilitators make explicit connections between personal goals and personal responsibility for learning (attributing performance appropriately). Students are reminded of the expectations for them in the context of the course, and are encouraged to discuss areas where they believe more or different goals and effort are required.

and that educators play a key role – through intentional practice – in helpings learners understand and master these habits.

Medical educators believe self-assessment is a vital skill in professional practice – particularly in light of its links to the quality of medical care; researchers connected with medical education have investigated this phenomenon inside and outside the classroom and clinic. They have, however, thus far been stymied in attempts to draw evidence-based conclusions that guide educators in how to help learners master the ability to self-assess themselves effectively. Perhaps this is because these efforts have been focused solely on self-assessment, and on measuring self-assessment accuracy.

In fact, practising professionals are not *just* self-assessing. They are self-regulating their learning through the decisions they make related to what to learn (goals), how to learn it (epistemology, styles, strategies, methods), whether or not they have learnt what they intended to learn (assessment) and what to do if they have not learnt what they intended to learn (adjustment). They are self-regulating, but perhaps not as effectively as they might if they had been trained to think about each of those steps consciously before they became habit.

The model proposed here takes a broader look at the self in the context of learning, beyond self-assessment as the 'driving force' in lifelong learning. Such a model gives us, as educators, a broader focus for helping our learners to become intentional self-regulators; within

this context self-assessment remains a key, but as a process interlinked with personal goals, actions and outcomes that reciprocally reinforce each other. It is within this broader context that learners can see and understand the importance of self-assessment in the process of learning, and the importance of assuming greater and greater responsibility for their own learning.

Acknowledgement

Casey White would like to acknowledge the significant contributions Joseph C Fantone MD made to this chapter. His feedback and suggestions were important, thoughtful and greatly appreciated.

References

1 Westberg J and Jason H (1994) Fostering learners' reflection and self-assessment. *Family Medicine*. **26**: 278–82.

2 Lowenthal W (1981). Continuing education for professionals: voluntary ormandatory? *Journal of Higher Education*. **52**: 519–38.

3 Miflin B, Campbell CB and Price DA (1999) A lesson from the introduction of a problem-based, graduate entry course: the effects of different view of self-direction. *Medical Education*. **33**: 801–7.

4 Ainoda N, Onishi H and Yasuda Y (2005) Definitions and goals of self-directed learning in contemporary medical education literature. *Annals of Academic Medicine Singapore*. **34**: 515–19.

5 Dornan H, Hadfield J, Brown M *et al.* (2005) How can medical students learn in a self-directed way in the clinical environment? Design-based research. *Medical Education.* **39**: 356–64.

6 White CB (2007) Smoothing out transitions: how pedagogy influences medical students' achievement of self-regulated learning goals. *Advances in Health Sciences Education.* **12**: 279–97.

7 Harvey BJ, Rothman AI and Frecker RC (2003) Effect of an undergraduate medical curriculum on students' self-directed learning. *Academic Medicine.* **78**: 1259–65.

8 Regehr G, Hodges B, Tiberius R and Lofchy J (1996) Measuring self-assessment skills: an innovative relative ranking model. *Academic Medicine.* **71**(10): S52–4.

9 Eva KW and Regehr G (2005) Self-assessment in the health professions: reformulation and research agenda. *Academic Medicine.* **80**(10): S46–54.

10 Davis DA, Mazmanian PE, Fordis M *et al.* (2006) Accuracy of physician self-assessment compared with observed measures of competence. *Journal of the American Medical Association.* **296**: 1094–103.

11 Pintrich PR (1995) *Understanding Self-Regulated Learning. New Directions for Teaching and Learning,* no. 63. Jossey-Bass, San Francisco, CA.

12 Evensen DH, Salisbury-Glennon JD and Glenn J (2001) A qualitative study of six medical students in a problem-based curriculum: toward a situated model of self-regulation. *Journal of Educational Psychology.* **93**: 659–76.

13 Zimmerman BJ (1989) A social cognitive view of self-regulated learning. *Journal of Educational Psychology.* **81**: 329–39.

14 Pintrich PR and Schunck DH (2002) *Motivation in Education: theory, research and applications* (2e). Merrill Prentice Hall, Upper Saddle River, NJ.

15 Locke EA and Latham GP (1990) *A Theory of Goal Setting and Task Performance.* Prentice Hall, Englewood Cliffs, NJ.

16 Bandura A (1994) Self-efficacy. In: Ramachaudran VS (ed.) *Encyclopedia of Human Behavior,* vol. **4**, pp. 71–81. Academic Press, New York, NY.

17 Ryan RM and Deci EL (2000) Intrinsic and extrinsic motivations: classic definitions and new directions. *Contemporary Educational Psychology.* **25**: 54–67.

18 Winne PH (1997) Experimenting to bootstrap self-regulated learning. *Journal of Educational Psychology.* **89**: 397–410.

19 Deci EL, Vallerand RJ, Pelletier LG and Ryan RM (1991) Motivation and education: the self-determination perspective. *Educational Psychologist.* **26**: 325–46.

20 Bloom B, Englehart M, Furst E *et al.* (1956) *Taxonomy of Educational Objectives: the classification of educational goals. Handbook I: Cognitive Domain.* Longmans, Green, New York and Toronto.

21 Driscoll MP (1999) *Psychology of Learning for Instruction.* Allyn and Bacon, Boston, MA.

22 Perry WG (1970) *Forms of Intellectual and Ethical Development in the College Years: a scheme.* Holt, Rinehart, and Winston, New York, NY.

23 Kegan R (1994) *In Over Our Heads: the mental demands of modern life.* Cambridge University Press, Cambridge, MA.

24 Kolb DA (1984) *Experiential Learning.* Prentice Hall, Upper Saddle River, NJ.

25 Zimmerman BJ (2000) Attaining self-regulation: a social-cognitive perspectives. In: Boekaerts M, Pintrich PR and Zeidner MH (eds) *Handbook of Self-regulation,* pp. 13–39. Academic Press, San Diego, CA.

26 Winne PH (1982) Minimizing the black box problem to enhance the validity of theories about instructional effects. *Instructional Science.* **11**: 13–28.

27 Butler DL and Winne PH (1995) Feedback and self-regulated learning: a theoretical synthesis. *Review of Educational Research.* **65**: 245–81.

28 Grow G (1991) Teaching learners to be self-directed. *Adult Education Quarterly.* **41**: 125–49.

29 Baxter Magolda MB (1999) *Creating Contexts for Learning and Self-authorship: constructive-developmental pedagogy.* Vanderbilt University Press, Nashville, TN.

30 King P and Kitchener KS (1994) *Developing Reflective Judgment: understanding and promoting intellectual growth and critical thinking in adolescents and adults.* Jossey-Bass, San Francisco, CA.

31 Balzer WK, Doherty ME and O'Connor R (1989) Effects of cognitive feedback on performance. *Psychological Bulletin.* **106**: 410–33.

32 Shokar GS, Shokar NK, Romero CM and Bulik RJ (2002) Self-directed learning: looking at outcomes with medical students. *Family Medicine.* **34**: 197–200.

33 Andrews GR and Debus RL (1978) Persistence and the causal perception of failure: modifying cognitive attributions. *Journal of Educational Psychology.* **70**: 154–66.

34 Sadler DR (1989) Formative assessment and the design of instructional systems. *Instructional Science.* **18**: 119–44.

35 Baker L (1984) Children's effective use of multiple standards for evaluating their comprehension. *Journal of Educational Psychology.* **76**: 588–97.

36 Rezler AG (1989) Self-assessment in problem-based groups. *Medical Teacher.* **11**: 151–6.

37 Das M and Mpofu D (1998) Self and tutor evaluations in problem-based learning tutorials: is there a relationship? *Medical Education.* **32**: 411–18.

38 Tousignant M and DesMarchais JE (2002) Accuracy of student self-assessment ability compared to their own performance in a problem-based learning medical program: a correlation study. *Advances in Health Sciences Education.* **7**: 19–27.

39 Fitzgerald JT, White CB and Gruppen LD (2003) A longitudinal study of self-assessment accuracy. *Medical Education.* **37**: 645–9.

40 Baliga S, Gruppen LD, Fitzgerald JT *et al.* (1998) Do personal characteristics and background influence self-assessment accuracy? Paper presented at the Eight Ottawa Conference on Medical Education, Philadelphia, PA, June.

41 The effectiveness of self-assessment on the identification of learner needs, learner activity, and impact on clinical practice: BEME Guide no. 10. (2008). *Medical Teacher* **30**(2): 124–45.

42 Engel CE (1991) Not just a method but a way of learning. In: Boud B and Geletti G (eds) *The Challenge of Problem-Based Learning,* pp. 23–33. Kogan Page, London.

43 Berkson L (1993) Problem-based learning: have the expectations been met? *Academic Medicine.* **68**(10): S79–88.

44 White CB, Haftel HM, Purkiss JA *et al.* (2006) Multi-dimensional effects of the 80-hour work week. *Academic Medicine.* **81**: 57–62.

45 Irby DM, Aagaard E and Teherani A (2004) Teaching points identified by preceptors observing one-minute preceptor and traditional preceptor encounters. *Academic Medicine.* **79**: 50–5.

46 Aagaard E, Teherani A and Irby D (2004) The effectiveness of the one-minute preceptor model for diagnosing the patient and the learner. *Academic Medicine.* **79**: 42–9.

47 Greenberg LW (2004) Medical students' perceptions of feedback in a busy ambulatory setting: a descriptive study using a clinical encounter card. *Southern Medical Journal.* **97**: 1174–8.

48 McIlwrick J, Nair B and Montgomery G (2006) 'How am I doing?' Man problems but few solutions related to feedback delivery in undergraduate psychiatry education. *Academic Psychiatry.* **30**: 130–5.

49 Meyers C and Jones TB (1993) *Promoting Active Learning: strategies for the college classroom.* Jossey-Bass, San Francisco, CA.

50 Chi MTH (1996) Constructing self-explanations and scaffolded explanations in tutoring. *Applied Cognitive Psychology.* **10**: 1–17.

51 Schön DA (1987) Teaching artistry through reflection-in-action. In: Schon DA (ed.) *Educating the Reflective Practitioner*, pp. 22–40. Jossey-Bass, San Francisco, CA.

52 Wiener B (1972) Attribution theory, achievement motivation, and the educational process. *Review of Educational Research.* **42**: 203–15.

53 Prawat RS (1998) Current self-regulation views of learning and motivation viewed through a Deweyan lens: the problems with dualism. *American Educational Research Journal.* **35**: 199–224.

54 Paris SG and Paris AH (2001) Classroom applications of research on self-regulated learning. *Educational Psychologist.* **36**: 89–101.

Further Reading

There is a substantial body of research and relevant literature on self-regulated learning. Although a fair amount of the work was done in kindergarten to 12th grade contexts, there is some evidence reported at the college level. As with any body of scholarly work in an academic field, some of this work is theoretical, some is quite complex, written in disciplinary vernacular and designed to inform researchers about the work that has been done and the evidence it has yielded, and some is practical, written in terms that help educators understand how theory has been applied effectively in classroom contexts. The reference list includes a lot of this work, across these various domains.

Thinking about research: frameworks, ethics and scholarship

Jan Illing

KEY MESSAGES

- Research is concerned with critical or scientific enquiry. It differs from audit, as research is concerned with discovering the right thing to do, and audit, with ensuring that it is done right. Evaluation aims to assess the worth or value of something.

- Theoretical perspectives provide the framework for research and inform the basic assumptions that guide the research. A theoretical perspective encompasses important elements: ontology, epistemology and methodology.

- Can research combine qualitative and quantitative research methods? One perspective is that the

- ontological and epistemological assumptions of these approaches are incompatible, and therefore it is not feasible to combine methods. An opposing view sees the two approaches as compatible, and combined approaches become feasible

- Researchers are expected to minimise the risk of harm or discomfort to people. Harm from educational or social research is more likely to take the form of psychological distress than physical injury. Research that aims to be published requires an ethical review.

Introduction

Quantitatative, qualitative, positivism, post-positivism, post-modern, naturalistic, interpretivism, constructionism, participatory, grounded theory, ethnography, phenomenology, hermeneutics, conversation analysis and narrative. A plethora of research approaches and methods; words that may leave the novice researcher feeling rather overwhelmed; that it's all 'too heavy'.

To make matters worse, authors will often confuse the use of terms,(1,2) sometimes relabelling research approaches(3) themselves. Without a map to organise and sort the labels into meaningful groups it can be quite a challenge to make any sense of these theoretical concepts at all. This chapter aims to provide such a map and will focus on the fundamental theoretical concepts associated with research and practical issues for the researcher to consider before starting out on their project.

What Is Research?

Research has been defined as 'a search or investigation directed to the discovery of some fact by careful con-

sideration or study of a subject; a course of critical or scientific inquiry'.(4) This definition may sound straightforward, in that most researchers would agree that they are involved in a critical inquiry of something, but some would argue that their aim is not to establish facts but to increase or change understanding about something.

How does research differ from audit?

Research is concerned with discovering the right thing to do, and audit, with ensuring that it is done right.(5) Following this definition, audit focuses on what is given and asks questions about the given, while research has the freedom to ask questions about the given, including 'Is this the best or only way to do something?'

How does research differ from evaluation?

According to Clarke,(6) what differentiates evaluation from research is the question of purpose. 'An evaluation is action orientated. It is conducted to determine the value or impact of a policy, programme, practice, intervention or service, with a view to making recommendations for change'. Robson(7) states that 'to evaluate is to assess the worth or value of something'. Following this definition, evaluation is about setting out to make a judgement. Going back to our definition of research, there is no mention of research leading to judgement, but to the discovery of findings by critical inquiry. Evaluation research is part of research, but in evaluation the aim involves assessing the worth of something.

Understanding Medical Education: Evidence, Theory and Practice. Edited by T Swanwick. © 2010 Association for the Study of Medical Education.

Theoretical Frameworks in Education and the Social Sciences

Kneebone(8) published a personal view about his attempt to engage with the education and social science literature. He wrote, 'At first and to my great surprise I found this literature almost impenetrable, of course it was peppered with unfamiliar words … I had the disquieting sensation of moving into alien territory, where familiar landmarks had disappeared'. Kneebone came to the realisation that all his medical training had been based within one view of science, the positivist paradigm, and that this was a very narrow and limited view. He ended with a plea to include an exploration of what the humanities have to offer the medical curriculum, and also with explicit guidance on how to gain access to this world. The aim of this chapter is to make this other 'world' penetrable.

The focus of this section is to present some of the frameworks within which quantitative and qualitative research is conducted in education and the social sciences. Quantitative research in education and social science is typically represented by the social survey and experimental methods, whereas qualitative research uses techniques such as observation and interview. Deciding on which method to choose is integral to the research question being posed, but each type of approach signals to the reader the framework within which the research is expected to be read and judged.

In the past, the scientific method applied to the study of the natural sciences was considered appropriate and desirable for the study of education and the social sciences. Early textbooks focused on the scientific method, and other methods such as participant observation were deemed less scientific and weak by comparison, and consequently of lower status. From the 1970s, the debate over the appropriateness of the natural science model for social sciences enquiry gained momentum. Arguments centred on the differences in focus: people in education and the social sciences, and objects in the natural sciences. There was an increase in philosophical ideas and debate on the key issue of whether scientific method was appropriate for the study of people. The terms 'qualitative' and 'quantitative' signified more than different methods of collecting data, they indicated different assumptions about research in the social world.

The debate may have gathered momentum following Kuhn's(9) work on the history of science. Of particular importance is Kuhn's idea of a *paradigm*: a set of beliefs and dictats that influence what should be studied, how the research should be conducted and how the results should be interpreted. Here, a paradigm is a set of basic beliefs or assumptions about the social world. It can be compared to viewing the social world through a particular lens and encompasses ontology, epistemology, theory and methods. Paradigms cannot be proven but rely on argument, persuasion and usefulness. A paradigm is defined as 'a conceptual or methodological model underlying the theories and practices of a science or discipline at a particular time; (hence) a generally accepted world view'.(4)

Apart from positivism, all the other paradigms discussed below are still in their formative stages of development, hence some of the changes in nomenclature referred to above. So from this point on I shall refer to theoretical perspectives rather than paradigms. Each perspective has important consequences for the research that follows in terms of procedure and interpretation of findings, and suggests to the reader how the research should be read and in which framework it sits.

Theoretical Perspectives in Research

Theoretical perspectives are taken here to mean the philosophical stances that lie behind the research methodology. The theoretical perspectives are the starting point from which assumptions about the research are based; they influence how the study is conducted, the researcher's role and the type of knowledge that is produced. Each perspective will also have a particular set of criteria to be used in evaluating a piece of research. There has been a great deal written about the different perspectives, and much of it has focused narrowly on only one perspective without guiding the reader on where each perspective sits in relation to others. What is offered here is an overview in which I will cover the conventional positivist and post-positivist perspectives, and then other, more emergent, perspectives. For more detailed exposition, see Guba and Lincoln,(1,10) Heron and Reason,(11) and Crotty.(12)

Each theoretical perspective takes a particular *ontological* and *epistemological* position that informs the resulting research methods. *Ontology* is the study of being, and is concerned with the nature of existence and the structure of reality. It raises questions about the nature and form of reality and what can be known about it. In the social world is there a 'real' and single reality? Are there multiple realities dependent on whose view is taken? *Epistemology* focuses on the nature of the relationship between the researcher and what is to be known. The epistemological question is dependent on the answer to the ontological question. For example, when reality is assumed to be 'real', then what can be known about it can be independent of any relationship between the researcher and the subject of enquiry, and knowledge can be said to be objective. Therefore, the concept of objectivity in research assumes the existence of a 'real' world. However, if the answer to the ontological question is that reality is

BOX 20.1 'Heavy' words

- *Epistemology:* the theory of knowledge, its origins and nature, and the limits of knowledge.
- *Ontology:* the study of being. It is concerned with the nature of existence and the structure of reality. With regard to social enquiry, this is often taken to mean the assumptions that a particular theoretical perspective makes about the nature of social reality.
- *Methodology:* the research design or plan that shapes the methods to be used in the study. The methodology provides a rationale for the choice of methods used in a study.
- *Methods:* the techniques used for data collection.
- *Theoretical perspective:* the philosophical stance that lies behind the methodology.

socially constructed and there is no 'real' version, then the answer to the epistemological question becomes subjective, as each researcher has his or her own version of reality and there is no true version, only a socially constructed reality. The methodological approach taken comes secondary to the answers to the ontological and epistemological questions (and focuses on the methods by which knowledge can be acquired on the subject of enquiry). If a 'real' reality is assumed, then this implies that the researcher can collect objective data and the ability to control variables becomes feasible (*see* Box 20.1).

Positivism

Positivism has been the dominant perspective in the physical and social sciences, going back to the Enlightenment in the seventeenth century, and is identified with quantitative methods. Positivism is linked to empirical science, offering assurances that knowledge is unambiguous, accurate and certain. 'Positive' comes from '*something that is posited*', a science that is firmly grounded, not something that is arrived at from speculation. Auguste Comte (1798–1857) is attributed as the founder of positivism, although the ideas on establishing scientific laws from observation and experiment are reported much earlier in the work of Francis Bacon (1561–1626). What is posited in positivist science is what is scientifically observed following use of the scientific method. Comte's positivism bids us to look for regular characteristics, constant relationships to facts and to laws that can be scientifically established using the scientific method of observation, experimentation and comparison. The 'verification principle', which became a central tenet of positivism, is attributed to Ludwig Wittgenstein (1889–1951). The verification principle focuses on the importance of verifying statements via the experience of the scientific

method. Today, positivism is still linked to empirical science. The confidence in science is reflected in the belief that science is both accurate and certain, in contrast to values, opinions and feelings, which are empirically unverifiable and of no interest to positivism.

Ontology, epistemology and methodology

The ontology of positivism is realism. Reality is assumed to exist and the aim is to explain the social world in terms of laws, often including cause and effect. The epistemology of positivism is objectivism. Positivism maintains that objects in the world have meaning both prior to and independently of any consciousness of them. Positivism maintains that there are 'facts' that can be accurately collected about the social world, which are independent of individual interpretation and are 'true'. Researchers can be objective in the collection and interpretation of data. It is assumed that the researcher is capable of investigating the object of study without influencing it or being influenced by it. This differs from our subjective understanding, which constitutes a different form of knowledge from knowledge made up of scientific facts.

Positivist methodology is usually deductive and the aim is often concerned with the prediction and control of phenomena, and involves testing hypotheses to support or disprove a theory. Research procedures need to be followed rigorously to prevent values and biases from affecting the data. Methods are reported in detail to enable others to repeat the study and show that the results are reproducible by others. The methods used are mainly quantitative, involving experimental or manipulative research designs. Results are generally reported using statistics to show that any differences are beyond mere chance. The aim is to generalise findings to a larger population than the study sample.

For positivists (and post-positivists), the important aspects of research are:

- the aim
- testing hypotheses
- cause and effect
- generalisability
- adding to existing knowledge
- research rigour, in particular validity and reliability.

These are the main areas where research rooted in other perspectives is attacked. Quality is assessed by internal (findings are congruent with reality) and external (findings are generalisable) validity, and reliability (findings are stable) and objectivity (researcher has not influenced findings).

Knowledge, values and ethics

Knowledge from positivist research is built up like building blocks, by adding new knowledge to old. Knowledge is viewed to identify patterns and determine where new knowledge fits with existing old knowledge, and frequently aims to form rules and laws such as cause and effect. While the reporting of scientific knowledge is acceptable, criticisms focus on claiming that scientific knowledge is the only valid form of knowledge and that it is completely objective and accurate. Ethics and values are important for all types of research although treated differently by them.(1) Values are excluded in positivism. Positivism claims to be value-free as a result of its epistemological position that research can be objective if rigour is applied. Positivists view values as confounding variables that need to be controlled and excluded from the study. The methodology is designed to isolate and remove subjectivity and bias. Research ethics, although of importance in positivism, is largely viewed as something external to the research itself. Ethics is seen as something that would be applied to the research, possibly by an external research ethics body or a professional body that may advise on the professional conduct of researchers.

The positivist researcher

The researcher is often in the role of 'expert'. The researcher takes on the role of independent observer, who is impartial to the study findings and reports them objectively, using them to inform decisions and recommendations. Positivists maintain that research is a specialist activity that needs to be carried out by trained and qualified 'scientists'. The novice researcher is trained in quantitative methods, research design and measurement. The aim is to be objective and any personal bias has no part in the research.

Is there conflict with other perspectives?

Proponents of positivism take a *reductionist* stance, in that it is assumed that at some point in the future a structure will be identified on which questions of difference can be considered and explained. This position assumes that the other perspectives are measurable or can be measurable by the same standards and therefore comparison can be made. There is much disagreement about this from proponents of critical theory and constructivism. Positivists would see action research as a contamination of both the research process and research findings.

Post-Positivism

Post-positivism emerged following a realisation that the scientific method couldnot be applied to all scientific theory and much of what was accepted as 'fact' was theory and had not been observed at all or the act of observation hadchanged the subject. The work of the physicist Heisenberg (1901–1976) highlights this. He claimed that it was impossible to determine the position and momentum of a subatomic particle with any real accuracy, as the very act of observing it changed it. Popper (1902–1994) introduced the princi-

ple of *falsification*, where the emphasis moves from proving a theory is correct to being unable through repeat testing to prove it is wrong. Popper maintained that no theory could ever be proven, only disproved, and if a theory or hypothesis was not open to refutation from experimentation or observation, then the claims or theories made were not truly scientific.

Kuhn (1922–1996) identified a disparity between Aristotelian and Newtonian physics and noted that the differences were so extreme that a revolution in scientific thinking must have occurred. Kuhn questioned the objectivity and value neutrality of the scientific method and findings that could not be explained within the positivist paradigm, which led him to question the adequacy of the paradigm and call for a 'paradigm shift' and a shift in the way scientists view reality. The post-positivist perspective is less absolute; probability has replaced certainty; a level of objectivity has replaced absolute objectivity; and approximate truth has replaced absolute truth.

Ontology, epistemology and methodology

The ontology of post-positivism is critical realism. Like positivism, reality is assumed to exist, but unlike positivism, reality cannot be truly 'known'. Access to reality is imperfect due to weaknesses in the human as researcher and the complexity of the enquiry. Post-positivist epistemology is objectivist; objectivity is the ideal, but the data are subject to critical review. The post-positivist perspective acknowledges that no matter how much rigour is applied to the scientific method, research outcomes are never totally objective or certain, and claims are tempered. Emphasis is placed on collecting more than one type of data (triangulation) and on the falsification of hypotheses rather than confirmation. Post-positivism aims to address some of the problems of positivist research by collecting data in natural settings and collecting the insider views. Aims are achieved by using both quantitative and qualitative methods. Like positivism, quality is assessed by internal validity (the findings are congruent with reality), external validity (the findings are generalisable), reliability (the findings are stable) and objectivity (the researcher or the study procedure has not influenced the findings).

Knowledge, values and ethics

Knowledge consists of hypotheses that thus far have not been falsified and is made up of facts and laws that are probably 'true'. But as with positivism, knowledge is built by adding new knowledge to old to fit into existing patterns and form generalisations or rules such as cause and effect. As in positivism, post-positivist values are excluded and claim to be value neutral. Values are perceived as confounding variables that need to be excluded from the study. Research ethics is again an area of importance but is viewed as something largely external to the research itself.

The post-positivist researcher

The post-positivist researcher is more often in the role of 'expert', and the aim of the study is to provide an explanation and, when possible, prediction and control of phenomena. Again the researcher takes on the role of independent enquirer, who is impartial to the study findings and reports them objectively, using them to inform decisions and recommendations. Positivists maintain that research is a specialist activity that needs to be carried out by trained and qualified 'scientists'. The novice researcher is trained in the same way as the positivist researcher, but with the addition of qualitative methods, so that more detail is added to the meaning of the data, and data are no longer 'context stripped' but put in context. The minority and the individual voice is presented as well as the majority voice.

Is there conflict with other perspectives?

Proponents of this perspective take the same reductionist stance as positivism. It is assumed that at some point in the future a structure will be identified upon which questions of difference can be considered and explained. This position assumes that the other perspectives are measurable by the same standards and therefore comparison can be made. There is much disagreement about this from proponents of critical theory and constructivism.

Critical Theory and Related Ideological Positions

In contrast to positivist or post-positivist perspectives oriented to understanding or explaining the world, critical theory is oriented towards critiquing and changing society as a whole. Critical theory is used here as a blanket term, which includes, among others, the feminist and Marxist perspectives.

Feminist research starts with criticism of science, stating that it is incomplete and reflects a male distortion of the social world. Although it is more accurate to talk of feminisms, as there is not one unified body of thought, Tong(13) categorises seven forms of feminism. However, there is agreement that society has marginalised women and that this is reflected in research practice. Science perpetuates the myth of the superiority of men to women. Gender, as a significant issue in dealing with explanations of social phenomena, has largely been absent. The feminist perspective maintains that perpetuating a male view of science narrows ideas and limits understanding of the social world, and that if the male viewpoint was not dominant, a different research model would be dominant. Positivist research has stressed the importance of emotional separateness of researchers from their research participants to maintain objectivity. The feminist perspective maintains that research is a two-way process and detachment and objectivity are impossible. It does not acknowledge how the researcher is affected by the research and how the researcher's own biography becomes a fundamental part of the research process.(14)

The Marxist perspective, like the feminist, is not merely seeking to understand and accept the status quo, but to challenge, to recognise conflict and oppression, and to bring about change. Marx perceived a basic conflict between capital and labour between the bourgeoisie and the proletariat, and believed similar class struggles were part of earlier society. Marx maintained that economic forces determine how we think. Thoughts and consciousness come from our social being, itself the result of economic forces. Marx maintained that those who held economic power also held the intellectual power. The ruling classes ruled as thinkers, producers of ideas, and regulated the production and distribution of ideas.(15) He described an oppression that penetrated deep into human life, resulting in the alienation from work and finally from others. The proposed solution was for the proletariat to emancipate itself in a revolt, destroying their inhuman existence and all other inhuman conditions in society.

Ontology, epistemology and methodology

The ontology of critical theory is historical realism. Reality is assumed to be capture-able, but has been shaped over time by social, cultural, gender, ethnic, political and economic factors, and changed into a reality that 'has set' over time. The epistemology is transactional and subjectivist: the researcher and the object of the research are assumed to be linked by the values of the researcher and relevant others who influence the study. Findings or knowledge are value dependent; they are mediated by the values of the researcher and the relevant others. It is the epistemological position that sets it apart from positivism and post-positivism. Methods require a dialogue between investigator and the subjects of enquiry. The aim of the research is to critique and change factors that constrain and exploit individuals. Quality is assessed by the historical context of the study, that is, whether it takes account of social factors of the studied situation and the extent to which the study acts to remove a lack of knowledge, and acts as a stimulus for action in the sense of bringing about a change in the existing structure.

Knowledge, values and ethics

Knowledge is made up of historical or structural insights that will transform with time. Transformations occur following informed insight. Knowledge grows and changes with historical revision as ignorance is eroded. Generalisations occur when the mix of social demographics, circumstances and values are similar. Values play a central role in critical theory and are important in shaping research outcomes. Excluding values would go against the interests of any minority or powerless group who were part of the study. The aim is to give the weak and powerless groups a platform and let their voice be heard along with any others who may be more dominant. Unlike the positivist and post-positivist perspectives, ethics is more internal than external to the research study. The critical theorist takes more of a moral standpoint in revealing full details about the study to ensure the study participant can be fully informed prior to consent and with no deception.

The critical theorist researcher

In critical theory, the researcher takes on the role of facilitator, raising not only their own level of consciousness about the object of study but also that of others. The researcher may facilitate change in the study group by providing greater insight into their situation and provide a stimulus for members of the community to take control of their future and initiate action and change. The novice critical theory researcher must first be 'resocialised' from previous exposure to the positivism. This involves conscious re-educating about positivism and post-positivism and its limitations. New researchers need to understand the perspective differences and understand both quantitative and qualitative methods so that they can understand how the perspectives differ and how the research is conducted. New researchers also need to understand the role that social issues have in the research context and structure and uphold the values of empowerment and altruism in their work.

Is there conflict with other perspectives?

Critical theory and constructionism (see below) agree that they are in conflict with positivist and post-positivist perspectives. The epistemological position of critical theory sets it apart from the positivist and post-positivist perspective; research can be value-free or it cannot; and a single model could not support both tenets.

Constructivism

Guba and Lincoln's(1) constructivism is a broad eclectic framework that embraces interpretive, phenomenology and hermeneutic perspectives (*see* Box 20.2). Space does not permit me to cover each of these, and for more detail I recommend Guba and Lincoln,(10) Crotty(12) and Schwandt.(16) Constructivism is the view that knowledge, and therefore all meaning, is not discovered but socially constructed. Meaning is not created but constructed out of the world that is already there, and objects in that world. The world and its objects may have no intrinsic meaning, but they are partners in the generation of meaning. Crotty(12) states that constructivism mirrors intentionality (meaning reaching out into directedness) in that con-

> **BOX 20.2 Focus on: Hermeneutics**
>
> The word 'hermeneutics' derives from the name of the Greek god Hermes, the messenger and interpreter of the gods. Hermeneutics is a branch of philosophy concerned with the understanding and the interpretation of texts, although the concept of 'text' has, in recent years, been extended beyond the written word to speech, performances, works of art and even events.
>
> A hermeneutic defines a method for interpretation, or a specific theory of interpretation. In contemporary usage it has been widely used to denote the study of the general principles of biblical interpretation. Hermeneutics assumes that the text remains as written, painted or recorded but that its interpretation changes with time and across contexts.
>
> In critical hermeneutics the interpreter constructs the context as another form of text, which can then, of itself, be critically analysed so that the meaning construction can be understood as an interpretive act. In this way, the hermeneutic interpreter is simply creating another text on a text, and this recursive creation is potentially infinite. Every meaning is constructed, even through the very constructive act of seeking to deconstruct, and the process whereby that textual interpretation occurs must be self-critically reflected upon.(18)

sciousness is directed towards an object such that the object becomes shaped by consciousness and what comes to the fore is the interaction between subject and object. From this, meaning is born. The acceptance of intentionality therefore means the rejection of both objectivism and subjectivism.

It is accepted, even by the positivists, that social realities are socially constructed. The difference between constructivists and positivists is that the former maintain that all meaningful reality is socially constructed. A table may have a real existence irrespective of whether anyone is consciously aware of it. However, it exists as a table only if it is recognised as a table by our consciousness. The table is also constructed through social life, and our culture informs how we see these objects and in some cases whether to see them at all. Throughout our lives we learn about the social and natural worlds and interpret them, not as separate worlds but as one human world. Schwandt(16) draws the distinction between constructivism, meaning that the individual mind constructs the meaning, and constructionism, meaning the society or culture the individual belongs to has constructed the meaning. This highlights the depth of human social constructions.

Ontology, epistemology and methodology

The ontology of constructivism is relativism; this assumes multiple and sometimes conflicting realities that are socially and experientially based and dependent on individuals for their form and content. There is no 'real' world that pre-exists and is independent of human consciousness. People could therefore inhabit very different worlds based on different sets of meaning. Constructions change as their associated realities change and become more informed rather than 'true'. The ontological position of constructivism is crucial in terms of separating it from other perspectives. The answer to the epistemological question of 'How do I know what I know?' is that reality is subjective. The researcher and the research object are assumed to be related, such that the research findings or knowledge are created from the relationship between the researcher and the subject of study. It is the epistemological position of constructivism that sets it apart from positivism and post-positivism. Guba and Lincoln[17] maintain that the enquiry methodology is a two-way process of listening to the constructions of both the researcher and the research participant. The optimum process of developing joint constructions is via 'hermeneutic–dialectic', meaning that the researcher compares and contrasts different constructions to achieve a consensus. For Guba and Lincoln, the researcher cannot and should not be separated from the research participant, and hence the research outcomes are a joint construction of the research process. The aim of the research is understanding or reconstruction of the constructions that are held by the subjects and the researcher about the study topic. Two sets of criteria are used to assess quality: *trustworthiness* (which parallels internal validity), *transferability* (which parallels external validity), *dependability* (paralleling reliability) and *conformability* (paralleling objectivity) make up the first set. These criteria are analogous to those used to judge quality in positivist research. The second set consists of authenticity criteria of fairness: *ontological authenticity* (develops and enhances personal constructions), *educative authenticity* (leads to improved understanding of others), *catalytic authenticity* (provides the stimulus to action) and *tactical authenticity* (the research empowers action) [see Guba and Lincoln[17]]. The second set of criteria share some common ground with critical theory.

Knowledge, values and ethics
Knowledge consists of constructions about which there is relative consensus. Multiple constructions can coexist and be of equal weight, depending on interpretation and factors that influence interpretation such as social, political and gender issues. For constructivism, values play a central role in creating and shaping the research outcomes. Constructivism views the role of researcher as the producer and facilitator of the research and acknowledges their central role in the research process. The role of ethics, like values, is central to constructivism. The researchers' role is to recognise their own constructs and values and, as in critical theory, inform the study participants fully about the research prior to taking consent, work towards uncovering the constructs of the study participants and work towards improving constructs. The methodology involves close personal interactions and as a result may raise some difficulties with confidentiality and anonymity (Box 20.2).(19)

Constructivist as researcher
The researcher takes on the role of participant or facilitator. Increasingly, constructivists aim to involve research participants to take an active part in the study, that is, by suggesting questions and outlets for research findings. The researcher is both facilitator and participant, who uncovers the constructs of self and others and reconstructs the 'multivoice' into more informed constructs. Change is facilitated when the reconstructions are formed and participants are stimulated to act on them. As in critical theory, the new researcher must first be 'resocialised' from previous exposure to the dominant perspective of positivism. Again this involves re-educating about positivism and post-positivism and the limitations of these perspectives. New researchers need to understand how this perspective differs from others, and be trained in quantitative and qualitative research methods to be able to understand how the research is conducted within this perspective.

Is there conflict with other perspectives?
The ontological stances of constructivism and critical theory are in conflict with the positivist and post-positivist perspectives. Either there is a 'real' reality or there is not; it is value-free or it is not. The concept of reconciling both of these positions in one system seems impossible.

Participatory Action Research

Participatory action research is a form of action research that involves practitioners as both subjects and co-researchers. It is based on the proposition put forward by Kurt Lewin (1890–1947) that causal inferences about human behaviour are more likely to be valid if the relevant humans participate in building and testing them. Participatory action research arose partly out of recognition that a gap often exists between the completion and publication of high-quality research and the implementation of findings. Researchers do their job and wait for the findings to be acted on by someone else. The view espoused by participatory action research is that it is important for the advancement of science to devise strategies in which research and action are closely linked. Participatory action research involves research participants in the research process working alongside the researcher from the first steps of designing the study through to research outcomes.(19) The participatory perspective was added by Heron and Reason(11) to Guba and Lincoln's(1) lists of the major paradigms that frame research, and was later included by Guba and Lincoln themselves.(17) The participatory perspective underpins forms of action research.

Ontology, epistemology and methodology
The ontology of participatory action research is subjective-objective. Heron and Reason explain this: 'When I hold your hand, my tactual imaging both subjectively shapes you and objectively meets you. To encounter being or a being is both to imagine it in my way and to know that it is there'.(11) In the participatory perspective, the mind is actively participating in a primordial reality, such that what emerges as reality is the result of an interaction and how the mind has engaged with it. The epistemological position of participatory action research is that the knower participates in the knowing in at least four different ways:

- *experiential* knowing – by direct encounter with feedback from the real world in real time
- *presentational* knowing – the artistic rehearsal process through which we craft new practices
- *propositional* knowing – knowing in conceptual terms that something is the case
- *practical* knowing – knowing how to do something.

The methodology is a collaborative form of action enquiry and is explained in terms of knowing:

> people collaborate to define the questions they wish to explore and the methodology for that exploration (propositional knowing); together or separately they apply this methodology in the world of their practice (practical knowing); which leads to new forms of encounter with their world (experiential knowing); and they find ways to represent this experience in significant patterns (presentational knowing) which feeds into a revised propositional understanding of the originating questions.(11)

Heron and Reason argue that cooperative enquiry has two participatory principles: first, that the research outcome is grounded in the researcher's own experiential knowledge, and second, that research participants have a right to participate in research that is about them. They argue that researchers are also research participants and vice versa, and the co-researchers are also the co-subjects. These two principles do not apply within constructivism (where there is no identified epistemological role for experiential knowing); researchers are not also subjects and the findings are grounded in the experiential knowing of others. Heron and Reason argue that participatory research differs from other forms of qualitative research in that research participants inform the research design and inform how knowledge is generated about them. They also argue that the purpose of research within the participatory perspective is closer

to the purposes of critical theory – 'the critic and transformation of social, political, economic, ethnic and gender structures that constrain and exploit humankind' – than constructivist, where the aim is about 'understanding and reconstruction'. The aim therefore is to create a situation in which participants give and receive valid information and are committed to the outputs of the study.

Social scientists are frequently faced with the dilemma of rigour or relevance. From the participatory action research perspective the aim is to define the standards of appropriate rigour and then meet them without loss to the relevance of the study. Validity is enhanced by the research process of participation and cycling several times through the four forms of knowledge in order to enrich congruence in articulating a subject–object reality.

Generalisations do occur, but they remain within local contexts, such as describing the thematic patterns in one context and suggesting how they might apply in a similar context, but would require a further study to confirm their relevance.

Knowledge, values and ethics
Knowledge is the result of collaboration and is built up from this collaborative relationship. Participatory action research emphasises the importance of a 'living knowledge' that is linked to practical knowing (how to do something) that comes from being grounded in the situation within which an action occurs. Participatory action research maintains that research subjects have a basic human right to be engaged in research that intends to gather knowledge about them. The roles of values and ethics are embedded into the study; the subjects are also the researchers and the researchers also the subjects.

The participatory action research researcher
The research voice is the result of 'aware self-reflective action'. The participatory action research researcher takes on the role of collaborator engaged with the practitioners and may need training to understand the relevant issues involved in the research. The researcher can act as research trainer to the practitioners to facilitate the research process. The novice researcher needs to acquire facilitator skills to work alongside their co-researchers. The researcher needs to acknowledge the skills and knowledge of the practitioners in the working partnership and, where appropriate, use this knowledge to understand the ongoing research. Participatory action research researchers need to be trained in both qualitative and quantitative research methods.

Is there conflict with other perspectives?
Participatory action research relates closely to both critical theory and constructivism but uses the same

type of measurement and standards as positivism and post-positivism. Arguably, the movement towards action research has come about as a result of non-utilisation of research findings and a desire to conduct research that will result in recommendations being implemented.

Reconciling and Combining Research Frameworks

The type of framework in which a piece of research is conducted has implications for how the research is conducted, who has control of the study, how quality is assessed, how values and ethics are viewed, and, ultimately, the type of knowledge that is produced and what is done with that knowledge. The researcher's role differs depending on the perspective influencing the study.

Guba and Lincoln(10) point out that: 'Within the last decade the borders and boundary lines between these paradigms and perspectives have begun to blur'. Rather than theoretical perspectives working in competition, they are more often combined into one study to inform the arguments of another perspective. It is more useful to identify how the enquiry perspectives are similar and how they differ. Perspectives can be blended together into two main groups: first, the positivist and post-positivist, who share important elements; and second, the critical theory, constructivist and participatory perspectives, which also share important elements. However, these two main groups are not easily combined into one model as their assumptions about reality and objectivity are contradictory.

Positivism has been the dominant research perspective for many centuries. However, in more recent years the superior status of quantitative research approaches within education and the social sciences has been challenged. Criticisms of quantitative approaches have included arguments about 'context stripping' (taking data out of context and thereby removing much of the associated meaning), that the focus is on the majority or dominant view and important messages from the minority are ignored, and that even in well-controlled experiments researchers and subjects can influence each other and bias the results. In 1994, Guba and Lincoln reported that the dominant perspective was the post-positivist perspective. Post-positivists tend to have power and influence in numerous professional decision-making processes, namely, research funding, journal publications and committees for promotion. Proponents of critical theory and constructivism have gained ground and recognition over the past 20 or so years, with more journal publications, journals and qualitative research. Participatory action research is emerging as a perspective. In 2005, Guba and Lincoln acknowledged that 'the number of qualitative texts, research papers, workshops, and training materials has exploded', and pointed out the distinct turn towards the emerging perspectives.

Writers such as Guba and Lincoln suggest that the use of a particular method implies commitment to a particular perspective and its associated ontology and epistemology. This position assumes that a methodology is necessarily indicative of particular assumptions about knowledge. This position is challenged by Bryman,(20) who suggests:

> if we accept that there is no perfect correspondence between research strategy and matters of epistemology and ontology the notion that a method is inherently or necessarily indicative of certain wider assumptions about knowledge and the nature of social reality begins to founder.

Bryman argues that research methods are more 'free-floating' in terms of ontology and epistemology than is often proposed. Bryan quotes the work of Platt, who conducted historical research on American sociology and reported no clear association between positivism and the social survey. Platt stated:

> research methods may on the level of theory, when theory is consciously involved at all, reflect intellectual *bricolage* or *post hoc* justifications rather than the consistent working through of carefully chosen fundamental assumptions … in many cases general theoretical/methodological stances are just stances: slogans, hopes, aspirations, not guidelines with clear implications that are followed in practice [Platt 1996, quoted in Bryman(20)].

Bryman continues that the link from methodology to certain assumptions is not absolute and suggests that research that combines both qualitative and quantitative approaches in one study illustrates that these research methods can be autonomous. Patton(21) concurs with the views of Bryman, commenting first on the parallel status of qualitative to quantitative research and on the increased use of multiple methods.

> Signs of détente and pragmatism now abound. Methodological tolerance, flexibility, eclecticism, and concern for appropriateness rather than orthodoxy now characterize the practice, literature and discussions of evaluation. Several developments seem to me to explain the withering of the methodological paradigms debate.(21)

Patton goes on to list several developments that explain the change towards combined methods. For example, the importance of methodological appropriateness rather than paradigm orthodoxy, that the strengths and weaknesses of both qualitative and quantitative approaches are better understood, advances in methodological sophistication, support for methodological eclecticism and increased advocacy for combing approaches (*see* Box 20.3).

The competing theoretical perspectives associated with *grounded theory* make for an interesting example.

BOX 20.3 How to: Combine qualitative and quantitative research

- *Triangulation:* use qualitative research to cross check finding from quantitative findings or vice versa.

- *Provide hypotheses:* use qualitative research to identify hypotheses that can be tested using quantitative research.

- *Aid measurement:* use qualitative research to inform survey questions.

- *Screening:* use quantitative research to screen for people with specific characteristics for in-depth qualitative study.

- *Fill gaps:* one methodology will not provide all of the needed information.

- *Snapshot versus process:* quantitative research will provide a single snapshot of the social, whereas qualitative research provides information on process.

- *Where two types of data are required:* sometimes both data about meaning and data about a set of issues are required.

- *Quantification:* use qualitative research to identify problems and quantitative research to quantify the problem.

- *Explaining the relationship between variables:* quantitative research frequently needs to explain the relationship between variables; this can be explored further by a follow-up qualitative study.

- *Exploring the micro and macro:* use of both methodologies allows a study to explore the different levels of a problem.

- *Solving a problem:* a different research strategy to the one already employed to explore unexpected or puzzling outcomes.

See Bryman(20) for further details.

Grounded theory methods were based on the work of Glaser and Strauss.(22) Glaser applied his positivistic methodological training from Columbia University to the development of qualitative data analysis, while Strauss brought symbolic interactionism following Blumer, from his training at the University of Chicago. Hence, Glaser brought epistemological assumptions and methodological terms, and Strauss brought the study of process and meaning.(23) Charmaz *et al.* (1,23,24) place grounded theory in the post-positivist perspective. Charmaz argues that Glaser's position comes close to a traditional positivist stance with assumptions of an objective, external reality and a researcher who remains neutral and discovers data. The position of Strauss and Corbin is considered post-positive as they propose giving a voice to the respond-

ents. Yet Strauss and Corbin(25) comment on the study by Orona, which is constructivist in stance, as 'a text-book' example, suggesting Strauss has a constructivist stance, which Bryman reports is evident in Strauss's earlier work.(20) Charmaz suggests that researchers can develop a constructivist ground theory by seeking the meaning of both respondents and researchers and by looking more for beliefs and values as well as acts and facts.

This example highlights that the linkage of perspective to methodology is not always clear, and if certain changes are made to the methodology, then it can become compatible with another theoretical perspective.

Box 20.4 illustrates how two contrasting research perspectives can illuminate the same research area, and provides a summary of two papers by O'Caithain *et al.*(26) and Stapleton *et al.*(27) These abstracts show quantitative and qualitative methods both being used within the same study and highlight some of the differences behind the qualitative and quantitative traditions.

It is possible to identify the post-positivist stance of the quantitative study, which attempted to control variables while manipulating others. There was concern with numbers and measurement and reporting findings in terms of statistical differences. There was also concern about using the 'correct' measurement, and fears were expressed about contamination of the intervention by earlier exposure to the leaflets.

The qualitative study referred to grounded theory, which originates from symbolic interactionism,(29) leans towards critical realism, with the researcher seeking the meaning in the data. However, grounded theory acknowledges that reality cannot be known but is interpreted, shifting towards relativism [Strausserian approach(28)], and shares a constructivist epistemology. The qualitative study was less concerned with numbers and measurement and more concerned with gaining a wider range of views and identifying all of the issues related to the intervention from many viewpoints. Observed behaviour was used to identify how the intervention was implemented, and findings were generated from observer notes. Analysis was conducted by looking for common themes in the data. The quantitative study reported that the intervention was not effective, and the qualitative study explained why.

Practical Considerations When Starting Research

The research question

Most researchers have little problem identifying the general field in which they wish to conduct their research, but have more difficulty finding a focus and pinning down a research question. Punch(30) makes a

BOX 20.4 Comparison of two linked studies

Quantitative study

O'Cathain A, Walters SJ, Nicholl JP, Thomas KJ and Kirkham M (2002) Use of evidence based leaflets to promote informed choice in maternity care: randomised controlled trial in everyday practice. *British Medical Journal.* **324**: 643–6.

This study was a randomised controlled trial with the aim of assessing the effect of leaflets on promoting informed choice in women using maternity services. The sample was clearly defined as women reaching 28 weeks' gestation before the intervention took place. Outcomes were assessed using a postal questionnaire. Various means were used to test the validity of the questionnaire, and a power calculation was used to identify the sample size needed to detect a 10% difference between the intervention and the control groups. Results included response rates (reported in numbers and percentages) and further analysis to identify any differences that could be related to age, social class, parity, pain relief and type of delivery. There was an attempt to examine confounding factors that would bias results, such as having been given the leaflets on another occasion prior to the start of the study.

The conclusion was that the evidence-based leaflets were not effective in promoting informed choice in the women. The authors reported on the limitation of the study and expressed concerns over their measurement of informed choice and the power of the study to detect a difference. Authors referred to the qualitative findings below for further explanation.

Qualitative study

Stapleton H, Kirkham M and Thomas G (2002) Qualitative study of evidence based leaflets in maternity care. *British Medical Journal.* **324**: 639.

The stated aim was to examine the use of evidence-based leaflets on informed choice in maternity services. The design involved both non-participant observation of antenatal consultations, and in-depth interviews with both the expectant mothers and the health professionals. The sample was initially opportunistic (depending on which staff were doing the clinic and which women agreed to be involved) but progressed to be more selective to ensure that women from all childbearing ages, social class, minority groups and current and past obstetric histories were represented. Observations were used to help identify how the leaflets were used, and field notes made on the setting, actions, words and non-verbal cues. Semi-structured interviews were conducted using an interview guide. A grounded theory approach was used(25,31) so as the interview progressed, interviewees were selected to help confirm or refute emerging theory, until no new information was gathered (theoretical saturation). Validity and reliability were said to be ensured by using several researchers and experts, to 'guard against any researcher dominating the analytical process'. Results were reported in terms of emerging themes, and quotes were used to illustrate them.

The qualitative study revealed that time pressures and competing demands within the clinical setting undermined the intervention. The observations revealed that health professionals rarely differentiated the leaflets from other information that they offered or discussed them. The interviews identified that the women confused the leaflets with other information they had been given or denied having received them. The midwives reported that hierarchical power structures resulted in obstetricians defining the choices possible, resulting in informed compliance rather than informed choice.

distinction between general research questions and specific research questions and offers the following hierarchy. This can be illustrated using the study by O'Caithain *et al.*(26) which can be summarised as follows (*see also* Box 20.4).

Research area	*Maternity care*
Research topic	*Informed choice*
General research question(s)	*Does informed choice change behaviour?*
Specific research question(s)	*To assess the effects of leaflets on promoting informed choice in women using maternity services*

Data collection question(s)	*Do women who receive the intervention answer 'yes' more often to the question 'Have you had enough information to make choice on …?'*
	Do the women who receive the intervention report greater satisfaction with antenatal information
	Do the women report being given at least one leaflet?

Novice researchers sometimes confuse data collection questions and research questions.(33) A research question is the question that the research is attempting to answer, whereas the data collection question is asked to collect data that will be used to answer the research question.

Coming up with a research topic is about following your interests (it is difficult to sustain interest if it is not there from the start). Looking around, listening or experiencing something or being aware of current issues are all sources of inspiration. Think about what is known and what is not known about something. O'Leary,(2) in her book for novice researchers, suggests the use of concept maps to help identify an area of interest. Once identified, the general area of interest needs to be narrowed down. A good research question needs to be feasible; this relates to the research expertise and resources available and, indeed, whether the question is capable of being answered at all. This last point involves checking with those who have more expertise in research and knowledge of the field of study.

Bell,(31) in her guide, advises that a good first step is to simply talk over your research ideas with a colleague. Gaining another perspective early on can be very valuable. A good research question not only gives the research focus and direction, but also sets boundaries. Boundaries are particularly important for novice researchers, who have more difficulty estimating how much research time is required to undertake a study and may need to limit both the size and the focus more than anticipated. Defining the terms used within the research question identifies the criteria of concern and by exclusion sets some boundaries on the study. Specifying a research question involves identifying the concepts or variables of interest and, where possible, identifying suitable indicators for the variables of interest. It is important to check that any assumptions made by the question are correct. Getting to the stage of identifying a good research question involves exploration of the topic in the literature to gain knowledge on what is already known (although for some study designs familiarity with the literature may come later, so that the researcher does not limit his or her view of the research area) and where the gaps are, or asking questions in a new context. Deciding on whether you need to frame your question as a hypothesis depends on the theoretical perspective the research will be framed in, and on the type of question being asked. Research within the positivist and post-positivist perspectives are more likely to contain a hypothesis, but the key question is whether the research question forms a testable statement about the relationship of one or more variables to others. Research that is exploratory or framed within the new perspectives is unlikely to start with a hypothesis. The research question should be a pointer to the methods to be used and indicate what type of data will be needed to answer the question.

The research proposal

All research should start with a proposal, also referred to as a *protocol*. Again, like the application for ethical review, it can be helpful for novice researchers to see another research protocol first to identify what is required.(30) A proposal is a plan of action, a communication on which approval to commence the study is given, and is a contract between the researcher and supervisor, university, any funding source and ethics committee.(31) The proposal describes the research background, including relevant literature, the research question, methods, and details about recruitment of the intended sample and how the data will be analysed. All applications for ethics review will also need a proposal. The protocol starts with the relevant literature by 'setting a scene' or 'telling a story' of what is known, how the knowledge built up to form our current understanding. The research question follows; this should extend that understanding.

Ideally, the background literature should present the context of the study, what is known already and what is needed – ideally this will match your study aim, but it could provide part of a much larger question. Literature searches are mainly conducted online using databases such as Medline, Education databases and Ovid, and key articles selected following searches on keywords or authors. Punch(30) reports that two common criticisms of literature reviews in dissertations are that they are not thematic, tending to be chronological or presented serially, and they are not properly integrated with the study. These criticisms can be addressed by creating a conceptual framework into which the literature can be organised.

The research question should suggest the types of method needed to collect the data required to answer the question. The two studies presented in the O'Caithain paper had the research question: 'To assess the effects of leaflets on promoting choice in women using maternity services'. The question suggests measurement in the use of the term 'assess', the leaflets were defined as '10 pairs of Informed Choice leaflets', the women were defined as 'women reaching 28 weeks gestation' and so on. 'Effects' were measured using a questionnaire. Assessment came in the design of comparing a control group with the women who received the leaflets. For the qualitative part of the study the research question was: 'To examine the use of evidence-based leaflets on informed choice in maternity services'. The term 'examine' suggests 'look at' rather than 'measure', and again the leaflets and maternity service were defined. Outcome measures were views and responses from the expectant mothers and the staff. Exactly how the methods are arrived at will be influenced not only by the research question, but also by the interest and expertise of the researcher, supervisor and team.

The protocol should include details about who will be recruited into the study and from where, how recruitment will take place and the numbers involved (this may require a power calculation for research designs). This should be followed by a detailed description of the research procedure. A plan or flow diagram will be useful if the procedure is complex. Details of how the data will be collected and analysed, and any planned statistical tests, should be included, and a timeline or gantt chart is useful to work out when each activity is planned to start and finish. A breakdown of the costs involved in the study for staff and research activities, among others, is also needed, as well as plans for the dissemination of findings(2,30,35) (*see* Box 20.5).

Ethics in Research

What is ethics?

Ethics is concerned with rules of conduct and principles relating to moral behaviour. Researchers are responsible for ethical decisions from formulation through to the dissemination of research. As discussed above, the type of research framework influences how ethics is regarded in the study, as well as appreciating other 'realities' and empowering voices otherwise not heard. All types of study involve making ethical decisions about what is right for the research participant, as well as considering the interests of the researcher, the funding body and the study itself. Ethical decisions are based on the values of the researchers and the research community, and those who hold access to the data the researchers hope to gather. Although there are codes of ethics covering all types of professional research, it is not possible to provide a list of rules that should be applied to every study as each piece of research will be individual and will require different solutions.

The emergence of research ethics came about after the end of the Second World War, when details of horrific medical experiments came to light during the Nuremberg trials. The Nuremberg Code (1947) was published two years later, followed by the Declaration of Helsinki (1964) and the World Medical Association(33) (which amended the declaration of Helsinki), which established ethical principles for research involving humans.

Social research has proceeded in two ways:
- deontological approaches to morality (Immanuel Kant 1724–1804)
- consequentialism (Jeremy Bentham 1748–1832).

Deontological approaches to ethics follow a set of principles that guide research. One such principle is that of 'informed consent', which was enshrined in the Nuremberg Code. Informed consent includes providing all relevant information about the study and what taking part will involve, including risks. The research subject must be able to comprehend the information and be competent to make a decision about involve-

> ### BOX 20.5 How to: Write a research protocol
>
> **Title**
> Relevant background literature
> Research question
> - general and specific questions
> Methods
> - study design (e.g. randomised trial, grounded theory)
> - sample
>   - sampling strategy (e.g. opportunistic, purposive)
>   - define target sample, i.e. demographic details, how selected and recruited to study
>   - sample size (reason for size, is it informed by power calculation)
> - data collection procedures
> - details of any instruments to be used
>   - references to existing tools
>   - details about validity, reliability
>   - outline stepwise procedures including pre-testing and piloting of tools
> - data collection methods (e.g. via postal questionnaire, field notes, interviews)
> Data analysis
> - details of how data will be analysed (e.g. statistical tests, type of qualitative analysis)
> - computer programs to be used in analysis
> How will quality issues be addressed
> - details of randomisation, piloting of questionnaires
> Ethical considerations and how these will be responded to
> - state if approval from ethics committee has been received or is in progress
> Plans for dissemination of findings
> References (e.g. from literature review, methods, instruments, etc.)
> Appendices
> - costings
> - research instruments (e.g. questionnaire, interview schedule, consent forms)
> - flow chart summarising study plan

ment, and agreement to take part should be voluntary, free of coercion or influence. This also involves taking steps to ensure the participant is protected from any consequences of being in the study by ensuring that the research protects the identity of the participant. Deontological approaches reject the notion that what is morally right can be considered by assessing consequences.

Consequentialism is not concerned with whether an act is morally right, but with the consequences of the act. For research this translates to potential ethical dilemmas that the researcher may have to respond to and the consequences of their actions. Classic utilitarianism is a form of consequentialism. Classic utilitarianism is consequentialist rather than deontologist because it denies that moral 'rightness' depends on anything except the consequences of an act. The consequences, not the intention, of an action determine its merit. Critics of consequentialism have commented on the difficulty of anticipating all the potential outcomes that might result from an act. Important areas to be considered are:

- informed consent
- confidentiality
- anonymity.

Informed consent has two components: the research participants need to understand what taking part will involve; and agreement to take part needs to be voluntary. Generally, consent will be obtained by asking the research participant to confirm their consent by signing a consent form, by giving recorded verbal consent or by returning a questionnaire. Gaining consent may involve gaining approval from many more people than those directly involved in the study, that is, the host care organisation, in order to access patients. Consent needs to be voluntary, free from coercion, manipulation and any threat. There is also some evidence that response rates improve as interviewees are given more details about what the study involves.(34) Gaining consent can provide an important part in negotiating the researcher's relationship with participants. This should involve participants being told about any risks of taking part and having the opportunity to ask questions about the study.

Consent to take part in research may be given on the basis that the information obtained about the participants will only be used by the researcher and only in particular ways. The information is offered to the researcher in confidence. Beauchamp and Childless(35) argue that the right to privacy rests on the principle of respect for autonomy. On this basis people have the right to decide who knows what about them. Research should uphold this principle. Confidentiality means protecting the identity of those who agree to take part in research, maintaining the data in a form such that the identity of the participant is protected. This implies keeping names and data separated by using a code that is only accessible to the researchers, and reporting data in a format that does not lead to individuals being readily identifiable. For example, it may involve removing or changing details to protect individuals who would otherwise be identifiable because of their unique characteristics or experiences.

Anonymity goes further than confidentiality, as the researchers do not collect named data at all. This means the researcher cannot identify which respondent gave the data (e.g. postal survey). This type of data allows participants to make any negative comments more freely without fears or concerns that anything they do report might be attributed to them with unknown consequences. For researchers, this might be difficult or impossible to achieve if the methods involve interviewing, and problematic if they wish to send reminders only to those who have not already agreed to participate. For a full discussion on ethics in research, see Israel and Hay(34) and Punch,(36) and for ethical dilemmas in qualitative research, see Welland and Pugsley.(37)

Returning to our example, ethics questions that may have been addressed before the Stapleton *et al.* study was carried out include:

- Will the midwives and expectant mothers be given all the information they require to give their informed consent?
- Is there any pressure or coercion to take part?
- How will consent be taken?
- How will confidentiality of the interaction of midwife and mother be assured?
- How will collected data be anonymised, particularly with reference to the use of quotes?
- Who will have access to the data?
- Have the researchers anticipated all that could go wrong? How would they respond if they did?

In conclusion, researchers are expected to minimise the risk of harm or discomfort to people, to conduct research in a manner that upholds certain principles such as informed consent and to consider any consequences or harm that may result from the research. Harm from educational or social research is more likely to take the form of psychological distress than physical injury. Conversely, many researchers aim to provide benefit by conducting research that empowers participants, such as in feminist research.

Statutory ethical review

Israel and Hay(34) commented that novice researchers rarely seriously consider the ethical implications of their research and that it is only when compelled to respond to the research ethics committee requirements that any detailed consideration is given to ethical issues. It is at this point that the novice researcher may confront considerable ethical difficulties. The formal mechanism can offer the opportunity to consider ethical issues, and this process can be helped by adapting tools that are available as guidance. Novice researchers may falsely anticipate that gaining approval for a study necessitates conforming to certain procedures, that is, written consent and providing a written participant information sheet, even when their study may not require such documentation, effectively making the study more difficult to conduct.

In the UK, it is necessary to make an application to a National Health Service (NHS) Research Ethics Committee (REC) before starting research, if the research involves NHS patients and/or staff.(38) Ethics review is one of a series of safeguards intended to protect individuals, and these are described in the Research Governance Framework for Health and Social Care. The primary function of a REC, when considering a proposed study, is to protect the rights, safety, dignity and well-being of all actual or potential participants. The remit of a REC is described in the Department of Health guidance, Governance Arrangements for Research Ethics Committees on the NHS National Research Ethics Service (NRES) website.(38)

Completing a REC application for the first time may seem rather daunting. I suggest that you gain sight of a couple of successful applications first – having a worked example can be helpful. The number of additional supporting documents (i.e. the protocol, contact letters, consent forms, any questionnaires, etc.) may seem burdensome because they are required upfront rather than developed at each stage of progress. However, this is all documentation required to proceed with the study. There are some advantages in preparing supporting documents early and getting feedback on them. The NRES regulations state that the time from receiving a valid application to notification of final opinion from the committee must not exceed 60 days. The biggest hold-up is the time taken for applicants to respond to the questions raised by the committee. All applicants are invited to attend the committee meeting. This can be very useful, as it provides the opportunity for the committee to ask questions and clarify points that have not been fully understood. This can speed up the process by reducing the need to ask further questions later.

In addition to a REC application, an application must also be made for research management and governance approval (this is usually referred to as R&D approval) to each NHS organisation in which the research will be carried out. As there is no time limit set for R&D approval, this could take longer than the REC application. Researchers are strongly advised to submit the R&D application in parallel with the REC application to reduce the time delay. The NRES website has a link to the online standard R&D application form. This was devised by the R&D forum,(39,40) but currently only about half of all R&D offices accept the standard form, and when this is the case, you will need to complete the relevant R&D office's own form. Each individual R&D office will need to be contacted to find out its requirements. The R&D form asks questions about funding, management and governance within each NHS organisation where the research will take place.

Ethical approval of research in medical education

In 2001, Morrison and Prideaux(41) asked whether research in medical education should be exempt from the ethical considerations that govern other research involving humans. The authors argued that it may be ethically wrong not to evaluate educational interventions, but then questioned at what point evaluation becomes research. They suggested that the crucial point is if the study is aimed at producing generalisable results with the intention of publishing in refereed literature. It is at this point that ethical approval must be gained and the following statement now makes this very clear. This journal conforms to contemporary standards on ethical publication. It requires evidence of approval by an appropriate human research ethics committee for all papers that report research involving human subjects.(42) However, with regard to journals accepting research from an international community, this requires accepting local standards of ethical review, which will mean accepting a variable ethical standard.(42) There has been a debate about the appropriate place to review educational research. This stemmed from a recognition that educational research does not incur the same level of potential risks as biomedical research, and from a concern that ethics committees that were originally established to review biomedical research may not fully comprehend educational research.(42,43) This concern has already been realised from educational research submitted to statutory ethics committees who reclassed the study as audit and therefore not requiring ethical review.(42) There are problems when submitting research classed as audit rather than research to journals, as there is no ethical review of the study. Possible solutions to the problem include gaining retrospective ethical consent and having studies reclassified as research(44); embedding consent into the delivery of the curriculum; and providing independent evidence that participants gave informed consent to data collection and that risk of harm to the participants was unlikely.(42,44) Another way of avoiding this problem would be by ensuring that researchers from the field of educational research are members of statutory ethics committees or by setting up alternative ethics committees within faculties to monitor educational research.(41,43,44)

Scholarship

Boyer(45) discussed the trend towards a singular view of scholarship as research and publication, and proposes reconsidering the priorities of the professoriate by broadening the definition of scholarly work. He argues that the definition of scholarship should be wider and proposes three additional areas of endeavour that should be viewed as scholarship, in addition to the discovery of new knowledge. These are:
• the integration of knowledge, by placing isolated research into a larger context and making connections within or between disciplines

- the teaching of knowledge, stimulating others to become active learners and encouraging students to be critical, creative thinkers, with the capacity to go on learning after their college days are over
- the application of knowledge – how theory and practice vitally interact to inform each other.

Discovery of new knowledge

This chapter has focused on scholarship as discovery of new knowledge. The first section explained how the framework in which the research is set influences the type of knowledge that is created and how it should be evaluated. Power is still held by the post-positive perspective, although over the past 10 years or so there have been more studies from the new perspectives and more that are informed from more than one perspective. The critical theorists inform us that other knowledge has been dominated by evidence from positivism and post-positivism perspectives, which has been influenced by men in positions of power, but that other forms of knowledge are valid. The two studies used to illustrate a quantitative and qualitative approach highlight the importance of using different approaches to the discovery of new knowledge.

Integration of knowledge

Integration of knowledge can be achieved by collaboration across disciplines in primary research, but equally important is the appraisal of existing knowledge to evaluate progress in a particular field or inform another. Unless literature reviews are conducted in a standardised way, they run the risk of being subjective and biased. To address these weaknesses, there has been increased interest in conducting literature reviews in a systematic way.

A systematic literature review is conducted using a transparent process such that the reader could replicate the study and arrive at the same findings. Far greater precision is required in a systematic review, which requires definitions of terms used, clearly written research questions, publication of the search strategy used, including search terms and databases used, and the incorporation of a complete list of inclusion and exclusion criteria. Papers initially selected by the search but excluded from the review are also listed with reasons for exclusion.(46,47)

Teaching of knowledge

Scholarship in teaching is the legacy of handing on knowledge to the next generation. Scholarship is said to occur when it is public, open to evaluation and presented in a format that others can build on.(48) However, while a clinical teacher may be informed about contemporary research in their area of clinical expertise, this is less common with regard to education, where change is more opinion than evidence led.(32)

Best evidence medical education (BEME)(49) is a collaboration of individuals and institutions that support the need to develop a systematic approach to the review of evidence about clinical teaching. The website shares information about completed and ongoing systematic reviews. Mennin and McGrew(50) stress that research in teaching and learning as applied to the clinical setting is in the early stages of development. BEME and the recent work on scholarship in teaching represents an opportunity for medical education to become more evidence based.

Application of knowledge

The application of knowledge is a crucial part of scholarship; otherwise research becomes an end in itself. There has been recognition that there is a delay from research findings to implementation, which evidence-based medicine in particular has tried to address.(51) The participatory action research perspective recognises the delay in implementing research findings and has resolved this problem by making the research part of the change programme.(19)

Implementation is the end point of research, but as Boyer(45) reminds us, this is only until new issues arise and are fed back into research and the cycle begins again.

Conclusions

Theoretical perspectives determine the assumptions that are made about reality and what can be known. Positivism became the dominant perspective after the Enlightenment, but following the realisation that all research did not fit into this paradigm, a shift in thinking occurred. This brought about a new way of thinking about social science, and new and competing theoretical perspectives emerged.

The arguments against combining qualitative and quantitative research centre on the acceptance that research strategies are committed to particular theoretical perspectives(2) or the view that they are autonomous.(20) A growth in the preparedness to view research methods as techniques for data collection and a movement away from concerns about ontology and epistemology has resulted in more research using a combination of both qualitative and quantitative research methods.(21)

Getting started in research involves identifying a good research question. After this, consideration needs to be given to the type of data that need to be collected to answer the question. A plan or proposal needs to set out how the research will be conducted, with milestones. Consideration needs to be given to ethical questions that affect the research and how these can be dealt with. Educational scholarship brings it all together. New knowledge is created, integrated and applied. And through dissemination, discussion and critical appraisal, new questions are generated. This in turn leads to the formulation of new research questions and the circle of scholarly enquiry is complete.

Acknowledgements

I would like to thank my colleagues for their helpful comments on earlier drafts: Prof. Tim van Zwanenberg, Dr Bryan Burford, Ms Charlotte Kergon and Dr Gill Morrow.

References

1 Guba EG and Lincoln YS (1994) Competing paradigms in qualitative research. In: Denzin DK and Lincoln YS (eds) *Handbook of Qualitative Research*, pp. 105–17. Sage, Thousand Oaks, CA.

2 O'Leary Z (2004) *The Essential Guide to Doing Research*. Sage, London.

3 Ivesson M (2002) *Postmodernism and Social Research*. Open University Press, Buckingham.

4 *Oxford English Dictionary* (http://www.oed.com).

5 Smith R (1992) Audit and research. *British Medical Journal*. **305**: 905–6.

6 Clarke A (1999) *Evaluation Research*. Sage, London.

7 Robson C (2000) *Small-scale Evaluation: principles and practice*. Sage, Thousand Oaks, CA.

8 Kneebone R (2002) Total internal reflection: an essay on paradigms. *Medical Education*. **36**: 514–18.

9 Kuhn TS (1970) *The Structure of Scientific Revolutions*. University of Chicago Press, Chicago.

10 Guba EG and Lincoln YS (2005) Paradigmatic controversies, contradictions and emerging confluences. In: Denzin DK and Lincoln YS (eds) *Handbook of Qualitative Research* (3e), pp. 191–215. Sage, Thousand Oaks, CA.

11 Heron J and Reason R (1997) A participatory inquiry paradigm. *Qualitative Inquiry*. **3**: 274–94.

12 Crotty M (2003) *The Foundations of Social Research: meaning and perspective in the research process*. Sage, London.

13 Tong R (1995) *Feminist Thought: a comprehensive introduction*. Routledge, London.

14 Steier F (1991) Introduction: research as self-reflectivity, self-reflexivity as social process. In: F Steier (ed.) *Research and Reflexivity*. Sage, London.

15 Marx K (1961) *Selected Writings in Sociology and Social Philosophy* (2e). Bottomore TB and Rubel M (eds). Penguin, Harmondsworth.

16 Schwandt TA (1994) Constructivist, interpretivist approaches to human inquiry. In: Denzin DK and Lincoln YS (eds) *Handbook of Qualitative Research*, pp. 118–37. Sage, Thousand Oaks, CA.

17 Guba EG and Lincoln YS (1989) *Fourth Generation Evaluation*. Sage, Newbury Park, CA.

18 Ricoeur P (1974) *The Conflict of Interpretations: essays in hermeneutics*. Northwestern University Press, Evanston, IL.

19 Whyte WF (1991) *Participatory Action Research*. Sage, London.

20 Bryman A (2001) *Social Research Methods*. Oxford University Press, Oxford.

21 Patton MQ (2002) *Qualitative Research and Evaluation Methods*. Sage, London.

22 Glaser B and Strauss A (1967) *The Discovery of Grounded Theory*. Aldine, New York.

23 Charmaz K (2003) Grounded theory: objectivist and constructivist methods. In: Denzin DK and Lincoln YS (eds) *Strategies of Qualitative Inquiry*, pp. 249–91. Sage, Thousand Oaks, CA.

24 Harris I (2002) Qualitative methods. In: Norman GR, van der Vleuten C and Newble D (eds) *International Handbook of Research in Medical Education*, pp. 45–96. Kluwer Academic, London.

25 Strauss A and Corbin JM (1997) *Grounded Theory in Practice*. Sage, Thousand Oaks, CA.

26 O'Cathain A, Walters SJ, Nicholl JP et al. (2002) Use of evidence based leaflets to promote informed choice in maternity care: randomised controlled trial in everyday practice. *British Medical Journal*. **324**: 643–6.

27 Stapleton H, Kirkham M and Thomas G (2002) Qualitative study of evidence based leaflets in maternity care. *British Medical Journal*. **324**: 639–42. (doi:10.1136/bmj.324.7338.639).

28 Strauss AL and Corbin J (1990) *Basics of Qualitative Research: grounded theory procedures and techniques*. Sage, London.

29 Blumer H (1969) *Symbolic Interactionism*. Prentice Hall, Englewood Cliffs, NJ.

30 Punch K (2000) *Developing Effective Research Proposals*. Sage, London.

31 Loche LF, Spirduso WW and Silverman SJ (1993) *Proposals That Work* (3e). Sage, Newbury Park, CA.

32 Tarling R (2006) *Managing Social Research: a practical guide*. Routledge, London.

33 World Medical Association (2002) *World Medical Association Declaration of Helsinki: ethical principles for medical research involving human subjects* (http://wma.net/e/polcy/b3.htm).

34 Israel M and Hay I (2006) *Research Ethics for Social Scientists*. Sage, London.

35 Beauchamp TL and Childless JF (2001) *Principles of Biomedical Ethics* (4e). Oxford University Press, New York.

36 Punch M (1994) Politics and ethics in qualitative research. In: Denzin DK and Lincoln YS (eds) *Handbook of Qualitative Research*, pp. 83–98. Sage, Thousand Oaks, CA.

37 Welland T and Pugsley L (2002) *Ethical Dilemmas in Qualitative Research*. Ashgate, Hampshire.

38 NHS National Research Ethics Service (NRES) (http://www.nres.npsa.nhs.uk).

39 R&D Form (http://www.r&dform.org.uk).

40 R&D Forum (http://www.rdforum.nhs.uk).

41 Morrison J and Prideaux D (2001) Ethics approval for research in medical education. *Medical Education*. **35**: 1008.

42 Prideaux D and Rogers W (2006) Audit or research: the ethics of publication. *Medical Education*: **40**: 497–9.

43 Evans A (2002) Ethics approval for research in medical education. *Medical Education*. **36**: 394.

44 McLachlan JC and McHarg J (2005) Ethical permission for the publication of routinely collected data. *Medical Education*. **39**: 944–8.

45 Boyer EL (1990) *Scholarship, Reconsidered: priorities of the professoriate*. Princeton University of New Mexico, Princeton, NJ.

46 Albanese M and Norcini J (2002) Systematic reviews: what are they and why should we care? *Advances in Health Sciences*. **7**: 147–51

47 Reeves S, Koopel I, Barr H et al. (2002) Twelve tips for undertaking a systematic review. *Medical Teacher*. **24**: 358–63.

48 Hutchings P and Shulman LS (1999) The scholarship of teaching: new elaborations, new developments. *Change*. **Sept/Oct**: 11–15.

49 Best Evidence Medical Education (http://www.bemecollaboration.org).

50 Mennin SP and McGrew MC (2001) Scholarship in teaching and best evidence medical education: synergy for teaching and learning. *Medical Education.* **2**(5): 468–72.

51 Sackett DL, Rosenberg WMC, Gray JAM *et al.* (1996). Evidence-based medicine: what it is and what it isn't. *British Medical Journal.* **312**: 71–2.

Further Reading

Introduction to research

Bell J (1999) *Doing Your Research Project: a guide for first-time researchers in education and social science* (3e). Open University Press, Buckingham.

Green J and Browne J (2005) *Principles of Social Research.* Open University Press, Buckingham.

Punch K (2000) *Developing Effective Research Proposals.* Sage, Thousand Oaks, CA.

Theoretical perspectives

Burr V (1995) *An Introduction to Social Constructionism.* Routledge, London, New York.

Cuff EC and Payne GCF (1979) *Perspectives in Sociology.* Unwin Hyman, London.

Gergen K (1999) *An Invitation to Social Construction.* Sage, London.

Kemmis S and McTaggart R (2003) Participatory action research. In: Denzin DK and Lincoln YS (eds) *Strategies of Qualitative Inquiry* (2e), pp. 271–330. Sage, Thousand Oaks, CA.

Kincheloe JL and McLaren PL (1994) Rethinking critical theory and qualitative research. In: Denzin DK and Lincoln YS (eds). *Handbook of Qualitative Research*, pp. 138–57. Sage, Thousand Oaks, CA.

May T (2001) *Social Research: issues, methods and process.* Open University Press, London.

Quantitative research methods in medical education

Geoff Norman and Kevin W Eva

KEY MESSAGES

- There is much more to good research than rigorous design.
- The appropriateness of a particular research design is dependent on the question to be addressed.
- The hierarchy of research methods commonly applied to clinical studies is inappropriate when judging the strength of research strategies in educational domains.
- The value of critical, synthesising, theoretically oriented and empirically based reviews of the literature cannot be overstated.

The Quantitative Paradigm

Quantitative research methods have been central to physical science for centuries, dating back as far as the astonishing developments in astronomy in the 1500s. Indeed, it is difficult to envision natural science without quantification, and it is even more difficult to delve into some of these accomplishments without feeling an overwhelming sense of wonderment at the ability of the scientist, whether we ponder on our understanding of the very big (e.g. cosmology) or the very small (e.g. particle physics), or closer to home, as we reflect on the rapid evolution of digital electronics in our lifetime. For those old enough to remember a computer card, a 1Gb flash drive contains as much memory as 10 000 000 computer cards – about the volume of a one-car garage. But quantitative methods are not a panacea. Many would claim that social scientists have been too quick to adopt the methods of natural science unquestioningly, perhaps to acquire a guise of scientific respectability, and have not given adequate recognition to the complexity of social situations, which are not evidently reducible to a few numbers. In an earlier chapter, Illing has reviewed the history of the adoption of quantitative methods into social science, and the subsequent uneasy integration (or partitioning) with qualitative methods. It is not surprising that the quantitative 'dust bowl empiricism' led to a counter reaction. It is embarrassingly easy to find examples in medical education that, on a moment's reflection, exemplify the silliness of attempts to reduce the complexity of human interaction in an educational setting to a 'treatment' that half receive and half do not, and an 'outcome' such as pass or fail on an examination.(1) Although we are personally wedded to quantitative approaches to social science research, such studies, which, as Illing points out, reduce the people in the study to 'objects' that are supposed to absorb exactly the same dose of the educational drug, amount to little more than unintended *'reductio ad absurdum'*.

Little is served by identifying specific examples. The larger question is the extent to which quantitative methods have been aligned with recognised progress in the field. There is simply no dispute that the methods of the natural sciences, from the electron microscope to the wet lab and the clinical trial, have led to enormous advances in medicine with direct consequences for human longevity and welfare. Clearly, it would be specious to try to make similar claims in the small and impecunious field of medical education. Nevertheless, the past three decades of research have seen substantial advances in medical education, much of it directly related to the application of sophisticated quantitative methods,(2) particularly in the area of student assessment.

Lost in the qualitative–quantitative debate is the complexity of both qualitative and quantitative methods. As Bordage notes,(3) the community should move on because 'this oft-repeated debate is not productive…each approach is useful in its own right and is often most productive when complementary'. In writing a paper on quantitative methods our goal is not to promote these methods over qualitative research strategies or even to contrast the two, but rather, to provide some guidance for those trying to better understand the variety of quantitative methods available.

Much is written about the various schools of qualitative research; Illing, as one example, cites

Understanding Medical Education: Evidence, Theory and Practice.
Edited by T Swanwick. © 2010 Association for the Study of Medical Education.

post-positivism, critical theory, constructivism and participatory action as various *genres* in qualitative research. To our knowledge, no similar taxonomy exists for quantitative research. Indeed, many critics of quantitative methodology appear to presume that educational research is about testing hypotheses using randomised experiments that are proven or disproven by application of statistical methods. This is a woefully inadequate description of, for example, the psychometric methods that have led to such significant advances in assessment methods.

In this chapter, we will distinguish four research traditions – experimental, epidemiologic, psychometric and correlational – exploring some basic principles of measurement and statistical inference along the way. Finally, we will describe the methods of meta-analysis and systematic reviews, and contrast these strategies with those of generating reviews that are better defined as critical and theory-oriented. We begin, however, with a commentary on the importance of precisely focusing one's research question, emphasising that while good studies require good methods, the quality of a study is not completely defined by its methodological rigour (Box 21.1).

The Research Question

In the previous section, we noted that many authors equate quantitative research with hypothesis testing. In our view, not only is this association simplistic, but it gives insufficient attention to the nature and adequacy of the research question. Far too frequently, when students do discuss the research question, much effort is expended in learning how to convert a practical, commonsense question into a formal research hypothesis or, even better, a 'null hypothesis' that frames it as no difference. Such efforts, by promoting precision of planning, can enable one to ensure that the research question is ultimately answerable. Much of that precision, however, becomes evident in any case as the research design and methods are devised, thereby leading us to believe that much of this effort is stylistic and does little to fundamentally improve the research. It really is of little consequence if a question is framed as a question, a research hypothesis or a null hypothesis.

BOX 21.1 A taxonomy of quantitative research traditions
- Experimental
- Epidemiologic
- Psychometric
- Correlational
- Reviews and meta-analyses

In any case, the idea of a research hypothesis only applies well to some kinds of quantitative research. The development of a new evaluation instrument will proceed by a very different route, with studies of reliability and validity. To frame a reliability study as a null hypothesis would look something like:

The reliability of the new written test of reflective practice will be less than 0.5.

This framing simply does not adequately capture the goal of the research. While our views may not represent a majority position, we believe that we should focus effort on an adequate research *question*, and forget about the niceties of null hypothesis creation. In the end, the goal of the research question is to reduce the possibility of post hoc explanations and to specify or constrain the methods used to answer the question. As human beings we are remarkably good at generating explanations for any pattern that is presented to us, so scientists try to avoid drawing conclusions without some *a priori* reason to have predicted the result. That is not to say that post hoc speculation is not useful when unanticipated findings arise, but it is to say that further study should be engaged to confirm the result before running to the printers. Style is unimportant, but precision is invaluable to avoid wasting time and resources in pursuit of ultimately unanswerable questions.

So how do we ensure that the research question is good? In contrast to the many approaches that exist to determine if the research methods are good, there is little written about what constitutes a good research question. What does exist tends to focus on the technicalities of what information should be present in the question.(4) There is a good reason for this. The worth of a research question cannot be judged in the abstract, but can only be viewed in the context of the specific research domain in which it arises. Research is about discovery, and there is little point in discovering what is already known (Box 21.2).

'Discovery' is a useful way to think about the potential contribution of a research study, but the word implies such large leaps from current understanding that we prefer to think of the act of discovery in terms of knowledge building. Arguably, the value of a study is directly related to the extent to which it reveals some new understanding of the world – it 'discovers' some new insight or builds on existing knowledge in a meaningful way. Quantitative research is judged, in large part, by the extent to which the lessons learned can be generalised to other contexts. But what advice can we give the beginning researcher to help him or her identify research studies that are most likely to yield knowledge-building discoveries? Very simply, this is the role of the literature review.

The latter point is worth reinforcing – this emphasis on using the literature is not meant to imply that there are not practical (potentially atheoretical) questions that need to be addressed; rather our view is that

BOX 21.2 How to: Select an issue worthy of research

When contemplating which research ideas are worth developing into more fully fledged projects, there are a variety of criteria that should be used. Here are just a few guiding principles.

- *Novelty:* Has the study been done before? It is insufficient to say 'to our knowledge this has never been done' without a concentrated effort to determine whether or not it has been done. Talk with experts, be they local or international, and scour the literature for other studies aimed at similar issues. Only after doing so can you make a compelling argument for how your particular study could advance understanding in some meaningful way beyond what's already been done.

- *Importance:* Medical education is an applied field. As a result, while any given study might not yield immediate practical implications, it should be possible to conceive of ways in which the research efforts might beneficially impact on the field in the future.

- *Programmatic:* Too often we in applied fields think of research in terms of projects as opposed to programmes. The later term, put forward by the Hungarian philosopher of science Imre Lakatos, should draw attention to the fact that real advances are typically made through systematic and long-term study of a particular issue.(5)

- *Guided:* What is the conceptual framework within which your study fits? Which theories speak to the issue you are trying to grapple with? Do they contradict one another in a way that you could shed insight into through your research efforts? Is your theory/hypothesis falsifiable (i.e could your study design yield an answer that would counter the theory you are using to guide your study design)?

- *Grounded:* Related to some of the previous points, we use the term 'grounded' to indicate that the study should be grounded in the context of what is already known such that that the context is used to determine which of the various possible research directions is most appropriate (i.e most likely to provide meaningful results to the community) at this point in history. One may not be able to predict this with perfect accuracy, but the issue should be considered through broad consultation and reflection.

grounding one's study in the existing literature is a valuable strategy for ensuring that even purely practical research projects have a decent chance of being successful and contributing to the generalisable knowledge base of the community. Too frequently, the literature review reads like a child recounting a playground fight: 'Johnny did this. Then Sally did that. Then Bob came along and said this other thing.' The literature review is not, and should not be, a chronological recounting of who did what to whom, but rather, should establish a conceptual framework within which the present study will reside.

It should clearly identify knowledge gaps, and the gaps should be substantive; statements such as 'this study has never been done in our country/city/university/discipline' are weak justification. The conceptual framework should be such that it helps the researcher and eventual readers focus on the bigger picture (i.e. the 'state of the art'), and it should clearly delineate how the present study adds to this knowledge. This implies that the researcher should begin every study with a formal literature review, from which all unanswered questions will become as evident as a full moon on a clear night. Of course, research does not proceed in such a linear fashion, but one characteristic of mature research programmes (i.e. long-term and systematic exploration of a domain) is that situations where a study is created *de novo* from a literature review are the exception. When a programme of research is ongoing, new study questions arise from existing study findings. So what can be done to ensure the quality of the question? One way to answer this question is to draw on the notion of 'theory'. In contrast to a research hypothesis, which ultimately leads to only two conclusions: (a) it worked, or (b) it did not, a research theory involves an understanding of the interaction of multiple variables. Such theory-based research is conspicuously in the minority within our field,(6) only about half the articles in a recent review being identified as having a conceptual framework(7) let alone a testable theory. Yet another 'study' showing that students gave your new course in anatomy an average rating of 3.5/5 is unlikely to provide any new insights into teaching and learning. But application of a novel theoretical perspective may alter the way the community thinks about the issue and reveal insights that are relevant to various curricular strategies. Although educational theories typically do not make quantitative predictions, they nevertheless often involve the interplay of several variables and may get people thinking about the problem in a more refined manner. That is the importance of theory; by the time the theory has been subjected to a critical test, inevitably involving a few to a few dozen studies, we can gain good insight into the limits and generality of the findings, thanks to an accumulation of evidence, rather than being stuck with a series of only superficially related results.

It is worth noting here that a defining property of scientific theory is, to use Popper's words,(8) that it is falsifiable (i.e. it can be proven wrong). As such, studies that use theory as a basis for knowledge building have a more dynamic quality than typical invocations of theory as context. Scientific theories are not permanent and immutable; we expect them to change and evolve (and increase in explanatory power) as new evidence arises. This stands in stark contrast to the use of theory as justification implied by statements such as: 'The curriculum was designed to be consistent with adult learning theory.' Such statements are not terribly useful, as adult learning theory can be implemented in countless ways and other theoretical positions might also promote the same types of learning activities.(9) More critically, adult learning theory is framed in such sweeping generalisations as to be virtually unfalsifiable. Just because a set of data 'is consistent with' one theory does not in any way amount to an accumulation of knowledge unless the data can be shown to be inconsistent with some alternative theory or unless they lead to revision and refinement of the theory being utilised.

It might also be noted that, while some notions of theory building remain firmly rooted in a positivist tradition, theory is probably best used when it moves some towards the recognition that the world is not adequately described by a single 'it worked/it did not' reductionistic package.(10) Further, as alluded to above, the fact that research is theory-based does not mean it is irrelevant to practice. On the contrary, as Stokes(11) has convincingly described, theory-based basic science and practically oriented research efforts should not be construed as lying on separate ends of a continuum. Rather, he argues, the two agenda should be considered orthogonal continua in their own rights, with the best researchers lying in what he called 'Pasteur's quadrant', to reflect the great strides Louis Pasteur made in advancing fundamental knowledge while simultaneously having practical, real-world, impact.

Research Designs

When the phrase 'research design' is mentioned, individuals who grew up in an educational research environment automatically think about experimental designs, quasi-experimental designs, and Cook and Campbell.(12) Those who are closer to clinical research are more likely to think of the epidemiological classifications of case-control study, cohort study and randomised trial. Both are inadequate taxonomies. Within medical education, much of our quantitative research, in particular psychometric and correlational research methods, does not fit neatly into any of these pigeonholes. Furthermore, which tradition one adopts should be tailored to the specific research questions one is trying to address.

In addition, different research design traditions arise from different kinds of question. In the remainder of this chapter we will examine various issues related to selecting a particular research design. The next section deals with the experimental tradition by exploring a set of methodologies primarily aimed at testing questions of causality (e.g. 'Does increasing test frequency cause better retention of studied material?'). A related tradition that we will then examine briefly is the epidemiologic approach. Because many methodological reviews address research design on the continuum of case-control study, cohort study and randomised trial, we will define these terms and show some (limited) applications in medical education.

The subsequent section will focus on the psychometric tradition, a method of study primarily directed (at least within educational circles) at the development of better measures of various aspects of competence or other outcomes of the educational process. These studies do not speak of interventions, control groups, outcomes and the like. Instead, the preoccupation is with issues of reliability and validity, which are indices of the ability of the instrument to differentiate between individuals in a defensible manner.

Finally, we will look at correlational research designs that tend to be used when the desire is to seek understanding by examining relationships among measured variables. As these measurements are frequently gathered from surveys and rating forms, we will also examine some basic principles of questionnaire design.

As can be seen from this introduction alone, each tradition has different aims, and the design conditions necessary for one may be exclusionary of another. As one example, which we will elaborate on later, correlational research requires individual variation in order to see relationships, while experimental research does its best to eliminate individual differences in order to detect treatment effects. There are other differences: experimental research is almost by definition prospective, whereas correlational research is often conducted on existing databases. Use of existing data, while often necessary, can encourage an attitude where the questions are driven by the available data, rather than the reverse, adding little in the way of advancing understanding. That danger noted, it is certainly true that prosaic questions are not proprietary to any one research approach, and conversely, some of the most interesting research has arisen from retrospective analysis of large institutional databases.(13,14)

The Experimental Tradition

The act of discovery, which is central to science as we discussed earlier, is usually, although not entirely, directed to discovering causal relationships among things (variables). The experimental tradition exemplifies this agenda. The basic notion of an experiment is that there is a relationship between the independent variable, which is usually, but not always, under the control of the experimenter, and the dependent variable, which is observed to change as a consequence of the intervention. Many methodological discussions focus on devising studies that can allow one to unambiguously infer causal relationships between experimenter-controlled independent variables and observed dependent variables.

Statements like:

- the absorption of a neutron by the P_{32} nucleus decreases its stability, making it radioactive and leading to decay to S_{32} by emission of a β particle
- excess sodium chloride in the diet leads to hypertension that results in increased risk of stroke
- a half-day nutrition workshop given to patients with transient ischaemic attacks increased compliance with a restricted salt diet

exemplify the causal goal of the experimenter. Yet while all these statements imply causation – an independent variable that 'causes' a change in a dependent variable – the meaning of causation is very different as we proceed from top to bottom, and the steps one must take to ensure a valid test of the inference are correspondingly more and more complex. For the neutron, there is no ambiguity. Everyone in atomic physics knows what a neutron is, how to 'make' one and how to get a phosphorus nucleus to absorb it. It is relatively easy to create a neutron target that is 100% phosphorus. The methods to detect β particles are clear and well understood. Further, the relationship is absolutely causal – if the P nucleus absorbs a neutron, it will eventually emit a β particle (with a known half-life of 14.28 days); if it does not, it will not. No control group of other phosphorus atoms that do not receive neutrons is necessary. While philosophers of science may challenge the reality of a neutron or a β particle, physics practitioners are unlikely to share their concern. However, there is much more uncertainty in the second statement. 'Excess' is not defined, nor is stroke, although there are probably fairly unambiguous criteria for the latter. 'Hypertension' has a definition, but this has drifted lower over the years and is somewhat cohort-dependent.(15) Nonetheless, it is not simply a definitional problem. The causal relationship in this example is far more probabilistic; reduction of salt intake has a fairly small effect on blood pressure, and hypertension is only one contributor to stroke, so excess salt may only 'cause' a small proportion of strokes.

The final causal statement is even more vague. It is difficult to unambiguously define compliance with a diet, and it is more difficult to attempt to define a cut-off point that unambiguously separates 'compliant' from 'non-compliant' patients. Further, it is well nigh impossible to identify what aspect of the workshop was the causal variable in inducing change, nor, for that matter, is it even likely that any single variable was causal for everyone in the workshop. If the 'causal' relationship is confirmed, this may simply be a stimulus for more research to establish the 'active ingredient' (or combination of ingredients) that led to change.

Of course, much of educational research resembles the final rather than the first example. This has two critical implications for our understanding of the role of experimental research in education. First, in contrast to physical sciences, the relationships we seek are inevitably probabilistic, and the signal of a causal relation is almost always swimming in a sea of noise. It is for this reason that we must impose such strategies as control groups, randomisation and inclusion criteria. Second, the complexity of the relationships may well stifle any serious attempt at understanding processes and mechanisms. To the extent that experiments are directed at, and useful for, discovering lawful causal relationships, it may well be the case that experimental methods like randomised controlled trials (RCTs), which tend to focus on curriculum-level interventions, are over- rather than underused in education.(16) That is, although many recent reviews have decried the paucity of good randomised trials in education,(7,17) it makes little sense to conduct elegant studies of interventions that are so complex in their idiosyncracies as to be unreplicable.(18) Still, much can be learnt from good experimentation in appropriate settings.

Study designs

The essence of the experimental approach is a comparison – between one group of individuals who received an intervention and another who did not. In an ideal situation, the participants in the two groups are as alike as possible before the intervention (which is why randomisation is used to ensure equivalence), so that any differences observed later can be unambiguously attributed to the intervention and nothing else.

However, although the two-group, intervention–control study design is ubiquitous, it is far from unique. Books on research design dating back over several decades have described many increasingly complex designs,(19) and we will discuss some of the more common variants.

One group: pre-test–post-test and post-test only

A recent review in medical education showed that a single-group pre-test–post-test design was the most commonly reported experimental methodology (32% of 105 studies) followed by a one-group post-test-only design (26%).(6) It is easy to see why this is the case. These designs can easily be incorporated into an ongoing curriculum or course change. All one needs to do is teach something to students taking the course and measure them at the beginning and end of the course. By contrast, comparisons with a control group require identification of a comparable control group of participants who will volunteer to be tested but will only receive a sham intervention or none at all. Regrettably, one-group designs, labelled 'pre-experimental' by Campbell and Stanley,(19) have very limited scientific value. The problems are myriad.

Logically, there is no way that whatever changes are observed from beginning to end can be ascribed to the intervention as opposed to competing hypotheses such as maturation, co-intervention or any number of other plausible explanations.

Further, while the logical flaws may appear parochial, there is a more fundamental educational problem.

If one shows a change in performance before and after an intervention, the comparison is against zero change, which implies a comparison against no education at all. While it may well be useful to determine whether, for example, a homeopathic remedy has any effect whatsoever [which is frankly not a question worth asking(20)], we can pretty well assume that an hour or two of education is going to result in more learning than none [although not always(21)]. In the end, a demonstration that students learnt something after a course reveals nothing about the contribution of any specific aspect of the course.

Two groups: randomised controlled trials and cohort studies

This difficulty with identifying a causal agent in one-group designs naturally leads to RCT. The standard RCT involves randomising participants to two groups, so that at the end of the study the only difference between the two groups (except for chance variation) should be that one group received one intervention and the other did not (or received a second intervention). Randomisation is intended to ensure equivalence at inception, standardisation of interventions facilitates interpretation, blinding avoids bias as does complete follow-up, and so on. In this manner, if a difference is observed, it can unequivocally be attributed to the intervention alone.

The criteria in Box 21.3 are easy to understand but much more difficult to put into practice. Some aspects,

---

BOX 21.3 Focus on: The randomised controlled trial

The randomised controlled trial has only a few critical elements:

- it has two (usually) or more (occasionally) groups
- participants are randomly assigned to each group
- the study is conducted prospectively
- all study participants are blinded to what group they are in
- the intervention(s) are standardised and under experimenter control
- outcome assessment is performed blind on all participants (i.e the person collecting the data does not know to which group the participants were assigned)
- complete follow-up of participants is achieved.

---

such as random assignment, are not too difficult. Blinding of participants, however, so they do not know what educational intervention they received, is effectively impossible. Indeed, if a student does not know whether he or she received problem-based learning (PBL) or lectures, one would worry about the student, the intervention, or both. Standardisation is much easier with drugs than curricula – what does 300 mg of PBL t.i.d. look like? We might recall that teacher differences typically account for twice as much variance in learning as curriculum differences, and it is not clear how one standardises teachers.(22)

Let us critically examine these aspects in more detail, and in doing so, identify the art of the possible.

Randomisation, quasi-randomisation and intact groups

One methodological *sine qua non* is randomisation, assignment to groups using a random process. But randomisation is difficult to achieve at times – a student may sign up for the Tuesday tutorial because he or she plays piano on Monday, and may not take kindly to a Monday tutorial assigned by a random number. We forget that randomisation is a means to an end; if students select a tutorial or a hospital rotation in some manner that is highly unlikely to have an impact on their ultimate performance, what we might call 'quasi-randomisation', that may well be good enough. Further, safeguard against bias must scale against the likely size of the treatment effect; if the treatment effect is large, concern about bias can be reduced. Lipsey and Wilson(23) analysed 319 systematic reviews of educational and psychological interventions and showed: (a) an average effect size of 0.45 (effect sizes of clinical interventions are much smaller; one study of aspirin in preventing myocardial infarction had a computed effect size of 0.02)(24) and (b) no influence of randomisation on effect size; the effects were of equal magnitude (on average) whether randomisation took place or not. Under some circumstances, the potential bias from 'quasi-randomisation' is negligible. Sometimes randomisation of individuals is just not possible. Students are in one section or another of the course; they are assigned to one hospital or another. A variant of randomisation to deal with this situation is called 'cluster randomisation' – where clusters (e.g. classes) are assigned to one treatment or another. Note that the analysis must account for clusters, and this may have an impact on sample size.

On the other hand, many studies use *intact* groups – what epidemiologists would call *cohort* studies (which we will discuss later). As one example, many studies have looked at PBL versus lecture-based curricula. Most of these studies involved between-school comparisons. A few, usually from the 1970s, involved within-school comparisons, where the school ran a parallel track. Fewer still randomised students to the two tracks. In considering any differences that emerge, between-school comparisons must be viewed with caution, since different schools differ on myriad variables, from the admissions criteria to the cost of tuition. Within-school comparisons may be better, although often students were selected using different criteria in the two tracks or may have self-selected one track or another. Thus, the finding that PBL students have better interpersonal skills(25,26) must be tempered by the likelihood that the PBL school may well select students for interpersonal skills, or that students with good interpersonal skills may prefer the small group focus of the PBL track.(27) The conclusion about allocation is a conditional one. In some circumstances there is a good likelihood that non-random assignment can be viewed as equivalent. In others, this may lead to serious confounding. To make an informed decision about which is most likely to be the case, researchers should gather as much information as possible on dimensions relevant to the question of interest from both groups and judge whether or not differences exist that are strong enough to account for differences observed in the outcome.

Placebo or usual care

The choice of control group in educational research is rarely given sufficient attention. This is hardly surprising. Programme evaluation is often initiated by someone who has put time and energy into a new curriculum, course or learning module. It hardly seems worth the effort to now put equal time into a second intervention that is only there for comparison. Consequently, it is often the case that students receiving the innovation are compared with students at another hospital, say, who receive the regular instruction – what epidemiologists may refer to as 'usual care'.

Such a comparison may be of limited value, regardless of how well other methodological criteria are accomplished. If usual care consists of, for example, lectures that are examined to ensure that the same content is covered, this is fair. If, however, the intervention amounts to a greater amount of time spent studying the to-be-learnt material relative to the control group (a situation that often arises when one simply adds the innovation, such as a high-fidelity simulation, to the curriculum in the treatment arm), then we again find ourselves in the awkward situation of concluding simply that the more they study, the more they learn. From a scientific perspective, a 'usual care' group is about as valuable as none at all, unless the specific aspects of the control intervention can be described as accurately as the experimental arm. It is far more informative to compare two experimental interventions where it is possible, for example, to standardise for total time of instruction or other confounders. As one excellent example of how this strategy would work, Cook(28) has discussed the many studies of e-learning and argued for studies within

medium (e.g. both arms of the study use the computer) so that pedagogical variables can be systematically manipulated (i.e. controlled) and the specific medium is not confounded. In deciding on a comparison, one must be careful also to avoid over-controlling the study by equating the two groups with respect to the very variables that are likely to make a difference. The literature on class size, in trying simply to test the impact of size, is guilty of this to some extent, as many studies control the very features of small class discussions (e.g. the opportunity to interact with the professor) that may yield benefits.(29)

Blinding

One criterion of a good RCT is that all participants – teachers, students and researchers – are 'blind' as to who is in which group. Of course, in education, this is simply farcical. While it may be possible to have outcome measurement performed with blinded assessors or with objective tests, it seems highly unlikely that students and teachers will be blinded. But the issue is broader than that. Implicit in the experimental method is that the participant is an 'object', whose motivation and ability is under experimental control. Orwell's vision of 1984 was never achieved, fortunately, and we are left with students who are unlikely (in the extreme) to knuckle under to a researcher's whims. Does this negate the experimental agenda? Not necessarily. But it does ring a cautionary note. To ensure the validity of the study we must make some calculated guesses about the effect of the inevitable unblinding. Failure to do so may lead to false interpretation. As one example, all medical students in North America are highly motivated to pass the licensing examination, for obvious reasons. Consequently, it makes little sense, in our view, to use a licensing examination as a criterion to evaluate a PBL curriculum since student performance on the licensing examination is likely to reflect many hours of study activity unrelated to the curriculum. The outcome may be of interest if it shows a difference, but the numerous studies showing no difference add little to our understanding, and are certainly no basis for any claim of equivalent curricula.

The perils of pre-tests

One variant on the RCT is a two-group, pre-test–post-test design. The usual reason for considering a pre-test, to correct for baseline differences, turns out to be not logically defensible, and the potential side effects of a pre-test often go unrecognised. The issues surrounding use of change scores are quite complex, and we can only highlight some.(30)

The problem with baseline differences is this. If the two groups were created by random assignment, then any difference between groups arose by chance, and to some extent can be adequately dealt with by statistical procedures, which explicitly examine the role of chance in any observed difference. Pre-tests *may* serve a useful role in identifying whether or not there are baseline differences that should factor into one's interpretation; however, if this is a consequence of non-random allocation, no amount of pre-test correction can control for such differences, simply because any correction involves strong assumptions about the relation between pre-test and post-test. This is described in *Biostatistics*.(30) In education, pre-tests have one further serious liability. There is no better way to inform students about what the final test will look like than to give them a parallel pre-test. The pre-test becomes part of the curriculum and has the potential to completely eliminate curriculum differences. Obviously, using exactly the same test both pre- and post-intervention simply magnifies the concern, as highlighted by Larsen *et al.*'s findings,(31) which suggest that the material one is tested on becomes particularly memorable. One solution that explicitly recognises this issue is called the Solomon Four Group Design. In this design there are four groups:

- pre-test, intervention, post-test
- pre-test–post-test
- intervention–post-test
- post-test.

It is then theoretically possible to disentangle the effect of pre-test from the intervention itself.

Outcomes: self-assessed versus performance-based, and short term versus long term

The choice of the appropriate outcome is perhaps the most difficult part of study design. It almost inevitably represents a compromise between what would be assessed in an ideal world and what can reasonably be assessed with the inevitable constraints of time, money and acceptability. Of course, we would like to show that ultimately the educational innovations we are studying have an impact on patient outcomes, and editors of three journals in the field have argued that this is a goal to be seriously entertained.(32–35) But realistically, with rare exceptions,(13,36) few studies will last long enough to examine patient outcomes. In any case, we agree with Gruppen(37) that such a quest is ill-advised for the more fundamental reason that there are so many intervening variables that it is unlikely any educational intervention will lead to detectable differences.

There is, however, another reason to seek more immediate measures, which aligns with the philosophical commitment to theory-based, programmatic research. While a demonstration that an intervention leads to a (small) increment in performance in, say, a final exam or a licensing examination may be of some practical value, even these outcomes are subject to so many confounders that they are unlikely to reveal a cause–effect relationship with the intervention. It is more profitable to think of a causal chain where an intervention at each level will have maximal effect on proximal outcomes, and less impact as the chain lengthens. (It is possible that the effects are additive or even multiplicative – the rich get richer – but this appears less likely in the situations we have examined.) For example, if an intervention can be shown to improve knowledge levels in the first year of medical school and first-year performance is shown to be predictive of clerkship performance, clerkship performance is found to relate to scores received on a national licensing exam, and so on, then we can develop a richer picture of what variables have an impact at each stage and make more informed decisions regarding the educational activities that should be undertaken. Our recent work on testing the validity of various admissions procedures provides an example of this approach.(38) As an aside, while it is difficult to show enduring effects of curricula, some recent studies have shown that individual differences in students, either in performance or ethical behaviour,(13,39) may have long-term effects that are not inconsequential.

A second issue to consider when deciding on outcome measures is the source. Satisfaction scales, completed by learners, are ubiquitously used as measures of programme effectiveness, probably because of their ease of administration. However, it is difficult to imagine how someone who has spent the time and money to take a course would perceive that they had learnt nothing and it was all a waste [even though some highly touted courses are exactly that(36)]. Satisfaction with teaching is moderately related to performance gains,(40) however, this may be a chicken–egg phenomenon as the strongest relations result when students know their scores. Worse still, self-reported judgements of competence have been shown repeatedly to have minimal relationship with observed competence,(41–43) thereby making it important that self-assessments are not used as surrogate markers of performance.

The optimal choice must be a measure that, on the one hand, is sufficiently close in time and context to be sensitive to intervention effects and to permit causal inferences, but is sufficiently relevant, in some absolute sense, to be viewed as a valid and important outcome. This latter point requires careful consideration, consultation and pilot testing to ensure that one is looking at outcomes that are likely to represent the changes that could conceivably be occurring. Again, one should use both theory and experience to interpret whether the intervention is likely to impact upon measures of affect, behavioural outcomes or cognitive indicators of ability (the ABCs of outcomes). Finally, note for now that the measures must be psychometrically sound, with proven evidence of reliability and validity. We will have more to say on this topic in the next section.

Three or more groups, and factorial designs

While a two-group comparison is undoubtedly the most common experimental design in the literature, there is rarely any reason to restrict a study to only two groups. Certainly, when one abandons the simplistic approach of a placebo or usual care control and seeks better explanation through systematic manipulation of a number of independent variables, there is good reason to consider multiple groups. Analytical methods are straightforward, analysis of variance (ANOVA) followed by some post hoc procedure. The primary disadvantage is that each additional group requires an additional sample of participants. However, an alternative design strategy, using 'factorial designs', has the remarkable property that one can address multiple hypotheses with very small penalty in sample size. An example is a study of e-learning in brain anatomy by Levinson *et al.*(44) There were two variables: key views (front, back, top, section) versus multiple views (where the visualised brain could assume multiple positions) and active versus passive control over the presentation (one group had control over the time the computerised image was presented in each of the various orientations, the other did not). This made four groups:

- active–key
- active–multiple
- passive–key
- passive–multiple.

These four groups can be thought of as lying within a 2×2 table (Figure 21.1).

Now, suppose that 25 students are in each group. The data would be analysed with a two-way ANOVA, giving a significance test for active versus passive based on two groups of 50, key versus multiple based on two groups of 50, and the interaction between them (i.e. whether or not the effect of active versus passive control is the same for both levels of the views variable), based on four groups of 25. In terms of the two main hypotheses, the comparison is virtually as powerful as the test using only two groups with 50 subjects per group.

Further, one cannot assess an interaction without including both variables in a single research study, and the interaction is often where the most interesting findings lie. Such was the case in the Levinson study in that the best group was the passive–key view participants, the worst was the passive–multiple view participants, and the two active groups were intermediate with respect to their performance at test.

This is the simplest of factorial designs. In our view, these designs, with their capability to examine multiple hypotheses simultaneously and to explore interactions among variables at almost no cost in sample size, are underutilised in education research.

Sample size and effect sizes

Given that the previous section argued for the value of multifactorial designs, in part on the basis that one can get more information with very small penalty in terms of sample size, it would be remiss of us not to include an answer to the ubiquitous question of 'How many people do I need?'. Of course, questions are usually ubiquitous when the answer is 'it depends', but we will provide an indication of what it depends on by highlighting issues that should be considered when engaging with experimental research paradigms.

There are two central issues to take into account in determining the required sample size. The first is statistical and is related to the concept of 'power' alluded to in the last section. In educational research, there is always variability related to differences among learners. Some students will learn more than others. Regardless of whether one is learning via large-group lecture or small-group tutorial (to name one example of a comparison that has been made *ad nauseum*) there will be variability in the amount learnt, and the distribution of one group is likely to overlap (often substantially) with the distribution of the other group. As such, statistics are required to determine the probability that the differences observed in the mean scores achieved by both groups could not have arisen simply by chance. The standard of '$P < 0.05$' means that the likelihood that an observed difference (or association as we will discuss later) arose due to chance is less than 5%, so the odds are good that the intervention, and not random variation, resulted in the differences between the groups. Because it is based on probabilities, the conclusion is fallible – one can falsely conclude that there is a difference when there is none, or that no difference exists when in fact there is an underlying effect of the intervention.

'Power' is the extent to which the study has a large enough sample to avoid making the latter mistake – assuming there is no difference when there is. Specific calculations for sample size are beyond the scope of this monograph as the formulae differ depending on the statistical test one needs to perform, but it should be noted that in all cases sample size calculations are dependent on predictions of how large a difference and how much variability in the sample one would expect. The predictions should be based on the best information available, but inevitably the calculations will be guesstimates to some degree. If one is able to find a statistically significant difference, however, then by definition the study was sufficiently powered (i.e. had a large enough sample size). One could debate the representativeness of the sample and whether or not

	Key views	Multiple views
Active control	(a)	(b)
Passive control	(c)	(d)

Figure 21.1 Example of two group comparison: elearning in brain anatomy.(44)

the effect might disappear with greater sampling, making replication an invaluable strategy for confirming the accuracy of the results, but whether or not the study had sufficient power (i.e. was statistically 'big enough') is not debatable. Power calculations are only relevant when significance was not obtained, but like sample size calculations these require an assumption of the magnitude of difference one wanted to detect. Big differences require smaller samples than small differences.

The second issue to consider is implicit in the preceding discussion. Very large samples can yield the opposite problem to small samples. An intervention can have a statistically significant effect even if it is of no practical importance, simply because the study had a very large sample size. For this reason, it is wise to consider not only the statistical significance, but also the size of the effect, typically defined as the difference between group means divided by the standard deviation (see any statistical text for more detail). The larger the effect size, the easier it is to argue that the findings are 'clinically important'. By convention, effect sizes of 0.2, 0.5 and 0.8 (i.e. differences that amount to 20%, 50% and 80% of the standard deviation) are considered small, medium and large.(45) Typical effect sizes observed in educational and psychological interventions are about 0.45, averaging across 319 meta-analyses.(25) Any one study might be misleading, so one often has to consider the average effect size by looking across many studies (a topic we will consider again in the section on meta-analysis).

Summary

For many, experimental research is held up as the gold standard for which we should strive when addressing all research questions. Clearly this is simplistic, but it is true that experimental designs, when applied appropriately, can have great impact on our ability to understand the extent to which causal relationships exist between variables (i.e. if one variable changes does it cause another to change?). However, curriculum-level interventions are vulnerable to many biases, and it is often more useful to design a series of small-scale experiments that tease apart the active ingredients, thus building knowledge of which elements are critical for learning. However, when one is interested in testing the relationship between naturally occurring variables that cannot easily be manipulated, then methodologies drawn from the epidemiologic or correlational traditions may be more appropriate, as discussed in the following sections.

The Epidemiologic Tradition

The term RCT has been used repeatedly in this chapter, referring to what is commonly viewed as the optimal experiment, in which subjects are randomly assigned

BOX 21.4 Randomised controlled trial study design

	Outcome	
	Present	*Absent*
Intervention		
Control		

to different groups that receive different treatments, and are then compared on some outcome measure. The RCT has a position of honour at the top of a hierarchy of research designs derived from epidemiology. While other designs in this hierarchy are rarely explicitly used in educational research, they may occasionally have a very useful role, as we shall point out.

Because many epidemiological investigations are based on a dichotomous outcome (dead or alive, improved or worsened, diseased or disease-free) as well as a dichotomous classification at inception (drug/placebo, risk factor present/absent, e.g. smoker/non-smoker), the easiest way to think about these designs is as a 2 × 2 table.

We have already discussed the RCT, the design of which is shown in Box 21.4. Respondents are randomised to rows (i.e. to the drug or placebo group) and the outcome (the columns) is tabulated. A *cohort* study looks the same, excep that subjects are not randomised to the two groups; rather, they are members of each cohort as a result of processes beyond the experimenter's control and, as such, the word 'intervention' should be replaced by 'exposure' or some other descriptor appropriate to the particular focus of the study.

Many studies of PBL versus lecture-based curricula can be classified as cohort studies, because students are in one cohort or the other through non-experimental factors such as self-selection or differential admissions policies. They may then be followed forward to determine, for example, success rates on licensing examinations or acceptance into primary care residency programmes. One example is the study by Woodward *et al.*(25) of billing patterns of McMaster graduates matched to graduates from the rest of Ontario.

A case-control study can be illustrated the same way, but the method of allocation runs in the opposite direction. Cases are selected by the outcome – they had the disease, or they failed the examination – and controls are selected who did not have that outcome. The study then looks back to determine whether the cases were more likely to be exposed to some risk (e.g. smoking or PBL). A case-control study, therefore, looks the same as the RCT with the exceptions that:

- the rows are better labelled as risk factors (present/absent)
- subjects are assigned by the columns rather than by the rows as the researcher looks for different rates of risk factor across the columns.

The important study by Papadakis *et al.*(13) of predictors of disciplinary action by a medical board is a good example of a *case-control* study. They identified a group of *cases*: 235 graduates from three medical schools who had some kind of disciplinary action as physicians and matched them to 469 *controls*, who were comparable demographically (i.e. were matched), but who had no record of disciplinary action. She then looked back at both groups' undergraduate records to determine whether they had episodes of unprofessional behaviour in medical school, and found that 92/235 cases (39%) revealed problems as a student, whereas only 90/469 controls (19.2%) revealed similar issues. One must consider base rates to determine the impact of acting on such differences,(46) but these compelling findings draw appropriate attention to the types of behaviour that should be considered in the context of professionalism.

Summary

Perhaps ironically, the most applicable study design from this hierarchy is the last. There are many examples of studies that resemble cohort studies or RCTs, and it is not particularly helpful to single these out with a new label. However, the case-control study is uniquely useful in situations analogous to its application in clinical medicine, where the outcome is categorical (disciplinary action yes/no), the prevalence of the outcome is low and the time delay until it occurs is long. Because it is usually retrospective, the case-control study may well be the only, or at least the most efficient, response to the concern to link educational interventions to patient outcomes; any alternative is likely to be too large, too costly and too inefficient to show any yield (Box 21.5).(39)

The Psychometric Tradition

As alluded to in the last section, the RCT is frequently held up as the 'best' research design with accompanying consternation regarding how few studies in medical education use an RCT. Such an attitude is, in our view, amazingly myopic.(16) One need not leave the quantitative domain to recognise that many of the most important questions and issues in the field cannot, *and should not*, be addressed with an RCT or, for that matter, any other experimental or quasi-experimental design.

> ### BOX 21.5 Focus on: Quasi-experimental designs
>
> Quasi-experimental designs including cohort and case-control studies have the following characteristics:
>
> - they include two (usually) or more (occasionally) groups
> - they enrol participants who are assigned to each group based on some predetermined characteristic on which it is not possible to randomise (e.g presence of disease or risk factor)
> - they are conducted retrospectively
> - participants are not blinded to the group they are in
> - complete follow-up of participants is rarely achieved.

Arguably, the most significant advances in our field have been in assessment, where medical education has, quite literally, led the world(47) in developing authentic, yet psychometrically defensible, measures like the Objective Structure Clinical Examination (OSCE).(48) Assessment methods are analogous to diagnostic tests, designed to identify those who have a lot or a little of the characteristic of interest, and perhaps to eventually create a cut-off to label a disease, in this case, 'incompetence'. Just as the starting point in developing a diagnostic test (e.g. a new radiographic procedure) is to assemble a group of patients, administer the test and look at (a) inter-rater agreement and (b) relation to some other measure of the same characteristic, we would set about testing a new assessment method by assembling a group of students, administering the test and examining reliability and then validity. Any radiologist who introduced a new diagnostic procedure by conducting a multi-centre trial to see whether patients who had the test lived longer before they first proved that radiologists had adequate inter-rater agreement and that the test results converged on other measures of disease would be at risk of psychiatric referral. Similarly, while we might like to eventually use an experimental method to show that students who get a new assessment method eventually perform better than those who are assessed using some conventional method, this is hardly the first step.

Because so much research in medical education is directed towards the development and testing of assessment methods, this section is devoted to a discussion of basic issues in psychometric methods. The discussion is necessarily brief; for a substantial elaboration, we refer you to Streiner and Norman.(49)

Basic concepts

Psychometric methods are designed to ensure that data are sufficiently trustworthy to enable appropriate interpretations and accurate decision making. Medical educators and the lay public are bombarded with 'databased' claims every day, but it goes without saying that not all such claims should be treated equally. Most threats to validity require us to formalise this intuitive skepticism and devise ways to test whether or not our measurement instruments are indeed measuring what we intend them to be measuring.

These strategies can be applied to any number of domains, including but not limited to assessments of the quality of admissions decisions,(50) research into the relation between personality and professionalism(51) or use of a questionnaire to measure the extent to which learners demonstrate self-directed learning.(52) In each case it is easy to collect information and make decisions, but much more is involved to determine whether or not those conclusions stand up to proper scrutiny. To understand this statement it is of course necessary to define 'proper scrutiny'.

For any measurement instrument to provide useful information, be it an objective indication of some physical state as would be measured with thermometers or a subjective claim about a more ethereal construct like one's perceptions of one's own abilities, it is necessary to ensure that the tool satisfies the four '-*ities*' of good measurement:

- feasibility
- acceptability
- reliability
- validity.

The first two need no explanation in that it seems fairly straightforward to suggest that a tool should only be used to the extent that it can be used (feasibility) and to the extent that people will use it (acceptability), but the latter two require elaboration. Before we begin, a disclaimer: while we will discuss *the* psychometric properties of measurement instruments, we do so simply for the sake of useful shorthand, as it is inaccurate to make acontextual claims about such properties in relation to any instrument. That is, the utility (see Chapter 14) of an instrument is based entirely on the population and context within which the instrument is to be used. While a grading system based on smiley faces might be appropriate for school-age children it is unlikely to be accepted in the context of national licensing exams in medicine; a survey that asks people to answer questions about their sexual activity levels may elicit accurate responses in some respondent cohorts, but may not be answered (and may cause offence) in others; a clinical skills examination that requires blood pressure to be taken may discriminate among beginning medical students but may be useless with medical residents. As we will see, these contextual variables can have significant impact on the assessment of reliability and validity.

Reliability

Reliability may be the most misused word in all of medical education. It does not mean agreement (although agreement is relevant), it does not mean variability (although variability is relevant) and it is not indicated by consistency of mean scores calculated for a group of individuals (although one would expect such consistency if the tool is reliable). Reliability is a statistical term indicating the extent to which a measurement instrument *consistently differentiates* between *individual* subjects of interest. The subjects may be learners, teachers, courses, schools, survey respondents or any other group of individual entities. As attempts to differentiate between students are most common within our community, we will use that domain as an example. Were one interested in developing a tool to assess knowledge of professional responsibilities, it would not be hard to generate items that result in variability of responses. That, in fact, would be a predominant goal as, presumably, if everyone were to provide the same responses there would be little reason to administer the test. That variability, however, could be attributable to any number of factors. Our hope is that scores on the test reflect true or consistent differences between students, with respect to their knowledge of professional responsibilities. Some portion of the variability, however, will be attributable to error of measurement because systematic biases and random forces can be expected to impact on the scores assigned to students.

While there are an infinite number of sources of error, the primary question is how much of the variability in scores can be attributed to error in relation to actual differences between the students? In other words, if we were to re-administer the test (or have different examiners rate the responses or use a parallel test), how consistent would individuals' scores be from one administration to the next? Mathematically, the simplest way to represent this concept is with the following equation:

$$Reliability = \frac{\sigma^2_{subjects}}{\sigma^2_{subjects} + \sigma^2_{error/n}}$$

σ^2 is the conventional symbol used to express variance, such that the numerator indicates the amount of variance attributable to differences between the students themselves and the denominator represents the total variability observed in the scores. This equation is not presented to scare away the innumerate, and we will not elaborate here on how one would calculate reliability. Rather, the formula is presented because it enables us to illustrate some fundamental points about reliability and, in turn, research in the psychometric tradition (*see* Box 21.6).

Within the psychometric tradition readers of educational journals will also encounter the notion of *generalisability*, a close cousin of the concept of reliability. Generalisability theory is a way of expressing the extent to which the scores assigned to individual subjects generalise to the scores assigned in another

BOX 21.6 Focus on: Reliability

- *Reliability is not a fixed property of the measurement instrument.* If a test of professionalism knowledge, as described above, is designed to provide an assessment of second-year residents, then its reliability (i.e its ability to consistently differentiate between subjects) must be tested on a sample of second-year residents. To recruit a more heterogenous sample (e.g. by enrolling first-year undergraduates and practising ethicists) will result in artificial inflation of the numerator, and as a result, artificially inflated estimates of the reliability of the tool. Researchers must make a concerted effort to specify the context within which they want to use their instruments and test by recruiting a sample of respondents representative of those working in that context.

- *Repeated measurement across the variables of interest are required to estimate the reliability of a tool.* If raters are liable to disagree about the strength of a student's performance, then multiple raters should be asked to rate the student's performance. If performance varies across the cases (content specificity) then students should be assessed on multiple cases. Simply administering a test and revealing that the scores are normally distributed tells us absolutely nothing about the extent to which the tool consistently differentiates between subjects because the variation can result from true differences between students or measurement error.

- *The more observations per individual one is able to average across, the more reliable the instrument will tend to be.* The *n* under the error term represents the number of observations collected (be they from multiple test questions, multiple raters, multiple administrators of the exercise or some other source of error variance). An average over multiple observations provides a better estimate of the amount of the construct held by the individual than any one score because random positive sources can cancel out random negative forces. Of course if a particular source of variance does not contribute error to a particular measurement, averaging across multiple observation collected across that source

  will have no impact (dividing zero by anything still leaves one with zero). An important aspect of psychometric analysis, therefore, is to determine how many observations one must collect for the total to achieve reasonable levels of reliability – if the answer is too many to be feasible, it suggests that the tool should be modified or abandoned.

- *A tool that does not discriminate is useless for assessment.* There may be other aspects of utility (specifically, motivating individuals to engage in desired study behaviour – educational impact) that warrants use of a particular measurement instrument, but generally, claim for utility rely on evidence of reliability and if everyone receives the same score, from an assessment perspective one may as well assume the result and do something better with one's time than administer the test.

- *Claims that the mean score of a group did not change over time (or across raters) provide no evidence of reliability.* One would find a stable mean even if the rank ordering of individuals within the sample perfectly reversed from one test administration to the next (i.e if there was absolutely no consistency in the scores assigned and, as a result, all variance could be attributed to error). A random number generator can be expected to result in equivalent means on different occasions, but random number generators can hardly claim to provide reliable measures of performance.

- *Occasionally, the claim is made that reliability of a measure is irrelevant because validity is more important.* Such a statement is simply illogical. One can view reliability as the correlation between a measure and itself (on repeated occasions). Validity expresses the correlation between a measure and some external (preferably 'gold') standard. It is axiomatic that a measure cannot correlate with something better than it correlates with itself. Hence, reliability is not dissociated from validity; instead, it sets an upper limit or possible claims to validity.

context (with another rater, at another time, etc.).(52) If that sounds familiar, it is because generalisability theory is simply an extension of reliability theory that provides the mathematical infrastructure to enable multiple sources of error variance to be considered simultaneously. The fundamental advantages are that one need not complete multiple studies to assess the relative error contributions of multiple variables and that, as a result, one can determine the relative benefits of increasing the number of observations collected across one variable relative to the benefits that can be gained by increasing the number of observations collected across another.

Validity

Historically, most descriptions of validity have used one taxonomy or another to differentiate various ways in which one can consider the trustworthiness of a set of ratings.(53) *Content validity* is considered the extent to which the items in a tool adequately sample the domain of interest without extending beyond it (i.e. are the questions sufficient and relevant?); *criterion validity* refers to the extent to which the measure correlates well with another measure of the same underlying construct; and *construct validity* indicates the extent to which the scores derived from the instrument align with expectations based on understanding of the underlying construct that the tool was intended to measure (e.g. a new measure of height should result in higher scores for basketball players relative to jockeys). Other taxonomies have been used, but in our minds it is all just validity (i.e. an indication of whether or not the scores derived from the use of the instrument vary in conjunction with the extent to which the amount of construct in the individual being measured varies). In fact, some have argued that reliability is simply one aspect of validity rather than a separate concept, the argument being that if the amount of underlying construct is not expected to have changed across administrations of the instrument, then the scores should not change either.(54) The various taxonomies that have been published may be useful to generate ideas as to how the validity of an instrument can be tested, but one should not allow the taxonomy to distract from awareness that proper validity testing requires systematic study, preferably with a variety of methodologies.

That said, one aspect of what Messick calls '*consequential validity*' is worth highlighting.(53) Any time we put in place an instrument to assess students, we must worry about the extent to which the measurement instrument has an impact on behaviour. Assessment has long been known to have a steering effect on the learning activities of students.(55) As a result, to ensure the utility of an assessment instrument it is necessary to engender a match between the learning activities one hopes to promote and the learning activities stimulated by the tool.(55) As these five principles of good measurement (the four '-*ities*' and educational impact) that form a tool's utility do not always align (and, in fact, often run counter to one another) it is almost inevitably necessary to decide on an appropriate compromise, the balance of which should be determined by the specifics of the situation.

Most will start their study of the validity of an instrument by testing its reliability as described above, for the simple reason that if a tool is not reliable, it cannot be valid. For example, in studying the consistency of ratings provided to medical school applicants during panel-based interviews, Harasym *et al.*(56) noted that over 50% of the variance in scores could be attributed to the person doing the interview, thereby fundamentally calling into question both the reliability and the validity of the panel-based interview process, as that process is intended to provide information on the quality of applicants, not the stringency of the interviewers.

However, reliability is insufficient. Just because something can be measured consistently does not mean that the measurements are valid. It is easy to measure the circumference of an individual's head in a consistent and reliable manner. Those data, however, are completely useless if one is trying to assess the empathy levels of the subjects – phrenology was dis-

credited a century ago.(57) A more direct example comes from the literature on OSCE testing formats. As most readers of this chapter will be familiar with the OSCE, we will note simply that it is a 'bell ringer' type of examination in which examinees interact with multiple patients in sequence while striving to demonstrate their clinical skills. The 'O' in OSCE stands for objective, to indicate the initial idea that one could evaluate performance by generating a checklist of appropriate behaviours and noting which were undertaken by the examinee. Indeed, such checklists have been shown to robustly provide very reliable measurements of individuals' performance.(58) In various studies, however, they have been seen to bear no relation to experience, an important variable if one wants to make claims about measuring ability. In contrast, global ratings of performance do tend to correlate with experience levels, suggesting that while checklists may provide a valid measure of comprehensiveness, subjective judgement provides a more valid measurement of clinical expertise in many domains.(59)

One could go on *ad nauseum* about the variety of methodologies that can be used to study validity. Comparing average scores received by different groups that can be anticipated to differ in amount of the construct, correlating individual scores with other continuous variables that are expected to be related to the underlying construct, and examining the change in scores that takes place after an intervention expected to change levels of the underlying construct provide three broad classes of approach that might be adopted. Interesting examples include the work of Tamblyn *et al.* who revealed a relationship between performance on the Canadian licensing examination and professional behaviours during practice as a physician,(39) the work of Ramsey *et al.*(60) who revealed that specialist certification based on multiple-choice testing is predictive of peer ratings 10 years into practice, and the work of Davis *et al.*(61) who has continued a line of inquiry that casts doubt on the validity of self-assessments as indicators of performance. In fact, many of the methodologies included in other sections of this chapter (as well as those not included) could be deemed strategies for testing validity.

Instead of trying to generate a comprehensive list of strategies we will close this section by simply noting that one can rarely expect to prove validity in any absolute sense. It is important to test validity because claims that a measure provides information that should be allowed to guide decision making rest on the balance of evidence. In essence, validity testing is theory testing; each new test that reveals a positive result supports both the theory and the validity of the instrument, but each new test that reveals a negative result should lead one to question (and study) whether the theory is incorrect or the tool provides an inadequate measure of the construct.

Summary

The overarching theme of research undertaken within the psychometric tradition is that researchers, educators, clinicians, and the lay public for that matter, need to strive to be sure that the data that guide our thinking and decision making are sufficiently trustworthy to warrant using them to draw conclusions. This is not simply an academic issue, as too often people's lives are altered (by admittance to/rejection from/advancement within their chosen profession, by decision making within the legal system, or by personal life/marriage counsellors) on the basis of 'data' of dubious validity. Ensuring the validity of one's research instruments and assessment strategies is an ethical imperative.(62) It is not easy and there are certainly factors that need to be considered beyond psychometric properties, but the methods and concepts outlined here hopefully provide a good start and, if nothing else, should provide a basis for reasoning about these types of problem.

The Correlational Tradition

A significant proportion of research in medical education is derived from survey questionnaires. These may cover a potentially vast array of topics, from intrapersonal issues such as learning styles or emotional intelligence, to observer ratings of achievement or other aspects of observable behaviour, to satisfaction measures. It would be unrealistic to attempt to cover this vast, heterogeneous and complex field; instead this section will be devoted to a number of common issues related to scoring, research design and analysis. Questionnaire 'design' is addressed by Wall in Chapter 23, but we would remind the reader that proper questionnaire-based research is not easy, and reliability and validity must still be ensured. In general, questionnaires are useful for systematically determining a large group of individuals' perceptions and attitudes towards a particular issue they have experienced. Beyond that, however, one must always be aware of the limitation that people are notoriously bad at accurately judging the cause of their behaviour,(63) or the adequacy of their own performance.(42,43)

Scoring

Quite commonly, responses from individual items are to be summed into a score. Much effort is sometimes expended to decide what weight should be given to each item comprising the score. As it turns out, an extensive literature dating back to at least 1976 is absolutely consistent – an equal weighting model, where each item is simply summed, is as reliable and valid as *any* alternative.(65) There is one cautionary note: a simple sum assumes that the items are similar in means and standard deviations. It would be no more appropriate to add together items, some of which are binary (0 or 1) and some of which are on seven-point scales, than it would be to add an interview score based on seven-point scales to grades out of 100, or for that matter, to add weight in kilograms to height in metres as a measure of overall size. When the individual items are on different scales, the correct approach is to convert to Z scores [(score – mean)/ standard deviation] before combining scales.

One other point about scoring is that there is extensive debate about whether the scores assigned to the sorts of scale described here should be summed to calculate a mean given that, technically, the data are ordinal in nature (i.e. they indicate rank order without any guarantee of there being equal intervals between all pairs of sequential points).(64) In practice the parametric statistical tests that require interval-level data tend to be quite robust to deviations from normality(66) and their ease of application provides great advantage in most situations.

Validation

The validation methods described in the section on psychometric methods are appropriate for survey instruments and should be considered carefully to avoid making decisions based on survey data that might not be trustworthy for the purpose for which they were intended.

Analysis

The correlational approach is based on a search for relationships among variables, and analysis typically begins (and all too often ends) with every variable being correlated with every other, and then post hoc stories being constructed around the few 'significant' correlations. The problem with the strategy is researchers appear to forget the meaning of '$P < 0.05$' – the likelihood that an observed relationship of this magnitude could have arisen by chance *if there was in fact no relationship*. In other words, for every 20 correlations that are calculated, one will be significant by chance at the 0.05 level. It is worth noting here that this applies to any statistical analyses, including ANOVAs, *t*-tests and other strategies that rely on *P*-values to determine whether or not the data can be accounted for by chance alone. An obvious solution to this 'data dredging' is to begin with a substantive theory about what relationships are expected. At a minimum, this can direct attention to specific correlations rather than using a 'shotgun' approach. Further, as it is likely that the researcher will still be interested in more than one correlation, the critical *P*-value should be set at $0.05/n$ where 'n' is the total number of statistical tests – a 'Bonferroni correction'(67).

A more sophisticated approach than correlations involves multivariate methods such as multiple regression, factor analysis and structural equation modelling. Strictly speaking, the term 'multivariate' should only apply to a situation with multiple *dependent* variables. So multiple regression is a univariate procedure, factor analysis and structural equation modelling are multivariate. Multiple regression involves predicting a single dependent variable with multiple independent variables [e.g. predicting licensing exam performance with a combination of variables like undergraduate grades, gender, Medical College Admission Test (MCAT) score]. Factor analysis seeks underlying associations among clusters of variables, which are called 'factors'. More sophisticated is the family of multivariate methods including confirmatory factor analysis, hierarchical linear models and structural equation models. In all these methods, the researcher begins with a theory about the relationship among variables (e.g. *good tutors* succeed by increasing *motivation* of students, and this, in combination with their *prior achievement*, predicts their *final exam performance*). Different causal models are fitted to the data set and the degree of fit computed. Challenges for these approaches include: (a) that all of these methods are sample intensive, and the rule of thumb is that the sample size should be at least 5 to 10 times the number of variables; (b) as the complexity of the model increases, it becomes less and less clear what it actually means to say that this model fits the data but that model does not; and (c) because it is unlikely that any two studies will use the same combination of variables, the concern remains that the causal theory, whatever it may be, is unique to the data set on which it is based.

Nevertheless, these approaches do represent a considerable advance over the mindless cranking out of dozens of correlation coefficients that is all too frequently the norm in correlational research. As in the discussion on effect size presented in the experimental studies section, we urge a focus on the correlation coefficient, not the associated P-value. With large samples even minute correlations (e.g. $r = 0.1$) can be statistically significant. The coefficient of variation (r^2), however, reveals that $r = 0.1$ describes a relationship that accounts for only 1% of the variance in the data. As a result, r^2 should always be used to judge the 'clinical' importance of a correlation. We will return to this issue in the final section (Box 21.7).

Cronbach's 'Two Disciplines'

At the outset of this chapter, we pointed out that many research questions cannot *and should not* be answered with experimental designs. The methodology that is most appropriate (whether choosing between quantitative and qualitative designs or between experimental and correlational methods) is dependent on the question the researchers want to address. In promoting theory-based and programmatic research efforts, we advocate using a variety of methods to enable triangulation on a problem, thereby developing a richer

---

BOX 21.7 Focus on: Common statistical tests
Statistical tests are based on two broad classes.

Parametric tests
Used for measured data on which it makes sense to calculate means and standard deviations.

Used for comparing means

- **t-test:** one independent variable with two groups, or two related observations (such as before–after).
- **Analysis of variance (ANOVA):** one or more independent variables, each containing two or more groups ('levels').
- **Repeated measures ANOVA:** a special case of ANOVA in which repeated observations are taken within an independent variable on the same subjects. Also used for reliability and generalisability studies.

Used for examining relationships

- **Pearson's correlation:** provides relation between two measured continuous variables.
- **Multiple regression:** provides relation between multiple predictor variables and a single *continuous* dependent variable.
- **Factor analysis:** provides relations (underlying factors) for a large number of related variables.

Non-parametric tests
Used for frequency counts

- **Chi-squared:** compares proportions in two or more related categories (e.g. 2 × 2 tables).
- **Logistic regression:** provides relation between multiple predictor variables and a single *dichotomous* independent variable.

---

understanding of the underlying issue than any one methodology would allow. However, the choice is not quite as value-free as might be imagined. Lee Cronbach first recognised a fundamental duality in a classic paper published in 1957(68) called the 'The two disciplines of scientific psychology'.

The essence of the dichotomy is this. Correlational methods, including psychometrics, are critically dependent on individual differences. It begins with the reliability coefficient, which is zero if everyone is alike. If we want to examine the relation between some individual attribute such as intelligence quotient or premedical grades and some outcome such as licensing examination performance, unless some students are high or low on each measure there can be no correlation. By contrast, if we were to do an experiment to see whether a supplementary course can help students achieve higher scores on a standardised admissions test, ideally we would like to begin with a cohort of students whose abilities, as measured by undergraduate grades, are exactly the same. To the extent that some students are already very good at biology, physics, etc., and others in the course have little knowledge or aptitude, this will lead to large variability in the scores of students in the experimental and control groups. This variability will, in turn, end up in the denominator of any statistical test designed to show that the treatment was statistically significant.

To the experimentalist, any variation between people will dilute the chances of finding a treatment effect. To the correlationalist, the goal is explicitly to understand the differences between people. Thus it is literally the case that one person's signal is the other's noise.

Given this dichotomy, it makes no more sense to argue which is 'better' methodologically than to try to find evidence that red is better than blue, respective of the use to which the colours are to be put. They are not better or worse, except in relation to what one is trying to achieve; they are just different. The situation was nicely summarised recently by a wag who declared that, 'Randomised controlled trials are the best design of all to find out if a treatment works, and the worst design to find out who it works for.'

Reviews

As mentioned earlier, any primary research study will have flaws; even if the perfect study could be designed, there is no way to completely control for the powerful forces of random variation. As a result, it is important to consider the balance of evidence available when deciding how to use the information that has accumulated in the literature. This is the key reason that scholarly reviews of a field are so valuable – when done well, they synthesise the available evidence in a way that can refine the readers' understanding of the focal problem and help them better understand the implications of the literature for their own practices or their own knowledge-building research efforts. We have already noted that every research effort should be informed by a review of existing literature. Here we provide some insights into the creation and interpretation of more formal efforts, starting with systematic reviews, as they represent a form of review on which emphasis has been growing in recent years.

Systematic reviews and meta-analysis

In part as a consequence of the Best Evidence Medical Education (BEME) movement, initiated by Harden et al.,(69) systematic reviews have become increasingly popular in the medical education literature. To some degree they epitomise the reductionistic approach to quantitative research – the goal is to determine the one number that best specifies how well 'it' works. Although many might assume that medical education has adopted the technology of systematic reviews

from clinical research, where systematic reviews of, for example, the risk reduction for stroke from beta-blocker therapy are commonplace, in fact the path is more tortuous than that. The first proponent of systematic reviews and the accompanying meta-analyses were educational statisticians Smith and Glass, whose 1977 article in *American Psychologist*(70) is usually cited as the first publication of the type.

What is a systematic review? The goal is, more or less, to identify *all* of the empirical literature on a particular question, and to then use statistical methods to best estimate the effect (or non-effect) of a particular intervention in a way that is relatively free of bias compared with less comprehensive strategies. There are, therefore, three aspects of 'systematic':

- a systematic search for all the literature relevant to a topic
- a systematic review to select the subset of articles achieving at least minimal quality and relevance
- a systematic summary using specific statistical methods to arrive at the best estimate of the effect in question.

It is clear that these aspects, while equally important, are separable. First, careful computer algorithms to search electronic databases must be devised and then supplemented with manual searches. Once the key articles have been located they must be reviewed in detail to ensure methodological rigour, often using a detailed reporting form that enables a quality score for each study. Finally, each study is typically analysed to estimate an 'effect size' indicating the strength of the intervention in each instance in which it was used.

In meta-analyses these effect sizes are then combined, using a weighting by sample size, to arrive at an overall (i.e. average) effect size and a statistical test of significance. It is at this point that the second 'systematic' emerges – a systematic statistical averaging of all the individual effects into an overall unbiased estimate. This is the whole point of the exercise: to determine whether a particular intervention affected a particular outcome. One example might be the effect of PBL on national licensing examinations.(71) Another is the recent BEME review of the predictive validity of undergraduate measures predicting licensing examination performance.(72)

Problems with systematic reviews

While wonderful in theory, there are at least three problems with trying to put these methods into practice.

Quality of the evidence

It seems that an inevitable consequence of the methodological review is a note of despair about the poor quality of the studies, based on the number of criteria that were not fulfilled. It has almost reached the point of there being a standard disclaimer in systematic reviews: 'The authors take no responsibility for any personal damage resulting from the quality of the studies that went into this review.'

This disparaging of the quality of published papers seems a bit strange because, for the most part, the articles had all satisfied peer reviewers. Either the peer reviewers are not very good at their jobs, or they are basing their judgements on different criteria altogether than the systematic reviewers. We sense the latter; as editors, we rarely judge the worth of a paper by the number of methodological criteria it fulfilled and, indeed, Bordage(73) has shown the same to be the case on the part of peer reviewers. Just as the OSCE literature has found that global judgements are superior to checklists, Bordage's examination of the peer-review process suggests that the methodological components of a paper provide a poor indication of its overall value. Further, a preoccupation with quality might be tempered by the finding of Lipsey and Wilson,(23) mentioned earlier, that there was no relation between judged study quality and treatment effect, nor did randomised trials yield systematically different treatment effects than non-randomised studies.

Heterogeneity of the outcome

While the use of effect sizes enables putting various measures *of the same construct* on a common metric, it appears that systematic reviews are rarely able to reduce the outcome to one measure such as examination performance. In fact, in the recent review of learning portfolios(74) there was commonality among studies only at the broad level of classification (e.g. learning versus assessment) and no attempt was made to try to average outcomes across studies. Instead, the review reported findings along the lines of 'two studies reported that portfolios contributed to reflective learning'.

Undoubtedly the most careful and comprehensive approach to systematic reviews in medical education has been mounted by the BEME group. Very careful quality control is exercised at every step of the process, and the group of collaborators go to enormous lengths to ensure consistent quality. The first review, of high-fidelity simulation, by Issenberg *et al.*(75) began with over 600 abstracts that were then reduced to 109 studies for detailed analysis. The review concluded: 'Heterogeneity of research designs, educational interventions, outcome measures, and time frame precluded data synthesis using meta-analysis.' The authors then went on to describe the conditions that led to effective use of simulation. This approach, where a systematic search on many abstracts yields a small number of suitable studies, which in turn are combined with too many potential outcomes to permit any quantitative synthesis or meta-analysis, emerges as the norm for these reviews.

Low yield of studies

Systematic reviews can be enormously labour-intensive, primarily because the yield of useful articles is so low. As some examples, again drawn from the BEME monographs, the study of early community experience(76) catalogued 23 outcomes from 73 studies (out of 6 832 abstracts) and no quantitative synthesis was possible. Perhaps the worst example of 'needle in a haystack' was the synthesis of inter-professional education(77) that began with 10 495 abstracts and ended with 12 worthy detailed review. Interestingly a hand search added a further 9, despite beginning with only 46. Again, the results consisted of counts of what kind of intervention led to what kind of result. To avoid some of these problems, while admittedly creating others, many scholars choose to engage in generating critical rather than systematic reviews. In the following section we will strive to compare the two strategies, highlighting strengths and weaknesses of both approaches.

Critical reviews

In our initial discussion of the research question, we described the characteristics of a good literature review, namely, that it represents a critical synthesis of a literature, identifying what is well established, what is only poorly understood and what remains to be understood. It may, when done well, bring together several disparate literatures and, as a result, offer a new perspective. It should *not* end up as a chronological 'blow-by-blow' account, with one paragraph per study and no real synthesis. There is no pretense in a critical review that the cited literature represents all the relevant literature in the field, so there may be less of a tendency to provide a one-paragraph summary of every related study; the author is bound by an unwritten moral code to represent the various perspectives fairly, but that is all.

To our knowledge little is written about how to go about such reviews, which is somewhat strange, as there is little doubt that some of these papers become, over time, the 'citation classics' of the field. Far and away the most cited papers in the area of PBL are three old chestnuts: Albanese and Mitchell,(78) Vernon and Blake,(71) and Norman and Schmidt;(79) two of the three are critical reviews. What distinguishes a good critical review from a poor one? One expects that it has little to do with comprehensiveness or systematicity. Instead, the cited reviews appear to be those that present unique perspectives and marshal evidence convincingly to support the claims. Rather than scouring the nooks and crannies of the literature for every paper that is relevant to a narrow question, successful critical reviewers explore a variety of literature, mining for gold nuggets that often alter the way the community fundamentally defines the question.

In practice, in fact, critical reviews and systematic reviews in education have often led to similar conclusions, in part because, while no one would debate that the goal of systematicity – to eliminate bias in the data one draws on – is laudable, to some extent the mantle of systematicity is just a guise of credibility. If one cannot combine the findings in some systematic way as a result of heterogeneity of outcomes to the point of having to describe each study independently, then the only thing separating systematic reviews from critical narrative reviews is the amount of time and resources spent searching for information. Given the typical low yield of studies, it is questionable whether or not that effort proves a worthy use of resources. Again, this is not meant to imply that systematicity is bad or that all systematic reviews have been thoughtless – the examples used in this chapter make it clear that is not the case. It is to say though, that too often the claim of systematicity is applied thoughtlessly as a criterion by which quality is judged, when in fact true advances in the field are as often gained from critical syntheses of diverse ideas rather than systematicity itself. That said, critical reviews are clearly not without their own problems.

Problems with critical reviews
Author bias
The strengths of critical reviews are also their weaknesses. When literature is marshalled to support a unique perspective, there is the vague disquiet that the literature used may be, consciously or unconsciously, biased in favour of the claim. The author is under no explicit mandate to present all the evidence for and against, only to be unbiased in their conclusions. But such a stricture may not be realistic; if we were aware of our biases, we may well not be biased, so it is not uncommon for two critical reviews to come to diametrically opposite conclusions. Such is the fodder for academic debate.

Biased sampling of literature
A second problem is that if the purpose of the review is really to obtain a best estimate of the value of something (the 'truth'), for example, the predictive value of standardised aptitude tests like MCAT, or the effect of PBL on outcomes such as standardised examinations, or the effectiveness of faculty development programmes in changing faculty teaching competence, the synthesis methods used in critical reviews, if used at all, are primitive at best. They often reduce to a summary like '22/30 studies showed a positive effect'. That is precisely what systematic reviews do best – sometimes.

Finally, critical reviews can also assume a mantle of academic dithering. Such reviews rarely conclude with a final 'It works–it does not work', instead providing far more nuanced discussion than purely systematic reviews, with an inevitable self-fulfilling call for more research. Again, however, we would emphasise that where one might call this a weakness we consider it a strength, as this sort of academic dithering can enable much more refined appreciation for issues than was available in the field before the review was generated.

Summary
In the examples cited, the distinction between systematic review and critical review becomes vanishingly small. While each type of review may be stimulated by differing goals (Does it work? versus How does it work?), inevitably, as the systematic review identifies subgroups and subgoals, the additional knowledge is more of the form of revealing how different circumstances may influence the results. And while the critical review may be directed at advancing a theory, the reality is that there are very few theories in this field, so it is more likely that it will be focusing on the various things that may influence the effect under review. So it would seem that the ecology of the domain may be forcing a convergence between the two approaches.

Discussion

For about three decades, educational research has been embroiled in the 'qualitative–quantitative' debate, to the detriment of both. A careful read of this chapter and the chapter on qualitative methods by Lingard and Kennedy reveals that there is probably as much divergence in goals, design and methods within each tradition as there are differences between the two camps.

Is there any way to resolve the differences? The insight was, we believe, again provided by Lee Cronbach. In his 'Two disciplines' paper that we described earlier,(68) he advocated a search for aptitude–treatment interactions – using more complex quantitative methods such as analysis of covariance to relate aspects of the individual learner (aptitudes) to curriculum design factors (treatments). As one recent example, a series of studies of learning anatomy from a computer showed that students with high spatial ability had a small benefit from multiple views, but that students with poor spatial ability were seriously handicapped by multiple views.(80) The current use of methods such as confirmatory factor analysis and structural equation models is a logical extension of this approach. However, after two decades failures far exceeded successes, and in our view, the more powerful methods now in vogue follow in this tradition, yielding little in the way of substantive theoretical explanation.

Cronbach's resolution in a later paper(81) was to abandon attempts at greater experimental control in favour of more careful observation:

> [This paper will] explore the consequences of attempting to establish in psychological experimentation, empirical generalizations in a world in which most effects are interactive. While the two scientific disciplines of experimental control and systematic correlation are designed to answer pre-stated formal questions, the time has come for more open-ended, inquisitive investigation that will more fully explore the richness of scientific reality.

Another way to think about the goal of an individual study is a categorisation developed by Schmidt,(82) who described three goals for studies.

- *Description*, which focuses on the first step of the scientific method – observation. An approach is described, but no comparison is performed.
- *Justification* represents the opposite extreme, where the goal is to justify a particular approach by a careful experimental study showing it is superior to some alternative. The problem, as identified by Cook *et al.*,(83) is that without sufficient theory specification the results may have limited application.
- *Clarification* studies are modelled on the scientific method, beginning with observation, proceeding to careful theory building, testing and elaboration.

In an initial study, Schmidt found that 64% of 850 medical education studies reviewed were description studies, a further 29% were justification studies and only 7% were directed at clarification.(82) Cook *et al.* looked at a different database of experimental studies only and found that 16% were description, 72% justification and 12% clarification.(83) However desirable theory-based research is, it is a small minority of educational research studies. We hope that by drawing attention to these issues, this chapter may, in some small way, help to redress the balance.

References

1 Dolmans D (2003) The effectiveness of PBL: the debate continues. Some concerns about the BEME movement. *Medical Education.* **37**: 1129–30.

2 Norman G (2002) Research in medical education: three decades of progress. *British Medical Journal.* **324**: 1560–2.

3 Bordage G (2007) Moving the field forward: going beyond quantitative-qualitative. *Academic Medicine.* **82**: S126–8.

4 Meltzoff J (1998) Research questions and hypotheses. In: *Critical Thinking About Research*, pp. 13–30. American Psychological Association, Washington, DC.

5 Eva KW and Lingard L (2008) What's next? A guiding question for educators engaged in educational research. *Medical Education.* **42**(8): 752–4.

6 Albert M, Hodges B and Regehr G (2007) Research in medical education: balancing service and science. *Advances in Health Sciences Education: Theory and Practice.* **12**: 103–15.

7 Cook D, Beckman TJ and Bordage GE (2007) Quality of reporting of experimental studies in medical education: a systematic review. *Medical Education.* **41**: 737–45.

8 Popper K (1959) *The Logic of Scientific Discovery.* Hutchinson and Co., London.

9 Norman GR (1999) The adult learner: a mythical species. *Academic Medicine.* **74**: 886–9.

10 Regehr G (2010) It's NOT rocket science: rethinking our metaphors for research in health professions education. *Medical Education.* **44**(1): 31–9.

11 Stokes DE (1997) *Pasteur's Quadrant: basic science and technological innovation.* Brookings Institution Press, Washington, DC.

12 Cook TD and Campbell DT (1979) *Quasi-experimentation: design and analysis for field settings.* Rand McNally, Chicago, IL.

13 Papadakis MA, Teherani A, Banach MA *et al.* (2005) Disciplinary action by medical boards and prior behavior in medical school. *New England Journal of Medicine.* **353**: 2673–82.

14 Hojat M, Paskin DL, Callahan CA *et al.* (2007) Components of postgraduate competence: analyses of thirty years of longitudinal data. *Medical Education.* **41**: 982–9.

15 Rose G (2001) Sick individuals and sick populations. *International Journal of Epidemiology.* **30**: 427–32.

16 Norman GR (2003) RCT = results confounded and trivial. *Medical Education.* **37**: 582–4.

17 Schuwirth LW and van der Vleuten CP (2006) Challenges for educationalists. *British Medical Journal.* **333**: 544–6.

18 Norman GR, Eva KW and Schmidt HG (2005) Implications of psychology-type theories for full curriculum interventions. *Medical Education.* **39**: 247–9.

19 Campbell DT and Stanley JC (1963) *Experimental and Quasi-experimental Designs for Research on Teaching.* Rand McNally, Chicago, IL.

20 Goldacre B (2007) A kind of magic? (www.guardian.co.uk/science/2007/nov/16/sciencenews.g2; accessed 26 February 2008).

21 Norman GR and Shannon SI (1998) Effectiveness of instruction in critical appraisal (evidence-based medicine) skills: a critical appraisal. *Canadian Medical Association Journal.* **158**: 177–81.

22 Schmidt HG and Moust JHC (1995) What makes a tutor effective? A structural equations modeling approach to learning in problem-based curricula. *Academic Medicine.* **70**: 708–14.

23 Lipsey MW and Wilson DB (1993) The efficacy of psychological, educational, and behavioral treatment. Confirmation from meta-analysis. *American Psychologist.* **48**: 1181–209.

24 Meyer GJ, Finn SE, Eyde LD *et al.* (2001) Psychological testing and psychological assessment: a review of evidence and issues. *American Psychologist.* **56**: 128–65.

25 Woodward CA, Cohen M, Ferrier BM *et al.* (1989) Correlates of certification in family medicine in the billing patterns of Ontario general practitioners. *Canadian Medical Association Journal.* **141**: 897–904.

26 Koh GC-H, Khoo HE, Wong ML and Koh D (2008) The effects of problem-based learning during medical school on physician competency: a systematic review. *Canadian Medical Association Journal.* **178**: 34–41.

27 Colliver JA and Markwell SJ (2007) Research on problem-based learning: the need for critical analysis of methods and findings. *Medical Education.* **41**: 533–5.

28 Cook DA (2005) The research we still are not doing: an agenda for the study of computer-based learning. *Academic Medicine.* **80**: 541–8.

29 Ehrenberg RG, Brewer DJ, Gamoran A and Willms JD (2001) Does class size matter? *Scientific American.* **285**: 79–84.

30 Norman GR and Streiner DL (2007) *Biostatistics: the bare essentials* (3e). BC Decker, Hamilton, ON.

31 Larsen DP, Butler AC and Roediger HL (2008) Test-enhanced learning in medical education. *Medical Education.* **42**: 959–66.

32 Whitcomb ME (2002) Research in medical education: what do we know about the link between what doctors are taught and what they do? *Academic Medicine.* **77**: 1067–8.

33 Bligh J (2003) Editorial. *Medical Education.* **37**: 184–5.

34 Colliver JA (2003) The research enterprise in medical education. *Teaching and Learning in Medicine.* **15**: 154–5.

35 Norman GR (2006) Outcomes, objectives and the seductive appeal of simple solutions. *Advances in Health Sciences Education.* **11**: 217–20.

36 Werner LS and Bull BS (2003) The effect of three commercial coaching courses on Step One USMLE performance. *Medical Education.* **37**: 527–31.

37 Gruppen L (2007) Improving medical education research. *Teaching and Learning in Medicine.* **19**: 331–5.

38 Eva KW, Reiter HI, Rosenfeld J and Norman GR (2008) Predictive validity of the multiple mini-interview for selecting medical trainees. *Medical Education.* **43**(8): 767–75.

39 Tamblyn R, Abrahamowicz M, Dauphinee D *et al.* (2007) Physician scores on a national clinical skills examination as predictors of complaints to medical regulatory authorities. *Journal of the American Medical Association.* **298**: 993–1001.

40 Cohen PA (1981) Student rating of instruction and student achievement: a meta-analysis of multisection validity studies. *Review of Educational Research.* **51**: 281–309.

41 Eva KW and Regehr G (2005) Self-assessment in the health professions: a reformulation and research agenda. *Academic Medicine.* **80**: S46–54.

42 Gordon MJ (1991) A review of the validity and accuracy of self-assessments in health professions training. *Academic Medicine.* **66**: 762–9.

43 Davis DA, Mazmanian PE, Fordis M *et al.* (2006) Accuracy of physician self-assessment compared with observed measures of competence: a systematic review. *Journal of the American Medical Association.* **296**: 1094–102.

44 Levinson AJ, Weaver B, Garside S *et al.* (2007) Virtual reality and brain anatomy: a randomised trial of e-learning instructional designs. *Medical Education.* **41**: 495–501.

45 Cohen JJ (1988) *Statistical Power Analysis for the Behavioral Sciences.* Erlbaum, Hillsdale, NJ.

46 Colliver JA, Markwell SJ, Verhulst SJ and Robbs RS (2007) The prognostic value of documented unprofessional behavior in medical school records for predicting and preventing subsequent medical board disciplinary action: the Papadakis studies revisited. *Teaching and Learning in Medicine.* **19**: 213–15.

47 Swanson DB, Norman GR and Linn RL (1995) Performance based assessment: lessons from the professions. *Educational Research.* **24**: 5–11.

48 Harden RM and Gleeson FA (1979) Assessment of clinical competence using an objective structured clinical examination (OSCE). *Medical Education.* **13**: 41–54.

49 Streiner DL and Norman GR (2003) *Health Measurement Scales: a practical guide to their development and use* (3e). Oxford University Press, Oxford.

50 Eva KW, Rosenfeld J, Reiter HI and Norman GR (2004) An admissions OSCE: the multiple mini-interview. *Medical Education.* **38**: 314–26.

51 Hodgson CS, Teherani A, Gough HG *et al.* (2007) The relationship between measures of unprofessional behavior during medical school and indices on the California Psychological Inventory. *Academic Medicine.* **82**: S4–7.

52 Mamede S and Schmidt HG (2004) The structure of reflective practice in medicine. *Medical Education.* **38**: 1302–8.

53 Messick S (1989) Validity. In: Linn RL (ed.) *Educational Measurement*, pp. 103–4. Macmillan, New York, NY.

54 Downing SM (2003) Validity on the meaningful interpretation of assessment data. *Medical Education.* **37**: 830–7.

55 Newble DI and Jaeger K (1983) The effect of assessments and examinations on the learning of medical students. *Medical Education.* **17**: 165–71.

56 Harasym PH, Woloschuk W, Mandin H and Brundin-Mather R (1996) Reliability and validity of interviewers' judgements of medical school candidates. *Academic Medicine.* **71**: S40–2.

57 Paul A (2004) *The Cult of Personality: how personality tests are leading us to miseducate our children, mismanage our companies, and misunderstand ourselves.* Free Press, New York, NY.

58 Hodges B, Turnbull J, Cohen R *et al.* (1996) Evaluating communication skills in the OSCE format: reliability and generalizability. *Medical Education.* **30**: 38–43.

59 Hodges B, Regehr G, McNaughton N *et al.* (1999) OSCE checklists do not capture increasing levels of expertise. *Academic Medicine.* **74**: 1129–34.

60 Ramsey PG, Carline JD, Inui TS *et al.* (1989) Predictive validity of certification by the American Board of Internal Medicine. *Annals of Internal Medicine.* **110**: 719–26.

61 Davis DA, Mazmanian PE, Fordis M *et al.* (2006) Accuracy of physician self-assessment compared with observed measures of competence: a systematic review. *Journal of the American Medical Association.* **296**: 1094–102.

62 Norman GR (2004) The morality of medical school admissions. *Advances in Health Sciences Education.* **9**: 79–82.

63 Bargh JA and Chartrand TL (1999) The unbearable automaticity of being. *American Psychologist.* **54**: 462–79.

64 Jamieson S (2004) Likert scales: how to (ab)use them. *Medical Education.* **38**: 1217–18.

65 Wainer H (1976) Estimating coefficients in linear models: it don't make no nevermind. *Psychological Bulletin.* **83**: 213–17.

66 Glass GV and Stanley JC (1970) *Statistical Methods in Education and Psychology.* Prentice Hall, Englewood Cliffs, NJ.

67 Wikipaedia (2010) Bonferroni correction http://en.wikipedia.org/wiki/Bonferroni_correction Accessed 1st April 2010.

68 Cronbach LJ (1957) The two disciplines of scientific psychology. *American Psychologist.* **12**: 671–84.

69 Harden R, Grant J, Buckley G and Hart I (2000) Best Evidence Medical Education. *Advances in Health Sciences Education.* **5**: 71–90.

70 Smith ML and Glass GV (1977) Meta-analysis of psychotherapy outcome studies. *American Psychologist.* **32**: 752–60.

71 Vernon DT and Blake RL (1993) Does problem-based learning work? A meta-analysis of evaluative research. *Academic Medicine.* **68**: 550–63.

72 Hamdy H, Prasad K, Anderson MB *et al.* (2006) BEME guide no. 5: predictive values of assessment measurements obtained in medical schools and future performance in practice. *Medical Teacher.* **28**: 103–16.

73 Bordage G (2001) Reasons reviewers reject and accept manuscripts: the strengths and weaknesses in medical education reports. *Academic Medicine.* **76**: 889–96.

74 Driessen E, van Tartwijk J, van der Vleuten C and Wass V (2007) Portfolios in medical education: why do they meet with mixed success? A systematic review. *Medical Education.* **41**: 1224–33.

75 Issenberg SB, McGaghie WC, Petrusa ER *et al.* (2005) Features and uses of high-fidelity simulation that lead to effective learning: a BEME systematic review. *Medical Teacher.* **27**: 10–28.

76 Dornan T, Littlewood S, Margolis S *et al.* (2006) How can experience in clinical and community settings contribute to early medical education? A BEME systematic review. *Medical Teacher.* **28**: 3–18.

77 Hammick M, Freeth D, Koppel I *et al.* (2007) BEME guide no. 9: a best evidence systematic review of interprofessional education. *Medical Teacher.* **29**: 735–51.

78 Albanese MA and Mitchell S (1993) Problem-based learning: a review of literature on its outcomes and implementation issues. *Academic Medicine.* **68**: 52–81.

79 Norman GR and Schmidt HG (1992) The psychological basis of problem-based learning. *Academic Medicine.* **67**: 557–65.

80 Garg A, Norman GR, Spero L and Maheshwari P (1999) Do virtual computer models hinder anatomy learning? *Academic Medicine.* **74**: S87–9.

81 Cronbach LJ (1975) Beyond the two disciplines of scientific psychology. *American Psychologist.* **30**: 116–27.

82 Schmidt HG (2005) *Influence of research on practices in medical education: the case of problem-based learning.* Paper presented at the Association for Medical Education in Europe, Amsterdam, The Netherlands, September.

83 Cook DA, Bordage G and Schmidt HG (2008) Description, justification and clarification: a framework for classifying the purposes of research in medical education. *Medical Education.* **42**: 128–33.

Further Reading

Norman GR, van der Vleuten CPM and Newble DI (eds) (2002) *International Handbook of Research in Medical Education*, vol. 7. Springer International Handbooks of Education, New York.

Bowling A (1997) *Research Methods in Health: investigating health and health services.* Open University Press, Philadelphia, PA.

Chalmers A (1999) *What Is This Thing Called Science?* (3e). Open University Press, Buckingham.

Streiner D and Norman GR (2003) *Health Measurement Scales: a practical guide to their development and use* (3e). Oxford University Press, Oxford.

Qualitative research methods in medical education

Lorelei Lingard and Tara J Kennedy

KEY MESSAGES

- Qualitative research explores social, relational and experiential phenomena in their natural settings.
- Qualitative research methods can contribute to theory building and to the study of complex social issues in medical education.
- Qualitative research encompasses an eclectic group of research approaches, including case study, grounded theory, phenomenology, hermeneutics, narrative inquiry and action research.

- Qualitative data collection tools (including interviews, focus groups, observations and assembly of textual documents) and qualitative analysis strategies (including thematic analysis and discourse analysis) must be selected for their suitability to a particular research question.
- Principles of rigour specific to qualitative research have been developed and can be used in appraisal of the quality of a qualitative manuscript or as a framework on which to build a qualitative research study.

The Paradigm and Purpose of Qualitative Research

What is qualitative research in medical education?

Qualitative researchers study social, relational and experiential phenomena in their natural setting. For questions about group interactions, social processes or human experience, a qualitative approach is appropriate. *How* and *what* questions are particularly suited for exploration through qualitative research (*see* Box 22.1).

The term 'qualitative research' encompasses a broad range of approaches and methods, which the following sections will take up in detail. However, some generic principles maintain across these particularities. Qualitative research explores the object of study within its natural environment, by observing and interacting with the people experiencing the phenomenon. Qualitative research seeks to understand complexity, to offer a richly textured account of social or human phenomena. Also, qualitative research attends carefully to the role of context, to produce situated accounts that are anchored in space and time. As a consequence of these principles, the goal of qualitative research is the careful understanding of instances. It does not make claims to generalisability; rather, it values situated understanding and theory building.

What are the origins of qualitative research in medical education?

Qualitative research comes to medical education from the social sciences and humanities, from disciplines such as anthropology, sociology, education and history. At various points, each of these disciplines used medical education as a site for research shaped by their own disciplinary questions and theories. Now, medical education researchers use tools from these disciplines to explore questions arising in the domain of medical education.

According to Harris,[1] the importation of methods from these disciplines into medical education began in the 1980s amid calls for more prescriptive theory building to complement the dominant paradigm of controlled experiments. Interestingly, these calls persist as reviews of the medical education research field continue to identify a need for increased theory building and qualitative strategies of inquiry to grapple with complex social questions.[2]

What is the qualitative paradigm?

Discussions on qualitative research often begin with reference to 'the qualitative paradigm'. As Denzin and Lincoln[3] explain, paradigms are basic sets of beliefs that guide action; Harris describes them as 'cognitive road maps, taken-for-granted assumptions within communities of scholars'[1] that orient researchers towards meaning and the research endeavour. The concept of paradigm includes three elements according to Denzin and Lincoln: epistemology, ontology and methodology.[3] Epistemology refers to world

Understanding Medical Education: Evidence, Theory and Practice.
Edited by T Swanwick. © 2010 Association for the Study of Medical Education.

view, ontology to beliefs about reality, and methodology to tools for data collection and analysis.

The qualitative paradigm is, in fact, a misnomer, for qualitative research takes place within a vast spectrum of paradigms: positivism, post-positivism, constructivism, critical theory and post-modernism. In medical education, the dominant paradigms currently framing qualitative research tend to be post-positivism and constructivism. Post-positivism shares with positivism the belief that there is an objective reality that can be discovered if the correct research procedures are in place. What distinguishes post-positivism is the acknowledgement that complex human behaviour is shaped by individual motivations and cultural environments, and research must represent these complexities rather than elide them in search of a contextual 'essence' or truth. Irby's account of how clinical teachers make decisions about what to prioritise in their round exchanges with students represents the post-positivist paradigm in his seeking for the essence of teachers' decision making while paying attention to the contextual and individual features that shape this process.(4)

Constructivism departs from post-positivism in its acceptance of reality and meaning as relative, produced through the interaction between researcher and researched. Research in the constructivism paradigm acknowledges the subjectivity of the researcher, producing accounts of a social phenomenon that reflect the researcher's interaction with the phenomenon. Lingard's accounts of tension, collaboration and socialisation on operating room teams provide an example of this approach, as she views team communication through her training as a rhetorician and blends this perspective with those of study partici-

pants and 'insider informants' engaged in the collaborative analysis process.(5–8)

Also becoming apparent in medical education research is work within the critical theory paradigm, which is identifiable by its goal of revealing power dynamics in studied phenomena and fostering empowerment through the careful description and analysis of these dynamics. Albert's account of tensions within the medical education research community uses Bourdieu's theoretical notion of field to explore the configuration of power relations in this research community.(9)

The researcher's paradigm does not necessarily predict his or her research approach or methods. A case study (approach) may use interviews or observations or both (method), and it may take place within a constructivist or a post-positivist paradigm. Because of this flexibility in the selection of an approach and a method, the principle of 'best fit' is used to decide how best to approach or frame a research question. The best approach depends on the research question, the nature of the research setting and the objective of the research. These factors also determine what the best methods are. This flexibility of approaches and methods is a key difference from the quantitative paradigm, where the randomised controlled trial is widely accepted as the 'gold standard' research approach, and those researchers not engaged in this approach are likely to be working towards a point where they will be.

For a more detailed discussion of research frameworks and paradigms, see Chapter 20.

What is the relationship between qualitative and quantitative research?

Historically, qualitative and quantitative research has tended to be represented as a dichotomy in medical education discourse. This dichotomising probably arises from strong paradigm differences between researchers working within these two approaches. Experimentalists have tended to espouse a positivist belief system, thus the intent to control variables in order to see the essence of a phenomenon, and the use of statistical analyses to reveal and represent knowledge. By contrast, qualitative researchers in medical education have been more likely to adopt post-positivist and constructivist world views.

There has been a gradual recognition that such dichotomising is distorting and unhelpful. From Irby's invited address in 1990 (cited in Reference 1) to Norman's editorial in 1998,(10) the doctrine of best fit increasingly governs discussions about the uses and relationships of qualitative and quantitative research. Certain kinds of research question are suited to certain paradigms, certain approaches and certain methods, and while numbers are not central to qualitative research, their presence does not automatically 'disqualify' a study from inclusion in the paradigm.(11)

BOX 22.2 Qualitative research approaches
- Ethnography
- Grounded theory
- Case study
- Phenomenology
- Hermeneutics
- Narrative research
- Action research

Qualitative Research Approaches

The domain of qualitative research encompasses an eclectic group of research approaches, which are linked by their common aim to explore social processes through interpretation of qualitative data. These research approaches, or 'systems of inquiry', are, according to Denzin and Lincoln,(3) 'a bundle of skills, assumptions, and practices' that the researcher employs to generate and address qualitative research questions. The various qualitative research approaches stem from different philosophical and/or theoretical perspectives, with resultant implications for the research process. Although there can be a significant overlap between them, the following section provides a brief overview of seven major qualitative research approaches (summarised in Box 22.2), with examples of their contribution to medical education research.

Ethnography

The tradition of ethnography originates in the field of anthropology, in which a researcher would travel to study an 'exotic' tribe.(12,13) Current-day ethnography often rejects the traditional notion of a privileged researcher, and ethnographic studies are now more likely to occur in local subcultures (such as a medical school or an operating room) than in far-flung locations. However, ethnographic studies carry on the practice of long-term engagement in a study setting, and the collection, through observation and conversational interviews, of data that are analysed to understand the meaning inherent in the everyday activities of a particular social group.(14) There are a number of classic ethnographies in the domain of medical education, including Becker's *The Boys in White*,(15) a study of the nature of student culture in medical school, and Bosk's *Forgive and Remember*,(16) a study of the treatment of medical error in postgraduate surgical education.

Grounded theory

Grounded theory research explores social phenomena through the development of theoretical explanations that are 'grounded' in (i.e. derived from) the practical experience of study participants.(17) Grounded theory

was developed by two sociologists, Glaser and Strauss, in the 1960s, to provide a systematic approach to the analysis of qualitative data that would live up to the standards of 'rigour' imposed by the quantitative paradigm and that would focus on theory generation rather than theory testing.(17) Key elements of grounded theory methodology include:

- *iterative* study design (cycles of simultaneous data collection and analysis, in which the results of the ongoing data analysis inform the subsequent data collection)
- *purposeful* sampling (purposeful selection of data sources for their ability to provide data that would confirm, challenge or expand an emerging theory)
- *constant comparison* approach to data analysis (through which incidents or issues of interest in the data are compared against other examples for similarities and differences).(18–20)

In the domain of medical education research, Ginsburg has used grounded theory to develop a behavioural theory of professionalism.(21–26)

Case study

Case study research involves an in-depth analysis of a 'bounded system' (a programme, an event, an activity, a process, a group, etc.).(27) The case study can have intrinsic value or can be used as a means of gaining understanding of a larger process.(28) Case study research has roots in sociological tradition as well as in the medical case report.(27) One hallmark of case study methods is triangulation, which is the use of multiple data collection tools or data sources to gain rich insight into the study phenomenon from multiple perspectives (*see* Principles of rigour, below). An example of a qualitative case study in medical education is Perley's study of a group of primary care physicians to explore their use of the 'curbside consultation' with colleagues as a continuing education tool.(29)

Phenomenology

Phenomenology arose early in the 20th century from philosophical reflections on consciousness and perception. Phenomenological research aims to understand the essence of a social phenomenon from the perspective of those who have experienced it.(30) Phenomenology involves the 'bracketing' (or putting aside) of the researcher's own preconceptions and perspectives in order to understand the 'lived experience' of the research participants.(30) Phenomenological studies often involve an in-depth exploration of the experiences of a small number of individuals. Bearman has used phenomenology to explore the experiences of medical students during interactions with virtual patients.(31)

Hermeneutics

The term hermeneutics historically refers to the interpretation of biblical texts. In the domain of qualitative research, hermeneutics uses the lived experience of participants as a means of understanding their political, historical and sociocultural contexts.(32) Hermeneutic analysis involves a cyclical process called the 'hermeneutic circle': movement back and forth between the consideration of the meaning of individual parts of a data set and the meaning of the whole text.(33) Addison has explored how medical residents cope with their training through a hermeneutic approach in his chapter 'Grounded interpretive research: an investigation of physician socialization'.(34)

Narrative research

Narrative research stems from the ancient practice of storytelling as a method of communicating, arranging and interpreting human experience. Narrative inquiry is a qualitative approach that 'solicits and analyzes personal accounts as stories'(35), using these stories as a means of understanding or making sense of a particular experience or situation. Narrative analysis seeks meaning in the content, the structure, the context and the relational aspects of a story.(36) Narrative methods have been promoted recently as an educational tool for teaching empathy and communication skills to medical students(37) but are also being used to address research questions in medical education. Ventres has used narrative case reports of patient interviews conducted by residents to compare differences between patients' and physicians' perspectives.(38)

Action research

Action research has its roots in the social activism movements of the mid-20th century. Key principles of action research are the explicit aim of producing social change through the research process and the direct engagement of research participants in the research process.(39) Action research classically occurs through sequential cycles of planning a change, implementing the change while observing the process and reflection on the consequences of the change.(40) Participants collaborate with researchers to construct the results of the research and implement social change. An action research approach was employed successfully in the design and implementation of a new general practice curriculum in Dundee, Scotland.(41)

Qualitative Research Tools

Qualitative research studies are carried out through a set of tools for data collection and analysis. In the following section, methods for data collection and approaches to data analysis will be reviewed separately. This separation of data collection from analysis is somewhat artificial in qualitative research for two reasons. First, many qualitative studies employ an iterative study design,(1) in which cycles of data collection and analysis occur simultaneously. In an iterative research process, preliminary analysis of data collected early in the study process affects decisions about how to go about the next phase of data collection by revealing questions that require clarification or new ideas that require further exploration in subsequent data collection and analysis cycles.(17) The second way in which data collection and analysis are linked in qualitative research practice is the way in which the choice of data collection methods necessarily informs the choice of the analytical approach and vice versa. For example, an exploration of the educational impact of the choice of language used during case presentations (*see* Discourse analysis section) requires access to audio-recorded data that can be transcribed for analysis. For the sake of clarity, in this chapter, data collection methods (including interviews, focus groups, observations and assembly of textual documents) and data analysis methods (including thematic analysis and discourse analysis) are considered separately.

General questions relating to ethics have been dealt with in Chapter 20, but particular ethical issues arise in the collection and analysis of qualitative data. These include both procedural ethics (how the research is conducted to protect research participants from harm) and situational ethics (how the researcher conducts himself or herself in what Guillemin and Gillam call 'ethically important moments').(42) Reflexivity is asserted as a sensitising concept researchers can use as they negotiate ethical tensions that may arise in their interactions with participants in the field (*see* Box 22.3).

Data collection tools

The various qualitative research approaches have in common a set of data collection tools. Although certain qualitative approaches are classically associated with particular data collection or analysis methods (for example, ethnography with participant observation or hermeneutics with document analysis), contemporary qualitative researchers commonly choose from the available methods the one(s) that is (are) best suited to address the research question at hand (*see* Box 22.4).(3)

Interviews

Individual interviews are probably the most familiar and the most often used form of data collection in qualitative medical education research.(1,43) Interviews provide access to participants' personal perspectives and relevant experiences on an unlimited number of topics.(44) The qualitative interview standard is the 'depth interview',(44) which provides a rich and detailed exploration of a research question and generally lasts between 45 minutes and a few hours.(45) Qualitative research interviews often follow a 'semi-structured' format.(43) The semi-structured interview is guided by a predetermined set of open-ended questions, but the researcher and participant are free to

BOX 22.3 Focus on: Ethical issues in qualitative research

Subjectivity of the researcher
- Who are you in relation to your participants?
- What power dynamics are inherence in your relationship to your research subject and participants?
- How can these be managed appropriately to safeguard confidentiality and anonymity, and to avoid harm?

Emotionality of research participation
- Will your research provoke powerful emotions in participants sharing their stories and experiences?
- How can you provide appropriate support and negotiate the evolving balance between harms and benefits in individual research interactions?

Minimal disclosure
- Have you used minimal disclosure in your informed consent process (offering generic rather than specific study information to help minimise observer effect in field observations)? Such studies must include a mechanism for full disclosure when appropriate, and the ability to exclude data if participants decline participation following full disclosure.

BOX 22.4 How to: Choose a data collection tool

Consider a hypothetical research programme about professionalism in medical student. The following potential research questions are matched with an appropriate data collection tool.

1 How do medical students' characterise professional behaviour in themselves and other members of the interdisciplinary healthcare teams?

In-depth interviews could provide a rich understanding of the students' conceptualisations of professional behaviour in multiple contexts, derived from detailed descriptions of relevant personal experience.

2 What are medical students' impressions of the professional behaviour of their clinical supervisors?

Focus groups could provide an affirming environment where the accounts of other students' similar experiences might promote disclosure of relevant anecdotes. Discussion between students could make evident the range of relevant experience.

3 Do patient care discussions on medical teaching teams promote professionalism in novice physicians?

Observations of case presentations or teaching rounds could provide 'real-life' data that would permit analysis of the language used by medical students and their supervisors.

4 What messages about professionalism are being conveyed through the clinical evaluations of medical students?

Textual analysis of the narrative comments on clinical evaluation forms could provide insight into the types of behaviour that are being promoted through the evaluation process.

pursue additional relevant topics as they arise (*see* Box 22.5 for a sample interview script). Qualitative interviews are usually audiotaped and later transcribed to facilitate analysis, but recent advances in analysis software allow analysis directly from a digital audio or video recording.

The main disadvantage of the interview method of data collection is the fact that the information provided is filtered through the memory of the participant and is influenced by the social context of the interview.(46) Interview researchers must be careful to avoid leading questions (consider, for example, the potential difference in responses to the questions 'What barriers to the mentorship process have you encountered?' and 'What have your experiences with the mentorship process been like?'). Researchers must also attend to the power dynamics of the interview. For example, candid opinions from medical students about their experiences during clerkship are unlikely in an interview conducted by the clerkship director.

Focus groups

Focus groups have recently become well known as a marketing research tool, but they have a long history in the domain of social sciences research. Focus groups are sessions involving 4–12 participants and a moderator or facilitator who guides the group discussion of a topic relevant to the research question.(47) Focus

groups provide access to multiple stories and diverse experiences in an efficient manner. More importantly, focus groups provide a dynamic and interactive exchange that can stimulate exploration of contrary opinions, reflection on group norms and common practices and exposure of taken-for-granted values.(48) Like individual interviews, focus group discussions often follow a semi-structured format and are audiorecorded and transcribed for analysis. The focus group moderator also records notes on group dynamics and interactions.

Researchers using focus groups must consider whether their topic would benefit from exploration in the synergistic and spontaneous focus group format (for example, some deeply personal topics might be more safely or productively explored in an individual interview). Issues of power dynamics are also critical in focus group methodology: one influential, opinionated group member can derail the entire process.(47)

Focus groups have been useful in exploring medical education questions such as the ethical implications of

BOX 22.5 Sample semi-structured interview script

Research question: How do medical students characterise professional behaviour in themselves and other members of interdisciplinary healthcare teams?

1 Could you give me an example of a time when you acted professionally? *(prompt for rich contextual details)* What is it about this behaviour that was professional? *(elicit further examples as appropriate, for this and all subsequent questions)*

2 Could you give me an example of a time when you acted unprofessionally? What is it about that behaviour that was unprofessional?

3 Could you give me examples of times when your medical student colleagues acted professionally or unprofessionally?

4 Could you give me examples of time when a nurse working with your team acted professionally? Unprofessionally? *(repeat question for other members of the healthcare team: therapists, social workers, staff physicians, etc.)*

5 What, in your understanding, are the important elements of professional behaviour for a medical student? For a nurse? For a physiotherapist? *(repeat for other relevant members of healthcare team)*

BOX 22.6 Sample field note

Research question: Do patient-care discussion on medical teaching teams promote professionalism in novice physicians?

Reflective notes*	Observation notes*
	Morning rounds, 31 Jan, ward 5C nursing station
	Present: AP**, MS1**, JR**, SR**, CN**
MS2 is flustered, out of breath	MS2 arrives 5 minutes after rounds have started
AP – good natured sarcasm	AP: Nice of you to join us! (laughter)
MS2 doesn't appear upset by the comment	MS2: Sorry, I ran into the asthmatic's mom in the hall – she wanted to know about the chest x-ray
Note respect for patient through use of name rather than diagnosis	AP: You mean J's mom...
	MS2: Right
	AP: Did you tell her?
	MS2: Yeah, that it was clear.
	AP: Thanks ...

*Two-column format is often used to facilitate recording of observation notes (containing details of the observed events) and reflective notes (containing the researcher's comments about the context and process of the observation, as well as emerging analytic ideas)
**Abbreviations used to distinguish participants without identifying personal information AP = attending physician, MS = medical student, JR = junior resident, SR = senior resident, CN = charge nurse

providing medical education in public and private hospital settings.(49)

Observation

Observation of study participants as they go about their regular activities can provide powerful insights into social processes. Researchers conducting observations have access to data on what participants do and not just on what they say they do.(50) Qualitative researchers conducting observations make records called 'field notes' (*see* Box 22.6 for an illustrative example), which can be structured to capture details such as the content of conversations, the context of discussions, the participants and intended audience for relevant comments and the non-verbal nuances that accompany these interchanges.(51) Observations are sometimes accompanied by audio recording of 'naturalistic' conversations, which are later transcribed for analysis.

Observational researchers must deal with 'observer effect', which is the fact that the presence of the observer has an impact on the behaviours of study participants. There are a number of ways to deal with observer effect.(50) Some researchers will spend long periods of time in the field to allow participants to become accustomed to their presence. Others will not reveal the specific focus of their observations to prevent participants from altering specific behaviours (for example, a researcher might get consent to observe all

clinical teaching in an intensive care unit without revealing to participants that the research question related specifically to the teaching of technical skills).(52) Still, others will take care to document evidence of the impact of their presence and then reflect on and write about the significance of this impact on their results.

Another consideration in observational research is the likelihood that relevant data will be obtained. Observations are a useful tool for gathering data about common events and activities, but they are inefficient when the event in question is uncommon or difficult to predict. For example, observations of teaching clinics would be an inefficient way to collect data about failing students if only one or two students fail their clinical rotations each year.

Observational research has a long tradition in medical education. Observational researchers in medical education, as in other fields, must decide to what degree they will participate in the activities around them. The term 'non-participant observation' has been used to signify an observer who remains uninvolved in the activities of their study participants, taking the role of a passive observer. Stern used non-participant observation of internal medicine teaching teams to investigate the hidden ethics curriculum being taught on the wards.(53) Observational research in the ethnographic tradition takes the form of 'partici-pant observation', in which the researcher becomes fully engaged in the daily activities of the study par-ticipants: Sinclair, a sociologist from London, enrolled in medical school and completed a medical degree as he conducted his ethnographic research.(54)

Assembly of textual documents

In the domain of medical education, a myriad of docu-ments is created on a daily basis, many of which can yield important insights into educational processes. Sources of text for analysis include course curricula, assignments and examinations, student and faculty evaluations, clinical notes and policy documents. More recently, texts from websites, email correspondence and even digital images and video have been included in qualitative analyses.(55) Analysis of pre-existing documents can be a quick and inexpensive data collec-tion method, and because they were created for pur-poses other than research, the content of these data is not influenced by the research process.(56) Assembly of textual documents, however, does not allow the researcher to take advantage of the powerful qualita-tive process of iterative inquiry (see above), in which ongoing analysis informs the data collection process because the data collection occurs one step prior to the analysis.

Perhaps the most common use of textual documents for qualitative analysis in medical education is the analysis of documents produced as course assign-ments by students. For example, Olney analysed written 'experience summaries' created by medical student participants in a community service project to explore learning outcomes.(57)

Data analysis tools

Qualitative data analysis is the process of making sense of a qualitative data set. As previously empha-sised, qualitative data analysis does not often mean sifting through hundreds of pages of text in one sitting but is rather an ongoing process of reading, reflecting on and questioning the meaning of the data as they are collected. Qualitative data analysis can be conducted individually or as part of a research team that analyses as a group or meets to compare and discuss results of individual analytical work.

Although the different qualitative approaches involve somewhat different analytical procedures, there are some basic processes that are common to most qualitative analyses. The most common of these is coding. Coding is a process of sorting or organising the data into categories representing similar trends.(17)

The first step in the coding process is the selection of the unit of analysis. For example, analysis of medical student interviews about professionalism might involve coding for the settings in which professional lapses occurred, or for types of professional behaviour or for specific words or phrases used by participants to describe unprofessional acts. Coding for more than one of these different units of analysis might occur over time. As the data are being sorted into categories or codes, names or labels are created for the codes that describe the essence of the category, and memos or reflective notes are written to document the process of the analysis and record reflections and analytical ideas as they arise. Qualitative software can be used as a data management tool to keep track of the coding process as it proceeds, but the cognitive work of cat-egorising data, identifying trends and interpreting meaning is still done by the researcher.

The specific approaches to data analysis in qualita-tive research are wide ranging. They are illustrated below in broad clusters involving approaches to the-matic analysis and approaches to discourse analysis.

Thematic analysis

The most commonly used qualitative analysis approach in the domain of medical education is the organisation of data according to topics, ideas or concepts, often called themes. Variations of thematic analysis are used in many of the qualitative approaches, and a number of different systems of thematic analysis have been developed (for example, content analysis(58) and con-stant comparative analysis).(17,19) The basic process of thematic analysis is to identify in the data set instances that are similar in concept. As further related examples are identified, a progressively rich under-standing of the concept is developed, and as other important concepts are identified in the data, the rela-tionships between concepts or themes are explored. The set of themes can then be used for description, theory development or interpretation (*see* Interpretation, below). Thematic analysis has been used to explore many complex issues in medical education, for example, Burack's study of the process of medical stu-dents' decision making on specialty choice.(59)

Discourse analysis

Discourse analysis is an approach to qualitative research that analyses data at the level of language. Discourse is a term meaning 'socially situated lan-guage'.(60) The aim of discourse analysis is to make explicit what is normally taken for granted about lan-guage use or to show what talking accomplishes in a particular social context. Discourse analysis is an umbrella term that references a number of different approaches to the analysis of socially situated lan-guage use. Some discourse analysts, often in the domains of linguistics or conversation analysis, work to understand the complex mechanisms and structures of social language. Others, in fields like sociolinguistics or critical discourse analysis, use talk as a source of evidence about social processes. Discourse analysis has an extensive history in the study of physician–patient communication(61) but has been more recently applied to the domain of medical education. Hekelman *et al.* conducted a discourse analysis to investigate the changes in language use in the teaching encounters of a physician-teacher who was enrolled in a peer-coaching programme intended to improve clinical teaching skills.(62,63)

Interpretation

The final stage of qualitative analysis is the process of interpretation, or finding the central meaning in a data set. Without interpretive work, qualitative research produces merely a catalogue of ideas or themes. Important as those ideas may be, qualitative studies that do not take the next step of exploring the meaning at an interpretive or theoretical level have not fully exploited the power of qualitative research.

There are different approaches to interpretation in qualitative research. In some qualitative approaches, the production of a thick, rich description of a social phenomenon is the goal of the research process (e.g. phenomenology). In other approaches, the development of a novel theoretical explanation of a social process is the aim (e.g. grounded theory). In still other qualitative approaches, the meaning of a data set is considered through the lens of pre-existing theory, such as feminist, rhetorical or Marxist theory.

Principles of Rigour

Qualitative researchers both within and outside the domain of medical education have sought to articulate criteria for judging the quality of a qualitative report. Journals have published papers with checklists,(64–67) and qualitative leaders have offered overarching concepts such as 'trustworthiness',(68) 'utility'(69,70) and authenticity.(71). Position papers on the state of medical educational research assert a need for education and attention to rigour in qualitative research.(72,73)

While there is growing debate about the politics of such criteria and their feasibility given the vast spectrum of activity housed within the term qualitative research,(74) this debate will not be taken up here. Rather, this section outlines and illustrates, using positive examples, some basic principles of rigour to assist the newcomer in their appreciation of 'quality' in qualitative research. These principles are drawn from an extensive literature outlining guidelines for excellence in qualitative research. They can serve either as a framework for critical appraisal of qualitative research studies in the literature or as a starting point for considering how to design a qualitative project (*see* Box 22.7).

BOX 22.7 How to: Achieve rigour in qualitative research

Adequacy and appropriateness of the sample
- Are the right people/activities being sampled?
- Is the sample size likely to yield sufficient insight?

The quality of the data collected
- Is the researcher's relationship to the participants/setting considered?
- Are interview and observation techniques likely to capture naturalistic data?

The clarity of the analysis process
- Can the analysis be audited?
- Were member checking techniques appropriately considered?

Sampling: adequacy and appropriateness

Sampling in qualitative research is not just about 'how many' subjects to include in the study. Because qualitative research explores social and experiential phenomena, deciding whom to include and exclude is a critical step in the sampling logic. A social phenomenon often engages a wide variety of participants, and the researcher must justify their decisions about who best to observe/interview and who to leave out of their study boundaries. While studies of individual experience clearly direct the researcher to observe/ask the individual, individuals rarely function in isolation, so the researcher must determine what additional contexts are appropriate to a full exploration of the study questions.

The following questions can help in assessing the nature and extent of a study sample and evaluating its adequacy.
- Who?
  - Can this sample provide data that answer the research question?
  - Does the sample tap into all relevant participants in the research setting?
- Why?
  - The choice of subjects must be justified, particularly if it does not represent all potentially relevant groups.
- How much?
  - Sample size is not a matter of mere numbers: it is a matter of a thorough exploration of a culture or phenomenon. Often, such thoroughness is referred to as 'saturation', which means that data collection was considered complete when dominant themes/trends were recurrent and no new issues were arising from subsequent data collection. For instance, if after 10 interviews the researcher is not hearing anything new on the

topic and recurrent themes are similar across interviews, saturation is said to have been reached, and data collection may be stopped using this rationale.

Sample estimations may be justified by reference to:
- method-based estimates (e.g. in-depth interviews)(45)
- sampling strategy (e.g. theoretical, confirming/disconfirming, snowball)(75)
- past research findings.

Methods need to reflect sampling strategy (e.g. confirming/disconfirming sampling requires data analysis to proceed alongside data collection).

Box 22.8 illustrates a number of issues relating to sampling through an extended example. The nature of the sample is specified, and justification is provided for the types of participant sampled, which include various kinds of problem-based learning (PBL) tutors and students who may perceive conflict resolution from different perspectives. Sampling strategies are well articulated. There is no explicit reference to saturation, although reference to the dominant themes implies this. A range of perspectives in faculty and students appears to be explored, suggesting that triangulation is adequate.

Data collection: authenticity and reflexivity

Because the qualitative researcher engages with their research participants in the collection of data, their role in the construction of meaning must be considered. As part of this, their relation to the participants, and the ways in which that relationship may shape the data that are being collected, requires careful thought both when deciding how to collect the data and when considering constraints on their interpretation. In educational settings, hierarchical relationships between researchers, who may be medical faculty members, and participants, who may be trainees, can have a distorting effect on the authenticity of the data collection. Participants in vulnerable positions may alter their observed behaviour or tailor their interview responses to safeguard themselves, to please the researcher or to advertise their membership in a group. Data collection processes must take such participant motives and actions into account, and researchers must both strategise to maximise the authenticity of their data and reflect on the ways in which the data are a construction of a research relationship in a hierarchical situation.

A common strategy used by qualitative researchers to maximise the quality of their data set is 'triangulation'. Triangulation is a term from cartography, which refers to the process of finding one's position on a map with reference to multiple other mapped positions. In a qualitative research study, the process of triangulation involves collecting data from multiple 'positions', so that the researcher can gain insight on the studied phenomenon from multiple perspectives, thus realising a more refined and comprehensive understanding by the end of the research. Triangulation requires the selection of most relevant data sources and their integrated analysis, exploring how they confirm or disconfirm one another.

The following questions can help when considering the factors related to the quality of the data collected.
- Has the researcher considered his or her relation to the study setting and subjects?
- Are the interview script and processes non-leading?
  - How was the script developed?
  - Was it piloted?
  - Were questions appropriate to capture relevant insights?
- Has the Hawthorne effect been considered? The Hawthorne, or observer effect, is seen when observed participants act differently from how they would act if the observer were not present.(76)
  - Were mechanisms to minimise the Hawthorne effect used, for example, prolonged engagement in the field, time taken to establish trust and rapport, and observer comportment (e.g. dressing like an insider)?
  - Was there a process for recording/reflecting on the Hawthorne effect; for example, field notes should record any references to observer presence, such as jokes made about being observed.

BOX 22.8 Example: Sampling

To explore how conflict resolution is achieved in problem-based learning (PBL) groups in medical school, we conducted both individual interviews and focus groups in the final month of the 1999–2000 academic year. Faculty interviews were conducted with 15 PBL tutors with at least three years' experience in the tutor role, to ensure an information-rich population. Purposeful sampling of faculty was employed, in order to include both non-clinical tutors ($n = 5$) and tutors from a variety of clinical disciplines, including medicine ($n = 4$), paediatrics ($n = 2$), psychiatry ($n = 1$) and surgery ($n = 3$). Students were sampled using two strategies: convenience sampling for the first six students interviewed, and then a confirming/disconfirming strategy in which interviewed students were asked to recommend potential participants who might: (a) have a similar experience/viewpoint to their own; and (b) have a divergent experience/viewpoint from their own. Using this sampling method, 11 additional students were recruited for voluntary participation. Following preliminary analysis of the interview transcripts, dominant themes were returned for discussion to three student focus groups comprised of both interview participants and new subjects.

BOX 22.9 Example: Data collection

Eleven students and 10 faculty participated in the observational phase. Students included five women and six men, while faculty included five women and five men. Faculty experience ranged from those within their first 5 years of appointment ($n = 4$) and those with 20+ years of teaching experience ($n = 4$). Nineteen oral case presentations and the teaching exchanges related to them were observed and audio-recorded by trained research assistants during morning rounds. Observers had no prior relationship with the study participants. All participants were observed at least once, with repeat observations purposefully distributed across the sample to maximise its range and richness. A pocket-sized micro-disk recording system and clip-on microphone worn by the observer were used to record data, and written field notes were compiled. Attempts to minimise the Hawthorne effect included the unobtrusiveness of the recording equipment, the duration of the observation phase (four months) and the observers' abilities (through similar dress, age and comportment) to blend into the team on rounds. The notes that students created as they prepared for their case presentations were also collected, anonymised and transcribed. Individual interviews were conducted with all students and faculty, using open-ended questions and asking participants to comment on two case presentation scenarios derived from the observational data.

BOX 22.10 Example: Data analysis

All interviews were audio-taped and fully transcribed. Themes were identified and developed by both authors by reading and re-reading transcripts. These themes were further refined and clarified using the framework analytic approach. The framework approach is based on a grounded theory approach to data analysis whereby theories are generated from data. It is heavily based on and driven by the original accounts and observations of the people it is about. It is also systematic and comprehensive and allows a full review of the material collected. Interviews and analysis were conducted concurrently and continued until no new themes emerged and data saturation was felt to be complete. The trustworthiness of the data was enhanced by the transparent process of analysis, the involvement of two independent researchers who read and compared ideas on the transcripts, and by searching for disconfirming evidence during the analysis. An analytical journal was kept, to record memos of ongoing analytical decisions, definitions of themes and discussions of disconfirming evidence. All interviewees were sent a copy of the primary analysis and asked to comment on the themes and concepts.

- Are data triangulated for maximal richness?
- Are complementary data sets collected?
- Are different forms of data/subject populations accessed?

Continuing our worked example, Box 22.9 illustrates how rigour is achieved in data collection. The relationship of the observers to participants has been considered, and steps have been taken to minimise the impact of the observer on the observed activities. Triangulation among methods (observations, interviews and case note analysis) and groups (students and faculty) will assist in creating a more in-depth portrait of this activity.

Data analysis: clarity and audit trails

The analysis process in qualitative research should be described such that there is little or no 'mystique' surrounding how the researchers went from a pile of transcripts to a list of thematic categories. This is not to suggest that there is no 'art' to qualitative analysis; there is, of course, and it includes serendipitous, imaginative links, just as it may in the analysis of experimental data. However, on the whole, the steps involved in the analysis process can be made explicit, and they should be both in a published manuscript and in the researchers' own journals, which can form the basis of

an 'audit trail' to review their analytical journey. Questions to consider include the following:
- Is the analysis process well described?
  - Can you tell what was done, by whom and how?
  - Were insider experts used to verify coding samples?
- Were the following key aspects of analysis evident?
  - Is 'constant comparison' evident?
  - How were discrepancies resolved?
- Was an attempt made to engage participants in reflecting on the results of the analysis?
  - Was 'return of findings' conducted? How?
- Was a software program used?
  - Was its use appropriately described?

Box 22.10 and our worked example illustrate attempts to address these questions. The analytical process makes clear who conducted the analysis, the steps involved, the iterative process of data collection and analysis, the strategy in place for keeping an audit trail and the effort to engage participants in refining the analytical concepts.

As suggested earlier, some qualitative researchers would argue with the broad application of any of these proceduralist principles as a way of measuring quality. As Eakin argues, this approach can oversimplify and distort the complex and non-formulaic nature of qualitative inquiry. Instead, the notion of a paper's 'so what' factor – its ability to contribute to the understanding of a social phenomenon – is offered as the most important criterion.(77) Similarly, Sandelowski(70) has proposed a study's 'utility', its power to 'be of use' in the world, as another holistic principle for consideration when evaluating qualitative research. This more holistic approach integrates other principles, such as sampling and authenticity, while trying to avoid the pitfalls of a naive, checklist approach to quality in qualitative research.

Conclusions

Qualitative research has made important contributions to medical education research in the past few decades. This form of inquiry is situated within a particular set of paradigms and draws on recognisable approaches and methodological tools to build knowledge regarding the experiences of teachers, trainees, patients and team members in medical education settings. Particular ethical issues must be considered in a qualitative project, as well as appropriate criteria for determining the most rigorous path for each individual study. Used properly, qualitative research promises to offer profound insights into the complex social and human aspects of how health professionals develop their identity, expertise and practice.

References

1 Harris I (2002) Qualitative methods. In: Norman G, van der Vleuten C and Newble D (eds) *International Handbook of Research in Medical Education*, pp. 45–95. Kluwer Academic Publishers, Dordrecht, The Netherlands.

2 Shea JA, Arnold L, Mann KV, Shea JA, Arnold L and Mann KV (2004) A RIME perspective on the quality and relevance of current and future medical education research. *Academic Medicine*. 79: 931–8.

3 Denzin N and Lincoln Y (2000) Introduction: the discipline and practice of qualitative research. In: Denzin N and Lincoln Y (eds) *Handbook of Qualitative Research*, pp. 1–28. Sage Publications, Thousand Oaks, CA.

4 Irby DM (1992) How attending physicians make instructional decisions when conducting teaching rounds. *Academic Medicine*. 67: 630–8.

5 Lingard L, Espin S, Whyte S *et al.* (2004) Communication failures in the operating room: an observational classification of recurrent types and effects. *Quality & Safety in Health Care*. 13: 330–4.

6 Lingard L, Garwood S and Poenaru D (2004) Tensions influencing operating room team function: does institutional context make a difference? *Medical Education*. 38: 691–9.

7 Lingard L, Espin S, Rubin B *et al.* (2005) Getting teams to talk: development and pilot implementation of a checklist to promote safer operating room communication. *Quality & Safety in Health Care*. 14: 340–6.

8 Lingard L, Reznick R, DeVito I and Espin S (2002) Forming professional identities on the health care team: discursive constructions of the 'other' in the operating room. *Medical Education*. 36: 728–34.

9 Albert M (2004) Understanding the debate on medical education research: a sociological perspective. *Academic Medicine*. 79: 948–54.

10 Norman G (1998) Editorial. *Advances in Health Science Education*. 3: 77–80.

11 Sandelowski M (2001) Real qualitative researchers do not count: the use of numbers in qualitative research. *Research in Nursing & Health*. 24: 230–40.

12 leCompte M and Schensul J (1999) *Designing and conducting ethnographic research. An ethnographers toolkit.* Alta Mira Press Lanham, MD.

13 Hammersley M and Atkinson P (1995) What is ethnography? *Ethnography: principles in practice.* Routledge, London.

14 Atkinson P and Pugsley L (2005) Making sense of ethnography and medical education. *Medical Education*. 39: 228–34.

15 Becker H, Geer B, Hughs E and Strauss A (1961) *The Boys in White: student culture in medical school.* University of Chicago Press, Chicago, IL.

16 Bosk CL (2003) *Forgive and Remember: managing medical failure.* University of Chicago Press, Chicago, IL.

17 Glaser B and Strauss A (1967) *The Discovery of Grounded Theory: strategies for qualitative research.* Aldine Pub Co., Chicago, IL.

18 Corbin J and Strauss A (1990) Grounded theory research: procedures, canons, and evaluative criteria. *Qualitative Sociology*. 13: 3–21.

19 Strauss A and Corbin J (1998) *Basics of Qualitative Research.* Sage Publications, Thousand Oaks, CA.

20 Kennedy TJ and Lingard LA (2006) Making sense of grounded theory in medical education. *Medical Education*. 40: 101–8.

21 Ginsburg S, Kachan N and Lingard L (2005) Before the white coat: perceptions of professional lapses in the pre-clerkship. *Medical Education*. 39: 12–19.

22 Ginsburg S, Regehr G and Lingard L (2004) Basing the evaluation of professionalism on observable behaviors: a cautionary tale. *Academic Medicine*. 79: S1–S4.

23 Ginsburg S, Regehr G and Lingard L (2003) The disavowed curriculum: understanding students' reasoning in professionally challenging situations. *Journal of General Internal Medicine*. 18: 1015–22.

24 Ginsburg S, Regehr G and Lingard L (2003) To be and not to be: the paradox of the emerging professional stance. *Medical Education*. 37: 350–7.

25 Ginsburg S, Regehr G, Stern D and Lingard L (2002) The anatomy of the professional lapse: bridging the gap between traditional frameworks and students' perceptions. *Academic Medicine*. 77: 516–22.

26 Ginsburg S, Regehr G, Hatala R *et al.* (2002) Context, conflict, and resolution: a new conceptual framework for evaluating professionalism. *Academic Medicine*. 75: S6–S11.

27 Stake R (2005) Qualitative case studies. In: Denzin N and Lincoln Y (eds) *The Sage Handbook of Qualitative Research*, pp. 443–66. Sage Publications, Thousand Oaks, CA.

28 Aita V and McIlvain H (1999) An armchair adventure in case study research. In: Crabtree B and Miller W (eds) *Doing Qualitative Research*, pp. 253–68. Sage Publications, Thousand Oaks, CA.

29 Perley CM (2006) Physician use of the curbside consultation to address information needs: report on a collective case study. *Journal of the Medical Library Association*. 94: 137–44.

30 Creswell J (1998) *Qualitative Inquiry and Research Design: choosing among five traditions*, pp. 47–72. Sage Publications, Thousand Oaks, CA.

31 Bearman M (2003) Is virtual the same as real? Medical students' experiences of a virtual patient. *Academic Medicine*. 78: 538–45.

32 Miller W and Crabtree B (1999) Clinical research: a multimethod typology and qualitative roadmap. In: Crabtree B and

Miller W (eds) *Doing Qualitative Research*, pp. 3–32. Sage Publications, Thousand Oaks, CA.

33 Addison R (1999) A grounded hermeneutic editing approach. In: Crabtree B and Miller W (eds) *Doing Qualitative Research*, pp. 145–62. Sage Publications, Thousand Oaks, CA.

34 Addison RB (2006) *Entering The Circle: hermeneutic investigation in psychology*, pp. 39–56. State University of New York Press, New York.

35 Muller J (1999) Narrative approaches to qualitative research in primary care. In: Crabtree B and Miller W (eds) *Doing Qualitative Research*, pp. 221–38. Sage Publications, Thousand Oaks, CA.

36 Bleakley A (2005) Stories as data, data as stories: making sense of narrative inquiry in clinical education. *Medical Education.* **39**: 534–40.

37 Pullman D, Bethune C and Duke P (2005) Narrative means to humanistic ends. *Teaching & Learning in Medicine.* **17**: 279–84.

38 Ventres W (1994) Hearing the patient's story: exploring physician–patient communication using narrative case reports. *Family Practice Research Journal.* **14**: 139–47.

39 Thesen J and Kuzel A (1999) Participatory inquiry. In: Crabtree B and Miller W (eds) *Doing Qualitative Research*, pp. 269–90. Sage Publications, Thousand Oaks, CA.

40 Kemmis S and McTaggart R (2005) Participatory action research: communicative action and the public sphere. In: Denzin N and Lincoln Y (eds) *The Sage Handbook of Qualitative Research*, pp. 559–604. Sage Publications, Thousand Oaks, CA.

41 Mowat H and Mowat D (2001) The value of marginality in a medical school: general practice and curriculum change. *Medical Education.* **35**: 175–7.

42 Guillemin M and Gillam L (2004) Ethics, reflexivity and 'ethically important moments' in research. *Qualitative Inquiry.* **10**: 261–80.

43 Dicicco-Bloom B and Crabtree BF (2006) The qualitative research interview. *Medical Education.* **40**: 314–21.

44 Miller W and Crabtree B (1999) Depth interviewing. In: Crabtree B and Miller W (eds) *Doing Qualitative Research*, pp. 89–107. Sage Publications, Thousand Oaks, CA.

45 McCracken G (1988) *The Long Interview*. Sage, Newbury Park, CA.

46 Reeves S, Lewin S and Zwarenstein M (2006) Using qualitative interviews within medical education research: why we must raise the 'quality bar'. *Medical Education.* **40**: 291–2.

47 Barbour RS and Barbour RS (2005) Making sense of focus groups. *Medical Education.* **39**: 742–50.

48 Brown J (1999) Focus group interviews. In: Crabtree B and Miller W (eds) *Doing Qualitative Research*, pp. 109–24. Sage Publications, Thousand Oaks, CA.

49 Maa A and McCullough LB (2006) Medical education in the public versus the private setting: a qualitative study of medical students' attitudes. *Medical Teacher.* **28**: 351–5.

50 Hammersley M and Atkinson P (1995) *Ethnography: principles in practice*. Routledge, London.

51 Bogdewic S (1999) Participant observation. In: Crabtree B and Miller W (eds) *Doing Qualitative Research*, pp. 47–69. Sage Publications, Thousand Oaks, CA.

52 Bannister SL, Hilliard RI, Regehr G and Lingard L (2003) Technical skills in paediatrics: a qualitative study of acquisition, attitudes and assumptions in the neonatal intensive care unit. *Medical Education.* **37**: 1082–90.

53 Stern DT (1998) In search of the informal curriculum: when and where professional values are taught. *Academic Medicine.* **73**: S28–S30.

54 Sinclair S (1997) *Making Doctors: an institutional apprenticeship.* Berg, New York.

55 Heath C, Luff P and Sanchez SM (2007) Video and qualitative research: analysing medical practice and interaction. *Medical Education.* **41**: 109–16.

56 Creswell J (2003) *Research Design: qualitative, quantitative, and mixed methods approaches*, pp. 179–209. Sage Publications, Thousand Oaks, CA.

57 Olney CA, Livingston JE, Fisch S and Talamantes MA (2006) Becoming better health care providers: outcomes of a primary care service-learning project in medical school. *Journal of Prevention & Intervention in the Community.* **32**: 133–47.

58 Krippendorf K (2004) *Content Analysis: an introduction to its methodology.* Sage Publications, Thousand Oaks, CA.

59 Burack JH, Irby DM, Carline JD, Ambrozy DM, Ellsbury KE and Stritter FT (1997) A study of medical students' specialty-choice pathways: trying on possible selves. *Academic Medicine.* **72**: 534–41.

60 Cameron D (2001) *Working with Spoken Discourse*, pp. 7–18. Sage Publications, London.

61 Maynard DW and Heritage J (2005) Conversation analysis, doctor–patient interaction and medical communication. *Medical Education.* **39**: 428–35.

62 Hekelman FP and Blase JR (1996) Excellence in clinical teaching: the core of the mission. *Academic Medicine.* **71**: 738–42.

63 Hekelman FP, Blase JR and Bedinghaus J (1996) Discourse analysis of peer coaching in medical education: a case study. *Teaching and Learning in Medicine.* **8**: 41–7.

64 Mays N and Pope C (2000) Qualitative research in health care. Assessing quality in qualitative research. *British Medical Journal.* **320**: 50–2.

65 Mays N and Pope C (1995) Rigour and qualitative research. *British Medical Journal.* **311**: 109–12.

66 Inui TS and Frankel RM (1991) Evaluating the quality of qualitative research: a proposal pro tem. *Journal of General Internal Medicine.* **6**: 485–6.

67 Rowan M and Huston P (1997) Qualitative research articles: information for authors and peer reviewers. *Canadian Medical Association Journal.* **157**: 1442–6.

68 Lincoln Y and Guba EG (1985) *Naturalistic Inquiry.* Sage Publications, Thousand Oaks, CA.

69 Sandelowski M (2004) Using qualitative research. *Qualitative Health Research.* **14**: 1366–86.

70 Sandelowski M (1997) 'To be of use': enhancing the utility of qualitative research. *Nursing Outlook.* **45**: 125–32.

71 Lincoln Y and Guba EG (2000) Paradigmatic controversies, contradictions and emerging confluences. In: Denzin N and Lincoln Y (eds) *Handbook of Qualitative Research*, pp. 163–88. Sage Publications, Thousand Oaks, CA.

72 Wolf FM (2004) Methodological quality, evidence, and Research in Medical Education (RIME). *Academic Medicine.* **79**: S68–S69.

73 Britten N (2005) Making sense of qualitative research: a new series. *Medical Education.* **39**: 5–6.

74 Rolfe G (2006) Validity, trustworthiness and rigour: quality and the idea of qualitative research. *Journal of Advanced Nursing.* **53**: 304–10.

75 Kuzel AJ (1999) Sampling in qualitative inquiry. In: Crabtree BF and Miller WL (eds) *Doing Qualitative Research*. Sage, Newbury Park, CA.

76 Holden JD (2001) Hawthorne effects and research into professional practice. *Journal of Evaluation in Clinical Practice.* **7**: 65–70.

77 Eakin JM and Mykhalovskiy E (2003) Reframing the evaluation of qualitative health research: reflections on a review of appraisal guidelines in the health sciences. *Journal of Evaluation in Clinical Practice.* **9**: 187–94.

Further Reading

Britten N (2005) Making sense of qualitative research: a new series. *Medical Education.* **39**: 5–6.

Crabtree B and Miller W (eds) (1999) *Doing Qualitative Research.* Sage Publications, Thousand Oaks, CA.

Creswell J (1998) *Qualitative Inquiry and Research Design: choosing among five traditions.* Sage Publications, Thousand Oaks, CA.

Denzin N and Lincoln Y (eds) (2005) *The Sage Handbook of Qualitative Research.* Sage Publications, Thousand Oaks, CA.

Miles MB and Huberman AM (1994) *Qualitative Data Analysis: a sourcebook of new methods.* Sage Publications, Thousand Oaks, CA.

Strauss A and Corbin J (1998) *Basics of Qualitative Research.* Sage Publications, Thousand Oaks, CA.

Evaluation: improving practice, influencing policy

David Wall

KEY MESSAGES

- Evidence from educational evaluation is essential to enhance professional practice and to achieve the best medical education for students, trainees and doctors engaged in continuing professional development.
- Well-constructed evaluation is rigorous and defensible.

- The direct use of evaluation evidence in educational policy decisions is unusual.
- Good evaluation of medical education will ultimately improve patient care.

Introduction

This chapter covers the wide role of evaluation in medical education from micro to macro, from the evaluation of individual teaching episodes to entire curricula, for the purposes of improving pedagogy to influencing national policy.

We begin with some definitions and a discussion of the purposes of evaluation. Some conceptual models are then described including the evaluation cycle, a task-orientated model of evaluation and versions of the 'Kirkpatrick hierarchy'. This first, theoretical, section of the chapter concludes by exploring the differences between evaluation and research.

The chapter goes on to describe potential sources of evaluation evidence and a number of evaluation methods, including questionnaires, interviews, focus groups, site visits and some group evaluation activities. As much educational evaluation involves questionnaires, the next section describes the design and use of questionnaires in evaluation. It includes advice on writing your own evaluation tool, including writing the statements and the response options, putting the questionnaire together, using paper and online formats, response rates, piloting and field testing.

Finally, the all-important issue about whether evaluation results are acted upon is addressed. The paper discusses the role of evaluation in change management and the relationship between evaluation and educational policy. The concept of 'enlightenment' – a gradual seeping in and acceptance of new ideas, rather than a logical step-by-step incorporation of evaluation evidence – is introduced, along with some more covert purposes of evaluation, such as control. The paper concludes with examples of the range of evaluation tools that have been brought to bear on the important topics of curriculum, faculty development and educational climate.

What Is Evaluation?

Evaluation in medical education has been defined as 'a systematic approach to the collection, analysis and interpretation of information about any aspect of the conceptualisation, design, implementation and utility of educational programmes'.(1) Evaluation is generally understood to mean 'the process of obtaining information about a course or programme of teaching for subsequent judgement and decision making'.(2)

Evaluation questions we might therefore legitimately ask would include the following:
- What did the specialty registrars think of the cross-cultural communication skills course?
- What is the educational climate like for medical students in the operating theatre?
- Was the six-day faculty development course effective?
- How reliable was our shortlisting and interviewing for paediatric trainees?
- What do students and junior doctors think about the career advice provided?

Evaluation is then much more wide-ranging than merely about handing out questionnaires to students and trainees at the end of teaching sessions.

Definitions: Evaluation, Assessment and Appraisal

In everyday life the terms *evaluation*, *assessment* and *appraisal* are often used interchangeably. This confusion is compounded by international differences in

Understanding Medical Education: Evidence, Theory and Practice.
Edited by T Swanwick. © 2010 Association for the Study of Medical Education.

definitions. In North America, for instance, the word 'evaluation' is equated with the UK term 'assessment', to mean measurement of learners' skills.(2) An example of this is in the mini-clinical evaluation exercise – actually an 'assessment' tool for testing junior doctors' history-taking and examination skills.(3) Since this is primarily a UK publication I shall be using the English and European meanings for evaluation, assessment and appraisal. Evaluation has already been defined and stipulative definitions of assessment and appraisal are provided below.

Assessment is defined as 'the processes and instruments applied to measure the learner's achievements, normally after they have worked through a learning programme of one sort or another.(1) Assessment then is about testing the learners. This also appears to be the way that the word 'assessment' is used in mainland Europe.

Appraisal is 'a two-way dialogue focussing on the personal, professional and educational needs of the parties, which produce agreed outcomes'.(4) In the UK National Health Service all general practitioners and consultants now have annual appraisals, with an appraiser, using a structured format to the appraisal documentation based on the General Medical Council's (GMC) *Good Medical Practice* areas.(5)

Purposes of Evaluation

There are many purposes of evaluation. One way to conceptualise this is to think in terms of curriculum, teaching and learning, and assessment.

Evaluation is vital for curriculum development, in measuring if the curriculum is fit for purpose and in terms of curriculum outcomes.

Evaluation may also be used to ensure that the education provided is meeting the learners' needs. Did the learners learn from the teaching programme? It is often used to identify areas where the teaching (in its widest sense) needs to improve. It is used to see if an educational programme is of an acceptable standard so it may be approved for training and accreditation purposes. It may be used to give feedback to teachers, to managers and to faculty on the programmes being run in the organisation. It may be used as part of the information presented at the annual appraisal process for medical teachers, and for promotion and career development. In terms of assessments, it may be used to gather outcome measures on pass rates for qualifying and professional examinations.

And increasingly, evaluation is used in the area of assessment, evaluating the development, uses, reliability and validity of assessment tools. Often this has reached very sophisticated levels, using complex psychometrics and statistics (e.g. generalisability theory) to ascertain if assessment tools are fit for purpose. In addition, evaluation may be used to determine future

---

BOX 23.1 Purposes of evaluation

Curriculum
- Curriculum development
- Fitness for purpose
- Curriculum outcomes

Teaching and learning
- Meeting learners' needs
- Identifying poor teaching
- Approval of teaching programmes
- Feedback to teachers and the organisation
- Annual appraisal for teachers
- Promotion and career development

Assessment
- Outcome of assessments
- Development and use of assessment tools
- Appropriateness of assessment strategies

Policy
- Determining future medical education policy

Control
- Gaining compliance
- Instilling values
- Surveillance
- Management

---

educational policy in either curriculum, teaching and learning, or assessment. It may also be used as a tool to implement centrally determined policy through a number of covert and controlling processes (Box 23.1).

Conceptual Models in Evaluation

Conceptual models and frameworks may help to further our understanding of evaluation. Three of these, the 'evaluation cycle', Musick's 'task orientated' approach(6) and Kirkpatrick's hierarchy, are described below.

The evaluation cycle
A simple four-step model of the evaluation cycle is presented in Figure 23.1.(7) It begins with *planning and preparation*, then the *teaching and learning activity*, then the *collection of data about the activity*, and then *reflection and analysis*.

Task-orientated evaluation
Musick(6) provides a task-orientated model of programme evaluation, a model with five steps, outlined in Box 23.2.

Kirkpatrick hierarchy
The Kirkpatrick hierarchy was first described by Donald Kirkpatrick in 1967, as a series of levels of

Figure 23.1 A simple four-step model of the evaluation cycle.

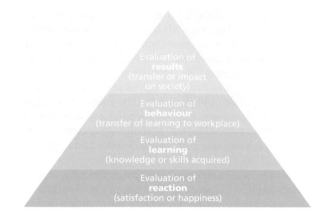

Figure 23.2 Kirkpatrick's hierarchy of evaluation.

evaluation on which to focus questions. These were, at the base (the lowest level), satisfaction with the teaching and learning, next if learning has taken place, then behaviour change and finally, at the top, results of the impact on society (*see* Figure 23.2).

Kirkpatrick's hierarchy(8) has been applied for use in medical education.(9) Here, the lowest level was defined as participation in or completion of the learning, followed by the reaction or satisfaction of participants, the learning or knowledge gained, the changes in health professionals' behaviours, performance or practice, and finally, at the top of the hierarchy, healthcare outcomes (*see* Figure 23.3). Many educational evaluations are at the lower levels of this adapted model. Belfield *et al.*(9) found that in a study of 305 papers, only 1.6% had looked at healthcare outcomes.

The Best Evidence Medical Education (BEME) collaboration has used this model in its various projects to evaluate particular educational strategies. Further information may be found on the BEME web site (http://www2.warwick.ac.uk/fac/med/beme), together with summaries of projects undertaken and in progress, coding sheets for evaluation, published papers and a wealth of other material. Several working groups, all involving multinational cooperation, have now reported.

Evaluation or Research?

Evaluation and research in education are similar activities, and may use the same research methods. Morrison(10) recently made a distinction between the two, claiming that research was aimed at producing generalisable results for publication in peer-refereed literature and needed ethical approval, whereas evaluation was carried out for local use. She also stated that evaluation was a continuous process whereas research may not be continuous if an answer were to be found. My personal view is that this is unhelpful. It is very important to produce well-designed evaluations for

BOX 23.2 Task-orientated model of programme evaluation in graduate medical education(6)

- Examine the evaluation need
  Why are you doing it, and for whom?
- Determine the evaluation focus
  What is to be evaluated?
- Determine the evaluation methodology
  When, where, how to be done and what analyses?
- Present the evaluation results
  Who are the key stakeholders to review results, and when should these be presented?
- Document the evaluation results
  How will the results be documented and used for programme improvement?

Figure 23.3 Kirkpatrick's hierarchy in medical education.(12)

publication, otherwise we may all be making the same mistakes over and over again in our local situations. For example, if we are to adopt a new assessment tool for 360-degree assessment, this needs to be piloted and properly evaluated in terms of validity, reliability, practicability and so on. Users will want to know how many raters need to be used for reliability, how many fails in any one domain is significant, who are the most appropriate people to fill in the form and so on. To evaluate the new instrument properly we may need to use interviews, questionnaires and focus groups, and analytical tests such as Cronbach's alpha(11) and generalisability theory(12) to answer these evaluation questions. This is exacting work, and not low-key activity purely for local use. Evaluation should be embedded in the culture of an organisation and used to provide feedback at all levels, but at its best, and arguably most useful, it should be conducted with the rigour of the best research project.

The overlap between evaluation and research causes most problems in the area of ethics. Bedward *et al.*(13) in their editorial in *Medical Teacher* in 2004, discussed the lack of clarity on what requires ethical approval, the reliance on one procedure for all applications, confusion over the scope of responsibilities within trusts and the scale of the work involved. In the UK, the National Research Ethics Service has published guidance differentiating research, audit and evaluation advising that only the former requires official research ethics committee approval. These guidelines can be found at http://www.nres.npsa.nhs.uk.

Despite the official view, there are some significant ethical issues in evaluation. In a recent review, Goldie(2) described some of these issues, including:

- doing what the client wants
- adhering to the written contract
- following a certain methodology
- giving equal weight to all opinion without bias
- elitism – allowing more powerful voices to be given greater weight.

Goldie cites seven ethics standards areas for evaluators, drawn from a number of national bodies by Worthen *et al.*(14) (*see* Box 23.3). Ultimately though, it is the individual evaluator's responsibility to work

ethically to bring to their work a principles- or virtue-based approach rather than to slavishly follow external codes.

Formative and Summative Evaluation

As with assessment, evaluation may be formative or summative in nature. *Formative* evaluation may be carried out by faculty to improve and shape the teaching, to gather evidence and to feed it back to those planning and carrying out the teaching in order to effect improvements.

Summative evaluation is used – often by powerful bodies with regulatory responsibility – for accreditation and reaccreditation purposes, and for promotion of individuals. These are often high-stakes decisions, such as the approval of the undergraduate curriculum of a new medical school, the accreditation of a training programme or the award of a professorship.

Regardless of the purpose of evaluation, the sources of evidence and methods used will largely be the same. And it is to these issues that we turn next.

Sources of Evaluation Evidence

In terms of evaluating teaching and learning, Berk(15) commented that student ratings have dominated as the primary measure of the evaluation of teaching effectiveness for the past 30 years. Berk(15) made a plea for '... a variety of sources to define the construct and to make decisions about performance ...'. Like him, I make a plea for the broadening and deepening of the evidence base with other sources of evidence, so that in any one evaluation we are able to use multiple sources of evidence. He suggested drawing on at least three sources of evidence, so that the strengths of one may compensate for the weaknesses of others (e.g. the different biases of peer ratings and student ratings). He suggested 13 sources of evidence, using a wide range of evaluation methods. These are listed in Box 23.4 and each is discussed in more detail below.

Student (learner) ratings
Here, students or learners evaluate the teaching programme, often by means of evaluation questionnaires. These have been used for many years and are a necessary and essential part of evaluating teaching effectiveness. Research confirms that student ratings are an excellent source of evaluation evidence.(16) However, they should not be relied on by themselves when making important decisions.

Peer ratings
With peer ratings, colleagues look at one's teaching programme, either by sitting in and observing, or reading and reviewing the teaching materials. Peer

---

BOX 23.3 Ethical standards in evaluation(14)

- Service orientation
- Formal agreements
- Rights of human subjects
- Complete and fair assessment
- Disclosure of findings
- Conflicts of interest
- Fiscal responsibility

BOX 23.4 Sources of evaluation evidence(14)

What	How	Who	Why
Student (learner) ratings	Rating scale	Students	Formative and summative
Peer ratings	Rating scale	Peers	Formative and summative
External expert ratings	Rating scale	Experts	Formative and summative
Self-ratings	Rating scale	Self	Formative and summative
Video recording of teaching	Rating scale	Self and peers	Formative and summative
Student interviews	Rating scale	Students	Formative and summative
Exit and alumni ratings	Rating scale	Graduates	Formative and summative
Employer ratings	Rating scale	Graduates' employer	Programme
Administrator ratings	Rating scale	Administrator	Summative
Teacher scholarship	Review	Administrator	Summative
Teaching awards	Review	Administrator	Summative
Learning outcomes measures	Exams	Administrator	Formative
Teaching portfolios	All above	Students' peers, administrator	Summative

review of teaching and peer review of teaching materials are useful, and cover aspects that the students as learners will not be in a position to evaluate. Since teaching is a scholarly activity, it should be subject to peer review (as with research). There is evidence that the results of peer review compare well with student ratings,(17) so peer ratings complement student ratings. Peer ratings are best used for formative rather than summative evaluation.(16)

External expert ratings

Here, an external expert will look at the teaching programme, as with peer evaluation. Such individuals will be very experienced and highly skilled with the ability to give really good and helpful feedback. This may be of great benefit to younger teachers, although in my own experience this is not always the case.

Self-ratings

Self-evaluation is an important part of the evaluation of a teaching programme. However, much like assessment, where there are differences between teacher and student assessment,(18) superior teachers provide a more accurate self-evaluation than do less highly rated teachers.(19) A highly effective, but rarely executed, evaluation strategy is to triangulate the three sources of evidence from students, peers and self.

Video recording of teaching

Berk(15) suggests that a video is one of the best sources of evidence for formative evaluation decisions. But who should evaluate it, and what methods and criteria should be used? A video recording of a teaching tutorial has been a requirement in UK general practice trainer approval for many years now. However, in hospital practice clinical teachers still seem to be wary of the video method, both in clinical work and in evaluation.

Student interviews

Interviews with groups of students are useful for evaluation purposes and may be considered more accurate and reliable than individual student ratings. Braskamp and Ory(20) suggested three types of group student interview:

- a quality control circle (perhaps what we would call a junior doctors' forum) that meets regularly to review the teaching and feedback comments and suggestions
- classroom group interviews (with someone other than the usual teacher)
- exit interviews with those who have completed the programme.

Exit and alumni ratings

A great strength of the alumni rating is that it can give valuable feedback but from a different perspective to that of current students. An example of the sort of question exit or alumni data can inform might be 'Was your medical school course for purpose?' We did precisely this study and found, perhaps not surprisingly, that it was good in some parts but not in others.(21) The young doctors and their consultant educational supervisors thought they were good at communication skills but less good at diagnosis, decision making and prescribing. Elsewhere, graduates' opinions have been shown to correlate very highly with current students' views, even up to four years later.(22)

Employer ratings

Is the young graduate fit to do the job? What is their performance like once qualified? Studies in this area can evaluate the strengths and weaknesses of the programme, and again can give valuable feedback from another, different perspective. In the study above(21) we also included the consultants. One common theme was that young doctors knew no anatomy, were good at communicating but lacked the basic knowledge with which to communicate with patients.

Administrator ratings

Deans and those in senior positions may evaluate faculty in terms of criteria for promotion, merit awards, discretionary points and so on, as well as for teaching excellence awards. Often they will rely on secondary evidence, rather than direct observation themselves.

Teaching scholarship

By this I mean the academic contribution that people make to the growing body of knowledge in medical education, in terms of development of teaching programmes, research, published papers, books and presentations at conferences. This can discriminate the key educators or star performers from others.(23)

Teaching awards

An example of reward for teaching excellence is the system of awards at Toronto General Hospital by Posluns *et al.*(24) The authors developed a programme to recognise teaching excellence, using evaluations from trainees and departmental administrators. Awards were presented to teachers at a ceremonial event.

Learning outcomes measures

Claims are often made that success in professional examinations are a measure of how good the teaching was in a particular hospital. Superficially this might seem attractive, in view of the present emphasis on outcomes-based curricula.(25) But can we really infer teaching excellence from student performance? In fact, the correlation is low to moderate, only 0.4 in meta-analyses.(26) The big problem is how we isolate teacher input as the sole cause of students' performance at the end of their programme of study. There are many variables in addition to the teaching (such as student ability, motivation, examination standards) that also have an impact on the achievement of outcomes. So in evaluating teaching effectiveness, learning outcome measures should be used with great caution.

Teaching portfolios

Currently portfolios seem to be everywhere in medical education, and increasingly these are 'electronic' and 'online'. Established practitioners use portfolios as collations of evidence towards an annual appraisal; doctors in the foundation and specialty training programmes use them as repositories for personal reflections and workplace-based assessments, and some medical schools have adopted portfolios as an integral part of the course. A teaching portfolio would ideally contain one's best work as a teacher, with evaluations from a variety of sources, and a reflective analysis on the different parts, together with appendices detailing some of the evidence. But how should such a portfolio of evidence be assessed? There are many approaches, with the assessment strategy chosen linked clearly to the portfolio structure. See Chapter 7 for further details.

Evaluation Methods

This section includes brief descriptions of several methods that may be used in educational evaluation:

- questionnaires
- interviews
- focus groups
- site visits
- examples of group methods.

In larger scale evaluations, such as those of nationwide educational programmes, several methods may be used serially, for example, in the case of a focus group being used to generate items for a questionnaire. Or they may be used in parallel where multiple methods are adopted to tap into different data sources in order to build the richest possible picture of the educational initiative under study.

Questionnaires

There are several advantages of using a questionnaire to evaluate a programme of teaching. The questionnaire is feasible and economical in terms of time and effort to collect a range of views from the whole population to be studied, rather than sampling some parts of the population. Questionnaire data (especially for closed rating scale questions) may be analysed using statistical testing for significance and associations between different data, including data reduction techniques such as factor analysis.(27,28) In addition, it may be necessary to use statistical testing to assess reliability of the data, for example, Kappa, Wilcoxon signed-rank test and repeated measures analysis of variance to assess test–re-test reliability, and Cronbach's alpha to assess internal consistency.(29) The questionnaire may also allow a search for new patterns, by two methods. One of these is the use of open-ended questions and free comments, analysed by qualitative methods, where one may catch the 'gem' of information that may be missed by the closed question.(30) The other is the method of principal component factor analysis, a data reduction method to reduce the quantitative data from the Likert questions to a small number of factors with common characteristics.

There are, however, some disadvantages to the questionnaire method. There is a well-recognised problem with pre-coded responses, which may not be sufficiently comprehensive to accommodate all answers, forcing the candidate to choose a view that does not represent their views correctly.(31) We make assumptions that all respondents will understand the questions in the same way, and there is no way of clarifying the question as in a one-to-one interview. Non-response affects the quality of the data and thus the generalisability of the results. Responders may differ from non-responders, in that non-responders may be of lower social class,(32) or older and more ill than responders.(31)

To overcome these problems, an evaluation questionnaire may be designed to include both open questions (to get at the gems), closed questions (yes/no), tick box questions with specified categories, scale items such as the Likert rating scale (agree to disagree points on a scale) and the opportunity for free comments to attempt to catch any other gems there may be.

Questionnaire design is covered in greater detail later on in this chapter.

Interviews

Cohen *et al.*(30) defined a research interview as a 'two-person conversation initiated by the interviewer, for the purpose of gathering research relevant information'.

The interview has several uses within educational evaluation and research. It can be used:

* as a way of gathering information about the evaluation questions
* to develop ideas for new hypotheses
* in conjunction with other evaluation methods in a study
* to validate
* to go deeper and explore new themes generated from other evaluation methods
* to test hypotheses that have already been generated.(30)

Also, the interview method is a powerful way to gain internal validity in case study work, to go deeper and explore new themes generated from other educational evaluation methods in this work.

Focus groups

The focus group is a form of group interview in which discussion and interaction within the group is part of the methodology.(33)

People are encouraged to talk, exchange ideas, tell stories, comment on each other's ideas and ask each other questions. The method is useful in evaluation in exploring learners' knowledge and experiences, and also in determining what they think about the course and why. The idea of a focus group is that it may help to clarify ideas and views that might be less accessible in a one-to-one interview.

Kitzinger(33) gives advice on group composition, running the group (with four to eight people as an ideal number), analysis and writing up. I believe it is essential to record such group activity and transcribe it for detailed analysis. Digital recording using a digital recorder and boundary microphone (for 360-degree capture of what people say) will give good sound quality. In addition, audio files may be stored on computer, burned onto compact disc and sent to participants and colleagues for further comments.

Site visits

This has been a traditional way to evaluate hospital posts and general practice training posts for many years. In general practice, Pereira Gray(34) advocated this in 1981 and remarked that '... some advisers and organisers have now visited as many as a hundred different practices and thus have built up a considerable experience of the characteristics of satisfactory and unsatisfactory training practices ...'. The visit to the organisation, speaking with the trainers and the trainees face to face, and seeing the working environment does still have a valuable place, but it is important the process is robust and reproducible, and that visitors are trained properly in their role.

Group consensus techniques

A number of consensus techniques have been developed for the evaluation of educational events involving medium to large groups. Two commonly used approaches are described here.

Snowball review

This is a group-based evaluation(1) that uses a series of steps where comment and opinion are suggested, discussed, shared and agreed, before going on to the next step, until a final list of good and not so good points about a course has been agreed. The steps are as follows.

* Each individual alone lists, say, three good and three not so good points about the course.
* Participants form pairs and discuss their suggestions then come to an agreement as a pair.
* Each pair then forms a group of four, and again debates the views and comes to an agreement.
* Two groups of four join up to form a group of eight. Again they debate and agree their conclusions.
* A reporter presents the group's views to the whole course.

This is a good method in that it involves everyone and ideally reaches a consensus and a conclusion, but it does take time.

Nominal group technique

This is another group-based consensus method. It differs from the snowball review (above) in that each person gives their views and then all the views are collected up and voted on. The steps are as follows.

- Each individual is asked in turn for feedback on the best and least good aspects of the course.
- Comments are collected and listed (once) on a flip chart, that is, if two members of the group thought that the catering was not very good, this is only listed once.
- The facilitator continues to go round the group until all (unique) comments have been exhausted.
- Group members are then allowed a set number of votes to distribute among the items listed.
- The result is a scored and ranked list of feedback comments to which all members of the group have contributed.
- An optional stage is to put people into groups to discuss some or all of the items derived from the voting.

Group consensus techniques carry a health warning. Both methods may achieve answers of good face validity but are of low order as far as Kirkpatrick's hierarchy is concerned and the results do not lend themselves to further analysis in terms of generalisability.

To defend what we do as educators, it is very important to conduct rigorous evaluations that are robust, well designed and measure what they are supposed to measure in a reliable way. The method that lends itself most easily to such an approach is the questionnaire, and we will now look at the design and use of questionnaires in greater detail. You may be fortunate to have a ready-made, valid and reliable tool available 'off the shelf', but you may need to design your own. If you do, here is some evidence-based advice to help you do so.

Designing Questionnaires for Evaluation

If you have decided on an evaluation questionnaire, then how should you proceed? You may know that there is already an existing evaluation questionnaire in use, validated, published in the medical education literature and in the public domain for you to use. You may wish to buy a commercially available rating scale from an organisation if this fits your purposes, and you have the funds to do so. Such scales have been developed and validated, and have good validity and reliability. A number are cited by Berk.(15) Or you may wish to pick statements already available in an item bank. One such source is Purdue University in the US, which has an item bank of over 600 evaluation question items. It may be accessed at the Purdue Instructor and Course Evaluation Service on http://www.cie.purdue.edu/data/pices.cfm.

Caution is needed when taking an off-the-shelf questionnaire and using it in your own organisation. The questionnaire may have been developed in another country, and terms used may have different meanings. The questionnaire may not really focus on what you need to evaluate in your own situation. If this is the case, you might have to develop your own questionnaire, as nothing already available will fit your purpose.

Developing your own evaluation tool

The process of developing your own evaluation instrument involves several steps. You will need to:
- decide what you are going to measure
- choose the right questions to ask
- write the statements
- design the response options (the anchors)
- put it all together and do field tests
- analyse the results.

Berk(15) describes all these steps in great detail. Similar information is given in the classic work on questionnaire design by Oppenheim.(27) The great detail in these texts is outside the scope of this chapter, but here are some general principles that may be of help.

Writing the statements
- Each statement should describe a particular idea.
- Use clear, simple language.
- Each statement should be grammatically correct, have the correct punctuation and avoid double negatives.
- Keep to one concept per question – do not ask two questions in one sentence.
- Avoid unfamiliar words.
- Avoid statements that suggest a single answer.
- Avoid abbreviations, as they may mean completely different things to different people.

Berk(15) provides a checklist of 20 questions to ask in relation to testing your rating scale statements.

Writing the response options – the anchors
One you have the statements, the next step is writing the response options. These may be structured in a number of ways as follows.
- *Likert scale:* a bipolar scale with positive and negative feelings towards the statement, 'strongly agree' to 'strongly disagree'. They may have even numbers, a two-, four- or six-point scale, or odd numbers, a three-, five- or seven-point scale with a middle point meaning 'not sure' or 'uncertain'.
- *Quality scale:* using terms such as 'poor' to 'excellent'.
- *Frequency scale:* asking how often something happens, such as daily, weekly, every two weeks or once a month.
- *Quantity scale:* using sometimes vague terms such as 'all', 'very much', 'often', 'a little' or 'not at all'. All points on the scale should be described.

How many points on the scale should there be? Increasing the number of points increases the reliability, but there is a point of diminishing return after five points,(35) so the nine-point scale we see on some current instruments may be difficult to justify.

Should there be a midpoint – an undecided or uncertain category? A midpoint score gives us little or no information. Berk(15) recommends a four- or six-point scale as these require the responder to come to a decision one way or another. There are inevitably biases in rating scales. A *halo effect* is seen where an overall impression will bias the score on each statement. *End aversion* is where responders avoid the extreme ends of the scale for a question. *Extreme response* bias is the opposite of the previous bias. *Positive response* bias is where responders agree irrespective of the question being asked. Also there may be *gender*, *age* and *racial* biases. Some or all of these may need to be addressed.(15)

Assembling the questionnaire

It is helpful to have a framework to follow when putting together a questionnaire. A list of the main points to consider is provided in Box 23.5.

Paper-based or online?

Although some prefer a paper-based questionnaire, the use of online questionnaires is increasing. Advantages for an online format include less cost(36) and some evidence of a higher response rate than in paper-based studies. There are good correlations between paper-based and online format.(37)

Pre-pilot testing

A pre-pilot is essential. Show the instrument to a few of your friends and colleagues. Can they understand the questions? A questionnaire I designed to evaluate our bursary scheme for university educational qualifications went through four versions before a pilot study was eventually undertaken, as problems were ironed out.

BOX 23.5 How to: Construct a questionnaire

Heading: what it is the questionnaire about?

Statement: what is the purpose of the evaluation?

Directions: for filling the questionnaire in.

Identification: of the course, the specialty, the grade of post (or other relevant identifiers), without which the evaluation may be meaningless.

Questions: a mixture of yes/no questions, tick box categories (such as gender, specialty, years qualified), Likert-type statements, open free text questions and free comment. It is usual to put personal information towards the end, and simple yes/no or tick box categorical questions near the beginning.

Return of the questionnaire: instructions for where to send the completed questionnaire, and by when.

Pilot study

The next step is a pilot study on a small sample, perhaps 5–10 people. Modifications may still need to be made after this stage. This is also an opportunity to check if you can code in the responses and put these into a form for analysis, perhaps with SPSS, a powerful statistical program used worldwide for statistical calculations, and NVivo, a programme for the qualitative analysis of free text (both written and spoken) into themes and concepts.

Field testing

Next would be a field test on a larger sample. Following field testing the questionnaire is now ready to be launched.

Response rates

The response rate is an important source of bias, so efforts need to be made to maximise the number of respondents. Methods known to increase the response rates to postal questionnaires include:

- designing and using a short, simple questionnaire
- providing a covering letter on headed notepaper
- including a reply paid envelope
- following up non-responders with a further questionnaire, covering letter and reply paid envelope.(31)

These procedures were much in line with a recent Cochrane review of the evidence by Edwards *et al.*,(38) which indicated that a short questionnaire, first class post, personalised letters, follow-up contact with a further questionnaire and a letter on university or other headed notepaper were all of value in increasing the response rate.

The judgement about what constitutes a good response rate is not clear cut. Suggestions about response rate in the educational literature vary somewhat. Edwards and Talbot(39) suggested a response rate over 60%. Cohen *et al.*(30) suggested at least 40%, and ideally up to 70–80%. Bowling(31) suggested that a response rate of 75% was generally accepted as good, since above this figure of response the biases from the non-responders assumed much less effect on the results as a whole.

Evaluation Results: Implementation and Influence

No matter how beautifully designed the evaluation strategy, the key question for evaluators is can the results be fed back into the system and acted upon? Put another way, how do we manage change in a medical education system? There is a vast amount of literature in the area of change management that has been well summarised elsewhere.(40,41) Much of the early literature suggested a controlled way of proceeding through the change process in a controlled and logical way. For example, using a problem-solving approach we might identify a problem, agree the problem, suggest solutions, agree solutions, implement solutions and evaluate the changes. This is very logical and rational, but as recent educational reforms in the UK have demonstrated, rational concepts and models have not been the only ones at work.

The UK policy initiative *Modernising Medical Careers* (42,43) began as an attempt to improve the senior house officer grade. In 2005, a new Foundation Programme for newly qualified doctors was launched, and 2007 saw the introduction of new curricula and assessments for all specialties with a new run-through training structure and junior doctors applying through a national untried online application system. All this has happened with very few evaluations of pilots to test the new ideas, with the exception of the Foundation Programmes. Perhaps as a result, the introduction of reform of specialty training proved a disaster for thousands of junior doctors, and we have yet to experience the effects on patient care.

To try to explain such events it is helpful to rethink the linear model of change referred to above. Mintzberg(44) suggested that change can either be thought of as a pre-planned and logical series of steps or, perhaps more realistically, as an open-ended, ongoing and unpredictable process that aims to align and realign in response to change within society. Political power, the Royal Colleges, the Postgraduate Medical Education and Training Board, the GMC and the British Medical Association were all active players in the *Modernising Medical Careers* process, a massive piece of educational change underpinned [with one or two small exceptions(45)] by almost no evaluation evidence.

So what then is the relationship between evaluation and public policy? Weiss(46) and Swanwick(47) both discuss this interface and highlight that although researchers would wish for a direct and logical link, this is rarely the case. Policy makers rarely base their new policies directly on evaluation decisions. Organisations do not often use knowledge directly to help organisational change. In fact, policy makers tend only to cite evaluation studies that suit their particular line of policy. Direct influence of evaluation on policy is unusual. Instead, a more gradual process of change, the slow incorporation of ideas and methods into policy, is more common, a process that Weiss calls 'enlightenment'. New ideas seep in, percolate through the system, gain ground and may eventually become mainstream. Through this softer process, evaluation can have real and powerful consequences, challenging old ideas, offering new perspectives and helping to influence the policy agenda. Finally, evaluation may be used by policy makers for the less overt purpose of control. Here, evaluation can be used to ensure compliance with a policy, to force a set of values on the medical profession, for surveillance and to manage the whole process. Harland(48) described four aspects to this control function of evaluation: compliance, patterning, surveillance and management.

Pitfalls in Educational Evaluation

There are several common pitfalls to try to avoid in educational evaluation, some of which have been mentioned earlier. Here are some common problems I have encountered over a career of conducting educational evaluation.

Only measuring what is easy to measure
This may be related to following a certain methodology. It might be quite easy to send out a questionnaire and more difficult to do case studies where problems of bullying, negative feedback and so on are the main problem. It may also relate to gathering only one source of evidence, rather than trying to triangulate the evidence from three different areas.

Low response rates
This has already been discussed above. The lower the response rate, the greater the bias of what the non-responders think. This may have a serious effect. So it is important to get a good response rate, of perhaps more than 70%, and to state what the response rate is in any analysis of evaluations carried out.

Poor reliability
Some evaluation instruments have not been properly tested for reliability, or if they have, have been found wanting. The latter situation is very rare, and a lack of proper testing, or even lack of knowledge as to what should have been done, is far more common. It may then be impossible to derive any conclusions, or the conclusions obtained may be unreliable, which is worse when important conclusions are drawn from them. Recently, when I was explaining about reliability of shortlisting procedures, many consultants told me they had never heard of measures of reliability being applied to such situations and were unable to understand what was involved.

Taking your eye off the ball
In many evaluations of previously good hospital posts, by the next time we visited the situation had changed for the worse. This may be because of a change of programme director, changes in the hospital trust organisation and government targets (such as the four-hourly accident and emergency targets).

Taking too much notice of the individual with a misplaced grievance
I have certainly seen examples of this, even on national quality assurance visits. Everyone is happy with the teaching except for one disaffected and sometimes

dysfunctional individual. The visiting team takes all of the disaffected one's concerns seriously, to the exclusion of all other evidence. All this appears in the report and slants the conclusions one way. Further investigations later show much of this to be factually incorrect, the individual never turned up to the teaching, scored very poorly on their 360-degree assessment and later turned out to have a severe mental illness. However, all this is found out after the event – and by then it is too late.

Ethical issues

A number of ethical issues commonly arise, including:

- always doing what the client wants (including producing the desired results)
- slavishly adhering to the written contract
- allowing bias to creep in
- ignoring minority reports
- allowing powerful voices to be given greater weight.

Adherence to standards of good practice, such as those produced by the UK Evaluation Society (*see* Box 23.6), will help to overcome some of these temptations.

Expecting your findings to be implemented widely

Change happens slowly, organically and often unexpectedly. Your evaluation findings may take some time to seep into the ground water of educational practice, or they may be picked up by an enthusiastic policy maker and used as justification for wholesale system reform. Just do not expect rational step-by-step decisions to follow from your evaluation, no matter how robust the design and analysis.

Conclusion

Evaluation is an essential part of medical education, needs to be carried out rigorously and correctly, and is certainly not an inconsequential activity as some have claimed. A good knowledge of many different areas is needed if we are to be able to carry out meaningful evaluations, which can be fed back to improve learning and teaching. At the end of the day, the aspiration is that our evaluations will produce improvements in patient care, an outcome right at the top of Kirkpatrick's hierarchy.

Examples of Evaluations in Medical Education

Example 1: evaluation of a course or curriculum

A widely known method for looking at course or curriculum content in medical education is what many know as Harden's Ten Questions.(49) These questions

> **BOX 23.6 Focus on: Good practice in evaluation**
>
> A number of organisations have defined standards for good evaluation practice. The European Evaluation Society lists the standards laid out by a number of European countries. The UK version spells out what constitutes good practice for:
>
> - evaluators
> - participants
> - commissioners
> - institutions conducting self-evaluation.
>
> The UK Evaluation Society Guidelines for Good Practice in Evaluation can be downloaded from http://www.evaluation.org.uk
>
> The American Evaluation Association has also produced guiding principles; these are built around five areas.
>
> *Systematic inquiry:* evaluators conduct systematic, data-based inquiries about whatever is being evaluated.
>
> *Competence:* evaluators provide competent performance to stakeholders.
>
> *Integrity/Honesty:* evaluators ensure the honesty and integrity of the entire evaluation process.
>
> *Respect for people:* evaluators respect the security, dignity and self-worth of the respondents, programme participants, clients and other stakeholders with whom they interact.
>
> *Responsibilities for general and public welfare:* evaluators articulate and take into account the diversity of interests and values that may be related to the general and public welfare.
>
> The full guidance can be viewed at http://www.eval.org/Publications/GuidingPrinciples.asp

can be used both in planning a course or curriculum, and to evaluate the course in a systematic way. The 10 questions are described below.

1 What are the needs in relation to the product of the training programme?

   Is the programme or curriculum fit for purpose? To evaluate this, one may consult experts, errors in practice, critical incident reports, task analysis, morbidity and mortality figures, opinions and beliefs of star performers, looking at existing curricula and views of recent students.

2 What are the aims and objectives?

   What will the student be able to do at the end of the course of study? Is this borne out by evaluation data?

3 What content should be included?

   Content should be put into a course if it:
   - directly contributes to the course objectives
   - forms a building block of skill or knowledge needed to tackle a later part of the course

- allows development of intellectual abilities such as critical thinking
- aids the understanding of other subjects on the course.

4 How should the content be organised?

This relates to the order in which subjects are taught, and a theoretical plan of why the order is organised as it is.

5 What educational strategies should be adopted?

'Strategies' relate to the curriculum model being used, such as a spiral curriculum, an objectives model, a process model or an outcome-based model. Sometimes there is no obvious model at all.

6 What teaching methods should be adopted?

Student grouping may be one way, with, for example, whole class teaching by the lecture method, small groups, one-to-one bedside teaching and distance learning. Another way may be by teaching and learning tools, such as computer packages, web-based learning, simulators, skills laboratories and role play. The choice of methods needs to reflect the course aims and objectives. One would not choose to teach communication skills and breaking bad news to patients in a lecture-based course.

7 How should assessment be carried out?

This includes the choice of assessments used [such as essays, projects, portfolios, multiple-choice questions, Objective Structure Clinical Examinations (OSCEs), oral examinations, and long and short cases].

- Who will assess the work?
- Are there external examiners?
- Is there self-assessment?
- Will assessment be continuous throughout the course or at the end?
- What are the standards to be achieved?
- Are the assessment standards criteria referenced or norm referenced?
- How is the course evaluated? Is it by the students?
- Is there internal and external evaluation?

8 How should details of the curriculum be communicated?

Details have to be communicated to those teaching the course, the students attending the course, potential students and other bodies. How is this done? How do the subjects relate to each other and the final product?

9 What educational environment or climate should be fostered?

Does the environment encourage cooperation between students, students and teachers, scholarship, probity and support, or is it hostile, with teaching by humiliation, sexism and bullying?

10 How should the process be managed?
- Who is responsible for planning, organising and managing the process?

- Can changes be made?
- How does this course relate to others?
- Is there student representation?
- Do the teaching staff know what is going on?
- Is there a course committee?

Example 2: evaluation of faculty development programmes

Does faculty development – teaching the teachers – really work? What is the evidence for this? This summary illustrates many different methods of evaluation that have been carried out seeking to answer this question. There is now good evidence that these courses do improve teachers' ability to teach, and do improve learning by trainees. Researchers in medical and dental education have shown that teaching the teachers initiatives really do work.

One of the few studies that tried to do this was undertaken by Whitehouse,(50) who followed up participants who had attended a six-day educational teaching the teachers course. Participants did use the lessons learnt on the course and put many of these ideas into their own education practice. Indeed, the group formed on this course continues to meet more than 10 years on from the original course.

In Turkey, Yolsal *et al.*(51) reported the impact of their Training of Trainers courses since 1997. They used a questionnaire at the end of their six- to nine-day courses, and at six months post-course. Seventy-two per cent of their medical teachers said they had implemented the knowledge and skills acquired on the courses, and that students had given better feedback on their teaching. Many stated they now enjoyed their teaching more, and that they had set up a network of keen teachers after being on courses together. This study and these results are very similar to Whitehouse's study and results.(50)

Steinert *et al.*(52) at McGill University in Canada described a year-long faculty development programme to develop leaders in medical education. The course included educational knowledge and skills, in protected time, while maintaining the participants' other clinical, teaching and research responsibilities. A year after completing the programme, the authors found in a follow-up survey of 22 faculty members that many had joined new educational committees, taken up new leadership roles in medical education and developed new courses for students and doctors in training, and two had pursued further studies to Masters level. However, all three studies relied on self-reporting by the candidates rather than other evidence.

There are more recent studies that used different methodologies and end-point assessments to make similar points. Godfrey *et al.*(53) from Sheffield asked whether a teaching the teachers course did in fact develop teaching skills. They used a quasi-experimental design and compared a group of consultant teachers who underwent a three-day teaching the teachers course with a control group taken from the course waiting list. However, the candidates were not assigned to the taught group or the control group randomly. A questionnaire of teaching skills was applied to participants and controls before the course and at 8 to 10 months afterwards. Up to 63% of participants and 51% of controls replied to all aspects of this study. Candidates who had attended the course did significantly better and reported significantly greater improvements in self-reported teaching skills. These authors did discuss self-reporting as a source of bias, but argued that the control group in this research design did help overcome these issues.

In a Californian study, Morrison *et al.*(54) used an experimental design with an intervention group and a control group of medical residents to explore whether they could improve residents' teaching skills. Their research question was: 'Do trained teachers perform better then untrained control residents?' They ran a 13-hour teaching the teachers course over six months. This was a rigorously designed and carried out study. The two groups were similar in terms of gender, specialty and academic performance, and people were assigned randomly to each group, either to attend the course or be a control. The outcome measures included an eight-station, three-and-a-half-hour OSCE – previously validated – in which the participants were assessed by trained medical students. A subset of the participants were interviewed one year later by two educational researchers, who did not know in advance who had attended the course and who was a control. Those residents in the teaching the teachers course group did significantly better in all eight stations of the OSCE, and people who were required to attend did as well as those who volunteered. Also, the interviews showed that the taught group showed greater enthusiasm for teaching, used learner-centred approaches, had more elaborate understanding of pedagogic principles and planned to teach after finishing their training.

In Alberta, Panderchuck *et al.*,(55) in another quasi-experimental study, looked at the effects of a two-day teaching the teachers workshop. They compared a group of medical teachers who had attended the workshops with controls (who had not) by means of ratings by medical students on their teaching abilities before and after the workshops, using the standard University of Alberta student evaluation questionnaire. Their study used data from 1993 to 2002. Students' ratings of teachers' teaching abilities increased significantly for the teachers after the workshops, but remained unchanged for the control group, who had not attended the workshops.

Most recently, in November 2006, new evidence from the BEME review of faculty development initiatives by Steinert *et al.*,(56) which reviewed 2777 papers and selected 53 of these papers for detailed analyses, showed:

- overall satisfaction with programmes was high
- participants reported positive changes in attitude to teaching
- increased knowledge of educational principles and of gains in teaching skills
- changes in teaching behaviours
- greater educational involvement and establishment of collegiate networks.

Key strategies for effective interventions to improve teaching effectiveness in medical education included:

- experiential learning
- feedback
- effective peer and colleague relationships
- interventions that followed the principles of teaching and learning
- the use of a wide variety of educational methods.

In summary, much of the earlier literature is based on opinion from distinguished and senior individuals within the profession, both individually and in terms of organisations such as expert government committees, Royal Colleges and the GMC.(57,58) More recently there are examples of good evaluation studies that try to examine the effects of teaching the teachers courses by means of follow-up and self-reporting of changes, and of the effects of such initiatives on the learners, the medical students themselves. Here there is evidence that teaching the teachers courses do improve teaching ability, widen teachers' pedagogic approaches to teaching and increase enjoyment of teaching.

Example 3: evaluation of the educational climate

The educational environment variously referred to as climate, atmosphere or tone is a set of factors that describe what it is like to be a learner within that organisation. Chambers and Wall(59) considered the educational climate in three parts. These were:

- the physical environment (safety, food, shelter, comfort and other facilities)
- the emotional climate (security, constructive feedback, being supported, and absence of bullying and harassment)
- the intellectual climate (learning with patients, relevance to practice, evidence-based, active participation by learners, motivating and planned education).

The good clinical teaching environment(60) should ensure the teaching and learning is relevant to patients, has active participation by learners, and shows professional thinking and behaviours. There should be good preparation and planning of both the structure and content, reflection on learning, and evaluation of what has happened in the teaching and learning. Spencer also goes on to describe some of the common problems with teaching and learning in the clinical environment, including lack of clear objectives, focus on knowledge rather than problem-solving skills, teaching at the wrong level, passive observation, little time for reflection and discussion, and teaching by humiliation.

Teaching by humiliation, bullying and harassment is a big problem in the UK and other countries. Much of this relates to teachers' lack of awareness of educational skills and knowledge(61,62) and inability to promote a good, supportive educational climate for trainees in which to learn.(57,58) Lowry(61) described disenchantment with medicine in the words of a young doctor as 'It could have been such a wonderful thing to be a doctor – but it's not. It's just a disaster.'

Sadly, there are many examples in the literature of bullying and harassment of junior doctors and medical students. Such studies show the practice is widespread, and on the individual level illustrate how destructive to confidence and well-being bullying and harassment can be. Wolf *et al.*(63) carried out a questionnaire study of medical students in the Louisiana State University School of Medicine. Of these, 98.9% reported mistreatment, with shouting and humiliation being most frequent. Over half reported sexual harassment, which was reported mainly by women students. There was a high level of remarks degrading doctors and medicine as a profession. Increased mistreatment was associated positively with a perceived increase in cynicism.

In Manchester, Guthrie *et al.*(64) used a postal questionnaire to measure the psychological morbidity and the nature and sources of stress in first-year medical students. Half the students reported a stressful incident, most of which related to medical training and the styles of medical teaching. They described being upset by the attitudes of tutors, including humiliation, shouting, ridicule, ignorance exposed and a confrontational nature.

Metcalfe and Matharu(65) used a postal questionnaire study of medical students in Manchester to investigate student perceptions of good and bad teaching. Good examples were when there was active learning, and teachers let students 'run the session'. Bad examples were mainly examples of bad behaviour of staff towards students, such as humiliation, sexism and ridicule.

Is this all in the past? In the 21st century, are all these problems behind us? The answer is probably no. The medical literature still reports bullying and harassment. Doctors are still disillusioned. Bullying and humiliation are still common within the medical profession. An anonymous author(66) described repeated bullying of a junior surgeon by a consultant. A questionnaire study by Quine(67) of bullying of junior doctors shows how common such behaviours still are. Of 594 doctors, 37% identified themselves as having been bullied in the past year, and 84% had experienced one or more bullying behaviours. Black and Asian doctors fared worse than white doctors, and women fared worse than men. The most common bullying strategies were attempts to belittle and undermine work, unjustified criticism, humiliation in front of colleagues, and intimidatory use of discipline and competence procedures.

Despite this, the evaluations from the trainees at senior house officer level report good to excellent scores for induction, supervision and clinical experience in these posts. This is using the post-evaluation tool, developed and used every six months on all senior house officer posts within the West Midlands since 1997.(68) Also, evidence from our Deanery Quality Assurance visits to intensive care units has repeatedly shown that senior house officers value their time there very much, feel well supported and rate the jobs highly.

So can the education environment be measured using a practical, valid and reliable tool? The Dundee Ready Education Environment Measure was developed in Dundee by Roff *et al.*(69) It is a valid and reliable measure of the perceived education environment. It has been widely used in many countries throughout the world, including the Gulf States, Nepal, Nigeria, the West Indies, Thailand, China, Canada and the UK. It has been used for medical students, nurses, dentists, chiropractors and other professions allied to medicine.

From this original environmental measure, further postgraduate measurement scales have been developed. For the postgraduate medical education environment, the Dundee group has also developed a 40-item inventory for the various aspects of junior doctor training in the UK and Ireland, the Postgraduate Hospital Education Environment Measure.(70) The Anaesthetic Theatre Educational Environment Measure(71) has been developed and validated for teaching in anaesthesia in the operating theatre, and for junior surgeons in the operating theatre; the Surgical Theatre Environmental Educational Measure(72) has been developed and validated.

In anaesthetic trainees, Holt and Roff(71) showed that there was a better educational climate perceived by first-year senior house officers than by specialist registrars, and these results were statistically significant. In the operating theatre, Nagraj *et al.*(73) showed that the educational climate was reasonably good for medical students and slightly less so for senior house officers. Only at specialist registrar level did the climate improve significantly. So, educational climate can be measured using a variety of well-researched, valid and reliable tools that are available free of charge in the public domain. One of the great assets of using these tools is that comparisons may be made of your own evaluations with others throughout the UK and indeed other parts of the international medical education community.

References

1 Mohanna K, Wall D and Chambers R (2004) *Teaching Made Easy – a manual for health professionals* (2e). Radcliffe Medical Press, Oxford.

2 Goldie J (2006) AMEE guide no. 29: evaluating educational programmes. *Medical Teacher.* **28**: 210–24.

3 Norcini JJ, Blank LL, Duffy FD and Fortna GS (2003) The miniCEX: a method of assessing clinical skills. *Annals of Internal Medicine.* **138**: 476–83.

4 SCOPME (1996) *Appraising Doctors and Dentists in Training.* Standing Committee on Postgraduate Medical and Dental Education, London.

5 General Medical Council (2001) *Good Medical Practice.* GMC, London.

6 Musick D (2006) A conceptual model for program evaluation in graduate medical education. *Academic Medicine.* **81**: 759–65.

7 Wilkes M and Bligh J (1999) Evaluating educational interventions. *British Medical Journal.* **318**: 1269–72.

8 Kirkpatrick DI (1967) Evaluation of training. In: Craig R and Mittel I (eds) *Training and Development Handbook,* pp. 87–112. McGraw Hill, New York.

9 Belfield CR, Thomas HR, Bullock AD *et al.* (2001) Measuring effectiveness for Best Evidence Medical Education – a discussion. *Medical Teacher.* **23**: 164–70.

10 Morrison J (2003) Evaluation. *British Medical Journal.* **326**: 385–7.

11 Field A (2004) *Discovering Statistics Using SPSS for Windows* (2e). Sage Publications, London.

12 Brennan RL (2001) *Generalizability Theory.* Springer, New York.

13 Bedward J, Davison I, Field S and Thomas H (2005) Audit, educational development and research: what counts for ethics and research governance? *Medical Teacher.* **27**: 99–101.

14 Worthen BL, Sanders JR and Fitzpatrick JL (1997) *Program Evaluation: alternative approaches and practical guidelines* (2e). Longman, New York.

15 Berk RA (2006) *Thirteen Strategies to Measure College Teaching.* Stylus Publishing LLC, Sterling, VA.

16 Arreola RA (2000) *Developing a Comprehensive Faculty Evaluation System: a handbook for college faculty and administrators on designing and operating a comprehensive faculty evaluation system* (2e). Anker, Bolton, MA.

17 Murray HG (1983) Low inference classroom teaching behaviours and student ratings of college teaching effectiveness. *Journal of Educational Psychology.* **71**: 856–65.

18 Falchikov N and Boud D (1989) Student self-assessment in higher education: a meta-analysis. *Review of Educational Research.* **59**: 395–430.

19 Barber LW (1990) Self assessment. In: Millman J and Darling-Hammond L (eds) *The New Handbook of Teacher Evaluation,* pp. 216–28. Sage, Newbury Park, CA.

20 Braskamp LA and Ory JC (1994) *Assessing Faculty Work.* Jossey-Bass, San Francisco, CA.

21 Wall D, Bolshaw A and Carolan J (2006) Is undergraduate medical education fitting for purpose to be a pre-registration house officer? *Medical Teacher.* **28**: 435–9.

22 Overall JU and Marsh HW (1980) Students' evaluation of instruction: a longitudinal study of their stability. *Journal of Educational Psychology.* **72**: 321–5.

23 Harden RM (1986) Approaches to curriculum planning. *Medical Education.* **20**: 458–66.

24 Posluns E, Sharon Safir M, Keystone JS *et al.* (1990) Rewarding medical teaching excellence in a major Canadian teaching hospital. *Medical Teacher.* **12**: 13–22.

25 Harden RM, Crosby JR and Davis MH (1999) An introduction to outcomes based learning. *Medical Teacher.* **21**: 7–14.

26 Feldman KA (1989) The association between student ratings of specific instructional dimensions and student achievement: refining and extending the synthesis of data from multisection validity studies. *Research in Higher Education.* **30**: 583–645.

27 Oppenheim AN (1992) *Questionnaire Design, Interviewing and Attitude Measurement.* Continuum, London.

28 Field A (2000) *Discovering Statistics Using SPSS for Windows.* Sage Publications, London.

29 Howitt D and Cramer D (2003) *A Guide to Computing Statistics with SPSS 11 for Windows.* Pearson Education, Harlow.

30 Cohen L, Manion L and Morrison K (2000) *Research Methods in Education* (5e). RoutledgeFalmer, London.

31 Bowling A (1997) *Research Methods in Health.* Open University Press, Buckingham.

32 Cartwright A (1988) Interviews or postal questionnaires? Comparisons of data about women's experiences with maternity services. *The Milbank Quarterly.* **66**: 172–89.

33 Kitzinger J (1996) *Introducing Focus Groups.* In: Mays N and Pope C (eds) *Qualitative Research in Health Care,* pp. 36–45. BMJ Publishing Group, London.

34 Pereira Gray DJ (1982) *Training for General Practice.* MacDonald and Evans, Plymouth.

35 Myford CM (2002) Investigating design features of descriptive graphic rating scales. *Applied Measurement in Education.* **15**: 187–215.

36 Bothell TW and Henderson T (2003) Do online ratings of instruction make sense? In: Sorensen DL and Johnson TD (eds) *New Directions for Teaching and Learning,* no. **96**, pp. 69–80. Jossey-Bass, San Francisco, CA.

37 Johnson TD (2003) Online student ratings: will students respond? In: Sorensen DL and Johnson TD (eds) *New Directions for Teaching and Learning,* no. **96**, pp. 49–60. Jossey-Bass, San Francisco, CA.

38 Edwards P, Roberts I, Clarke M *et al.* (2002) Increasing response rates to postal questionnaires: systematic review. *British Medical Journal.* **324**: 1183–5.

39 Edwards A and Talbot R (1999) *The Hard-Pressed Researcher* (2e). Pearson Education, Harlow.

40 Handy C (1989) *The Age of Unreason.* Business Books, London.

41 Iles V and Sutherland K (1997) *The Literature on Change Management. Review for Healthcare Managers, Researchers and Professionals.* National Co-ordinating Centre for NHS Service Delivery and Organisation, London.

42 Donaldson L (2002) *Unfinished Business: proposals for the reform of the SHO grade. A Report by Sir Liam Donaldson, CMO for England.* Department of Health, London.

43 Department of Health (2004) *Modernising Medical Careers: the next steps.* Department of Health, London.

44 Mintzberg H (1987) Crafting strategy. *Harvard Business Review.* **65**(4): 66–75.

45 Walzman M, Allen M and Wall D (2008) General practice and the Foundation Programme: the views of FY2 doctors from the Coventry and Warwickshire Foundation School. *Education for Primary Care.* **19**(2): 151–9.

46 Weiss C (1999) The interface between evaluation and public policy. *Evaluation.* **5**: 468–86.

47 Swanwick T (2007) Introducing large-scale educational reform in a complex environment: the role of piloting and evaluation in modernizing medical careers. *Evaluation.* **13**: 363–73.

48 Harland J (1996) Evaluation as Realpolitik. In: Scott D and Usher R (eds) *Understanding Educational Research.* Routledge, London.

49 Harden RM (1986) Ten questions to ask when planning a course or curriculum. *Medical Education.* **20**: 356–65.

50 Whitehouse A (1997) Warwickshire consultants' 'training the trainers' course. *Postgraduate Medical Journal.* **73**: 35–8.

51 Yolsal N, Bulut A, Karabey S *et al*. (2003) Development of training of trainers' programmes and evaluation of their effectiveness in Istanbul, Turkey. *Medical Teacher*. **25**: 319–24.

52 Steinert Y, Nasmith L, McLeod PJ and Conochie L (2003) A teaching scholars program to develop leaders in medical education. *Academic Medicine*. **78**: 142–9.

53 Godfrey J, Dennick G and Welsh C (2004) Training the trainers: do teaching courses develop teaching skills? *Medical Education*. **38**: 844–7.

54 Morrison EH, Rucker L, Boker JR *et al*. (2004) The effect of a 13 hour curriculum to improve residents' teaching skills – a randomised trial. *Annals of Internal Medicine*. **141**: 257–63.

55 Panderchuck K, Harley D and Cook D (2004) Effectiveness of a brief workshop designed to improve teaching performance at the University of Alberta. *Academic Medicine*. **79**: 798–804.

56 Steinert Y, Mann K, Centeno A *et al*. (2006) A systematic review of faculty development initiatives designed to improve teaching effectiveness in medical education: BEME guide no. 8. *Medical Teacher*. **28**: 497–526.

57 SCOPME (1992) *Teaching Hospital Doctors and Dentists to Teach: its role in creating a better learning environment. Proposals for Consultation – full report*. Standing Committee for Postgraduate Medical Education, London.

58 SCOPME (1994) *Creating a Better Learning Environment in Hospitals 1. Teaching Hospital Doctors and Dentists to Teach*. Standing Committee on Postgraduate Medical Education, London.

59 Chambers R and Wall D (2000) *Teaching Made Easy: a manual for health professionals*. Radcliffe Medical Press, Oxford.

60 Spencer N (2003) The clinical teaching context: a cause for concern. *Medical Education*. **37**: 182–3.

61 Lowry S (1993) Teaching the teachers. *British Medical Journal*. **306**: 127–30.

62 Lowry S (1992) What's wrong with medical education in Britain? *British Medical Journal*. **305**: 1277–80.

63 Wolf TM, Randall HM, Von Almen K and Tynes LL (1991) Perceived mistreatment and attitude change by graduating medical students: a retrospective study. *Medical Education*. **25**: 182–90.

64 Guthrie EA, Black D, Shaw CM *et al*. (1995) Embarking on a medical career: psychological morbidity in first year medical students. *Medical Education*. **29**: 337–41.

65 Metcalfe DH and Matharu M (1995) Students' perceptions of good and bad teaching: report of a critical incident study. *Medical Education*. **29**: 193–7.

66 Anon (2001) Personal view. Bullying in medicine. *British Medical Journal*. **323**: 1314.

67 Quine L (2002) Workplace bullying in junior doctors: questionnaire survey. *British Medical Journal*. **324**: 878–9.

68 Wall DW, Woodward D, Whitehouse A *et al*. (2001) The development and uses of a computerised evaluation tool for SHO posts in the West Midlands Region. *Medical Teacher*. **23**: 24–8.

69 Roff S, McAleer S, Harden RM *et al*. (1997) Development and validation of the Dundee Ready Educational environment Measure (DREEM). *Medical Teacher*. **19**: 295–9.

70 Roff S, McAleer S and Skinner A (2005) Development and validation of an instrument to measure the postgraduate clinical learning environment for hospital based junior doctors in the UK. *Medical Teacher*. **27**: 326–31.

71 Holt M and Roff S (2004) Development and validation of the Anaesthetic Theatre Educational Environment Measure (ATEEM). *Medical Teacher*. **26**: 553–8.

72 Cassar K (2004) Development of an instrument to measure the surgical operating theatre learning environment as perceived by basic surgical trainees. *Medical Teacher*. **26**: 260–4.

73 Nagraj S, Wall D and Jones E (2006) Can STEEM be used to measure the educational environment within the operating theatre for undergraduate medical students? *Medical Teacher*. **28**: 642–7.

Further Reading

Here are some texts I have found useful, both as reference guides and for further information on a day-to-day basis.

BERA (2004) *Revised Ethical Guidelines for Educational Research (2004)*. British Educational Research Association, Southwell. (http://www.bera.ac.uk/files/guidelines/ethical.pdf; accessed 1 December 2006.)

Bowling A (1997) *Research Methods in Health*. Open University Press, Buckingham.

Brennan RL (2001) *Generalizability Theory*. Springer, New York.

Cohen L, Manion L and Morrison K (2000) *Research Methods in Education* (5e). RoutledgeFalmer, London.

Cramer D (2003) *Advanced Quantitative Data Analysis*. Open University Press, Maidenhead.

Dent JA and Harden RM (2005) *A Practical Guide for Medical Teachers* (2e). Elsevier Churchill Livingstone, Edinburgh.

Edwards A and Talbot R (1999) *The Hard-Pressed Researcher* (2e). Pearson Education, Harlow.

Field A (2004) *Discovering Statistics Using SPSS for Windows* (2e). Sage Publications, London.

George J and Cowan J (1999) *A Handbook of Techniques for Formative Evaluation*. Kogan Page, London.

Haig A and Dozier M (2003) BEME guide no. 3: systematic searching for evidence in medical education. Part 1: sources of information. *Medical Teacher*. **25**: 352–63.

Haig A and Dozier M (2003) BEME guide no. 3: systematic searching for evidence in medical education. Part 2: constructing searches. *Medical Teacher*. **25**: 463–84.

Howitt D and Cramer D (2003) *A Guide to Computing Statistics with SPSS 11 for Windows*. Pearson Education, Harlow.

Oppenheim AN (1992) *Questionnaire Design, Interviewing and Attitude Measurement*. Continuum, London.

Pell G (2005) Use and abuse of Likert scales. *Medical Education*. **39**: 970.

Pereira Gray DJ (1982) *Training for General Practice*. MacDonald and Evans, Plymouth.

Shavelson RJ and Webb NM (1991) *Generalizability Theory – a primer*. Sage Publications, London.

Selection for medical education and training

Fiona Patterson and Eamonn Ferguson

KEY MESSAGES

- Assessment for selection is significantly different from that in end point examinations.
- There is relatively little research investigating selection for medical education and training other than the prediction of exam performance.
- Best practice selection involves a thorough job analysis and the use of evidence from validation studies to continually improve accuracy and fairness.

- Establishing the predictive validity of a selection method can present many conceptual and practical problems. The validation process may take several years, and piloting is essential.
- At postgraduate level, selection ratios between specialties may differ. This has implications for the design of the selection system.

Introduction

Selecting the wrong person for a job can have serious consequences for an organisation, the employee involved and, perhaps of most importance in medicine, the patient. For many occupational groups, there exists a large body of international research investigating best practice selection. In medicine, there is a significant volume of publications exploring predictors of performance at medical school but little research literature exploring selection for entry into postgraduate training or, indeed, into senior medical appointments. This chapter outlines the key concepts associated with selection processes and the relative accuracy of selection methodologies for medical education and training. It is divided into three broad sections. The first suggests why medicine is a unique occupational context and summarises international perspectives on selection practices, referencing both undergraduate and postgraduate training. The next section introduces the key concepts underpinning selection research, and the third section summarises the evidence on the accuracy of selection methods. Finally, we present some considerations for a future research agenda.

Medicine as a profession

Compared with many other professions, the length of training required to practise as a clinician in any given specialty is long and costly (usually taking more than 15 years from medical school to senior appointments).

Understanding Medical Education: Evidence, Theory and Practice.
Edited by T Swanwick. © 2010 Association for the Study of Medical Education.

When reviewing selection issues within the training pathway, a distinction must be drawn between selection into medical school (*pre-employment*) and that into postgraduate training (*employment*). Importantly, the latter is governed by specific employment law, for which there are also significant international differences.(1,2)

The assessment paradigm in a selection context is different from that in, for example, professional college examinations. In professional examinations, the aim is to assess end-of-training capability, where judgements about an individual's capacity to perform a job with competence are made by trained examiners. In theory, all candidates can pass the assessment. By contrast, in selection settings, if the number of candidates outweighs the number of available posts, then the assessment is geared towards ranking individuals effectively. Potentially, if the competition is very high, competent candidates may not be awarded a post.

Undergraduate and postgraduate 'selection' may have different goals; undergraduate courses select primarily on academic ability, with a focus on passing the course, and postgraduate selection focuses more on job fit. It cannot necessarily be assumed that those with high academic ability alone can be turned into potentially good doctors via medical training; other skills and qualities may need to be present from the start. Although there are several similarities, the parameters for designing and validating a robust selection system and selection tools are different from other assessment settings. Importantly, the criteria used to judge the effectiveness of a selection system are potentially more complex. The core concepts underpinning best practice selection in both medical education and training are reviewed in this chapter.

International Perspectives on Medical Selection

Undergraduate selection

Recently, there has been much scrutiny of medical schools' admission processes, where policies vary internationally. Faced with limited student places and large numbers of applicants, most medical schools have traditionally relied on academic criteria in admission procedures. Almost universally, high academic achievement is a minimum entry requirement. This assumes that with good academic ability, other skills required to be a good doctor are then trainable. However, researchers recognise that future clinicians should be selected on criteria other than solely academic performance.(3–5) Conceptually, a key question is whether medical schools should aim to select for individuals who will make successful students, or should the focus be on selecting those who will make competent clinicians.(6) These are not mutually exclusive, and the former is not necessarily a precursor for the latter.

Around the world there is an increasing emphasis on assessing a candidate's personal characteristics (such as communication skills) for admission to medical school.(7) Examples are to be found in guidance from the General Medical Council in the UK, the American Board of Medical Specialties and the Accreditation Council for Graduate Medical Education in the US and CanMEDS 2000 in Canada. In the UK, for example, the majority of applicants are offered a place based on a combination of academic competence and an interview. In the US, Canada and Australia, aptitude tests are used, such as the Medical College Admission Test (MCAT),(8) the Graduate Australian Medical School Admission Test(9) and the Undergraduate Medical and Health Science Admission Test. However, with the possible exception of MCAT, there is relatively little published evidence on the reliability and validity of these tests.(10) Of the research available internationally, current selection practices in medical schools are shown in Boxes 24.1–24.4. Specifically, practice in the US, Canada, Australia and The Netherlands is explored to illustrate the similarities and differences.

Postgraduate selection

Of the limited research available, selection criteria used at postgraduate level varies not only within and between countries but also within and between specialties. In the US, medical students apply for residency positions in postgraduate specialty training through the National Resident Matching Programme.(24) Selection criteria usually comprise performance on the United States Medical Licensing Examination (USMLE), clinical rotation grades, class rank and interviews with faculty members.(25)

In the US, the selection tools used by admission panels have changed in the past 20 years.(26) In the

---

Concern about medical school admission procedures has been raised in the US recently.(11) In 2001, in his address to the Association of Medical Colleges, Cohen criticised the use of undergraduate grade-point averages (GPAs) and Medical College Admission Test (MCAT) scores as the principal method of selecting students. The MCAT is a standardised, multiple-choice examination designed to assess the examinee's problem solving, critical thinking, writing skills, and knowledge of science concepts and principles. Almost all US medical schools require applicants to submit MCAT scores. However, Cohen suggested using 'MCAT scores and GPAs only as threshold measures', or 'beginning the screening with an assessment of personal characteristics and leave the GPAs and MCAT scores till later'. He emphasised: 'admission committees might well find many instances in which truly compelling personal characteristics would trump one or two isolated blemishes in the academic record',(12) highlighting the importance of personal characteristics in the selection of medical students.

In a survey of admissions directors, Mitchell(13) reported that total undergraduate GPA, science GPA, quality of undergraduate institution, letters of evaluation, medical school interviews, involvement in relevant extracurricular activities, MCAT scores, relevant work experience and state of legal residence were all heavily weighted in selection decisions. In a similar study,(14) college GPA, medical school interviews and MCAT scores were established as the three most important variables considered in selecting a candidate for admission to medical school. Several studies(15–17) have shown that measures of academic performance, such as high GPAs and high standardised entrance examination scores, are good predictors of preclinical performance. However, many authors(4,11,15–20) have also argued that evidence for prediction of clinical performance is less compelling, and published evidence of GPA predicting competence as a physician is lacking.

There is substantial evidence that admission panels give considerable weight to information obtained in interviews. Puryear and Lewis(21) found that 61% of 107 medical schools responding to their survey regarded interview data as the most important in selection. Although admission panels appear to place great emphasis on the data obtained through the interview, the range of desirable qualities assessed varies widely. Albanese *et al.*(11) identified as many as 87 different qualities relevant to the practice of medicine. In addition, candidates are generally asked for letters of recommendation. Personal statements are also usually requested. References used in selecting students vary in terms of structure and in the type of instructions given to candidates concerning their choice of referees.

> ### BOX 24.2 Selection practices in medical schools in Canada
>
> Medical schools across Canada have devised various strategies for selecting students from a large number of qualified candidates. Most schools include non-cognitive assessments in their selection processes. Typical admission procedures include an assessment of the applicant's academic achievement and an attempt to assess non-academic qualities such as communication skills, empathy, altruism and reliability.

> ### BOX 24.3 Selection practices in medical schools in Australia
>
> In the past 20 years Australian medical schools have expended great effort in the way they select students. Currently, 10 of the 11 schools use an approach that considers both academic and personal characteristics.(22) Australian medical schools rely on a psychometric template for medical school selection. Often evidence of academic achievement is supplemented with tests of personal characteristics considered important in future doctors. In practice, most admission assessments for the purpose of medical student selection include a structured interview and a battery of aptitude tests such as the Graduate Australian Medical Schools Admission Test (GMSAT) or the Undergraduate Medicine and Health Sciences Admissions Test. Selection for medical schools with graduate-entry programmes is based on a combination of results from the applicant's undergraduate degree, a semi-structured interview and a psychometric test (the GMSAT).

> ### BOX 24.4 Selection practices in medical schools in the Netherlands
>
> Prior to 1999, medical students in the Netherlands were allocated to one of the eight medical schools by a national lottery procedure, which considered the students' high school subject report and grade-point average (GPA) and their preference for a particular medical school.(19) In 1999, the Dutch Higher Education and Scientific Research Act was changed in connection with the admission of students to university studies such as medicine.(23) With the new Act, a weighted lottery was introduced: candidates with pre-university GPAs ≥8 (1 = poor, 10 = excellent) are given unrestricted access; medical schools are allowed to develop local selection procedures for up to 50% of the number of students to be admitted. Following the Dutch government's request that medical schools experiment with qualitative selection procedures, a number of universities have piloted and tested new selection processes.

1970s, a survey of residency programme directors showed the interview to be the most important selection method.(27) Additional information used included the dean's letter, other letters of recommendation and honour grades in clinical clerkships. Scores on the national board examination and membership in Alpha Omega Alpha Honor Medical Society were given less consideration in selection. In a survey of programme directors conducted in the 1980s,(28) the interview was considered the most important criterion for selection. However, 46% of the directors indicated that evidence for academic achievement was essential for the candidate to be admitted to interview. In addition, 86% declared they would not consider a candidate who had failed part 1 of the national board examination and had not passed it prior to interview.

More recent studies show measures of academic performance, such as honours in the rotation of the chosen specialty or scores on USMLE Step I, are given substantial weight in both primary care and non-primary care residencies.(29–33) Emphasis on indicators of academic success is more pronounced in more competitive specialties, such as surgery.(31–33) Awareness that dean's letters and other letters of recommendation do not always contain 'valid' information has led many programme directors to place less emphasis on data gathered from References 33 and 34. In the US, Crane and Ferraro(30) investigated selection criteria used by emergency medical residency committees. Results showed that in order of reported importance, the interview was seen as the most important followed by clinical grades and recommendations. Moderately important determinants of candidates' eligibility for training included:

- elective completed at the programme director institution
- USMLE Step II
- interest expressed in programme director institution
- USMLE Step I
- awards/achievements.

In Canada, selection for admission to the various training programmes is made primarily on the basis of scholastic, personal and professional attributes, as determined by academic records, personal interviews, letters of reference, choice of electives and in-training evaluation reports. The selection process is determined by each particular training programme, and admission to the postgraduate training year 1 for most programmes is conducted through a matching system.(2)

The Selection Process: Design, Evaluation and Research

Design
The main elements in the design and implementation of a selection process are outlined in Figure 24.1. The process starts by conducting a thorough analysis of the

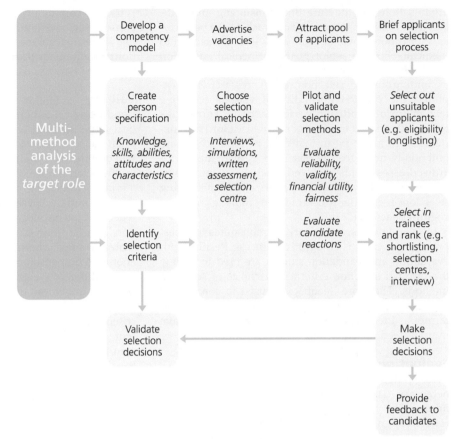

Figure 24.1 The selection process.

relevant knowledge, skills, abilities and attitudes associated with performance in the target role. This information is used to construct a person specification (and job description where appropriate). This is used to decide which selection instruments are best used to elicit applicant behaviour related to the selection criteria. In deciding to apply for a post (or a place at medical school), applicants will engage in *self-selection*, where they can make an informed judgement about whether the particular role suits their skills and abilities.

This in-depth analysis is the cornerstone to producing an effective selection process because the aim is to accurately identify appropriate selection criteria. In job analysis studies, researchers use various methods, such as direct observation and interviews with job holders and job incumbents.(35) Having defined these criteria at a level appropriate for the career stage (e.g. entry to specialty training), this information is used to guide choice of selection methods. Outputs from this analysis should detail the responsibilities in the target job and also provide information about the particular competencies and characteristics required of the job holder.

Once selection decisions are made and the accepted applicants enter training, information on the performance of trainees related to the original selection criteria

should be used to examine the predictive validity of the selection instruments (i.e. to what extent are scores at selection associated with assessment of in-training and work performance?).

Figure 24.1 also shows that best practice selection is a 'two-way' selection process. In other words, to attract the best trainees, both medical schools and hospitals have become increasingly aware that evaluating candidates' reactions to the selection process is essential, particularly in relation to perceptions of fairness. Since large resources are often spent on selection procedures, the utility should be evaluated. In addition, information collected at selection (i.e. entry point to training) can be used to design tailored development plans for trainees.

The basis for best practice selection is clear, and yet research shows that there are two core elements in the process that are often not conducted effectively. First, many organisations fail to conduct a thorough job analysis to precisely identify the key knowledge, skills and behaviours associated with competent performance in the target job role (and potentially these should be incorporated into undergraduate selection processes). This is particularly important when exploring potential differences between medical specialties. Second, validation studies are rarely conducted in organisations, as they are time-consuming and difficult to administer. It often means tracking the performance of trainees over several years – from selection to medical school to senior posts. In medical education and training, far more validation research has occurred in undergraduate selection. Here, research has explored the predictive validity of various cognitive factors (prior academic performance or knowledge tests) with respect to exam performance.(36) The criteria used to judge performance at medical school are potentially more readily observed as there are standardised assessments involved, such as examinations. By contrast, literature is sparse when considering selection for either postgraduate training or noncognitive factors.(36)

In overview, research clearly demonstrates that best practice selection is an iterative process. Results from evaluation and validation studies are used to review the original selection criteria and choice of selection methods. Therefore, feedback is used to continually improve selection systems to enhance accuracy and fairness. Ideally, a selection system should have mutual 'feed forward' and feedback connections.

Evaluation

Before judging how well selection methods work, it is necessary to understand the framework used for determining best practice. Box 24.5 lists 12 evaluative criteria for judging the 'quality' of selection procedures. This should be reviewed when designing and implementing any selection system.

When choosing the selection method, it is important that it is consistent/stable (*reliable*), relevant/precise/accurate (*valid*), *objective*, *standardised*, administered by trained professionals) and monitored. Evaluation of the system is essential to ensure that selection tools are also *fair*, *defensible*, *cost-effective* and *feasible*. Feedback

is used to continually improve the selection system to enhance accuracy and fairness. For postgraduate training, there are legal reasons for ensuring accurate selection procedures are used; this is essential for compliance with employment law.

Validity

Conducting validation studies is very complex in practical terms because researchers rarely use one single predictor to make selection decisions, and applicants will be judged on multiple selection criteria. Given the multifaceted nature of the role of a doctor, recruiters are likely to design multiple selection tools to assess these criteria. Therefore, recruiters must decide whether a job applicant must score highly on all selection criteria (non-compensatory) or whether high scores on some criteria can make up for low scores on another (compensatory). In practice, recruiters might assign different weightings to various selection criteria, depending on the nature of the job role. For example, if clinical knowledge is the most important criterion and an applicant does not achieve a certain score, he or she may not be considered further.

In theory, the way to collect criterion-related validity data (i.e. how well do scores on the selection measure predict some future outcome or criterion) is to use a predictive (or follow-up) design. This design involves collecting predictor information (e.g. interview ratings, test scores) for candidates and then following up (e.g. during their first year of employment or exams at medical school) to gather data on their performance. Predictive validity is assessed by examining the correlation between scores at selection (Time 1) and criterion data collected at Time 2 (perhaps through relevant work-based assessments, examinations, etc.). Research shows it is unusual in field studies to obtain validity coefficients greater than $r = 0.5$.(37) Validity coefficients of considerably less than +1.0 can provide a basis for improved selection practices.(38)

Conducting validation studies in practice presents a variety of problems. One major problem is with regard to accessing the appropriate criterion (outcome) data to validate the selection process. Often, the criteria used to measure performance in the job role do not match the criteria used for selection. Conversely, sometimes the criterion and predictor are very similar (e.g. using the MCAT or other knowledge-based tests to predict exam performance in medical school), which may lead to problems of common method variance and content overlap. Ideally, predictor scores should not be used to take selection decisions until after a predictive validation study has been conducted. Practically, this is difficult to achieve, and so piloting is essential to conduct an appropriate validation. Box 24.6 highlights three sources of error that are important to consider when conducting validation

---

BOX 24.5 Evaluative criteria for selection procedures

1 Reliability and validity of selection tools
2 Candidate/applicant reactions
3 Ease of interpretation
4 Generality of use
5 Cost
6 Practicality/administrative convenience
7 Legality
8 Availability of analytical expertise
9 Fairness
10 Educational impact
11 Mechanisms for obtaining feedback
12 Arrangements for ongoing evaluation and development

BOX 24.6 Focus on: Sources of error in validation studies

1 Sampling error
If relatively small samples are used in many validation studies, the results obtained may be unduly influenced by the effects of small numbers of people within the sample whose results may be unusual. As sample size increases, more reliable results are obtained.

2 Poor measurement precision
The measurement of attributes at both the predictor (i.e. selection method) and the (i.e. job performance) stage of the validation process is subject to unsystematic error. This error (unreliability) in the scores obtained will reduce the ceiling for the observed correlation between predictor and criterion: the error is unsystematic and random; thus this element of the predictor or criterion score will not correlate systematically with anything. This means that as reliability decreases, the maximum possible correlation between predictor and criterion will decrease.

3 Restricted range of scores
The sample of people used in a validation study may not provide the full theoretically possible range of scores on the predictor and/or criterion measures. A restricted range of scores has a straightforward statistical effect on limiting the size of the linear correlation between two variables. So, like unreliability, range restriction in a sample serves to reduce the magnitude of the observed correlation coefficient.

studies in selection, including sampling, measurement precision and restriction of range issues.

Any single validation study is unlikely to provide a definitive answer regarding the validity of any selection method. This is because any particular study can be conducted on only a sample of relevant people and, of course, has to be conducted at a particular time using particular measures. There are likely to be specific factors, such as the sampling, the measures and the timing of the study, that influence the results in some way. To estimate the validity of a particular selection procedure, more than one study design is needed to minimise error. Most selection systems combine several predictors (selection tools), such as an applicant's score on an interview and academic achievements.

In validation studies, a key question is how much adding another predictor increases the predictive power of the selection process. This is known as *incremental validity*. Specifically, recruiters want to know how accuracy is improved as a result of using a personality test (rather than relying solely on interview

scores). Information on the incremental validity of a specific selection tool is extremely valuable as it allows organisations to conduct a cost–benefit analysis of using additional tools. Types of validity are discussed in more depth in Chapter 14.

Candidate reactions
Of crucial importance in selection design are the *candidates' reactions* to different methods.(39) Considerable research has attempted to determine applicants' views on selection methods. Research has tended to explain the different factors that affect applicant reactions, using theories of *organisational justice*.

Distributive justice focuses on perceived fairness regarding equity (where the selection outcome is consistent with the applicant's expectation) and equality (the extent to which applicants have the same opportunities in the selection process). *Procedural justice* refers to the formal characteristics of the selection process, such as information and feedback offered, job relatedness of the procedures and methods, and recruiter effectiveness.(40) Four main factors seem to account for positive or negative applicant reactions where selection methods are:
* based on a thorough job analysis and appear more job relevant
* less personally intrusive
* do not contravene procedural or distributive justice expectations
* allow applicants to meet in person with the recruiters.

Other literature shows that applicants prefer multiple opportunities to demonstrate their skills (as in selection centres), and prefer selection systems that are administered consistently for all applicants. In particular, when competition ratios are high, applicant reactions and candidate expectations of 'fair play' are crucial.

Fairness
Fair selection and recruitment is based on:
* having objective and valid criteria (developed through an appropriate job analysis)
* accurate and standardised assessment by trained personnel
* monitored outcomes.

Research has explored the extent to which selection procedures are fair to different subgroups of the population (such as ethnic minorities and women). First, it is clear that a test is not unfair or biased simply because members of different subgroups obtain different scores on the tests. Men and women have different mean scores for height; this does not mean that rulers are unfair measuring instruments. However, it would be unfair to use height as a selection criterion for a job if the job could be done by people of any height since it is important for selection criteria to be job related.

Normally, of course, the extent to which a selection method is related to job performance can be estimated by validation research, and it is clear, therefore, that fairness and validity are closely related.

Selection ratios

Clearly, when the selection ratio is greater than 1 (i.e. there are more available jobs than applicants), the use of any selection procedure is likely to be of relatively little benefit. In this situation, an organisation must specify the minimal level of competence required of those applicants suitable for the post.

Clearly, an employing institution would not accept everyone who applies for a post. Even with a selection ratio of more than 1, stringent selection criteria must be applied, and there must be the potential to leave posts unfilled rather than recruit totally unsuitable candidates. When the selection ratio is less than 1 (i.e. more applicants than jobs), the choice of selection methods becomes very important. Consider the situation for two different selection ratios. If the selection ratio is 0.7 (i.e. seven jobs for every 10 applicants), the organisation can afford to refuse jobs to candidates with 30% of the lowest scores on the predictor. If, however, the selection ratio is 0.4, the bottom 60% of applicants can be rejected, and the group of applicants selected will have a much higher score. This illustrates how 'cut scores' in selection differ from standard-setting procedures in clinical examinations, for example.

Selection Methods

Many different selection methods have been reviewed by researchers in several different occupational groups.(41–43) Although some of these methods have been piloted for selection into medicine, the interview tends to be the most common method used for both undergraduate and postgraduate selection. Each of the methods is now reviewed in turn.

Interviews

Interviews are ubiquitous in the selection process in a variety of professions.(41) Interviews are used at different stages of the selection process, either as the sole method of selection or in conjunction with other methods. Interviews vary in terms of:

- purpose
- duration
- medium used to conduct the interview (telephone, face to face, video conference)
- number of interviewers (one to one, panel)
- degree of structure (unstructured, structured).

Research consistently shows that structured interviews (when based on thorough role analysis) with validated scoring criteria tend to have much higher criterion-related validity than unstructured inter-

---

> ### BOX 24.7 How to: Run a structured interview
>
> - Questions are directly related to the person specification, which is based on a thorough job analysis.
> - Ask the same questions of each candidate, limit prompting, use follow-up and probing questions to elicit evidence.
> - Use relevant questions and design as either situational, competency-based, biographical or knowledge questions.
> - Use longer interviews or a larger number of questions, control the input of ancillary information.
> - Do not allow questions from the candidate until after the interview (when the information to make selection decisions has been collected).
> - Rate each answer and use standardised rating scales (increase specificity).
> - Use detailed anchored rating scales and take detailed notes.
> - Use multiple interviewers where possible (but ensure efficiency).
> - Provide extensive interviewer training to enhance reliability.

views.(44–47) Box 24.7 provides a brief guide to structured interviewing.

Meta-analytical studies (i.e. identifying generalisable effects by statistically combining results from a number of studies) have found that structured interviews are valid predictors of job performance.(46,48) Evidence also suggests that structured interviews have incremental validity over cognitive ability tests(49,50) and that they generally yield smaller ethnic group differences.(51,52) Adding structure to an interview may also increase the chances of an organisation successfully defending a lawsuit.(53)

Unfortunately, unstructured interviews are still widely used for selection in a variety of industries, despite their low reliability and predictive validity, and thus their lack of legal defensibility in numerous countries.(1,54,55) Unstructured interviews are prone to potential biases and errors, including:

- stereotyping
- first impressions (e.g. making a judgement solely on first impressions – 'I know if they are the right person immediately' – rather than allowing the candidates a chance to demonstrate their skills)
- halo and horns effects (e.g. selectors are unduly influenced by one positive or negative characteristic of the applicant)
- leniency.

All of these are likely to distort ratings of candidates. (56)

References

Large-scale empirical studies consistently show that references tend to be unreliable and ineffective at predicting job performance.(57–59) Despite these rather pessimistic findings, references are widely used for selection in a variety of occupations, including medicine, and it is likely that they will continue to be used as an additional guide to the selection process.(60,61) In practice, employers tend to value references, but often ratings tend to be poor at differentiating between candidates fairly. Anecdotally, low scores on reference reports can be informative, and further research is warranted in this area.

In the UK, references for undergraduate applicants are used. However, the reliability is often questionable given recent changes in data legislation that remove the confidentiality that existed previously.(4) In studying predictive validity, Ferguson *et al.*(58) showed that references obtained through the University and Colleges Admissions Service (UCAS – the central organisation that processes applications for full-time undergraduate courses at UK universities and colleges) did not predict preclinical and clinical performances. However, medical schools differ in terms of the weight they place on references obtained through the UCAS application.(62)

Application forms

To 'shortlist' candidates, application forms are often used as an alternative to curriculum vitae. The information obtained through application forms is collected systematically, making it easier for employers to make an objective assessment of the candidates' suitability for a given post and compare across applicants.(63) Application forms may include questions on biographical information, educational background, previous work experience and competencies identified through a job analysis. Application forms are a crucial part of the selection process, and the quality of information obtained varies according to the design of the form. Research shows that structured application forms can provide valid information on a candidate as long as they are based on appropriate selection criteria obtained through a job analysis.

Academic record

Academic criteria are a major component of selection to medical school in several countries. Traditionally, in the UK, for example, selection for admission to medical school is based on predicted or actual A-level results (a school-end examination designed to assess knowledge in various chosen subjects). One problem associated with using A-level grades for selection is in discriminating among students who obtain similarly high A-level results.(64) One concern is that entry into medical school is socially exclusive, partly because A-level results might reflect type of schooling and 'social class'.(65) In the US and Canada, students apply to medical school at postgraduate level (graduate entry). However, academic grades, such as the GPA, remain the main criterion for selection, although they are usually considered in combination with other predictors, such as the MCAT.

Some authors have shown that academic criteria such as A-level grades correlate with dropout rates, career progression, postgraduate membership and fellowship exams.(36,66–70) These findings are in contrast with earlier studies that questioned the long-term predictive validity of academic ratings.(5) While pre-admission academic grades, such as A levels or GPAs, are undoubtedly related to academic performance at medical school, their relationship with long-term outcome measures of a doctor's performance is less obvious, partly because of the 'criterion problem' discussed earlier.(63,68)

General mental ability and aptitude tests

Tests of *general mental ability* (GMA) and tests of specific cognitive abilities (e.g. numerical, verbal, spatial) are increasingly popular in selection procedures both in the US and the UK.(37,61,71) Internationally, GMA and cognitive ability tests are robust predictors of job performance and training success across a wide range of occupations.(72,73) However, there are concerns regarding fairness because GMA tests can produce adverse impact, with marked racial differences in test performance.(74–76) Specific ability tests tend to show smaller group differences.(75)

Aptitude tests are typically defined as standardised tests designed to measure a person's ability to develop skills or acquire knowledge. They are used to predict future performance in a given activity.(77) Like tests of GMA, aptitude tests measure an individual's overall performance across a broad range of mental abilities. In addition, aptitude tests also often include items that measure more specialised abilities, such as verbal and numerical skills, which predict academic, training or job performance.

Aptitude tests that include specific ability tests and a knowledge component are increasingly popular in medicine. In the UK, concerns over the discriminatory power of A levels led to the introduction of additional selection methods, such as specific medical knowledge tests(62) and intellectual aptitude tests (e.g. the Oxford Medicine Admission test). The use of aptitude tests for medical school selection is increasing in several countries.(64) The outlook is somewhat different at postgraduate level, where aptitude tests are rarely, if at all, used. This is not surprising given that most applicants, in the US particularly, have already passed an aptitude test for entry into medical school, and there is a danger of obtaining redundant information. At this stage, arguably, cognitive ability is a necessary but not a sufficient condition for predicting who will be a competent physician.

In a selection context, especially with respect to widening access, it is important to assess GMA in terms of *crystallised* intelligence (i.e. knowledge based, acquired via schooling) and fluid intelligence (i.e. biologically based cognitive skills, such as processing speed and inductive reasoning).(78,79) It has been argued that tests of *fluid* intelligence should be used to select candidates for medical school to widen access, i.e. to identify 'raw talent' independent of education. There are, however, various problems with this approach. Research shows that most tests of 'intelligence' assess fluid intelligence(79) and that knowledge-based measures may be better predictors of exam performance.(64) In addition, assuming it is possible to assess raw talent, unless this is combined with an assessment of the desire to study medicine and the other necessary non-cognitive skills (as determined by a job analysis), a student may fail, drop out or underperform at medical school.

Personality inventories

The past 20 years have seen a substantial increase in the use of personality and related tests in personnel selection for a broad spectrum of jobs.(80) Over many decades of research, personality researchers have agreed on a general taxonomy of personality traits – the Big Five model, which is based on five factors or traits:

- extraversion (i.e. outgoing, sociable, impulsive)
- emotional stability (i.e. calm, relaxed)
- agreeableness (i.e. trusting, cooperative, helpful)
- conscientiousness (i.e. hardworking, dutiful, organised)
- openness to experience (i.e. artistic, cultured, creative).

Some research has shown that important relationships exist between measures of personality and job or academic performance.(80) Conscientiousness has been shown to be a positive predictor of preclinical medical school exam results(58,81,82) and shows incremental validity over knowledge-based assessments.(58,82) However, the use of personality tests to assess characteristics of job applicants remains controversial. Critics argue that the predictive validity of personality traits for job performance is often low and badly understood.(83) Furthermore, personality tests used by organisations are often poorly chosen,(84) and 'faking' can compromise the validity of personality tests.(85–87) However, there is also evidence to suggest that faking or responding in a socially desirable way does not compromise the predictive validity of personality tests.(88,89)

In medicine, concerns over the strong reliance on academic predictors have led to the search for alternative selection methods. Specifically, there is a growing interest in the role of personality tests in selection at the undergraduate level. A new psychometric test,

the Personal Quality Assessment, is being piloted for use in medical school selection in Australia and Scotland.(65) Best practice is to use personality assessment to drive a more focused questioning at interviews, where psychometric measures of this nature should not be used in isolation to make a selection decision.

Selection centres

A selection centre is a selection *method*, not a *place*. Selection centres, often called assessment centres, involve a combination of selection techniques, such as written exercises, interviews and work simulations, to assess candidates across a number of key skills, attitudes and behaviours (e.g. empathy) required for the job, as identified in the job analysis. Candidates are usually assessed in groups or individually by multiple assessors. The selection centre is different from an Objective Structured Clinical Examination (OSCE). In an OSCE, each station assesses a candidate on *one* key skill and is usually observed by one assessor. By contrast, the selection centre allows the candidate *multiple* situations (interview, work simulation, written exercise, etc.) in which to demonstrate a key skill and to be observed by a number of trained assessors. Thus, a fairer (multiple opportunities to perform) and more reliable (multiple observations of key behaviours by multiple observers) assessment can be made. With careful design, the increased reliability should equate to greater validity (maximum validity is a function of reliability – a test cannot be valid if it is not reliable) and more positive candidate reactions (*see* Box 24.8).

Selection centres were first used during the Second World War to select military personnel. However, it was not until the American company AT&T used selection centres to identify industrial managerial potential in the 1950s that the idea developed as a selection method. Since then, selection centres have become widely used as a tool for recruitment.(90) Selection centres are especially popular for graduate recruitment, with the IRS estimating that over half of recruiters and over 95% of large organisations employing more than 10 000 individuals use selection centres for graduate recruitment.(91) However, it is only recently that this approach has been used in medicine.(92) In the UK, Patterson *et al.* have pioneered the use of selection centres, initially used to select general practitioners. The results have shown good predictive validity.(35,93) This work has been extended to select doctors for postgraduate training in other specialties, such as obstetrics and gynaecology and paediatrics.(94,95) The design process followed a thorough multi-method job analysis study of the target specialty. Patterson *et al.* have also piloted the use of selection centres in the UK for graduate entry to medical school, in addition to other academic assessments.(96)

BOX 24.8 Where's the evidence: Predictive validity, acceptability and use of
selection method

Selection method	Evidence for criterion-related validity	Applicant reactions	Extent of use
Structured reviews	High	Moderate to positive	High
Cognitive ability	High	Negative to moderate	Moderate
Personality tests	Moderate	Negative to moderate	Moderate
Work sample tests	High	Positive	Low
Selection centres	High	Positive	Moderate
Handwriting	Low	Negative to moderate	Low
References	Low	Positive	High

Research shows that a carefully designed and well-run selection centre can be highly effective at predicting job performance across a wide range of occupations.(50,97–99) As described above, gains are made in reliability and validity because selection centres use a combination of different exercises (using a multi-trait, multi-method approach), and standardised scoring systems to measure the selection criteria. Scoring should be directly linked to the selection criteria (not the exercise scores) and the information gathered should be interpreted in context by appropriately trained assessors. Unfortunately, few understand this fundamental difference between OSCE-style examinations and selection centres, in a selection context (see earlier). Well-executed selection centres have incremental validity over cognitive ability tests,(100–102) and they tend to be viewed positively by candidates.(103,104) Careful design and implementation of a selection centre is crucial for the assessment to live up to its reputation and be cost-effective.(105,106)

Box 24.8 summarises the research evidence on the predictive validity of different selection tools. The evidence on each of the techniques listed also includes an estimate of extent of usage across all occupational groups, and likely applicant reactions to each. Note that there are international differences in the extent of usage for various techniques, which is also governed by international differences in employment law.

Recommendations for Future Research

In medicine, selection is a relatively new research topic, and there are many uncharted territories for exploration. The discipline of medicine is changing dramatically, and thus the skills relevant to many specialties are changing rapidly. For example, in surgery, the use of laproscopes and other technologies has transformed many surgical procedures. With international developments in technology and new treatment regimens, it is likely that the pace of change will increase in the future. As a result, since the career path for a physician is long and complex, defining appropriate selection criteria that are associated with the physicians of the future is difficult. In many countries, the enhanced focus on patient satisfaction has highlighted the requirement for empathy and communication skills, for example, where physicians work in partnership with patients. In this way, given that medicine involves a highly specialised career path, the demands on individuals entering a career in medicine are potentially high.

The selection gateways to progressing on the medical training pathway should be preceded by accurate career information for individuals. The process of self-selection is crucially important, and further research is clearly warranted in this area. When exploring selection literature, it is notable that very little exists at more senior-level appointments. Future research must address this area, particularly at the consultant level, where competencies required may also include leadership of teams, resource management and political awareness, among others.

More research is needed in the area of candidate reactions with respect to medical education and training. What combination of selection tests are seen as fair and valid by candidates? What is the effect of candidate reactions (emotional, anxiety, perceived justice and fairness) on test performance and test validity? While there is growing research literature on these topics in other professions,(39,107) it has not been explored within medicine.

Future research should explore how a selection system is best designed across the whole training pathway. There may be generic skills required across all specialties (i.e. the basic skills for being a doctor, including cognitive, non-cognitive and behavioural skills). These should guide the design of selection criteria used to recruit to undergraduate medical courses at the outset of training. It should not be assumed that one part of the medical career path (e.g. undergraduate to initial specialty training) should fully prepare an applicant with all the skills to progress from one stage to the next (e.g. from specialty training to senior appointments), especially if candidates are not selected to have the core aptitude at the outset. Indeed, a selection centre approach could be adopted for undergraduate selection, in addition to academic assessments, to address this issue.

Designing an accurate selection system is a complex process. It should be acknowledged that medical education and training is a continual process and that the predictive validity of selection tests may vary depending on the stage in the career pathway. In other words, a factor may be identified as an important predictor for undergraduate training but may not be predictive for aspects of specialty training. For example, conscientiousness is a positive predictor for undergraduate preclinical training but a negative predictor for undergraduate clinical performance.(58) Similarly, other evidence shows that openness to experience is important to general practice training performance but is not important for undergraduate training performance. The real challenge is to integrate this knowledge and to develop selection systems that are internally reliable from undergraduate selection to selection for specialty training.

Future research must account for contemporary theoretical models of adult intellectual development and skill acquisition, which attempt to integrate cognitive and non-cognitive factors. One such model is PPIK theory,(108) which asserts that adult intellectual ability is a function of process (basic mental capacities such as processing speed), personality (e.g. extraversion, conscientiousness), interests (e.g. preferences for science or art) and knowledge (e.g. factual knowledge as contained in A levels). PPIK theory specifically proposes a developmental trajectory to understand adult intellectual functioning, where personality, intellect and interests operate in tandem. For example, the interests that a person may express influence the types of knowledge he or she seeks out. This approach may help us understand what motivates people to study medicine and also their choice and aptitude for a specialty later in training. The idea of trait complexes (overlapping cognitive and non-cognitive traits) should be considered in medical selection.(78,108) Clusters of traits may be identified that overlap to define areas of competence and preference. In future, it may be possible to identify trait complexes that are unique to success in undergraduate medical education and in later specialty training.(82) In summary, there are many opportunities for research in this area. We propose that thorough job analyses, detailed validity studies, issues of organisational justice, the exploration of trait overlaps and the temporal dynamics of training are key topics for a future research agenda in selection to undergraduate and postgraduate medical educations.

References

1 Klehe UC (2004) Choosing how to choose: institutional pressures affecting the adoption of personnel selection procedures. *International Journal of Selection.* **12**: 327–42.

2 Jefferis T (2007) Selection for specialist training: what can we learn from other countries? *British Medical Journal.* **334**: 1302–4.

3 Greengross S (1997) What patients want from their doctors. In: Allen I, Brown P and Hughes P (eds) *Choosing Tomorrow's Doctors,* pp. 12–19. Policy Studies Institute, London.

4 Hughes P (2002) Can we improve on how we select medical students? *Journal of the Royal Society of Medicine.* **95**: 18–22.

5 Reede JY (1999) Predictors of success in medicine. *Clinical Orthopaedics and Related Research.* **362**: 72–7.

6 McManus IC (2003) Commentary: how to derive causes from correlations in educational studies. *British Medical Journal.* **326**: 432.

7 Eva KW and Reiter HI (2005) Reflecting the relative values of community, faculty and students in the admissions tools of medical school. *Teaching and Learning in Medicine.* **17**: 4–8.

8 Wiley A and Koenig JA (1996) The validity of the Medical College Admission Test for predicting performance in the first two years of medical school. *Academic Medicine.* **71**: S83–5.

9 Aldous CJ, Leeder SR, Price J *et al.* (1997) A selection test for Australian graduate-entry medical schools. *Medical Journal of Australia.* **166**: 247–50.

10 Tutton P and Price M (2002) Selection of medical students: affirmative action goes beyond the selection process. *British Medical Journal.* **324**: 1170–1.

11 Albanese MA, Snow MH, Skochelak SE *et al.* (2003) Assessing personal qualities in medical schools admissions. *Academic Medicine.* **78**: 313–21.

12 Cohen J (2001) Facing the future. President's address, 112th Annual Meeting of the Association of American Medical Colleges, 4 November, Washington, DC.

13 Mitchell KJ (1990) Traditional predictors of performance in medical schools. *Academic Medicine.* **65**: 149–58.

14 Arnold DM, Coe RM and Pepper M (1984) Structure and function of medical school admission committees. *Journal of Medical Education.* **59**: 131–2.

15 Kulatunga-Moruzi C and Norman GR (2002) Validity of admission measures in predicting performance outcomes: the contribution of cognitive and non-cognitive dimensions. *Teaching and Learning in Medicine.* **14**: 34–42.

16 Norman G (2004) The morality of medical school admissions. *Advances in Health Sciences Education.* **9**: 79–82.

17 Salvatori P (2001) Reliability and validity of admission tools used to select students for the health professions. *Advances in Health Sciences Education.* **6**: 159–75.

18 Harris S and Owen C (2007) Discerning quality: using the multiple mini-interview in student selection for the Australian National University Medical School. *Medical Education.* **41**: 234–41.

19 Hulsman RL, van der Ende JS, Oort FJ *et al.* (2007) Effectiveness of selection in medical school admissions: evaluation of the outcomes among freshmen. *Medical Education.* **41**: 369–77.

20 Silver B and Hodgson CS (1997) Evaluating GPAs and MCAT scores as predictors of NBME I and clerkship performances based on students' data from one undergraduate institution. *Academic Medicine.* **72**: 394–6.

21 Puryear JB and Lewis LA (1981) Description of the interview process in selecting students for admission to US medical schools. *Journal of Medical Education.* **56**: 881–5.

22 Turnbull D, Buckley P, Robinson JS *et al.* (2003) Increasing the evidence base for selection for undergraduate medicine: four case studies investigating process and interim outcomes. *Medical Education.* **37**: 1115–20.

23 Dutch Ministry of Education, Culture and Science [Dutch Higher Education and Scientific Research Act] (1999) Wet van 3 April 1999 tot wijziging van de Wet op het hoger onderwijs en wetenschappelijk onderzoek, houdende aanpassingen in het systeem van selectie voor opleidingen waarvoor een toelatingsbeperking is vastgesteld. *The Hague.* **170**: 1–8.

24 Miller JB, Schaad DC, Crittenden RA *et al.* (2003) Communication between programs and applicants during residency selection: effects of the match on medical students' professional development. *Academic Medicine.* **78**: 403–11.

25 Bell JG, Kanellitsas I and Shaffer L (2001) Selection of obstetrics and gynecology residents on the basis of medical school performance. *American Journal of Obstetrics and Gynecology.* **186**: 1091–4.

26 Brandenburg S, Kruzick T, Lin CT *et al.* (2005) Residency selection criteria: what medical students perceive as important. *Medical Education Online.* **10**: 1–6.

27 Wagoner NE and Gray GT (1979) Report on a survey of program directors regarding selection factors in graduate medical education. *Journal of Medical Education.* **54**: 445–52.

28 Wagoner NE and Suriano JR (1999) Program directors' responses to a survey on variables used to select residents in a time of change. *Academic Medicine.* **74**: 51–8.

29 Adams LJ, Brandenburg S and Blake M (2000) Factors influencing internal medicine program directors' decisions about applicants. *Academic Medicine.* **75**: 542–3.

30 Crane JT and Ferraro CM (2000) Selection criteria for emergency medicine residency applicants. *Academic Emergency Medicine.* **7**: 54–60.

31 Travis C, Taylor CA and Mayhew HE (1999) Evaluating residency applicants: stable values in a changing market. *Family Medicine.* **31**: 252–6.

32 Villanueva AM, Kaye D, Abdelhak SS and Morahan PS (1995) Comparing selection criteria of residency directors and physicians' employers. *Academic Medicine.* **70**: 261–71.

33 Grantham JR (1993) Radiology resident selection: results of a survey. *Investigative Radiology.* **28**: 99–101.

34 Wagoner NE and Suriano JR (1992) Recommendations for changing the residency selection process based on a survey of program directors. *Academic Medicine.* **67**: 459–64.

35 Patterson F, Ferguson E, Lane PW *et al.* (2000) Competency model for general practice: implications for selection, training and development. *British Journal of General Practice.* **50**: 188–93.

36 Ferguson E, James D and Madeley L (2002) Factors associated with success in medical school: systematic review of the literature. *British Medical Journal.* **324**: 952–7.

37 Salgado JF, Viswesvaran C and Ones D (2001) Predictors used for personnel selection: an overview of constructs, methods, and techniques. In: Anderson N, Ones DS, Sinangil HK and Viswesvaran C (eds) *Handbook of Industrial, Work and Organizational Psychology*, pp. 165–99. Sage, London, New York.

38 Anastasia A and Urbina S (1997) *Psychological Testing* (7e). Prentice Hall, Upper Saddle River, NJ.

39 Hausknecht JP, Day DV and Thomas SC (2004) Applicant reactions to selection procedures: an updated model and meta-analysis. *Personnel Psychology.* **57**: 639–83.

40 Anderson N, Born M and Cunningham-Snell N (2001) Recruitment and selection: applicant perspectives and outcomes. In: Anderson N, Ones DS, Sinangil HK and Viswesvaran C (eds) *Handbook of Industrial, Work and Organizational Psychology*, pp. 200–18. Sage, London, New York.

41 Campion MA, Palmer DK and Campion JE (1997) A review of structure in the selection interview. *Personnel Psychology.* **50**: 655–702.

42 Lievens F and Thornton III GC (2005) Assessment centers: recent developments in practice and research. In: Evers A, Smit-Voskuijl O and Anderson N (eds) *Handbook of Personnel Selection*, pp. 243–64. Blackwell Publishing, Oxford.

43 Salgado JF and Anderson N (2002) Cognitive and GMA testing in the European Community: issues and evidence. *Human Performance.* **15**: 75–96.

44 Campion MA, Pursell ED and Brown BK (1988) Structured interviewing: raising the psychometric properties of the employment interview. *Personnel Psychology.* **41**: 25–42.

45 Goho J and Blackman A (2006) The effectiveness of academic admission interviews: an exploratory meta-analysis. *Medical Teacher.* **28**: 335–40.

46 McDaniel MA, Whetzel DL, Schmidt FL and Maurer S (1994) The validity of employment interviews: a comprehensive review and meta-analysis. *Journalof Applied Psychology.* **79**: 599–615.

47 Wiesner WH and Cronshaw SF (1988) A meta-analytic investigation of the impact of interview format and the degree of structure on the validity of the employment interview. *Journal of Occupational Psychology.* **61**: 275–90.

48 Huffcutt AI and Arthur Jr W (1994) Hunter and Hunter (1984) revisited: interview validity for entry-level jobs. *Journal of Applied Psychology.* **79**: 184–90.

49 Cortina JM, Goldstein NB, Payne SC *et al.* (2000) The incremental validity of interview scores over and above cognitive ability and conscientiousness scores. *Personnel Psychology.* **53**: 325–51.

50 Schmidt FL and Hunter JE (1998) The validity and utility of selection methods in personnel psychology: practical and theoretical implications of 85 years of research findings. *Psychological Bulletin.* **124**: 262–74.

51 Bobko P, Roth PL and Potosky D (1999) Derivation and implications of meta-analytic matrix incorporating cognitive ability, alternative predictors and job performance. *Personnel Psychology.* **52**: 561–89.

52 Huffcutt AI and Roth PL (1998) Racial group differences in employment interview evaluations. *Journal of Applied Psychology.* **83**: 179–89.

53 Posthuma RA, Morgeson FP and Campion MA (2002) Beyond employment interview validity: a comprehensive narrative review of recent research and trends over time. *Personnel Psychology.* **55**: 1–81.

54 Terpstra DE, Mohamed AA and Kethley RB (1999) An analysis of federal court cases involving nine selection devices. *International Journal of Selection and Assessment.* **7**: 26–34.

55 Williamson LG, Campion JE, Malos SB *et al.* (1997) Employment interview on trial: linking interview structure with litigation outcomes. *Journal of Applied Psychology.* **82**: 900–12.

56 Edwards JC, Johnson EK and Molidor JB (1990) The interview in the admission process. *Academic Medicine.* **65**: 167–77.

57 McCarthy JM and Goffin RD (2001) Improving the validity of letters of recommendation: an investigation of three standardized reference forms. *Military Psychology.* **13**: 199–222.

58 Ferguson E, James D, O'Hehir F and Sanders A (2003) A pilot study of the roles of personality, references and personal statements in relation to performance over the 5 years of a medical degree. *British Medical Journal.* **326**: 429–31.

59 Muchinsky PM (1979) The use of reference reports in personnel selection: a review and evaluation. *Journal of Occupational Psychology.* **52**: 287–97.

60 IRS Employment Review (2002) Of good character: supplying references and providing access. *IRS Employment Review.* **754**: 34–6.

61 Ryan AM, McFarland L, Baron H and Page R (1999) An international look at selection practices: nation and culture as explanations for variability in practice. *Personnel Psychology.* **52**: 359–93.

62 Parry JM, Mathers JM, Stevens AJ *et al.* (2006) Admissions processes for five year medical courses at English schools: review. *British Medical Journal.* **332**: 1005–9.

63 British Medical Association Board of Medical Education (2006) Selection for specialty training (http://www.bma.org. uk/ap.nsf/Content/selectionforspecialtytraining; accessed 23 August 2007).

64 McManus IC, Powis DA, Wakeford R *et al.* (2005) Intellectual aptitude tests and A levels for selecting UK school leaver entrants for medical school. *British Medical Journal.* **331**: 555–9.

65 Nicholson S (2005) The benefits of aptitude testing for selecting medical students. *British Medical Journal.* **331**: 559–60.

66 McManus IC and Richards P (1986) Prospective survey of performance of medical students during preclinical years. *British Medical Journal.* **293**: 124–7.

67 Arulampalam W, Naylor RA and Smith JP (2004) A hazard model of the probability of medical school dropout in the United Kingdom. *Journal of the Royal Statistical Society: Series A (Statistics in Society).* **167**: 157–78.

68 McManus IC (1997) From selection to qualification: how and why medical students change. In: Allen I, Brown P and Hughes P (eds) *Choosing Tomorrow's Doctors*, pp. 60–79. Policy Studies Institute, London.

69 McManus IC, Smithers E, Partridge P *et al.* (2003) A-levels and intelligence as predictors of medical careers in UK doctors: 20-year prospective study. *British Medical Journal.* **327**: 139–42.

70 Lumb AB and Vail A (2004) Comparison of academic, application form and social factors in predicting early performance on the medical course. *Medical Education.* **38**: 1002–5.

71 Hodgkinson GP and Payne RL (1998) Graduate selection in three European countries. *Journal of Occupational and Organizational Psychology.* **71**: 359–65.

72 Bertua C, Anderson N and Salgado JF (2005) The predictive validity of cognitive ability tests: a UK meta-analysis. *Journal of Occupational and Organizational Psychology.* **78**: 387–409.

73 Salgado JF, Anderson N, Moscoso S *et al.* (2003) A meta-analytic study of general mental ability validity for different occupations in the European community. *Journal of Applied Psychology.* **88**: 1068–81.

74 Murphy KR (2002) Can conflicting perspectives on the role of g in personnel selection be resolved? *Human Performance.* **15**: 173–86.

75 Kehoe JF (2002) General mental ability and selection in private sector organizations: a commentary. *Human Performance.* **15**: 97–106.

76 Outtz J (2002) The role of cognitive ability tests in employment selection. *Human Performance.* **15**: 161–71.

77 Cronbach LJ (1984) *Essentials of Psychological Testing* (4e). Harper & Row, New York.

78 Ackerman PL and Heggestad ED (1997) Intelligence, personality, and interests: evidence for overlapping traits. *Psychological Bulletin.* **121**: 219–45.

79 Blair C (2006) How similar are fluid cognition and general intelligence? A developmental neuroscience perspective on fluid cognition as an aspect of human cognitive ability. *Behavioral and Brain Sciences.* **29**: 109–60.

80 Barrick MR, Mount MK and Judge TA (2001) Personality and performance at the beginning of the new millennium: what do we know and where do we go next? *International Journal of Selection and Assessment.* **9**: 9–30.

81 Lievens F, Coetsier P, De Fruyt F and De Maeseneer J (2002) Medical students' personality characteristics and academic performance: a five-factor model perspective. *Medical Education.* **36**: 1050–6.

82 Ferguson E, Sanders A, O'Hehir F and James D (2000) Predictive validity of personal statements and the role of the five factor model of personality in relation to medical training. *Journal of Occupational and Organizational Psychology.* **73**: 321–44.

83 Tett RP, Jackson DN, Rothstein M and Reddon JR (1999) Meta-analysis of bi-directional relations in personality-job performance research. *Human Performance.* **12**: 1–29.

84 Murphy KR and Dzieweczynski JL (2005) Why don't measures of broad dimensions of personality perform better as predictors of job performance? *Human Performance.* **18**: 343–57.

85 Birkeland SA, Manson TM, Kisamore JL *et al.* (2006) A meta-analytic investigation of job applicant faking on personality measures. *International Journal of Selection and Assessment.* **14**: 317–35.

86 Rosse JG, Stecher MD, Miller JL and Levin RA (1998) The impact of response distortion on pre-employment personality testing and hiring decisions. *Journal of Applied Psychology.* **83**: 634–44.

87 Scarpello VG, Ledvinka J and Bergmann TJ (1995) *Human Resource Management, Environments and Functions* (2e). South-Western College Publishing, Cincinnati, OH.

88 Hough LM, Eaton NK, Dunnette MD *et al.* (1990) Criterion related validities of personality constructs and effect of response distortion on those validities. *Journal of Applied Psychology.* **75**: 581–95.

89 Li A and Bagger J (2006) Using the BIDR to distinguish the effects of impression management and self-deception on the criterion validity of personality measures: a meta-analysis. *International Journal of Selection and Assessment.* **14**: 131–41.

90 Chartered Institute of Personnel and Development (2004) *Recruitment, Retention and Turnover 2004: a survey of the UK and Ireland.* CIPD, London.

91 IRS Employment Review (2004) Graduate recruitment 2004/05: upturn and optimism. *IRS Employment Review.* **811**: 40–8.

92 Patterson F, Ferguson E, Lane P and Norfolk T (2001) A new competency based selection system for general practitioners. Paper presented at the 10th International Conference of the International Society for the Study of Individual Differences, Edinburgh, July.

93 Patterson F, Ferguson E, Norfolk T and Lane P (2005) A new selection system to recruit general practice registrars: preliminary findings from a validation study. *British Medical Journal.* **330**: 711–14.

94 Randall R, Davies H, Patterson F and Farrell K (2006) Selecting doctors for postgraduate training in paediatrics using a competency based assessment centre. *Archives of Diseases of Childhood.* **91**: 444–8.

95 Randall R, Stewart P, Farrell K and Patterson F (2006) Using an assessment centre to select doctors for postgraduate training in obstetrics and gynaecology. *The Obstetrician and Gynaecologist.* **8**: 257–62.

96 Kidd J, Fuller J, Patterson F and Carter Y (2006) Selection centres: initial description of a collaborative pilot project. *Proceedings for the Association for Medical Education in Europe (AMEE) Conference*, Genoa, Italy.

97 Damitz M, Manzey D, Kleinmann M and Severin K (2003) Assessment center for pilot selection: construct and criterion validity and the impact of assessor type. *Applied Psychology: An International Review.* **52**: 193–212.

98 Lievens F, Van Keer E and De Witte M (2005) Assessment centers in Belgium: the results of a study on their validity and fairness [French]. *Psychologie du Travail et des Organisations.* **11**: 25–33.

99 Schmitt N, Gooding RZ, Noe RA and Kirsch M (1984) Meta-analyses of validity studies published between 1964 and 1982 and the investigation of study characteristics. *Personnel Psychology.* **37**: 407–22.

100 Dayan,K, Kasten R and Fox S (2002) Entry-level police candidate assessment center: an efficient tool or a hammer to kill a fly? *Personnel Psychology.* **55**: 827–49.

101 Krause DE, Kersting M, Heggestad E and Thornton GC (2006) Incremental validity of assessment center ratings over cognitive ability tests: a study at the executive management level. *International Journal of Selection and Assessment.* **14**: 360–71.

102 Lievens F, Harris MM, Van Keer E and Bisqueret C (2003) Predicting cross-cultural training performance: the validity of personality, cognitive ability, and dimensions measured by an assessment center and a behaviour description interview. *Journal of Applied Psychology.* **88**: 476–89.

103 Macan TH, Avedon MJ, Paese M and Smith DE (1994) The effects of applicants' reactions to cognitive ability tests and an assessment center. *Personnel Psychology.* **47**: 715–38.

104 Rynes SL and Connerley ML (1993) Applicant reactions to alternative selection procedures. *Journal of Business and Psychology.* **7**: 261–77.

105 Woodruffe C (2000) *Development and Assessment Centres: identifying and developing competence.* Institute of Personnel and Development, London.

106 Algera J and Grueter MAM (1989) Job analysis for personnel selection. In: Smith M and Robertson I (eds) *Advances in Selection and Assessment*, pp. 7–30. John Wiley and Sons, Chichester.

107 Skarlicki PD and Folger R (1997) Retaliation in the workplace: the roles of distributive, procedural and interactional justice. *Journal of Applied Psychology.* **82**: 434–43.

108 Ackerman PL (1996) A theory of adult intellectual development: process, personality, interests and knowledge. *Intelligence.* **22**: 227–57.

Further Reading

Ackerman PL (1996) A theory of adult intellectual development: process, personality, interests and knowledge. *Intelligence.* **22**: 227–57.

Arnold J, Silvester J, Patterson F *et al.* (2004) *Work Psychology* (4e). Financial Times: Prentice Hall, London.

Ferguson E, James D and Madeley L (2002) Factors associated with success in medical school: systematic review of the literature. *British Medical Journal.* **324**: 952–7.

Patterson F and Lane P (2007) Assessment for recruitment. In: Jackson N, Jamieson F and Khan A (eds) *Assessment in Medical Education and Training*, pp. 62–73. Radcliffe Publishing, Oxford.

Patterson F, Ferguson E, Norfolk T and Lane P (2005) A new selection system to recruit general practice registrars: preliminary findings from a validation study. *British Medical Journal.* **330**: 711–14.

Patterson F and Rowley D (2007) The right choice: a pilot selection centre to select future surgeons. *Surgeons News.*

Managing remediation

Deborah Cohen, Melody Rhydderch and Ian Cooper

KEY MESSAGES

- The first interview requires careful planning; be sure of your role, ensure you have all the necessary documentation to hand, set objectives and an agenda at the outset.

- Poor performance is a symptom, not a diagnosis. All relevant biopsychosocial factors should be considered.

- Moving into 'action' – providing solutions and fixing problems – too early may lead to disengagement, a loss

of ownership and reduced chance of successfully achieving change.

- There can sometimes be a tendency to continue with sessions when it might be more effective to stand back and allow the doctor to function independently for a while and practise their newly acquired skills, then bring them back for review at a mutually agreed time.

- Keep records to the same standard as clinical notes. They may come back to haunt you.

Introduction

The management of poor performance in doctors poses considerable challenges to both employing organisations and educational bodies. The problem is complex and goes beyond a simple question of *ability*, since personality, motivation and organisational factors all impact on individual performance.(1) Models of performance assessment are now well researched and have evolved with a consistent approach worldwide. Models of remediation, however, do not yet have a consistency of approach. Some examples of good practice do exist,(2–8) but evidence of long-term outcomes is harder to establish.

This chapter aims to provide a practical guide for educational supervisors and others faced with the challenge of remediating poor performance. It provides advice on how to navigate and manage the process of remediating underperformance among doctors and students. It addresses concerns in a qualified doctor; however, the same principles apply to personal tutors managing medical students who are found to be failing. Indeed, the problems discussed and the issues raised as causes of underperformance in doctors also hold true for students.

From Assessment to Remediation

Remediation is an intervention, or suite of interventions, required in response to assessment against

threshold standards of performance. In the UK, there has been an increase in threshold and aspirational standard-setting activity over the past 10 years at a professional level, care pathway level and organisational level. Assessment activity is the mechanism against which individual performance is judged.(9) Historically, the focus of standardised assessment has been targeted to the small minority of doctors whose performance gives substantial rise for concern. In the UK, such doctors were typically referred to the General Medical Council (GMC) and since 2001, the National Clinical Assessment Service (NCAS). However, with the arrival of *Modernising Medical Careers*(10) and *Good Doctors, Safer Patients*,(11) the rise in local routine performance assessments has increased further, paralleled by a decreased tolerance for poor performance. This situation has created a pressing need for educational supervisors to develop their remediation skills in order to respond effectively to the needs of doctors (and indeed students) for whom they are responsible.

To deliver effective remediation, educational supervisors must be sensitive to the assessment process and provide a flexible response. They must be able to offer personalised support and direction to the individual while being sensitive and responsive to the organisation(s) in which they work. The problem may often lie in the organisational structure and culture rather than solely with the individual referred.(12,13) The educational supervisor must also consider health and well-being, alongside personality, motivation to change, and organisational and social issues.(1,14,15) Rising to these challenges is no easy task (Box 25.1).

Perhaps the first and maybe most important task for supervisors is to consider the principles and beliefs that shape their chosen approach to working with

---

Understanding Medical Education: Evidence, Theory and Practice.
Edited by T Swanwick. © 2010 Association for the Study of Medical Education.

BOX 25.1 Focus on: Identifying the doctor in difficulty

The doctor who is struggling has many different faces. Paice describes certain 'early warning signs' of the trainee in difficulty.(17) Some of the attributes she describes include:

- the doctor who is often difficult to find (*The disappearing act*)
- the doctor who is always at work but achieves less than their colleagues (*Low work rate*)
- the doctor who is quick to lose their temper (*Ward rage*)
- the doctor who is inflexible and has difficulty prioritising (*Rigidity*).

Some doctors she describes as displaying problems with their career choice or having difficulty obtaining their required exams (*Career problems*), while others lack insight and reject constructive criticism (*Insight failure*). Finally, there are those who find ways of sidelining the difficult doctor (*Bypass syndrome*).

those doctors who require remediation. What follows are some principles that we believe to be fundamental to successful remediation.

Principles Underpinning Success

Personalised remediation: it's not about a standard prescription

The purpose of personalised remediation is to match provision closely to individual need and to take health, personality and motivation to change into account. This provides a more holistic approach to the problem. Personalised remediation can and should be tailored to different learning styles. Thus educational supervisors need to be aware of the ways in which other disciplines such as occupational health, occupational psychologists and language experts can contribute to remediation. A key skill for educational supervisors is knowing when and how to involve and seek advice from others.

Engagement and motivation: what is in it for me?

Goulet *et al.*'s work on personalised remediation within the Canadian health system suggested that a doctor's motivation may initially be low, but that the involvement of a licensing authority had a positive effect on the doctor's motivation and cooperation.(3) However, while the high stakes may motivate a person to agree to attend for remediation, it is not always enough to stimulate genuine engagement. Using techniques and a process to engage doctors and motivate

them towards change requires careful planning. Our own preferred evidence-based method for behaviour change is based on 'motivational interviewing' techniques.(16) The key message for educational supervisors is to highlight that you can and should access evidence-based methods for engaging and stimulating behaviour change when remediating doctors whose performance gives rise for concern.

Organisational issues: culture eats strategy for breakfast every time

Organisational factors may both trigger and perpetuate individual poor performance. Unsupportive work environments in the form of high work demands, role ambiguity, poor teamworking and punitive cultures can all serve to undermine a doctor striving to maintain newly acquired behaviours. In our experience, there is also a pattern of behaviour among a subset of underperforming doctors that demonstrates a tendency to 'rage against the machine'. This group continues to fight and blame the whole system rather than considering the relevant importance of each battle and indeed which battles are worth fighting. Organisational issues and the ways in which they enhance and inhibit individual performance present one of the greatest challenges for educational supervisors.

Independence: whose side are you on?

Finucane *et al.* have previously argued that performance assessment impacts upon three distinct groups: patients, doctors and employers.(9) He also argued that while these groups may have conflicting beliefs and expectations of assessment, the process must be acceptable for all. We believe that this also applies to remediation. While as an educational supervisor you are embedded in and part of a system, the ability to stand back and evaluate the issues surrounding underperformance and remediation is critical to what can be achieved. Independence is a mechanism for promoting acceptability by all stakeholders.(9) Acceptability by the underperforming doctor is key to them 'trusting and accepting the process'. This is by no means an easy line to tread and pressures to compromise your independence come from all directions. However, a commitment to taking an independent view may ultimately enable you to do the best for all relevant parties.

A key message at this point is that it is all about process. Adopting the correct process for assessing performance, planning remediation and evaluating outcomes is critical, whether you are working with a medical student or a doctor. The importance of adopting a rigorous process when managing underperformers must not be underestimated. Developing an effective process enables an educational supervisor or personal tutor to have confidence that they are doing the right thing for the underperformer, the patients, the service and the training system.

Getting Started

Providing support to a doctor who might be underperforming requires careful consideration. The doctor's career might be at risk and they may often be resentful of the predicament they find themselves in. They may lack insight into the issues raised or have underlying health, personality or social issues that may have precipitated the event. The aim for the educational supervisor is to help guide the individual through what can often be a painful and stressful process.

Identifying resources

Managing underperformance usually requires significant resources in a number of areas if it is to be successful. How those resources are accessed will be dependent on the organisation or organisations involved. The overarching principle, we believe, is to have continuity and careful liaison between all parties to provide the doctor with a flexible yet coherent programme of support. NCAS in its assessment processes recognises the benefit of a multidisciplinary approach with occupational psychologists working closely with occupational health clinicians and the workplace. We suggest that a similar approach is needed to manage remediation, whereby occupational psychology sits alongside occupational health and case management.(18) Thus before embarking on managing underperformance it is worthwhile considering how such services might be accessed.

Planning the first interview

Regardless of the resources available, conducting the first interview is likely to fall to the educational supervisor. The interview requires planning to ensure that all the information is at hand to manage the meeting with confidence. The information the interviewer requires includes a summary of the exact nature of the concern and evidence of significant events or complaints. Outline letters suggesting concern about performance without detail are unhelpful.

The first interview requires careful planning. Be sure of your role, ensure you have all the necessary documentation to hand, structure the interview and set your objectives before starting. Setting the agenda at the outset reduces misunderstandings and the interviewer should aim to cover the presenting problem, factors leading up to the referral, a review of any significant event(s) and relevant past workplace experience.

Exploring the problem

The aim of this first interview should be to develop a picture of the doctor, their views on the problems that have been raised and their understanding of how the problems might have arisen. Giving the doctor time to speak openly and without prejudice is an important part of the engagement process. Discussion about the details of critical incidents and the doctor's views on events starts to allow ownership of a process that the doctor often feels at odds with. This first encounter will need time and a slow pace. In our experience it can take two hours or more, and doctors sometime take a while to begin to relax and talk freely. An important factor at this stage will be your ability as an educational supervisor to demonstrate and remain independent in your role. Signposting the structure of the meeting at the beginning of the interview and sharing information helps provide clarity and a neutral position. This will enhance the move towards engagement. Emphasising that the first meeting is to understand the doctor's perspective allows the individual space to develop confidence in the process.

It is helpful at this stage for you to think of yourself as a 'case manager'. The role of the case manager is different from that of the line manager, human resources or the treating physician. As the case manager, the aim is to support and provide appropriate advice. It is not to offer 'treatment'. It is also, we would suggest, not to tell them what they 'must' or 'have' to do but to *guide* them towards a joint understanding of the problem and help them to arrive at solutions that have shared goals and objectives.

Allowing the doctor to tell their story is often the best starting point for the interview. The doctor will often describe strong feelings of injustice and misunderstandings, and have their own answers as to why and what happened. Active listening (*see* Box 25.2) will allow you to guide them through this process.(19) Engagement will then come with ownership of events and beliefs. Engagement is the first step towards a joint

---

BOX 25.2 Focus on: Active listening

Active listening is a client-centred technique expounded and developed by Carl Rogers(21) ensuring that cues are recognised and explored. Rollnick, Butler and McCambridge(19) describe 'three styles' of communication that can enhance this process.

Instruct: Give information or advice. Other activities associated with this style include directing, informing, leading, educating, telling and using one's expertise. It is used when there is information one wants to provide that hopefully the person wants to receive.

Guide: Encourage the person to set his or her own goals and find ways of achieving them. Other activities associated with this style include coaching, negotiating, encouraging, mobilising and motivating. It is used when the person is facing change, having to make decisions and to act upon them.

Follow: Understand the person's experience. Other activities used include gathering information, following, eliciting, attending and empathising. It is used when one wishes to understand how the person feels or what has happened to him or her.

understanding of the problem and a move towards behaviour change.(20)

Behaviour change counselling evolved from the work of Carl Rogers and was defined first by Miller and Rollnick.(16) Behaviour change counselling is a client-centred approach to discussing lifestyle changes. Rollnick describes it as: 'ways of structuring a conversation to maximise the individual's freedom to talk and think about change in an atmosphere free of coercion and the provision of premature solutions'.(16) By working carefully through a detailed history of events, a picture of behavioural patterns often starts to emerge. By allowing ownership of the story and the problems through the interview it is our experience that the doctor will often be quite open in providing you with information about difficulties and problems they have encountered in the past. The first interview can provide great insights into how and why the doctor might be struggling.

Obtaining significant background information

Having elicited from the doctor the presenting problem and their perception of the factors leading up to the referral, it is important to also gather information around previous significant events and the doctor's past workplace experience.

Significant event review

Significant events should be recorded in detail, continually checking your understanding of the doctor's perspective. Move away from confrontation. You may have details of some events from the referrer, but challenging the doctor with the content of these at this stage can lead to resistance and difficulty with engagement. Try and get them to recount any other past significant events. This should extend to previous employment and time as a student. Do not focus here just on the present situation. This often will help elicit an emerging pattern of behaviour. Useful questions to guide the review include:
- What led up to the event?
- What actually happened?
- Was the way you managed the interaction effective or ineffective and why?
- On reflection, how else could it have been handled?

Workplace behaviours

A more detailed picture of how the doctor interacts in the workplace is important. Information gained about how individuals recall their early school years can be invaluable. It can provide insight into how people naturally behave and often illustrates and confirms the behavioural patterns that are emerging. Once in medical school, exam achievements and topics enjoyed or disliked help build the picture further. Finally, postgraduate exams and previous posts, including any problems that have arisen during their training years, help complete the picture. Useful questions to guide understanding workplace behaviour include:
- What are your memories of school?
- What subjects did you enjoy most?
- Did you take part in team sports?
- How did you see yourself academically compared with your peers?
- What exam results did you attain at school and at the university?

What's Next?

The first interview is likely to provide a wealth of information about the events leading up to problematic performance. If conducted effectively, from a neutral position and with a commitment to explore the doctor's own perspectives without judgement, then the groundwork has been laid towards effective engagement. At this stage, as the educational supervisor you might suspect that you need more detailed information about one or more of the following:
- past medical history
- family history
- social history
- personality
- language skills
- cultural issues.

Some of the above information is sensitive to access. There is a strong argument that the educational supervisor might not be the right person to seek and discuss all the above factors with the individual doctor unless the doctor volunteers it freely. This may be a challenge for the educational supervisor whose everyday work as a clinician is to ask patients questions and for intimate details about their personal history. However, a key message at this point is to understand that there are experts whose legitimate professional role is to assess the potential relationship between each of the above factors and work performance. The Chinese wall created by referring an individual doctor to other professionals to discuss issues associated with health, personality, language and culture, which may or may not be related to performance, ensures that irrelevant but potentially deeply personal information can remain private to the individual doctor. The tension for the educational supervisor is attaining the right balance and knowing when to refer on.

From the above discussion it can be seen that underperformance is often multifactorial in nature: biological, psychological and social. This first interview allows the educational supervisor as a case manager to start to understand how each of these elements might impact on the doctor's performance. Therefore the first interview should tentatively explore whether the individual's health and social background merits review by an occupational health physician. The presentation as a doctor in difficulty can often mask underlying

BOX 25.3 Biopsychosocial factors and stages in a doctor's underperformance

Factors	Biological	Psychosocial	Social
Predisposing	Underlying mental or physical disease	Personality Family	Cultural Family
Precipitating	Acute ill health events	Interactions at work	Economic factors Social isolation The culture of the organisation
Perpetuating	Chronic disease	Lack of insight by organisation or individual	Economic Cultural Organisational

Adapted from Sharpe and Wilks(22)

BOX 25.4 Case Study 1

Dr X was in his second year of specialist training and was referred for support because of failure to progress. He seemed always to have an excuse for not being at case presentations and had poor team management skills. Dr X described how he enjoyed primary school. He had lived in a small village so knew everyone and was always top of the class. When he moved to the secondary school it was in the city and he did well and passed all his exams. He described himself as having a few close friends. He played chess for the school team but hated team sports. At medical school he did well in the written exams but failed a couple because he hated doing the oral presentations.

---

mental health problems. What at face value might present as aggressive or bullying behaviour might on careful evaluation suggest underlying depression, anxiety or bipolar disorder. Physical ill health may also be revealed. Finally, developing a clear understanding of the individual's social environment and placing this in the context of the problems that they are now facing is important in perhaps understanding *why* the doctor has started to develop difficulties at this point. Box 25.3 provides a framework for understanding how these potential factors may lead up to and perpetuate a doctor's underperformance.

Referring to our illustrative case study in Box 25.4, further questioning elicited evidence of some obsessive-compulsive behaviour where Dr X constantly checked the notes and would return to the ward repeatedly to check on patients. His mood was now low, as was his self-esteem. His lack of self-confidence led him to believe he would not be able to present an adequate case in front of his colleagues. When asked whether he felt there were any other factors that led up to his referral he offered the information that his father had died six months previously and he was now supporting his mother and his disabled sister who

lived abroad. He felt a great responsibility for his family and a sense of loss at being so far away.

Having obtained information on the presenting problem and some relevant biopsychosocial background, at the end of the first interview the educational supervisor was able to decide on the appropriate next assessment steps before going on to plan the remediation.

To conclude, the challenge for the educational supervisor is to determine through the first interview the nature of the problem and the likely causes leading to the referral. In addition, the educational supervisor at this stage will need to decide whether more information is required from other sources, such as occupational health, occupational psychology, psychiatry or communication and language skills assessment. What follows is a description of the kinds of information that you might expect other professionals to be able to provide.

Digging Deeper

Occupational health assessments

The impact that physical and mental ill health can have on a doctor's performance is well recognised.(14) The Chief Medical Officer's report on medical regulation, *Good Doctors, Safer Patients*, recognised deficiencies in the provision of care to doctors impaired by mental health and addiction problems, and recommended that services be created to offer appropriate support.(11) What is also accepted in this report is that doctors do present a special case in relation to the need for workplace support.

Employers and training organisations should look towards close collaboration with their occupational health provider for advice and support in the assessment and possible management of doctors who are seen to be underperforming.

An occupational health physician would perform a detailed medical history and look at that history in the context of the workplace and workplace issues that have been raised. For instance, a doctor who presented with poor team management and prioritisation might on detailed questioning admit to a previous head injury or cerebrovascular accident that could indicate a neuropsychological impairment. A doctor presenting with aggressive or inappropriate behaviour might display features suggestive of underlying mental health issues such as depression, alcohol or drug problems or personality disorder. Once a problem has been identified, onward referral for specialist opinion can be made where appropriate.

Management of health issues in the workplace requires specialist advice and support. So when constructing a remedial programme for a doctor with health issues, advice from an occupational health physician should be sought, alongside advice from any specialist that the individual might be seeing. Some doctors may have a disability that has impacted on their performance and relevant legislation, such as the UK's Disability Discrimination Act,(23) must be considered in supporting them back into the workplace. Once again, an occupational health physician can support any remediation programme in terms of providing advice on 'reasonable adjustments' to the workplace.

Advising the doctor to seek (or providing access to) appropriate medical support should always be considered. Liaising with the family doctor or a general practitioner (with the client's consent) can hasten recovery or, where possible, provide secondary opinions and advice. The educational supervisor working closely with the occupational health and other specialist can help coordinate, rather than *deliver* timely and appropriate interventions.

Behavioural assessments

Understanding individual behaviour is key to establishing effective individualised remediation. Behaviour is a function of personality, learnt behaviour and situational drivers in the organisation. The purpose of this section is to indicate to the educational supervisor the kind of information an occupational psychologist could bring to understanding the relationship between personality and performance. It also distils some key messages about the impact of personality on remediation.

The link between personality and performance has been studied for many years, and research has mostly been conducted in an attempt to help the selection procedures.(24) Research up to the late 1980s suggested that there was little if any association between personality and performance. However, this theory was dismissed with the emergence of the five-factor model of personality (*see* Box 25.5).

The GMC also stresses a number of different aspects that are required of a doctor, including the importance of good communication skills, being able to work well

---

BOX 25.5 Where's the evidence: Personality and performance

Since the early 1990s many different personality tests and performance in many different jobs have been investigated. Overall, it has been concluded that personality can be reliably measured using appropriate tests, and for most jobs, certain personality traits can predict job performance.(24) Research has shown that in a large number of occupations job performance can be predicted by the big five personality factors.(26) The big five factors are:

- extraversion
- agreeableness
- emotional stability
- openness
- conscientiousness.(27)

Barrick *et al.* suggest that although not all of the big five personality factors predict generalisable job performance, they do predict success in specific occupations.(28)

---

with colleagues and patients, technical competence and general skills.(25) General skills include managing one's time, effective prioritising, being self-critical, problem solving and analysing numerical data.(25)

A number of different personality characteristics are therefore required to fulfil the different aspects of the role of a doctor. In some specialties, doctors constantly have to interact with patients and other members of the healthcare team and thus being extraverted seems to enhance performance in this area.(17) A number of other personality traits have been investigated that could affect a doctor's performance; they include self-criticism, confidence, perfectionism and communication style.

How behavioural assessments can benefit the educational supervisor in planning remediation will again be considered using the case of Dr X.

The aim of a behavioural interview with an occupational psychologist is to clarify Dr X's behavioural patterns, to determine his beliefs about the organisation/teams he works within and to understand how much insight he has into his behaviour. In other words, to clarify Dr X's perspective and to establish how best to work with him.

Dr X agreed that he is viewed as quiet and somewhat reserved by his colleagues. He stated that he has high clinical standards and works hard on the ward and in clinics. He enjoys the busy nature of his clinical work and describes himself as liking to be organised. His personality questionnaire describes a number of strengths, including the ability to get things done and on schedule, and a capacity to concentrate on detail.

Discussing the positive aspects of the profile and allowing Dr X to talk about himself in a positive way first helped to engage him in reviewing how his behaviour might have contributed to the specific concerns about his performance.

The first interview with the educational supervisor documented significant events relating to attendance at case presentations and poor team management. These events were discussed in turn with the occupational psychologist. The resulting interview suggested that Dr X may have a tendency to neglect the emotional side of relationships at work, may be perceived as inflexible and can overlook the long-range implications of day-to-day actions.

During this part of the interview, Dr X disagreed that he overlooks interpersonal relationships, stating that he is always polite, but that service pressures are such that in order to be good at his job he has to be task-focused. In any case, in situations where he has been criticised for rudeness, his priority was patient care and the nurse who was angry about his attitude has never liked him. At this stage, it is not the behavioural interviewer's role to challenge that view, but rather to make a note of it, perhaps as an indicator of possible lack of insight. Moving on to discuss the lack of attendance at case presentations, Dr X acknowledged that he finds standing up and presenting to others very difficult. It is OK until the point where he receives questions and then he finds the spontaneous and unpredictable direction that the presentation takes quite uncomfortable. The behavioural interviewer notes that on this issue, there is some insight, but a lack of understanding about how to improve. Dr X then moved on to talk about the way in which he considers the case presentations to be a waste of time and the behavioural interviewer checks whether he understands the long-range implications of continuing with this approach. At this point the interviewer considers that Dr X may have some development needs around building an effective career development strategy.

The interview also provides a work sample where some of the behaviours cited in the original referral are observable, such as abrupt questioning, justifications and lack of rapport building.

Communication and language assessments
Communication
Poor communication with patients is frequently cited as a core indicator of underperformance. Assessment of communication skills is therefore a vital constituent of the remediation process. Using observed simulated patient consultations offers the opportunity for the doctor to evaluate their own consulting style and behaviour alongside models of good practice in a non-judgemental manner, hopefully allowing the doctor to develop some insight into their own practice.(29) We would suggest that it is invaluable for an educational supervisor to undertake this activity with all referrals.

It can provide a good baseline indicator of their active listening and shared decision-making skills as well as being an indicator of their likely approach to communicating with colleagues.

It is important to note that the object of the exercise is to continue to engage the doctor while making an assessment of their 'needs'. This exercise is not meant to serve as a challenge to the doctor, so it should not include challenging scenarios of, for instance, breaking bad news or dealing with someone who is angry. It is intended to provide a baseline only. In other words, the activity here is to understand which skills the doctor relies on in everyday situations.

Self-evaluation is intended to be descriptive and diagnostic rather than summative, and providing the doctor with some sort of structure for this is useful. This could, for instance, be a rating scale adapted from standardised forms used in an Objective Structure Clinical Examinations. Using something standardised also provides the opportunity to reflect on progress at a later stage by repeating the exercise.

Language
The assessment of a doctor's language skills is not a novel undertaking. In the UK it has been a requirement for international medical graduates for some years. However, understanding how an individual's language skills impact on a doctor's performance is a relatively new area.

For the doctor, assessing language may present certain problems with regard to engagement. They may have lived and practised in the UK for some time. They may have already jumped through the requisite hoops such as the International English Language Testing System, and Professional and Linguistic Assessment Board to demonstrate competence in communicating in English. In the case of doctors recruited from the European Union, they will not have been required to submit to a language competence test.

For some doctors, particularly those who qualified overseas, one of the factors linked to underperformance may be their use of language. Use should be understood differently from usage. The latter relates more to 'correctness': accuracy of grammar, spelling and pronunciation. Use relates more to the ability to communicate clearly, coherently and appropriately with another person with the range of language knowledge and skill at one's disposal. Of course, there may be some overlap between use and usage, for instance, in the selection of vocabulary.

It is important to look at language use in context: in the workplace, socially and in the UK in comparison to country of origin. To this end, the assessment needs to be open-ended, qualitative and exploratory. As with other areas of the assessment the objective is to agree with the doctor possible areas for remediation, and the assessor's role is to provide expertise in helping them to identify and address those areas.

In our experience, assessing language is a highly specialised field but adds significant value to the assessment and the remedial plan. If looking to develop assessment in language we would suggest that the interview comprise of two broad parts: a semi-structured interview and a task. The focus of the interview is the doctor's experience of language learning and language use. Here, it is important to explore the doctor's own perception of their language skills and language use, comparing what they learnt with experience 'on the ground' in this country. The tasks could involve the doctor performing some form of extended speaking, for example, explaining something or giving a presentation.

On occasions, the issues may be to do with written language. In this case, the doctor should bring samples of reports or correspondence.

During the assessment, the assessor observes the doctor's language use. The aim is to highlight evidence of fluency and disfluency, to explore the range and appropriateness of lexis used by the doctor. This assessment is also interested in phonological features (pronunciation, stress, rhythm and intonation, discourse management, grammatical range and accuracy). In particular, the purpose of the tasks is to enable an exploration of the doctor's ability to convey meaning clearly, to present complex information with suitable guidance following rules of coherence and cohesion, to guide the listener and to use appropriate rhetorical devices.

Delivering Remediation

By the end of the assessment stage, a picture of the doctor should have emerged that relates not only to the doctor's perceptions of the issues raised, but also their insight into any contributory factors that might have led to the referral. The process should have provided an understanding of the doctor's personality and the way they learn, thus paving the way for the development of a tailored programme of support.

A key challenge for you as the educational supervisor will be to consider your role in the remedial process. Depending on the services available, you may have to occupy a combination of roles. During the assessment phase you might be acting as the case manager, conducting an initial interview and then maybe referring on to some of the specialist services described above. However, as the case progresses, the educational supervisor may also have to take on the role of the remediator. This might also include acting as an assessor at the end of the process. We have written what follows with the idea in mind that you are likely to take all three roles in some form or other during the remediation process.

Case review
The remedial plan will undoubtedly be dependent on the complexity of the case. A complex case may require bringing together the individuals who have supported you in your assessment, such as the occupational health physician, occupational psychologist and language assessor (where services are available). These professionals will not only provide varying perspectives on the problems raised, but also bring robustness to the review. A multidisciplinary approach will enhance the rigour of the process. This becomes crucial in maintaining your independence if decisions are challenged at a later stage. If the case manager sources opinion from other individuals, such as a psychiatrist, then well-constructed reports are also useful in adding to the picture. Recording of all documentation should be rigorous.

In a more straightforward case, case review may simply involve discussing the findings with one team member and planning the next steps with the doctor and their workplace supervisors.

Once all the documentation is collated, the next stage is to discuss the evidence with the team and decide what the remedial plan should look like. In essence, what interventions are required, in what order they should be delivered, who should deliver them and finally the time lines for review. This is a process that will develop with case experience. Below we describe such a process with reference to the case of Dr J (*see* Box 25.6).

The remedial plan
The case review should give you as the educational supervisor an overall picture of the major issues that need to be addressed. So, in relation to Dr J, the team came to the conclusion that he was quite extrovert in nature, so 'spoke before he thought'. He had strongly held beliefs about what was right and wrong in terms of the quality of medical practice and felt he was justified in airing his views. However, he seemed to lack insight into organisational issues around his team and the hospital in which he worked. Finally, underlying this there were definite issues around lack of self-confidence both in the workplace and being able to support his wife with their son's disability.

Therefore for Dr J, the issues that required support were around learning to reflect on his practice, developing his negotiating skills and work on organisational issues. These three threads would aim to develop more insight into his behaviour and provide him with some skills and strategies to manage more challenging situations. Thus the interventions used are likely to require a blend of behavioural and cognitive approaches. This in turn might help him develop more confidence in thinking about how he might manage his personal situation.

Ordering the interventions
Once the remedial plan has been outlined the educational supervisor will need to decide which interventions to use and how to link them. Ordering the

BOX 25.6 Case study 2

Dr J is in his fourth year of specialist training in obstetrics and gynaecology and has been referred following his annual assessment. He was noted to have somewhat erratic and unpredictable behaviour. His referral described someone who shouted at the nurses and the junior staff when under stress and who most recently had thrown equipment around the operating theatre. On a day-to-day basis he was known for being a social and friendly character although in his 360-degree appraisal he has been criticised for being overly jocular with staff. An initial assessment was conducted. This reveals that Dr J is married with one child, a boy aged 5, who suffers with autism. Dr J moved schools five times as a child. He participated in team sports at medical school and was a high achiever. His father died when he was 16. When asked about his strategy for getting things done, his belief is that it is 'OK to tell it as it is'. His consultation video revealed a tendency not to listen to patients and there was also a lack of clarity in the way he gave and explained information. During his videoed doctor–doctor consultation where he was asked to provide feedback to a more junior trainee who had persistent performance problems, he became quite agitated when the junior doctor questioned his judgement. He gave an indication during all three assessments that he was angry to have been referred as he felt strongly that he was a good doctor, cared about his patients and had no problems with his clinical skills. He had to contend with a very difficult work environment that was riddled with poor practice.

interventions requires careful consideration. The correct order will allow the doctor to move forward in a manner that will build on ownership and sense of autonomy of the process. Therefore by allowing the doctor some feeling of control and ability to work in their comfort zone the process starts to move the doctor from engagement into action.

Mustering resources

A key decision at this point is to consider who will be involved in the remediation process and how that will be resourced. Those institutions responsible for medical education vary with regard to the specific arrangements that exist to undertake remedial work and thus what follows is a general description of remediation activity, some of which may be undertaken by you as their supervisor and some of which my be undertaken by others. However, if your role is that of case manager then you will be responsible for ensuring that continuity exists between remediation activities. In each of the activities described below, we use the term 'remediator' to cover the individual who is working with the doctor at that moment, acknowledging that a combination of different remediators may be used.

Starting out

Understanding the individual's personality and what is of 'high importance' suggests pathways for initiating the process. So for Dr J, starting with a session that explores real events in a way that might use role play and video feedback would probably feel acceptable given his preference for practical, action-based learning. Using actors who are trained in giving feedback is especially helpful in this role. Thus, setting up the actor as someone with a similar personality to Dr J would be a useful starting point. Dr J would probably not find this too stressful as like personalities often respond well to each other. The remediator can then coach Dr J around 'what he did', 'how it felt' and what he 'might want to do better'. The remediator might anticipate that reflection is less comfortable for Dr J. This would be predicted by personality questionnaire feedback and reinforced by work on learning styles. The actor can respond in role about how they felt, what worked and what did not work. This is often the first step for the doctor in gaining insight into their normal behavioural pattern. It starts the reflection into daily practice that might not come easily to someone like Dr J.

Coaching would follow on from such an activity. This session could focus on some of the activities and responses discussed in the first role-play session. Starting with such a session for Dr J may have led to resistance, as this is not a natural path for him. Finally, further interactive role play with a more difficult case and sessions building on organisational issues is a pathway we have found to lead to increasing self-confidence and change. Had Dr J been a more introvert individual, starting with reflection and critical incident analysis with a coach might have been a more natural pathway.

Coaching

Coaching in this context describes an activity whereby remediation is based on a method or methods for stimulating change. It is important that the methods and approaches chosen have an evidence base, and also that the acquisition of practical behavioural skills takes place within a wider framework whereby the individual is encouraged to think about their beliefs and strategies. It is our view that remediation has behavioural and cognitive components. The purpose of coaching is to create a context whereby the individual can acquire new behavioural skills and cognitive strategies side by side.

At this stage, active listening skills help guide the individual to discover insights into the conditions under which they might be prepared to change, and thus its emphasis is on the cognitive. Rooting the development of new skills in a context whereby the individual is discovering a new way of interpreting what is going on around them prepares the individual for getting ready to acquire new skills.

Role play

A typical tipping point comes with the realisation by the doctor that their current approach is not working or does not always work, or simply that they could become more effective. The question asked by the doctor then centres around how they can become more effective. If shouting at the nurses does not result in the correct equipment being given to Dr J when he needs it, what else can he do? One common pathway is that a doctor such as Dr J, who is usually extroverted and expressive, becomes uncharacteristically quiet and unsure about how best to assert himself. Equally he finds this strategy frustrating because it is not his preferred way of behaving and he feels it also achieves nothing, but at least he perceives that it keeps him out of trouble or beyond criticism.

Role play creates a situation whereby the new skills can be practised and improved. Using constructive feedback from the remediator and actor, combined with video review and self-assessment, can be powerful and effective in engaging the doctor. Some doctors question the extent to which role play in this context can really simulate the organisational context. Central to our approach is the use of events from their own occupational history, particularly those significant events that contributed to the referral. The doctor is asked to retell the story of the event. The actor will often be present to allow a picture to be constructed of both the events and the doctor. This type of intervention is used to explore memories of interpersonal interactions. It provides a structure to examine not just actual communication and language skills, but also beliefs about influencing, negotiation and leadership.

Setting goals and time lines

Remediation should be set apart from counselling or other forms of therapy that the individual may require and seen as a clearly defined set of interventions that have a manageable time line. Counselling or therapy might sit alongside the remedial process, but they are not one and the same thing.

Setting time lines should be seen as part of the agenda-setting process.

Consideration of how many sessions should be provided and when progress should be reviewed adds structure and helps guide the referrer, the remediator(s) and the doctor. Review dates should be considered at the outset. In our experience, setting three sessions and then a team review is often sufficient.

There are also external constraints to consider when setting time lines, such as in-training assessments, hospital reviews or GMC hearings. Sharing an understanding with the doctor that the remedial process sits alongside these time lines helps engagement and reduces anxiety. Thus when developing the remedial plan, these factors should be taken into consideration. Understanding the doctor's work and social environment is also important. For instance, if Dr J was a trainee working in a nearby hospital with a review of their progress in four months, then the majority of the work should be completed in three months and sessions might last two to three hours each time. If, however, Dr J was a consultant who has a long distance to travel, it might be more applicable to run a two-day intensive workshop for him with a review one month later, while keeping a reflective diary that he emailed to his supervisor every week. Setting clear objectives at this stage helps set out the plans and reviews that will guide the process at a later stage.

Reviewing progress

The amount of time taken to see progress appears to vary as a function of individual differences, reason for referral and grade. The proxy measures for progress in this context are as follows:

- engagement with the service, that is, turning up for appointments
- willingness and ability to engage in reflective conversation
- insight into the nature of the problem(s) and their causes
- ability to work with the remediator to generate alternative strategies and skills
- active participation in practising new skills
- ability to discuss the use of acquired skills and strategies and how these have been applied in the workplace.

With regard to the process of review, it is difficult to be prescriptive in setting review points for each doctor when the programme is individualised. However, the educational supervisor in the role of case manager should bring the remediation team together to routinely review progress and will need to be sensitive to particular tipping points, such as reaching a judgement about:

- when a doctor has made enough progress such that remediation can stop
- whether a doctor has reached a plateau in their progress such that further remediation is unlikely to achieve additional improvement
- whether the doctor is likely to benefit from individualised support at all.

Measuring success

Success is hard to measure and at present there are few validated tools that help provide hard evidence. Success might be seen as improved feedback from colleagues and the remediator(s). It may be passing exams that have been repeatedly failed. It might be achieving success at interview where the individual had failed for many months previously. It might also be an end to the patient complaints that had triggered the referral.

Success might also be the doctor recognising their own limitations, whether due to behaviour or underlying health issues, and leaving their specialty.

However, developing insight and changing behaviour takes time. The remedial process should give the individual space to move from an often resistant position to a place where they are ready to change. It should guide the doctor to develop an understanding of how his or her behaviour has impacted on his or her performance and offer solutions in the form of strategies and skills.

The role of insight

In our experience, underperformance is complex, such that it is not possible to conclude that any one personality profile is more at risk than any other. However, we have seen common patterns of behaviour that appear to trigger and perpetuate episodes of underperformance. More importantly perhaps with regard to remediation, some patterns of behaviour stand out as indicating the stage of development that a doctor may be at.

We have recognised the following specific patterns.

- The doctor recognises the problem behaviour as an area for development but does not know how to develop an alternative set of skills.
- The doctor recognises the problem but focuses on justifying why that behaviour pattern is important.
- The doctor does not recognise that a particular behaviour pattern is negative.

Kruger and Dunning(30) described how poor performers have less insight into their inadequacies than high performers. The more competent they become, the lower they self-rate their own performance. Kruger and Dunning conclude that perhaps insight in some doctors can be achieved with training.

Evaluation

Evaluation of the effectiveness of a remediation process can be guided by its design. As in other educational settings, such as assessment and development centres, evaluation is concerned to a large extent with the utility of the process. The reason evaluation in this context remains a challenge is that while multiple sources of evidence and/or methods are often used, they are typically fragmented and not always conducted in a pre-planned way in the workplace. Even where they are pre-planned, such as in the case of NCAS assessments, it can be difficult to bring together evidence conducted by different professionals, often over many months, even with the presence of a skilled case manager. Thus evaluation of remediation services across the UK is in its infancy and needs to be further developed. However, educational supervisors should strive to develop some system of evaluating the individual doctors they work with that fits within their organisational structure.

Pitfalls and Problems

The process of remediation is high stakes. Ensuring clarity at all stages is important.

Legal and ethical issues

The nature of the remediation service provided must be carefully considered prior to entering into any agreement with an individual or organisation. The ethical and legal implications of a training-led service providing support for a trainee will be different from a hospital offering independent services to an employed consultant. Understanding where the responsibilities to the individual doctor and the referring organisation may lie and the nature of the information that can be imparted to third parties should be carefully considered before entering into any process. Areas to review when setting up a service should include:

- written reports: confirming whether these fall within the Access to Medical Reports Act
- patient safety: if there is evidence of risk to patient safety then there must be a pathway in which serious concerns can be raised with the referring organisation
- consent: the individual doctor should be aware of the contract they are entering into when they attend for remediation
- case notes: ownership of the notes and how they are stored and held, along with access to the case files.

Blurring of boundaries

Good communication between stakeholders at the outset is key to a successful service. Managing the expectations of both the referrer and the individual doctor reduces the risk of misunderstanding later on. Such communication might include:

- outlining the roles of the remediation process for both the doctor and the referring organisation at the outset
- specifying what the process can offer and its limitations
- clarity of what the content of any report might look like
- patient safety and duty of care of the educational supervisor to the referring doctor and the organisation.

Record keeping

It is advisable to keep records to the same standard as any clinical records. They should be stored in the same manner, locked away in fireproof cabinets.

Inappropriate referrals

Setting referral criteria is crucial to reducing the risk of inappropriate referrals. The package of remediation offered should centre on the areas of expertise that you are able to offer. However, knowing where to refer on

BOX 25.7 Focus on: When to refer on (UK)

The General Medical Council's (GMC) key concern is whether a doctor is fit to practise. It is not involved with general complaints of a minor nature, nor of performance problems that are capable of being resolved locally. It can take action when:

- a doctor has been convicted of a criminal offence
- there is an allegation of serious professional misconduct
- a doctor's professional performance may be seriously deficient
- a doctor with health problems continues to practise while unfit and patient safety is compromised.

If there is evidence that patients may be at risk, the GMC can suspend or restrict a doctor's registration as an interim measure. See the 'Concerns about doctors' section of the GMC's web site (http://www.gmc-uk. org/concerns/index.asp).

A National Clinical Assessment Service (NCAS) assessment is likely to be appropriate where:

- concern(s) are substantiated: from the evidence available there is confidence that expressed concerns are accurate statements
- concern(s) are significant: the actions about which concerns are expressed fall well short of what would be expected from another doctor in similar circumstances
- concern(s) are repetitious: ongoing problems and/or problems on at least two separate occasions are identified
- concern(s) do not appear to be sufficiently serious to warrant an immediate referral to the GMC
- local procedures have failed to resolve the problem or are not appropriate
- a NCAS performance assessment appears to offer a likely way forward in enabling the case to move towards a resolution.

for further support is also a requirement of an efficient service (Box 25.7).

References

1 Cohen D and Rhydderch M (2006) Measuring a doctor's performance: personality, health and well-being. *Occupational Medicine.* **56**: 38–40.

2 Cohen D, Rollnick S, Smail S *et al.* (2005) Communication, stress and distress: evolution of an individual support programme for medical students. *Medical Education.* **39**(5): 76–81.

3 Goulet F, Jacques A and Gagnon R (2003) An innovative approach to remedial continuing medical education, 1992–2002. *Academic Medicine.* **80**: 553–40.

4 Joesbury H, Mathers N and Lane P (2001) Supporting GPs whose performance gives cause for concern: the North Trent experience. *Family Practice.* **18**(2): 123–30.

5 Bahrami J (1997) Remediation. *British Medical Journal.* **315**: 2.

6 Burrows P, Khan A, Bowden R *et al.* (2004) The fresh start simulated surgery. *Education for Primary Care.* **15**: 328–35.

7 Firth-Cozens J and King J (2006) The role of education and training. In: Cox J, King J, Hutchinson A *et al.* (eds) *Understanding Doctors' Performance*, pp. 61–77. Radcliffe Publishing in association with National Clinical Assessment Service of the National Patient Safety Agency, Oxford.

8 Paice E (2006) The role of education and training. In: Cox J, King J, Hutchinson A *et al.* (eds) *Understanding Doctors' Performance*, pp. 78–90. Radcliffe Publishing in association with National Clinical Assessment Service of the National Patient Safety Agency, Oxford.

9 Finucane PM, Barron SR, Davies HA *et al.* (2002) Towards an acceptance of performance appraisal. *Medical Education.* **36**: 959–64.

10 Department of Health (2003) *Modernising Medical Careers.* Department of Health, London.

11 Department of Health (2006) *Good Doctors, Safer Patients: proposals to strengthen the system to assure and improve the performance of doctors and to protect the safety of patients.* Department of Health, London.

12 Murphy KR and Cleveland JN (1995) *Understanding Performance Appraisal: social, organisational and goal-based perspectives.* Sage Publications, Thousand Oaks, CA.

13 Leape L and Fromson JA (2006) Problem doctors: is there a system level solution. *Annals of Internal Medicine.* **144**: 107–15.

14 Firth-Cozens J (2006) A perspective on stress and depression In: Cox J, King J, Hutchinson A, McAvoy P (eds) *Understanding Doctors' Performance*, pp 22–37. Radcliffe Publishing in association with National Clinical Assessment Service of the National Patient Safety Agency, Oxford.

15 Harrison J (2006) Illness in doctors and dentists and their fitness for work – are the cobblers children getting their shoes at last? *Occupational Medicine.* **56**: 75–6.

16 Miller W and Rollnick S (2002) *Motivational Interviewing: preparing people to change* (2e). Guilford Press, New York.

17 Paice E and Orton V (2004) Early signs of the trainee in difficulty. *Hospital Medicine.* **65**: 238–40.

18 Cohen D and Rhydderch M (2007) Assessment when performance gives rise for concern. In: Jackson N, Jamieson A and Khan A (eds) *Assessment in Medical Education and Training*, pp. 150–8. Radcliffe Medical Press, Oxford.

19 Rollnick S, Butler CC, McCambridge J *et al.* (2005) Consultations about changing behaviour. *British Medical Journal.* **331**: 961–3.

20 Rollnick S, Mason P and Butler C (1999) *Health Behaviour Change: a guide for practitioners.* Churchill Livingstone, Edinburgh.

21 Rogers CR (1951) *Client Centered Therapy.* Houghton-Mifflin, Boston.

22 Sharpe M and Wilks D (2002) ABC of psychological medicine: fatigue. *British Medical Journal.* **325**: 480–3.

23 Disability Discrimination Acts (1995, 2005) Crown Copyright, UK Government.

24 Kierstead J (1998) Personality and job performance: a research overview (http://www.psagency-agencefp.gc.ca/research/personnel/personality_e.asp).

25 General Medical Council (1993) *Tomorrow's Doctors*. GMC, London.

26 Dudley N, Orvis KA, Lebiecki JE *et al.* (2006) A meta-analytic investigation of conscientiousness in the prediction of job performance. *Journal of Applied Psychology*. **91**: 40–57.

27 Ferguson E, James D and Madeley L (2002) Learning in practice: factors associated with success in medical school. *British Medical Journal*. **324**: 952–7.

28 Barrick M, Mount M and Judge T (2001) Personality and performance at the beginning of the new millennium. *Personality and Performance*. **9**: 9–30.

29 Lane C and Rollnick S (2007) The use of simulated patients and role-play in communication skills training: a review of the literature to August 2005. *Patient Education and Counselling*. **67**: 13–20.

30 Kruger J and Dunning D (1999) Unskilled and unaware of it: how difficulties in recognising one's own incompetence lead to inflated self-assessments. *Journal of Personality and Social Psychology*. **77**: 1121–34.

Further Reading

Cox J, King J, Hutchinson A *et al.* (eds) (2006) *Understanding Doctors' Performance*. Radcliffe Publishing, Oxford.

Firth-Cozens J (2006) A perspective on stress and depression In: Cox J, King J, Hutchinson A, McAvoy P (eds) *Understanding Doctors' Performance*, pp 22–37. Radcliffe Publishing in association with National Clinical Assessment Service of the National Patient Safety Agency, Oxford.

Jackson N, Jamieson A and Khan A (eds) (2007) *Assessment in Medical Education and Training: a practical guide*. Radcliffe Publishing, Oxford.

The National Clinical Assessment Service (www.ncas.npsa.nhs. uk) provides advice to trusts and training organisations. The web site is packed with comprehensive and informative resources, including toolkits, publications and practical advice.

Quality in medical education

Oonagh Corrigan, Kate Ellis, Alan Bleakley and Julie Brice

KEY MESSAGES

- High-quality medical education is crucial to the delivery of high-quality patient care.

- Quality improvement is a dynamic and continuous process where the aim is the achievement of excellence rather than mere fitness for purpose or competence.

- A commitment to quality improvement is a lifelong obligation that starts at medical school, continues through training and forms an essential component of a doctor's professional practice.

- Medical educators may have many and varying roles in supporting teaching and learning at all stages of a

doctor's education, but whatever an educator's role, there are endless opportunities to reflect on and improve quality in practice, by studying, contributing to and making use of the best evidence currently available.

- Quality may be considered in terms of discourses: scientific, aesthetic, managerial, economic, ethical, professional and political. It is important for medical educators to be aware of these discourses if they are to be pro-active and imaginative in developing a culture of quality in their own fields of practice.

Introduction

Medicine and society have undergone enormous changes in recent decades, with significant consequences for medical education. Advances in science and technology mean that doctors need to be able to use complex equipment, keep up to date on the growing range of modern drug treatments and deal with the ethical dilemmas posed by both the fast pace of scientific transformation and changing societal expectations and values. Delivering high-quality patient care also relies on an understanding of the wider context of healthcare delivery and the varying needs of patients. Responding to the changing conditions in the healthcare delivery system and the needs and expectations of societies is a challenge for medical education.(1) The pursuit of quality in medical education is crucial to meeting this challenge; however, although high-quality educational processes and outcomes are commonly desired, their achievement is far from easy. We can often recognise when quality is absent, and we may know when we experience its presence, but describing it, explaining it and ensuring that we contribute towards it are difficult for all involved in medical education.

In the following pages, we will attempt to answer the following questions:
- What is meant by 'quality'?
- How might we recognise it?
- How might we achieve it?

Understanding Medical Education: Evidence, Theory and Practice.
Edited by T Swanwick. © 2010 Association for the Study of Medical Education.

We begin by examining the nature of quality in medical education. We then present a series of examples based on actual learning and teaching experiences to illuminate quality standards in medical education. Finally, we discuss a number of discourses that currently frame notions of quality, and examine how such discourses can both facilitate and constrain the pursuit of excellence in medical education.

Importantly, we suggest one main framework for ensuring quality in medical education: the application of best available evidence. As doctors are encouraged to pursue evidence-based medicine, medical educators should also be drawing on the evidence base derived from education and medical education research. What is considered quality research and what counts as evidence in medical education are both contested, but medical educators who are interested in continuous quality improvement will be engaging with these debates.

Our focus here is on high-quality medical education in terms of teaching and learning, and how this translates into practice to improve patient care and safety. We also recognise the importance of quality in governance and the wider political environment in medical education, but do not discuss such issues in depth.

Quality in Medical Education

Quality can be said to exceed initial purposes. Asked 'what is the purpose of medical education?', many would answer that it is to produce competent generalist and specialist doctors. But high quality goes beyond mere competence or 'fitness for purpose'. If the role of a doctor is 'the pursuit of health in the service of society',(2) then excellent doctors will not only show expertise in clinical medicine, but will also set up excellent relationships with patients, practise ethically, research their practice, teach others, engage in public health activities, take on management and leadership roles, act as valued citizens and, importantly, reinvent these roles and activities over time. In other words, a quality medical education will expand the role of the doctor to educate for continuous quality improvement of medical education itself. The dynamic nature of medicine and society means that quality is not something that remains fixed. Processes that are designed to assure high-quality outcomes must instead be constantly reviewed as to the extent to which they exceed initial purposes.

Preparation for Practice

There is a growing global consensus on the essential knowledge and skills that medical students need to acquire before they are fit to practise as junior doctors.(3–5) There is less consensus on quality education and training as doctors enter specialties. The historian Kenneth Ludmerer(6) suggests that there are two pressing issues for medical education to address: first, to heal a social breach, or regain public confidence; and second, to educate medical students to tolerate uncertainty and to discuss uncertainty openly with patients. These two imperatives readily apply to medical education in the 'post-industrial' world and are central to developing quality in medical education.

To provide a firm foundation for early practice, an initial medical education seeks to move beyond knowledge and skills acquisition to emphasise identity construction and values. A quality undergraduate medical education should produce 'rounded' graduates, who have not only sound knowledge and understanding of the clinical and basic sciences and their application in clinical contexts, but also a reflexive understanding of their 'cognitive apprenticeship'(7), that is, of how they are making the transition from novice to early expertise – from 'thinking as a student' to 'thinking like a doctor' as preparation for 'thinking as a doctor'.

The rounded graduate will have learnt from exposure to both relevant and meaningful aspects of the behavioural and social sciences, arts and humanities applied to medicine, and medical ethics and law. The acquisition of knowledge and understanding of the natural history of human disease mechanisms, disease presentation and responses to illness are essential. However, better medical school graduates will, for example, understand the difficulties in drawing a line between the 'pathological' and the 'normal', and will appreciate the strategies of preventive medicine. Medical students will need to develop an array of clinical and practical skills, including the taking of a patient's history and the ability to interpret this.

By the time they have graduated, medical students in transition to junior doctor status will need to have the ability to make clinical decisions based on the evidence they have gathered, and to assess a patient's problems and make plans to investigate and manage these. Furthermore, the medical student will have learnt how to work collaboratively in a clinical team (to work and learn with, from and about other professionals) and to appreciate the importance of coordinated, cross-team work around a patient on a care pathway. A quality undergraduate medical education then produces the identity of a 'professional' (a doctor) and an 'interprofessional' (a team worker). In an excellent, or high-quality, medical education, doctors of the future will be educated to address Ludmerer's key issues – to practise patient-centred medicine with a social awareness, and to manage uncertainty and share this with patients in a productive way.(6)

The acquisition of good communication and teamwork capabilities is essential to a quality medical education. The evidence base suggests that doctors are still, in general, not good enough at communicating with patients(8) and that poor communication with colleagues can put patients at risk. Those graduating in medicine must be able to communicate clearly, sensitively and effectively with patients and their relatives, and with colleagues from a variety of health and social care professions. Ideally, they should display knowledge and understanding of relevant medico-legal and ethical issues in performance, as well as promoting systems of quality assurance and safety. A high-quality undergraduate curriculum will not only meet these learning needs, but will also seek to promote reformulation of such learning over time, aiming for a 'value added' curriculum that is focused on capability rather than on competence – not just retrospective assessment of the 'good enough' graduate, but also prospective evaluation of excellent doctors. A high-quality medical profession is of course not simply achieved by focusing on medical students at the undergraduate level, as this tells us about medical graduates but not about doctors in practice. Quality must permeate the entire spectrum of medical education.

Postgraduate Medical Education

While the contexts and systems that are in place to deliver postgraduate and continuing education differ from those of university-based medical schools, improved healthcare and patient safety depend on quality education at all levels of training. In recognition of this, the World Federation for Medical Education has established standards on postgraduate medical education and continuing professional development in addition to those in basic medical education.(1,7,9)

Furthermore, it has framed its standards to specify attainment at two levels: one based on basic standards or minimum requirements; and the other based on standards for quality development.

In the UK, a number of initiatives to improve the quality of postgraduate medical education and training have been established. *Modernising Medical Careers* (MMC),(10) a government programme of reform, was established in 2003 with the aim of 'improving medical education' and providing 'a transparent and efficient career path for doctors' (p. 310). A new two-year Foundation Programme, followed by a number of broad-based specialist training programmes running through to consultant level or general practice, has since been established. For the first time clearly defined curricula are available defining clinical competencies that must be achieved in all specialties and at all stages of training. A new (but short-lived) regulatory body, the Postgraduate Medical Education and Training Board was established in 2002 and now merged together with the General Medical Council (GMC) is responsible for a host of published standards for curricula, assessments, training posts, trainers and deaneries, as well as the first national trainee survey and a UK-wide process of quality assurance.(11)

Continuing Medical Education

Medical education is a lifelong process and does not end once doctors have finished their specialist training. Qualified doctors are largely responsible for directing their own learning. Professionals' reflection on their practice as a means of continuous change and learning is an essential component in the achievement of high-quality standards. In some countries it is mandatory for doctors to provide evidence of participation on courses in order to be recertified for continuing medical practice. In the US, for example, most licensing authorities issue specialists time-limited certificates requiring doctors to be recertified every few years to retain their 'board certified' status. The aim of recertification is to encourage doctors to learn and keep up to date, as well as to identify those doctors who do not continue to meet the specialty boards' standards. Although such processes may be useful in identifying poor quality, it has been suggested that the multi-billion dollar enterprise of didactic courses that have arisen to meet the needs of doctors requiring credit hours for recertification purposes is not necessarily the best means to achieve high quality.(12) Doctors may prefer peer appraisal methods for revalidation.

In Europe, participation in programmes of continuing medical education (CME) is mostly voluntary. However, the European Union of Medical Specialists and the Standing Committee of European Doctors have adopted charters stating that doctors have an ethical duty to undertake further education, but recognise that they may need be given incentives to participate in CME activities.(13) In the UK, the government, along with the GMC and the Royal Colleges, has begun to develop plans for a revalidation process to be introduced. The aim is to support doctors in meeting their personal and professional commitment to continually sustain and develop their skills, and enhance public confidence in the profession as a whole by providing periodic assurance that doctors continue to be fit to practise. It is further proposed that such processes include a strong element of patient and carer participation and evaluation.(11,14)

The issue of CME or continuing professional development is one that is likely to be further debated in the pursuit of high-quality professional conduct and patient care, not least as the relationships between the various stakeholders, such as the individual doctor, the employer, the profession and the patient, must been taken into account. The most important issues in CME are the professionals' quality of reflection on practice as a means of continuous development and the quality of the education programmes on offer rather than whether these programmes are voluntary or mandatory.

Experiences in Teaching and Learning

In this section, we provide six illustrative examples based on reports provided by a number of medical educators, medical students and junior doctors, with a view to raising some quality issues for consideration in your own educational practice. These case studies are structured around the areas of activity set out in the UK Higher Education Academy's *UK Professional Standards Framework for Teaching and Supporting Learning in Higher Education*(15) (*see* Box 26.1). Notably, a similar framework has been developed by the Academy of Medical Educators,(16) reflecting a national consensus on what constitutes quality in medical education today. In our discussion, we draw on research evidence to reflect further on ways to achieve high-quality educational processes and outcomes. Award-bearing teacher education programmes in medical or clinical education offer intensive introductions to the culture of medical education research, theory and practice. Pursuit of such qualifications will raise quality within the culture of medical education.

Design and planning of learning activities

It is widely recognised that one of the main challenges of medical education, for both those delivering it and those undertaking it, is the requirement to consolidate a vast amount of knowledge into a coherent and cohesive whole, continually updated and relevant to contemporary clinical practice.(17,18)

BOX 26.1 Focus on: The Higher Education Academy

The role of the UK Higher Education Academy (HEA) is to work with the higher education sector in the UK to enhance the quality of students' learning experiences. It aims to:

- identify, develop and disseminate evidence-informed approaches
- broker and encourage the sharing of effective practice
- support universities and colleges in bringing about strategic change
- inform, influence and interpret policy
- raise the status of teaching.

Founded in 2004, the HEA is supported by the four Higher Education Funding Councils in the UK and provides services to individual academics, staff in subject communities and also to universities and colleges. It administers the UK's National Teaching Fellowship Awards scheme, which recognises best practice in teaching in higher education. The HEA recognises individuals' commitment to enhancing the student learning experience through its professional recognition scheme.

Services to medical educators are provided by the Academy Subject Centre for Medicine, Dentistry and Veterinary Medicine, one of the 24 subject centres covering all disciplines within the HEA.

For more information about the Higher Education Academy, see http://www.heacademy.ac.uk. For more information about the Academy's Subject Centre for Medicine, Dentistry and Veterinary Medicine, see http://www.medev.ac.uk.

BOX 26.2 Example 1: Design and planning of learning activities

'At the start of this year's small group session, the students discussed what they had learned as a result of their small group work in previous years. Several students argued that they had not really learned anything. When I asked "how would things have been if you hadn't had any small groups?", they listed a range of benefits, including peer support, developing skills in group work and learning new ways of looking at issues, including the appreciation of others' views. What became clear was that students did not see these benefits as "learning". Learning, one student said, "is about facts".'

Small group lead facilitator

Careful curriculum design, revisiting subjects in increasing depth and complexity as the programme progresses, thereby encouraging deeper learning, has been shown to be an effective way of doing this, but it brings many challenges for students who have not worked in this way before.(19) Activity-based and problem-based learning, self-directed learning and student-selected components encourage both independent and collaborative learning. These methods lead to linking concepts as principles, which, once understood, can be applied across contexts, rather than to memorising information by rote. Social learning approaches prepare students for working in team settings, where knowing how to access knowledge is as important as having that knowledge yourself. Recent research suggests that medical students, whether mature students or school leavers, need to adopt new learning approaches. If they resist this process, relying instead on the techniques they developed before joining medical school, they impose barriers to learning and may be left ill equipped to deal with the demands of the curriculum. This, in turn, increases anxiety expressed by students concerning workload, further impeding a high-quality learning experience.(19) Nevertheless, it is unlikely that even the well-educated post-school student arrives at medical school fully equipped with expert strategies that will enable him or her to learn by looking for patterns and underlying principles, and integrating the task with existing awareness. As Tamsin Haggis reports in her study of approaches to learning in higher education,

> Arguably, students cannot integrate, and therefore be successful, unless they understand what it is that they are expected to do. Discussing with students what a 'deep approach' might mean could be one form of explicitness(20) (p. 100).

As the quote in Box 26.2 illustrates, explaining to students what learning means, and getting them to understand their own learning experiences more fully, can help develop these skills. In addition to students, teachers and tutors have a significant role in a student's engagement with 'deep learning'.

Teaching and support of learners

Student barriers to high-quality learning are perhaps more difficult to anticipate than regulatory, financial or other external obstacles. In the example, in Example 2, lack of enjoyment of the learning activity prevented the students from recognising its educational value until the group feedback was restructured (Box 26.3). Active engagement with the student body is crucial and the 'student voice' has long been viewed as an essential quality assurance mechanism, providing feedback on satisfaction levels about everything from university sports facilities to the ease with which students can contact their academic tutor. However, as Example 2 shows, not only do these data provide invaluable insights into students' perceptions of their experiences, but that these perceptions also have an inherent impact on the provision of high-quality learning, often in unexpected ways.

Therefore, listening to the student voice is important not only in terms of ascertaining satisfaction levels, but also to feed into the development of learning strategies and the shaping of the curriculum. In other words, to minimise the number of student-imposed barriers to high-quality medical education, it is crucial to know what these barriers are, how they obstruct the aims of the learning activity and ways in which to manage them. The UK Quality Assurance Agency for Higher Education has recognised this, and recently recruited students to become full and equal members of their audit teams. The pilot was extended to the wider higher education sector and, after an evaluative review of the exercise, reported: 'It has been positive in terms of feedback from students and from staff who have been involved, who appreciate the students' input and them bringing a fresher perspective and challenging academic perceptions and assumptions about students' experiences'.(21) In medical education, student engagement in quality assurance processes goes some way to ensure that potential barriers to the learning experience are anticipated and addressed as far as possible.

Assessment and feedback to learners

What implications does Example 3 in Box 26.4 have for the quality of the junior doctor's learning experience? Although the example describes a clinical tutor's experience of assessing the student summatively. Perhaps the most striking issue to arise is the importance of the formative feedback preceding this assessment, and an apparent slippage in medical education between what kind of feedback students find most effective to aid their learning and what extent of feedback teachers consider to be sufficient. This has substantial implications for the perceived and actual quality of the learning experience. The student in this scenario had been told repeatedly that his performance was satisfactory, despite the fact that several members of the clinical team had identified to one another that he was struggling, under the illusion that identifying areas of weakness to the student would undermine his confidence.

A recent Malaysian study has demonstrated that this apparent mismatch is not confined to medical education in the UK.(22) The study, which investigated 'the relationship and degree of correspondence between perceptions of teachers with student perceptions and expectations, with regard to feedback received during learning', demonstrated that students expected formative feedback to be integrated into every learning activity from the beginning of their study, and that they viewed it as an invaluable tool in identifying and remedying poor performance. In contrast, most of the tutors surveyed believed that model answers supplied by non-specialist facilitators provided adequate feedback. In other words, whereas students would appreciate a dialogue with their teacher, with some opportunity for reflection, the feedback meted out in a number of cases may provide the 'right' solution, but no further discussion about where the student's performance stands in relation to that solution, or the steps the student needs to take to address identified improvement areas.

To return to the case outlined in Box 26.4, had the student received constructive and honest comment on his performance in the clinical environment, this, combined with his engagement with a curriculum designed to foster a deeper learning approach, would have better equipped him to direct his independent learning objectives accordingly. Instead, without having all the relevant information on his own performance, he has had to set personal objectives that may not necessarily reflect or address all issues arising from his practice.

The discussions surrounding formative feedback, and the most effective way to deliver it, suggest that sometimes barriers to a high-quality learning experience are created by the gap between the expectations of the student, and student and tutor perceptions of that learning experience. In our work-based assessment scenario, the student's perception of formative feedback as an invaluable learning tool conflicts with the healthcare team's perception that negative feedback, albeit constructive, would be detrimental in some way to the student. Moreover, student perceptions construct the reasons for adopting specific studying techniques and so their importance cannot be underestimated in creating a high-quality learning environment. Indeed, recent research into this gap between expectation and experience indicates that this extends beyond the provision of feedback to other areas of the learning experience, including the design of the curriculum itself.(19)

Developing effective environments and student support and guidance

Medical training must at some point use 'live' patients to develop the skills of health professionals. As Pugsley and McCrorie note, 'the best possible learning resources for medical students to learn and practise all these skills are the patients on the wards and in general practice/family medicine. Students are encouraged to check and examine patients as much as possible, preferably under supervision. It is only through practice that the skills are learnt'.(17) However, a high-quality outcome of a patient-centred learning experience is not necessarily one in which no mistakes are made, but one in which a safe environment has been provided to allow students to make mistakes and identify areas of weakness in their own practice.

In the case related in Box 26.5, the safety of the environment was compromised, apparently by a lack of prior communication to ensure that the student was fully prepared for the clinical encounter. In this instance, insufficient attention to the intellectual and emotional well-being of the student affected a potentially high-quality educational experience for both the student and the patient. However, had inadequate preparation resulted in poor physical rather than mental student performance, the consequences for the safety of the learning environment could have been far more serious.

The pursuit of excellence in medical education has the patient at its centre. Other means to bring the

> **BOX 26.5 Example 4: Developing effective environments and student support and guidance**
>
> 'A medical student encountered a patient in palliative care. The student felt intimidated by entering an environment of peace and tranquillity, where she was the outsider. This had inhibited the student's learning. Why was this? On further exploration, the student had not been given prior warning of the situation of this patient with motor neurone disease or had any debrief following this encounter. It seemed to me that a powerful educational opportunity had been lost, where the patient and the family may have provided many issues to consider, including medical management, end-of-life care and the ethical issues of euthanasia. It demonstrated that the environment is of paramount importance to provide a safe and effective learning environment where clinical teaching is enhanced by prior preparation, teaching with patients and providing clear, immediate feedback'.
>
> *Clinical teacher*

patient experience into the learning frame have been developed in places such as Africa and Latin America. Here 'expert patient-trainers' (EPTs), often recruited from groups of people living with HIV/AIDS, have been introduced as a learning intervention.(23) A recent report by Seung *et al.* of such an intervention describes how EPTs lead classroom discussions on living with HIV to help healthcare workers understand HIV as it affects patients.(23) Special 'skill stations', consisting of one-to-one encounters with EPTs and health workers where the EPTs portray a standardised case but then uses their own life experiences to fill in emotional details, have been developed as part of the learning process. Although health workers were initially sceptical about EPTs, 'this generally turned to enthusiasm after participating in the skill stations and intervention benefited from the sense of being part of the training team, the satisfaction of improving the skills of health workers, and learning more about their illness'.(23)

Integration of scholarship, research and professional activities with teaching and supporting learning

To be an excellent teacher one must involve and integrate scholarship and research into one's professional practice (Box 26.6). Yet teaching and research are often viewed as distinct from each other, occupying opposite ends of a spectrum of scholarly activity.

Fincher and Work(27) argued that teaching and research are also part of a continuous whole, characterised as 'scholarly teaching'. For these authors, teaching and research shade into one another and

An enthusiastic consultant and an orthopaedic team who were willing to experiment thought that they might be able to improve the quality of their post-take trauma meetings. They particularly wanted to increase the diversity of contributions to the multi-professional meetings and to move away from traditional doctor-orientated meetings. They wanted to incorporate four key principles for teaching and learning into their revised approach:

1 active rather than passive learning should be encouraged

2 teaching should be at a level appropriate to knowledge and ability

3 cognitive overload should be avoided

4 threatened self-esteem diminishes learning.(24)

They worked with medical educators to develop a more structured approach to meetings using the five teaching micro-skills developed by Neher *et al*.(25) (sometimes known as the 'One Minute Preceptor'). They experimented with the model in a controlled environment, observed the sessions, sought feedback and evaluated the responses. The medical educators found that the new-style meetings resulted in more involvement from the whole team. They discerned a clear shift in the meeting dynamics 'from the didactic parent–child relationship towards professional adult peers searching together for the best possible patient care'. They knew the study had limitations because it was small, and they realised that there was more that they could do to continue the work, but they reported their findings in a peer-reviewed journal aimed at practising clinical teachers in order to encourage colleagues in the field to consider undertaking similar interventions.

Project reported in Atkinson and Spencer(26)

---

there is an enormous area of overlap where scholarly teaching and the scholarship of teaching may be found.

Any conscientious teacher designs and implements activities designed to maximise students' learning – but good teachers are not necessarily scholarly teachers. To develop excellence, medical education practitioners must deliberately improve their teaching by engaging with the educational literature to design, apply and evaluate the methods and interventions they use in their professional practice, seeking feedback from colleagues and students on their work, and then making use of the results. By undertaking this process, they become scholarly teachers.

As they broaden the range and scope of their scholarly teaching, some medical educators develop a peer-reviewed and published product (such as a poster, website, conference presentation or paper) designed to help others to build on their work, and which advances the whole field rather than just a single individual's practice. This is the scholarship of teaching. The scholarship of teaching shades into the classic definition of research – the type of 'blue skies' thinking that increases and extends our knowledge and understanding of the world and is so highly valued in research assessment terms.

What Example 5 in Box 26.6 shows us is an excellent example of scholarly teaching and the scholarship of teaching in action. The group made use of the education literature to theorise the ways in which an intervention could be developed; they designed it, applied it in a controlled and safe environment, evaluated it and published it for the benefit of the community. In many ways, this small study is typical of the work that is being done by medical educators in a variety of teaching and learning settings across the world, and it shows what can be done, even on a small scale, to use research and scholarship to develop excellence in teaching and learning.

However, what makes this intervention of particular interest is the emphasis it places on the professional values that should underpin any scholarly effort in teaching and learning in medicine. There is clearly no doubt in the minds of anyone who was involved in the project that good practice and scholarship in medical education are absolutely critical to patient care; and the emphasis throughout the project is to ensure that patients receive the best possible outcome.

Evaluation of practice and continuing professional development

Medical education must at some point use real patients to develop the skills of health professionals but there is also an obligation to provide optimal treatment and to ensure patients' safety and wellbeing.(28) New skills and techniques involved in technological advances, such as those in micro-surgery, must be practised to increase levels of dexterity and precision. Increasingly, simulators are used to develop medical students' and junior doctors' knowledge, skills and attitudes while protecting patients from unnecessary risks. Simulation training can be used to introduce the learner to less-common conditions and to allow more experienced practitioners to keep their skills up to date.

As Example 6 in Box 26.7 illustrates, this form of training is welcomed by the newly qualified doctor. Nevertheless, for simulation to be used as a good-quality educational intervention, it must conform to a high degree of 'psychological or functional fidelity'.(29) This is the degree to which the skill or skills in the real task are captured in the simulated task. Furthermore, for the learning tool to be effective, it needs to involve deliberate practice, reflection and

BOX 26.7 Example 6: Evaluation of practice and continuing professional development

Newly qualified doctor: When you start working and especially when you're just doing ward jobs a lot, you kind of sometimes feel like, you know, knowledge-wise and clinically you think 'oh goodness, am I really progressing here?' After the exams, when you start working you know you're less sharp in terms of the factual things than you were when you finished finals. I think you tend to know more of the relevant stuff in what's relevant to what you generally do on a day-to-day basis, but small print things, you know, you generally forget so I think it's important to still have that teaching element. So far the teaching I've been to has actually been quite useful, so I think that's something that's good that we're having. And we had an acute, like acute-case scenario teaching session with the manikin, which is you know …

Interviewer: … the simulation man?

Newly qualified doctor: Simulation, yeah, which was really good. I thought that was really good because it was much more hands-on and true to life and what have you, and real situations, so that was really good and I hope we'll get some more of that.(30)

feedback, with any differences between the execution of a skill on the simulator and in the clinical environment made clear to the learner. Research shows that sustained and deliberate practice, using set aims and objectives with specific informative feedback, improves long-term skills acquisition.(31)

Technology must not be used to drive the educational agenda, but rather the development of technology should assist in identified training. Simulation does not replace the need for learning in the clinical environment but can provide the means to develop preparation to enhance the clinical experience and improve patient care.

How, then, may the quality of the simulation experience be improved? Noting that simulation deprives learning of real-time context (such as the hustle and bustle of the ward), and that learning skills in one context does not guarantee transfer to another context, Kneebone *et al.*(32) have devised a number of 'authentic simulation' learning experiences. For example, students can carry out an intervention on a simulated body part, but with an actor-patient in a real ward, to offer authentic context.

Discourses of Quality

Discourses are organised, culturally legitimated ways of knowing and doing. Discourses have been described as 'practices that systematically form the objects of which they speak'.(32) What Foucault means by this, for example, is that 'madness', or 'crime', or 'health', are not absolute or universal categories, but are 'produced' within a cultural setting and change historically. 'Quality' can be seen as a discourse, sensitive to historical and cultural production. A 'quality' medical education at the time of Abraham Flexner's influential report in 1910 would be different from a 'quality' medical education for the 21st century. Medical knowledge has grown exponentially since Flexner, and 'medicine' cannot now be taught in its entirety. Indeed, much of what is taught will be out of date in the very near future. So, medical students now have to learn to learn, and become both independent and collaborative inquirers. Furthermore in Flexner's day, students were almost wholly male and white. Now, women students are the majority and medicine shows a diverse ethnic mix. This raises very important quality issues – those of improving conditions of equity and equality of opportunity.

Historical and cultural discourses that produce the phenomenon we call 'quality' then fluctuate, so that views on quality are not fixed. What we mean by 'quality' at any one time (the dominant view) will come to marginalise other views. When Peter Fraser of the Chartered Quality Institute noted, 'there is a growing realisation that quality is multi-dimensional – things do not get done as a result of random acts and events, but rather as a sequence of interrelated actions which depend on resources being available and which are affected by a variety of influences',(34) we should note that quality as 'multi-dimensional' is a current popular, and dominant, discourse. Dominant discourses have gained 'legitimacy'. In the following section, we outline how 'quality' gains legitimacy from differing perspectives (Box 26.8).

Scientific

Scientific research approaches to medical education have become the most influential aspect of quality in medical education in recent years, as we move into an era of evidence-based practice. Since the 1970s, evaluation and research have become increasingly significant factors in the identification and measurement of quality. The randomised controlled trial (RCT), heralded as the 'gold standard' in clinical research, is often also promoted as the pinnacle method for gaining high-quality medical education research evidence. While the RCT and epidemiology studies have their place in medical education research,(35) the field is increasingly informed by research methodologies from the social sciences, which are aimed at gaining a richer, more complex understanding of educational processes. Experimental methods derived from cognitive and educational psychology have made substantial contributions towards an understanding of student learning, and qualitative research methods derived from sociology, anthropology and social psychology

BOX 26.8 Focus on: Learned societies in medical education

Professional development is crucial to the formation of high-quality medical educators, and if the quality of educational practice is to be continually improved, then all medical educators, whatever their professional background, discipline or specialty, need opportunities to:

• form and develop a sense of collective identity

• network

• update their skills and knowledge

• share ideas about best practice

• present their work for peer review and feedback

• reflect on their own practice as a means of continuous change and learning.

There are learned societies all over the world specifically set up to offer these opportunities. Most offer a variety of benefits to members, which are typically likely to include:

• meetings, conferences, short courses and workshops

• special interest groups

• training materials, bulletins, web sites and newsletters

• peer-reviewed journals

• grants, prizes and scholarships.

Space does not permit us to list all organisations that serve the medical education community, but they include:

Academy of Medical Educators (AoME) http://www.medicaleducator.org

Association for the Study of Medical Education (ASME) http://www.asme.org.uk

Association for Medical Education in Europe (AMEE) http://www.amee.org

Association of American Medical Colleges (AAMC) http://www.aamc.org

Australia and New Zealand Association for Medical Education (ANZAME) http://www.anzame.unsw.edu.au

Canadian Association for Medical Education (CAME) http://www.came-acem.ca

have provided frameworks that enable the interpretation of students' experiences as they undergo medical education. Furthermore, systematic reviews and meta-analyses of individual studies on particular issues, such as those conducted on behalf of the Best Evidence in Medical Education collaboration have produced forms of evidence that readily inform quality improvement.(36) However, scientific discourse remains dominant,(37) potentially marginalising other ways to gain evidence, such as narrative methods.

Aesthetic

Paradoxically, the *quality* of education is often measured using *quantitative* methodologies, allowing comparison of standards and experience through statistical analysis. However, as Eisner has shown, viewing the cognitive culture from a different, more aesthetically inclined viewpoint can provide a more generous conception of the practice of education.(38) Medicine has long been considered both science and art, and an aesthetic discourse on the 'quality' of medical education may view educational practice as a form of 'connoisseurship'.(38) This is embodied in the culture of 'expert review', rather than experimental evidence. It is common in medical education research to garner the views of high-profile figures in the field on any topic (such as 'what makes a "good" doctor?'). This is connoisseurship. 'Quality' is the central concern of an aesthetic outlook, as opposed to a technical outlook, which may see quality only in terms of 'efficiency'. At root, 'aesthetic' means 'sense impression', and medical education in its clinical aspect is largely about educating the senses as the basis for clinical judgement. The medical humanities can help to develop such acumen, where a 'quality' doctor is now one with added value, over and above technical competence.

Managerial

'Quality' for many is an issue of efficiency rather than aesthetics. This is especially true for providers of healthcare, be they commercial, insurance-based businesses such as in the US, or politicians in countries with a state-sponsored healthcare system, who see factors such as 'throughput' as vital to the efficient running of health services. Such values also permeate management of those services. The discourse of 'quality management' has increasingly become a significant feature of medical education.

The concept of 'quality assurance' first arose in the context of industrial manufacturing. In particular, a scientific approach to quality assurance arose in the context of mass production, as the 'skilled craftsman' was replaced by an assembly line of different workers responsible for the assembly of small segments of a given product. Procedures based on empirical measuring were introduced to assess the quality of the materials used, the process of manufacturing and the products produced. However, it became apparent that these procedures alone could not guarantee high quality. In the business world during the 1980s, the concept of total control quality management (TQM) came to be seen as an increasingly important framework in the drive to achieve excellence and success. TQM is based on strategies aimed at achieving excellence in business by building outstanding relationships with clients and employing visionary managers with 'hands-on' management styles to lead enthusiastic teams. While medical educators might not readily identify their field with that of business, such management discourse has undoubtedly influenced medical education and systems of quality assurance.

Economic

The managerial and business discourses are intimately bound to economic discourses. Doctors are increasingly being reminded that allocation of resources must be an important part of their decision-making processes. This is commonplace experience for general practitioners, who now run practices as businesses. It is acute where pressure is placed on medicine to utilise expensive, technologically sophisticated approaches that may only benefit relatively few, but high-profile, cases. Doctors have to be aware that a quality practice is also a fair practice in terms of limited resource allocation.

The world of medical education has necessarily been subjected to the demands of the marketplace, and these may undermine drives for improvement in quality. Economic discourses on the quality of education inevitably impose boundaries on its potential. Marketisation, governance and working conditions are forces that challenge the higher education sector and have an inevitable international impact.(39) Of these, perhaps the most pertinent to maintaining high-quality medical education is marketisation, in which the temptation to 'package' medical training for a global market, to global standards, may actually serve to lower standards. This has been recognised to a certain extent, with international and national regulatory bodies recommending a dual-layered process which both meets minimum standards and encourages enhancement. A high-quality medical education is one that needs to maintain awareness of these tensions.

Budgetary constraints and ever-decreasing funding mean that the ideals of high-quality teaching and learning have to be compromised, delivering instead the highest quality provision possible within the limits of money, time and resources. This is of particular relevance to medical education, where innovative new learning modes are replacing dissection as a means of learning anatomy, using high-tech, high-quality models and simulated systems in the life sciences and clinical skills environments. To remain at the forefront of medical education, these programmes are under pressure to keep up with, and where possible, anticipate, the latest technological developments and how these can be translated into a high-quality educational experience.

Ethical

The practice of medicine is seen an ethical endeavour requiring the highest possible standards in professionalism. Nevertheless ethical discourse often presumes a fixed set of ethical standards that can be universally applied. Patients and communities vary in their needs, and hold different cultural values and norms of health. We might assume that ethics quality is the same in all healthcare organisations, but as Wynia observes, 'anyone who's worked in more than one healthcare organization knows that the ethical culture of different organizations can vary dramatically'.(40) This is further exacerbated where the complexity and inherent contradictions of what might constitute 'ethics' quality is considered. Wynia questions, for example, whether concern for justice is more important than concern for autonomy, or whether it is ethically more commendable to fulfil a duty to community or to special relations. In a clinical environment, these issues are further compounded by competing ethical standards based on business, public health, and personal and professional ethics.

Ethical standards are not based on fixed objective principles but, rather, reflect the values of a given society. Sociologist Renee Fox and historian Judith Swazey(41) have shown that the conceptual framework of bioethics as espoused within the ethics curriculum has accorded paramount status to the value-complex of individualism, underscoring the principles of individual rights, autonomy and self-determination. After their 1981 visit to hospitals and clinics in China, they argued that the team of bioethicists who had previously visited and had mistakenly concluded that there were 'no medical ethics in China', were simply blinded by their own ethnocentricity. Indeed, they demonstrated that the kind of medical morality being practised by doctors and nurses in China was one that focused on sensitivity to the interdependency and relatedness of their patients to others. The same argument applies to the exportation of individualistic learning theories, and 'intimate' learning practices such as small group problem-based learning to cultures used to collectivist and authority-led practices. Bleakley *et al.* argue that the export of ideas from the West could be in danger of becoming a 'neo-colonialism'.

> How can we be sure that modern global initiatives in medical education, which are largely advocated and funded by those in the modern, metropolitan West who have the resources and influence to drive them through, are not just another type of domination by the advanced country over the developing nation?(42)

It is evident that a high-quality curriculum is one that needs to be sensitive to the varying needs of patients recognising the ethnic and cultural diversity that exists in many societies. However, alongside this, a drive for improvement in quality usually involves both standard setting and the standardisation of medical education. There is therefore an inevitable tension between the *universal* and the *particular*.

Professional

A discourse of professionalism has come to the fore in recent years. Medicine as a profession has long been identified with a series of traits and characteristic practices that include an altruistic orientation towards those served by the profession, and a code of ethics through which to define and monitor that service. However, during the 1970s and 1980s, Freidson developed a critique of professional dominance.(43) He argued that medicine, in common with other professions, is an organised occupation that seeks to control the conditions of its own work by developing and defining a relevant body of knowledge, and by educating, testing and credentialing practitioners. The medical profession is thus able to exercise autonomy over work undertaken by its members, control and manage the work of others in the healthcare field, evoke deference from patients and the wider public, and exercise institutional power, maintaining cultural and legal authority over its jurisdiction. Furthermore, Freidson argued that it was the ability of the medical profession to persuade successive governments to support them (for example, through legal recognition of the AMA in the US and the GMC in the UK) that helped them to secure their dominant position.

The status of the profession has been somewhat further undermined in recent years with well-publicised scandals relating to bad practice and poor regulation, along with changing societal expectations about the role of the doctor. Medicine is regarded as being less altruistic, of abusing its privileged position to advance the status of the profession and of failing to self-regulate effectively. The maintenance of quality standards has always been the province of the profession, but questions have arisen as to whether medicine and other professions are capable of self-regulation.

The profession has responded to such criticisms by setting in place more robust self-regulation mechanisms, ensuring:

- that errant doctors are detected and prevented from practising
- that measures are set in place to ensure the high-quality education of all doctors
- a growing realisation that professionalism must be taught explicitly to encourage the internalisation of the value systems of the good doctor.

Ethical norms underpinning professionalism are currently being debated. In the UK, the Royal College of Physicians has abandoned previous aspects of professionalism, in particular the notions of 'mastery, autonomy, and privilege, and self regulation', replacing them with increased emphasis on the patient, doctor–patient interaction and on securing public trust.(44) This echoes Ludmerer's (1999) suggestion that restoring trust between medicine and the wider community is a pressing issue for medical education as we enter the 21st century.(6) These new aspects reflect changing norms and values in contemporary society, where hierarchies of power have been challenged and more democratic forms of accountability have become the norm. The role of the doctor and what counts as high-quality medicine need to meet changing societal expectations and values.

Political

Given that most universities, medical schools and providers of healthcare around the world are at least in part state funded, it is not surprising the political discourse should shape medical education. The Flexner report at the beginning of the 20th century, for example, revolutionised the way American medical education was delivered. However, Flexner did not adequately judge the depth of the political paradoxes facing his recommendations. One of the most controversial of his recommendations was the consideration given to the medical education of women and black students in a time before women had the vote and bigotry was rife.(45) In 1908, this was ground-breaking. However, as Hodges(46) points out, the schools that Flexner recommended should be closed because of poor practices and under-resourcing included, understandably, those very schools that had committed to the intake of women and black students. A century later, equal opportunities are at the forefront of legislation and it is inconceivable that provision of medical education (or any education) would not be inclusive. In the UK, where most healthcare is provided by the state, the government has been influential in shaping medical education. As noted earlier, MMC,(10) for example, is a government programme of reform established with the aim of 'improving medical education' and providing 'a transparent and efficient career path for doctors'. Moreover, for the first time in the history of UK medical education, the training of doctors and their registration is not the sole province of the medical profession and medical schools.(47) The discourse of politics dominates quality debates in medical education, where it is intimately tied to the economic, managerial, and instrumental.

It may be that the key dilemma facing 'quality' improvement in medical education is the tension between the medical education community's long-term vision of developing an authentic patient-centred approach based on best evidence, and the demands of the political community for short-term efficiency in a complex system of healthcare.

Conclusion

In summary, while there are competing discourses of 'quality', continuous quality improvement in medical education is a pressing concern for the medical education community. Pro-activity is required in developing a coherent community as a vibrant culture of medical education. Key to this is to develop collaborative research between clinical and academic communities of practice. 'Quality' for the clinical communities of practice may differ from definitions proposed by academic communities of practice, and this dialogue must be pursued.

One way in which to encourage such a dialogue is for academic researchers to help clinical communities to better research their own practices, for example through collaborative inquiry. In turn, academic researchers will achieve a better quality of research through longer periods of socialisation into the medical and healthcare communities they study. A second encouraging development is an emerging structure that promotes academic medicine and medical education as legitimate specialties within medicine, with appropriate career paths.

Third, and finally, quality improvement will occur as medical education redefines its own purposes as an excellent example of an interdisciplinary culture. The culture of medical education must be fully professionalised, with transparent mechanisms for accreditation and recognition of achievement, such as the new schemes developed by the UK Academy of Medical Educators (Box 26.8).(48)

Acknowledgements

The authors wish to acknowledge the contributions of John Bligh, Julian Archer, Karen Mattick, Nick Cooper, Hilary Neve, Nick Toms and Nicola Brennan.

References

1 World Federation for Medical Education (2003) *WFME Global Standards for Quality Improvement: continuing professional development (CPD) of medical doctors*. WFME, Copenhagen.
2 Lewkonia R (2001) Medical revalidation and education; directed self-learning. *Medical Education*. 35: 426–7.
3 Brownell AM (ed.) (1998). *Learning Objectives of Medical Student Education: guidelines for medical schools*. Association of American Medical Colleges, Washington, DC.
4 General Medical Council (2003) Tomorrow's Doctors. GMC, London.
5 World Federation for Medical Education (2003) *WFME Global Standards for Quality Improvement: basic medical education*. WFME, Copenhagen.
6 Ludmerer KM (1999) *Time to Heal: American medical education from the turn of the century to the era of managed care*. Oxford University Press, New York.
7 Collins A, Brown JS and Newman SE (1989) Cognitive apprenticeship: teaching the craft of reading, writing and matematics. In: Resnick LB (ed.) *Knowing, Learning and Instruction: essays in honor of Robert Glaser*, pp. 453–94. Erlbaum, Hillsdale, NJ.
8 Roter D and Hall JA (2006) *Doctors Talking with Patients/Patients Talking with Doctors: improving communication in medical visits* (2e). Praeger, West Port, CT.
9 World Federation for Medical Education (2003) *WMFE Global Standards for Quality Improvement: postgraduate medical education*. WFME, Copenhagen.
10 NHS (2008) *Modernising Medical Careers Online* (http://www.mmc.nhs.uk/default.aspx?page=280; accessed April 2010).
11 GMC (www.gmc-uk.org; accessed April 2010).
12 Holm HA (1998) Continuing medical education: quality issues in continuing medical education. *British Medical Journal*. 316: 621–4.
13 European Union of Specialist Doctors (UEMS) (1994) *Charter on Continuing Medical Education of Medical Specialists in the European Union*. UEMS, Brussels.
14 Department of Health (2008) *Medical Revalidation – Principles and Next Steps: the report of the Chief Medical Officer for England's Working Group*. The Crown, London.
15 Higher Education Academic (www.heacademy.ac.uk; accessed April 2010).
16 Academy of Medical Educators (2009) *Professional Standards*. Academy of Medical Educators, London.
17 Pugsley L and McCrorie P (2007) Improving medical education: improving patient care. *Teaching and Teacher Education*. 23: 314–22.
18 Jolly B and Rees L (eds) *Medical Education in the Millenium*. Oxford University Press, Oxford.
19 Mattick K and Knight L (2007) High-quality learning: harder to achieve than we think? *Medical Education*. 41: 638–44.
20 Haggis T (2003) Constructing images of ourselves? A critical investigation into approaches to learning research in higher education. *British Educational Research Journal*. 29: 89–104.
21 Stothart C (2008) Watchdog adds students to audit teams to assess university quality. *Times Higher Education*. **24 July**, 2008.
22 Perera J, Lee N, Win K, Perera J and Wijesuriya L (2008) Formative feedback to students: the mismatch between faculty perceptions and student expectations. *Medical Teacher*. 30: 395–9.
23 Seung KJ, Bitalabeho A, Buzaalirwa LE *et al*. (2008) Standardized patients for HIV/AIDS training in resource-poor settings: the expert patient-trainer. *Academic Medicine*. 83: 1204–9.
24 Bandiera G, Lee S and Tiberius R (2005) Creating effective learning in today's emergency departments: how accomplished teachers get it done. *Annals of Emergency Medicine*. 45: 253–61.
25 Neher J, Gordon K, Meyer B and Stevens N (1992) A five-step 'microskills' model of clinical teaching. *Journal of the American Board of Family Practice*. 5: 419–24.
26 Atkinson S and Spencer E (2008) Structuring the orthopaedic trauma meeting to improve learning. *The Clinical Teacher*. 5: 213–17.
27 Fincher R and Work J (2006) Perspectives on the scholarship of teaching. *Medical Education*. 40: 293–5.
28 Bradley P (2006) The history of simulation in medical education and possible future directions. *Medical Education*. 40: 254–62.
29 Maran NJ and Glavin RJ (2003) Low- to high-fidelity simulation; a continuum of medical education? *Medical Education*. 37(s1): 22–8.
30 Brenan N and Corrigan O (2009) Longitudinal Evaluation of South West Peninsula Deanery F1 Doctors, Final Report (http://sites.pcmd.ac.uk/ice/; accessed 6th January 2010).
31 Liddell M, Davidson S, Taub H and Whitecross L (2002) Evaluation of procedural skills training in an undergraduate curriculum. *Medical Education*. 36: 1035–41.
32 Kneebone RL, Kidd J, Nestel D *et al*. (2005) Blurring the boundaries: scenario-based simulation in a clinical setting. *Medical Education*. 39: 580–7.
33 Foucault M (1972) *The Archaelogy of Knowldege*. Tavistock Publications, New York, London.
34 Fraser P. Concepts of quality, history and development (http://www.thecqi.org/knowledge/evolution.shtml; accessed 22 September 2008).
35 Torgerson C (2002) Educational research and randomised trials. *Medical Education*. 36: 1002–3.

36 Mufunda J, Chatora R, Ndambakuwa Y *et al.* (2007) Challenges in training the ideal doctor for Africa: lessons learned from Zimbabwe. *Medical Teacher.* **29**: 878–81.

37 Bleakley A (2005) Stories as data, data as stories: making sense of narrative inquiry in clinical education. *Medical Education.* **39**(5): 534–40.

38 Eisner EW (2004) What can education learn from the arts about the practice of education? *International Journal of Education and the Arts.* **5**(4): 1–13.

39 Gill J (2008) New AAUP chief to fight 'academic capitalism'. *Times Higher Education.* **1860**: 22.

40 Wynia MK (1999) Performance measures for ethics quality. *Effective Clinical Practice.* **1999**: 294–9.

41 Fox R and Swazey J (1984) Medical morality is not bioethics – medical ethics in China and the United States. *Perspectives in Biology and Medicine.* **27**: 337–61.

42 Bleakley A, Brice J and Bligh J (2008) Thinking the post-colonial in medical education. *Medical Education.* **42**: 266–70.

43 Freidson E (1970) *Profession of Medicine: a study of the sociology of applied knowledge.* Dodd, Mead, New York.

44 Royal College of Physicians (2005) *Doctors in Society: medical professionalism in a changing world.* Royal College of Physicians, London.

45 Meites S (1995) Abraham Flexner's Legacy: a magnificent beneficence to American medical education and clinical chemistry. *Clinical Chemistry.* **41**: 627–32.

46 Hodges B (2005) The many and conflicting histories of medical education in Canada and the USA: an introduction to the paradigm wars. *Medical Education.* **39**: 613–21.

47 Corrigan OP and Pinchen I (2010) Tomorrow's doctors, a changing profession: reformation in the UK medical education system. In: Bronson C and Turner B (eds) *Handbook of the Sociology of Medical Education,* pp. 242–60. Taylor and Francis, Oxford.

48 Bligh J and Brice J (2007) The Academy of Medical Educators: a professional home for medical educators in the UK. *Medical Education.* **41**: 625–7.

Further Reading

Best Evidence in Medical Education collaboration http://www.bemecollaboration.org

Gunderman RB (2006) *Achieving Excellence in Medical Education.* Springer-Verlag, London.

Sallis E (2002) *Total Quality Management in Education* (3e). Kogan Page, London.

Dealing with diversity

Antony Americano and Dinesh Bhugra

KEY MESSAGES

- Competence in diversity requires an awareness of differing styles, values, beliefs and practices.
- Diversity includes areas covered by legislation, other stratifications in society and the differences that make us all unique.
- Social inclusion is a key political priority.
- Understanding disability and different approaches to it is very important for clinicians.

- Barriers in diversity are linked to language, stereotypes and cultural bias.
- Lack of awareness of diversity affects all levels of training.
- Societies of origin influence personality traits and expectations.
- Training in diversity can be integrated with teaching and supervision.

Introduction

Theory and a growing body of evidence suggest that competence in diversity is central to the successful relationship between the clinician and patient. This interaction is based on a power differential that is reliant on education, social status and other factors, which will vary according to culture, gender, disability, location of the interaction (e.g. home visit or outpatient clinic) and geography (e.g. rural or urban). Similarly, belief systems, religious factors and cultural expectations play a role in acceptance of, and adherence to, treatment in which again the clinician–patient encounter becomes central. Paralleling this interaction in healthcare education is the relationship between clinician-teacher and learner. An understanding of diversity is therefore essential in the teaching and practice of medicine as well as for personal and professional growth. Diversity is not a straightforward concept, however, and confusion surrounds its meaning and aims. Diversity is complex, multifactorial and its value contested. The aim of this chapter is to help the reader understand this complexity, in particular as it relates to clinical education.

Defining Diversity

The terms *diversity* and *equalities* (sometimes *equality* or *equal opportunities*) often appear together and may be used interchangeably. But, while similar, the foci for these terms are different. The *diversity* approach is concerned with valuing the contributions of everyone in society, embracing individual differences and encompassing the full range of social groupings. It has a broad scope and covers issues such as personality traits and type, learning style, accent, class and professional background, as well as a number of societal subgroups recognised in law. While the diversity approach recognises *group* issues, the emphasis is on the *individual*.

Equalities, on the other hand, although concerned with the same general principle of inclusion, has a greater focus on legislation or groups experiencing officially recognised social exclusion or injustice. Because there is legislative force behind much of equalities, it has a greater emphasis on policies, monitoring and targets than diversity. The emphasis is on the level of the group.

The concepts of diversity and equalities are not fixed and immutable; they vary across geography: Northern Ireland, for socio-political reasons, addressed discrimination on the grounds of religion years before the rest of the UK, and across time, sex and race discrimination legislation have been on the statute in the UK for over 30 years, while age was not added until 2006. Similarly, the way diversity is medicalised (or pathologised) changes over time. For example, until the 1970s homosexuality was a mental illness to be found in the *Diagnostic and Statistical Manual (DSM II) of Psychiatric Disorders*. Once it was removed, homosexuality was no longer an illness and gay and lesbian people are now afforded legal protection from discrimination.

These examples demonstrate that the concepts of diversity and equalities are socially constructed and reflect the concerns of particular groups of people at particular points or periods in time.(1,2) As society is

Understanding Medical Education: Evidence, Theory and Practice.
Edited by T Swanwick. © 2010 Association for the Study of Medical Education.

heterogeneous, at any one time there will be dissent about what or who is to be included or excluded. It is nevertheless helpful to consider an illustrative taxonomy of diversity proposed by Jehn *et al*.(3)

Social category diversity

This is concerned with demographic differences like gender and ethnicity, core equalities concerns in medical education. Jehn *et al*. theorised that difficulties in this factor would impact on group communication and cohesion, which of course are essential to effective clinical practice.

Informational diversity

Also known as 'organisational diversity', this refers to background diversity such as knowledge, education, experience, tenure and functional background. Medicine is recognised as a distinct 'tribe' among other 'tribes' such as nursing and other healthcare professions. A similar situation is replicated within medicine itself, where there are many distinct subgroups. These types of difference were theorised by Jehn *et al*. to affect group communication and cohesion as well as generate higher task-related conflict.

Value diversity

This refers to differences in personality and attitudes. In some ways perhaps this is the richest source of difference but an area that has the potential to impact on individual, team and organisational life. This factor raises issues of 'team fit' and personality clashes, as well as fundamentally different belief systems. If this difference cannot be managed, it can lead to conflict within teams, across professional groups and with patients and carers.

Jehn's taxonomy helps us to understand the complexity of diversity, because no single element will define an individual's unique contribution as they will differ within and across the three domains.

Fairness

The complexity of different belief systems is then at the very core of diversity. But why is it necessary to take such an approach? Why, specifically, is the commonsensical notion of *fairness* not acceptable to all? We can see why not by looking at three different approaches to fairness: equity, equality and need. To illustrate these approaches we use the example of selection, which could be into training, or higher education.

Equity

An applicant considers his or her own merits and selection outcome compared with a referent other's input to output ratio. If the referent other is deemed to be getting more for the same input or the same for less input then unfairness will be perceived. This is in line with the principle of meritocracy and is individualistic in nature. Fairness is therefore judged by whether the person who has done most (studied, gained prizes, etc.) gets the job.(5)

Equality

Here, an applicant will take a more social view looking for equal chance and representation for groups within society. In particular, this has been relevant when considering the employment position of minority ethnic groups, women and disabled people, and more recently in relation to age, sexual orientation and religion. Fairness in selection is judged by the presence or absence of discriminated-against groups in the workforce, for example, at the consultant level or within training programmes.

Need

This approach goes further in applying the principle of social justice allocating employment on the basis of need, for example, economic in respect of the unemployed or social with regard to the child-rearing responsibilities of single parents. Fairness is judged by meeting the needs of those who have nothing or not enough, for example, refugee doctors needing support to restart their career.

These three different approaches help to explain why any move to make a given process fairer is likely to be met with approval from some and disapproval from others, depending on the values they bring(6) and their own conceptualisation of fairness. This analysis is applicable to any situation where access to limited resources or to desired goals are in play. At the same time, it should be recognised that human motivation can be more complex than this simple model proposes and that people can be more selfless and selfish than suggested.

Diversity in Organisations

Impact

How does diversity impact, positively or negatively, on group performance and behaviour? It has been theorised that effective management of diversity is good for group and organisational performance, and conversely that poor management of diversity is damaging.(7)

An evidence base for this assertion exists but is generally inconclusive. Different studies show a complex range of results that are hard to generalise, in part due to the limitations of the studies themselves and the difficulty in controlling for variables. Additionally, it is theorised that the value of diversity to group performance may depend on the type of task. The value may be particularly high when understanding of a particular social category is a benefit, but less, or negatively so, when tasks do not require such input.(3) One study proposing a positive benefit looked at 486 British companies and found that promoting diversity reduced recruitment costs, increased employee motivation and staff retention, and improved employer image.(8)

Whatever the questions about the evidence base, there is a socio-legal reality to be faced. A well-established body of legislation and new legal responsibilities for promoting race, gender and disability equality in the public sector make some aspects of diversity a must-do (*see* The socio-political context section).

Furthermore, bad publicity on diversity can be damaging to an organisation and may alienate sections of the community it serves. The findings of institutional racism (*see* Box 27.1 for definition) against the Metropolitan Police as a result of the Stephen Lawrence Inquiry(4) is a good example of the damaging impact of failing to manage diversity adequately.

Competence

There are five essential elements that contribute to a system's ability to become more diversity competent and compliant. These principles are based on those for organisational cultural competency. The system should:

- value diversity
- have the capacity for diversity self-assessment
- be conscious of the dynamics inherent when cultures and diversities interact
- institutionalise diversity knowledge about its client group

---

BOX 27.1 Focus on: The evolution of terminology

You can be forgiven for being confused about some of the terminology used when discussing diversity. The language used differs from place to place and has changed over time. For example, *Asian* in the UK refers to Indian, Bangladeshi, Pakistani and other similarly located peoples. In the US, this refers mainly to people of Chinese and Far Eastern origin.

While it is important to try and use acceptable terminology, particularly if the group concerned has requested this, using the correct terms does not, by itself, achieve equality, and using the wrong term unknowingly is not a cardinal sin. Otherwise fear of offending takes over from having an open dialogue on the issues. The dialogue is what matters. The following explains some terms and how they have evolved over time.

Black

A common term 20 years ago, 'black' was used as a generic, political term to describe all non-white minority ethnic groups. The aim was to emphasise solidarity among those who shared a common experience of discrimination because of skin colour. Currently, it is not common to describe skin colour in this broad way. Mainly this is because many people did not feel that this term adequately considered the diversity of culture and experience present. The term black and minority ethnic groups (BME) has come into common use recently.

Ethnic minorities

This term refers to groups that are not the major ethnic group in a country or particular geography. There is a growing preference for using the term *minority ethnic* group as opposed to ethnic minority group. The reason for this is that the former emphasises the minority aspect rather than the ethnicity. It reminds us that everyone has an ethnicity and therefore ethnicity should not be demonised or made to be exotic. Additionally, minority ethnic groups can be predominantly white, for example, Irish.

Disability

There are a number of conflicting models of disability (*see* Box 27.3). Disability is often used to refer to an individual's impairment – the medical model. However, many disabled people see their disability as being caused by the attitude of society and the organisational arrangements (services, etc.) made by society – the social model. Thus *disabled person*, rather than person with a disability, is preferred.

Equalities

Equalities are often misinterpreted as being concerned with treating everyone the same. In reality the equality, or *equal opportunities*, is concerned with 'opportunity' rather than treatment. Outcomes are the important measures of equal opportunities. We do not start on a level playing field and social exclusion is inevitable if differences are not recognised.

Institutional racism

New words and phrases emerge all the time from the general socio-political milieu, sometimes from a single event. One example is the term *institutional racism*, which was coined following an enquiry into the handling of the investigation (by the Metropolitan Police) of the killing of black teenager Stephen Lawrence. The Macpherson report(4) defined institutional racism as: 'The collective failure of an organisation to provide an appropriate and professional service to people because of their colour, culture or ethnic origin which can be seen or detected in processes; attitudes and behaviour which amount to discrimination through unwitting prejudice, ignorance, thoughtlessness and racist stereotyping which disadvantages minority ethnic people.'

Figure 27.1   The continuum of diversity competence. Source: Cross *et al.*(9).

- develop adaptations to delivering what is required and expected by reflecting an understanding of diversity.

These five elements must be manifested in every level of the organisation through policy, structures and services.

As cultural competence is a developmental process,(9) so diversity competence can be conceived along a continuum. These developmental stages of an organisation's competence in diversity are depicted in Figure 27.1. It is essential that organisations assess where they are on the continuum because it will allow them to put ameliorative measures, such as appropriate staff training, in place.

Clinical teachers may also need to determine where they are along the continuum of diversity competency so they can choose what steps are required to further develop their needs (*see* Box 27.2). The teachers should check their own responses to other cultures, strategies for coping with these and their ability to understand and help students from diverse backgrounds. The consequences of a lack of awareness of broad diversity-related issues are many and would mean, for example, that trainers are unable to train trainees properly, who in turn then ignore these issues in their patients and carers.

The Socio-political Context

Everyone in society will come into contact with the healthcare system whether directly or via family and friends. The effectiveness of that contact can make a difference in the quality and duration of a person's life. Healthcare is therefore rightly a political issue and at times, more problematically, an ideological battlefield. Medical education cannot shield itself from this reality and the current political priorities of ending social exclusion. This includes fair selection and promotion in the medical profession for people from all backgrounds, as well as fair access to healthcare and equality of outcomes. To this end, the UK Higher Education Funding Council has set clear targets to promote access to higher education. In some areas, such as gender, the student profile has changed dramatically, with many more women getting into medical school. In other areas, such as disability participation and social class, much work remains to be done.

As key political issues, diversity and social inclusion have seen themselves incorporated into plans to mod-

> **BOX 27.2 Diversity competence: A framework**
>
> *Knowledge*
> - Understanding of culture, conflict and potential problems
> - Knowledge of history, language, religion, customs, values
> - Knowledge of medical models predominant
> - Understanding of social, political, economic, institutional factors
> - Knowledge of support and services
> - Knowledge of local diversity and differences
>
> *Professional skills*
> - Techniques for learning and teaching about diversity
> - Ability to communicate clearly and accurately
> - Ability to openly discuss diversity issues
> - Ability to recognise issues to do with conflict
> - Ability to recognise and combat racism
> - Ability to plan culturally appropriate teaching
> - Ability to evaluate skills
>
> *Personal attributes*
> - Empathy and flexibility in attitudes
> - Acceptance of differences due to diversity
> - Openness to new experiences and people
> - Willingness to work with diverse clients
> - Awareness of differences and similarities across diverse groups

ernise the UK National Health Service (NHS). *The NHS Plan* states that:

> No injustice is greater than the inequalities in health which scar our nation. The life expectancy of a boy born into the bottom social class is over nine years less than a boy born into the more affluent social classes.(10)

Disparity between different groups, for example, gender, ethnic and social class, can be found in health, income, education, employment, housing and community safety, and in many aspects of day-to-day life. Health professionals should have an interest in all aspects of social inequality as they all have an impact on health.

Despite significant advances in medicine and higher spending on health, profound social inequalities persist in the UK. For example, there are marked differences between the health outcomes of people from different socio-economic groups and ethnic backgrounds on key health outcomes such as infant mortality and life expectancy.(11) For example, in London, there is a difference of seven years in life expectancy to be found by simply travelling eight stops on a local rail link.(12) Such differences in health outcomes are very real and demand attention.

Governments use the law as a key method of tackling these concerns. Accordingly, we have seen 40 years of developing law and case law concerning equality, inclusion and inalienable human rights. First tackling gender and race issues, legislation and case law has grown to include human rights, disability, age, religion, gender reassignment and sexual orientation. These have not only had a fundamental influence on organisational policy but also on clinical practice.

The influence on policy and behaviour in the public sector has recently been increased with the introduction of equalities duties, first covering race, closely followed by disability and gender. Legislation in 2010 should also add public sector duties around the promotion of diversity in areas of age, religion and sexual orientation. For example, the Race Relations (Amendment) Act 2000 has placed a new and important statutory duty on public bodies, whether NHS or higher education, to promote race relations. Key measures for this duty are as follows.

- Students from all ethnic backgrounds are equally satisfied with their education.
- Levels of educational achievement are high, with all students achieving their full potential.
- The trainees are representative of the relevant population from which the organisation recruits.
- Generally, the level of complaints is low, and there are no significant differences between ethnic groups in complaints about admission, training posts, teaching, assessment and support.(13)

Such legislative requirements apply across the board and in medical education will impact on the postgraduate as well as undergraduate arena. Both will need to show their ability to comply with this duty through strong leadership, clear policies and clear evidence of compliance. Education and training is central to managing this process successfully. This is particularly challenging for postgraduate medical education where trainees learn on the job and as employees. All organisations involved in postgraduate medical education must show leadership if the aims of diversity are to be achieved.

The regulatory framework mirrors these broader concerns. The General Medical Council's (GMC) foundation document *Good Medical Practice*(14) lays out the professional standards expected of all doctors. This includes a diversity statement in that doctors must not discriminate against colleagues because of their views on culture, beliefs, race or colour. To address this standard and ensure legal compliance, the teaching of cultural competence has become increasingly common in undergraduate medicine. Less is understood about cultural competence training in postgraduate education, where it competes with organisational and service priorities and training in clinical competencies.

More generally, concerns about *adverse impact* in medicine have been raised for over 25 years now. Adverse impact is where a particular group performs or succeeds noticeably below the norm. There have been concerns about the success rate of minority ethnic candidates gaining entry into medical school(15–17) and in relation to age and socio-economic background.(18) This concern about adverse impact extends to the career progression of women and minority ethnic groups through the junior doctor grades.(19,20) Black minority ethnic groups are most likely to end up working in unpopular specialties or in career-grade posts.(21) Further concerns encompass leadership and academic roles, with women and minority ethnic groups found to be under-represented in these areas too.(22,23)

A similar situation can be found in the US: 'Although minority groups comprise 30% of the US population, only 13% of medical students, 6% of practicing physicians, and 3% of medical school faculty are members of an underrepresented minority group'.(24) Similar international concerns regarding the representation of women are documented with horizontal (women concentrated in certain areas) and vertical (women under-represented in higher levels of the profession) segregation common.(25)

Adverse impact does not equate to unlawful discrimination. It does, however, challenge us to look at the reasons for the differences and consider the consequences for social equity that this disparity causes.

Disability

Among diversity themes, disability merits specific mention as it is frequently misunderstood.(26) Inevitably, the following section can only function as an overview of a complex area. The Medical Act 1983 has long allowed the GMC to tailor training to enable disabled students to become qualified. More recent moves to competency-based assessment will also help with this approach. The focus of training can change from an individual being required to carry out particular tasks/procedures in order to progress. Instead, the underlying competencies can be identified and demonstrated in alternative ways, where it is safe to do so.

More recently, the Special Education Needs and Disability Act 2001 (SENDA) was introduced to protect students, including higher education students, from disability discrimination. Its scope includes examinations and assessments, short courses, arrangements for work placements, and libraries and learning resources. SENDA has amended the Disability Discrimination

Act 1995 (DDA), which has a broader view of disability discrimination. Under the terms of the DDA it is illegal to treat people less favourably in the provision of goods, facilities and services; in offering and during employment; and in education. All three areas are key, as postgraduate medical education occurs in employment and while providing essential services to patients. To ignore these aspects is therefore to miss the reality of what the student is being trained to do.

In October 2004, the Act was further extended to cover organisations that confer, renew or extend a professional or trade qualification, for example, GMC and General Dental Council. It is therefore unlawful for a qualifications body to discriminate against a disabled person when it is awarding, renewing, extending or withdrawing a professional or trade qualification.

Despite the legislation, disabled people are underrepresented among medical graduates when compared with other disciplines. The number of disabled applicants accepted into degree courses rose from just under 5% to 5.5% between 2001 and 2006. The figure for medicine and dentistry stands at 2%.(27) There remains a significant stigma around disability in medicine, with a study suggesting that medical students associated disability with predominantly depersonalised or negative words.(28) These associations improved with training. This is an example of a medical model of disability that is often prevalent in healthcare. A social model is preferred by disabled people (*see* Box 27.3).

Cultural Diversity

The concept of *culture* cuts across all three categories of Jehn's typology,(3) referring to the 'inherited ideas, beliefs, values and knowledge which constitute the shared bases of social action'.(30) Often, we have inherited multiple cultures within us, for example, the culture of a particular university or organisation, and

values related to religion, gender or sexual orientation often compete within an individual and influence his or her net interactions with others. As a result, cultural identity is evolutionary, and changes with time and place. Diversity can be as great within a culture as it is across cultures, since not all beliefs, values, attitudes or behaviours will be shared, even within the same cultural group. Culture, again, needs to be distinguished from *race*, which is defined as a group of people with common ancestry with identifiable inherited physical attributes, and from *ethnicity*, which is usually a self-ascription reliant on common ancestral characteristics and cultural traditions, including religion and language.

Cultural competence

Cultural competence relies on a sophisticated awareness of these cultural beliefs, values and practices, yet cultural competence is somehow expected to emerge if the racial and ethnic mix of the workforce is representative of the local population. In reality this is not the case, and as the working practices of health professionals are theoretically the same, because of a common education or job description, understanding of differences in how those practices are acted out, through training in cultural competence,(31) becomes essential.

Training in cultural competence then bridges a number of social, cultural and economic factors. Undergraduate curricula often incorporate lectures and course work on cultural competency in healthcare provision. In a review, Bhui *et al.*(31) noted that the importance ascribed to training and education in cultural competence was high, but limited information was available on the contents or learning methods. Furthermore, there was no information on whether groups of health professionals required similar or different approaches. The authors also argued that cultural competence, including attention to organisational values, training and communication, must be embedded in the organisational infrastructure and ethos.

BOX 27.3 Models of disability

	Medical model	Charitable model	Social model
The individual	Individual is a patient/dependent	Individual is a charity case/ hero (dependent or exceptional)	Individual is a distinct member of society with rights/independent
Source of problem	Medical condition	Impairment	Attitudes in and organisation of society
Solution/approach	Medical intervention/conditions to be treated/controlled	Provide help. Cases to be pitied/made heroic	Change society, ensure individuals' rights
Locus of power	Responsibility held by clinical staff	Responsibility held by 'charitable' staff/volunteers	Responsibility held by disabled people

Source: Americano (29)

Cultural competence has been defined as the ability of the individuals to:

- look beyond their own cultural interpretations
- to maintain objectivity when dealing with individuals from other cultures
- demonstrate an ability to understand behaviours without passing judgement.

The acceptance of, and respect for, difference, coupled with self-assessment and an attention to the dynamics of difference and resources available, form part of the cultural competence. Culturally competent individuals incorporate skills, knowledge, attitudes and competencies to address the needs of service users, whose cultural values and expectations are different.

As doctors or other healthcare professionals, one of the main vehicles for the expression of cultural competence is how we communicate with others. And it is to issues of cross-cultural communication that we turn next.

Cross-cultural communication

Cultural communication refers to the process of exchanging ideas using culturally appropriate idioms that can be understood in the context of culture, gender, previous experience and education. Barriers to cross-cultural communication are linked to language, non-verbal communication, stereotypes of other cultures and the tendency to evaluate behaviour from the other culture as good or bad based on one's own cultural bias. Stress related to cross-cultural encounters and filters may prevent one from accurately understanding what others are trying to communicate and may lead to culture clash.(32) The key components of all interpersonal communication are verbal and non-verbal, the two working in synergy to convey a message.

Verbal communication

Both verbal and non-verbal types of communication are influenced by cultural norms and values. Culture has language as a key component and using verbal skills to communicate with those from different cultural and linguistic backgrounds may need adequate adjustment. Individuals who speak two or more languages may often have a primary language, which is the language they think in. They may hide communication problems in the guise of reverting to primary language or they may revert to it when feeling anxious or distressed. This may be particularly important at the time of examinations and assessments. It is worth bearing in mind that some words are particularly specific to some cultures, for example, *schadenfreude* (broadly interpreted as pleasure derived from the misfortunes of others), and cannot easily be translated. Thus concepts that are meaningful in one language may not exist in another. Poor skills in English language are sometimes mistaken for low intelligence

quotient or slowness. Furthermore, an understanding of English language in social settings may not translate into understanding medical terminology or vice versa.

Non-verbal communication

It has been argued that over two-thirds of communication is non-verbal. Non-verbal communication includes gestures, eye contact, touching, facial expressions, body language, proximity, style of speaking and emotional tone. Non-verbal communication refers to the way we look, move, feel, sound or smell.

Gesturing can vary across cultural settings and extra gestures should not be misinterpreted as agitation unless there are clear reasons for this assessment and other signs support this view. Similarly, in some cultures close proximity to the teacher may be sought, whereas in others it may be frowned upon, and therefore being close and making eye contact may be seen as hostile. In some cultures avoiding direct eye-to-eye contact and looking at the floor may be a sign of deference and respect rather than an insult or ignoring the individual. The physical distance between two people is also a result of cultural norms and values. Close proximity and touching may be a sign of warmth in some cultures, whereas in others it may be seen as a representation of sexual interest. Lack of close contact or touching may be seen as cold and hostile in some cultures. Similarly, speaking at a louder level is acceptable in some cultures but seen as aggressive in others. Furthermore, cutting across conversations is common in some cultures but not others, and thus may be interpreted as rude and intrusive. Silence, in some cultures, may be seen as approval and agreement, whereas in others it may be hostile. In summary, non-verbal communication:

- conveys personal attitudes – respect, being interested, liking the speaker or person being spoken to, etc.
- expresses emotional states – cultures determine when and how disappointment, anger, etc., are shown
- manages conversation – by encouraging or discouraging, exchanging rituals and regulating self-presentation.

Non-verbal communication can be improved by increased sensitivity to the student's body language, demeanour, eye contact, gestures, emotional tone, physical distance and an awareness of what may be normal in the culture.

Working with interpreters

Interpreters are generally professional individuals who are proficient in at least two languages and therefore can act as a bridge and a communicator between two individuals. Their task is to facilitate the exchange of information in a non-biased manner. Bearing in mind both verbal and non-verbal communication, a good interpreter should be able to interpret both without taking sides. Frequent errors in interpretation include distortion, deletion, omission, blocking of messages that may be seen as against the culture, incorrect translation, inadequate interpretation and difficulty in finding equivalent words for concepts that cannot be translated. Translation can be literal or conceptual. There is an equal danger in underestimating someone's language skills as in overestimating them. The gender and age of the interpreter may be important, as is preparation before any teaching session, especially in relation to difficult words. In the session, ensure that their roles are clearly defined, with plenty of time and written materials and verification that the message is understood.

After the session, a period of debriefing with the interpreter would be very helpful to explore technical problems, cultural nuances and share information on the session, and this will make teaching for the next session easier (Box 27.4).

Diversity in Medical Education

Students and trainees in the healthcare professions come from a variety of cultural backgrounds and bring their own set of experiences, prejudices and expectations with them. In teaching and training, these can be worked with to develop diversity awareness and overcome prejudice. This is (literally) vital as patients' exposure to actual and 'perceived' beliefs about prejudice and related acts influences their own and their carers' expectations of healthcare professionals and the health service. A patient's readiness to seek help from any particular healthcare professionals will depend on their overt or tacit appraisal of the professional's competence and knowledge,(35) and that will include their assessment of the individual's cultural competence. On the other side of the desk, insensitivity to diversity in the process of diagnosis and management has been often blamed for over-diagnosis of certain conditions(36,37) and pathways to care experienced by ethnic minority patients.(38)

The training of students can take place in different settings using different models. Training in diversity can be delivered by students themselves, the voluntary sector, academics, professional experts from different backgrounds using experiential, cognitive or knowledge-based models in small groups, lectures, large groups or through policy changes.

Training and education in diversity can also be provided in the postgraduate sector through in-service training. This will include knowledge-based learning – keeping up to date with changes in local laws pertaining to equalities – but to develop and improve the coordination of agencies and professions, a team-based learning approach is required, allowing team members to learn from each other and hone their own skills. Core skills may be shared across disciplines within the team; the training is therefore both multi- and interdisciplinary.

Similarly, although clinical teachers in medical schools may be aware of cultural and diversity issues, social services and the voluntary sector appear to be much better at training their staff for cross-cultural (and diversity) encounters and in the implementation of equal opportunities practice.(39) Theoretical models used for training can be reflexive, experiential, motivational change, cognitive or based on belief systems. Role play, small groups, observations, knowledge and attitudes can be used to explore learning.

The exact formats for teaching diversity can be multi-level and multifaceted. These can be developed according to the interest and resources available. Courses may be day release or weekend, organised in teams or groups, and at the local, regional or national level. Further top-up sessions can be provided by e-learning or distance-learning packages. Each student can thus work at both an individual and a group level.

It will be apparent from the above that diversity is a subject that is best dealt with in groups. This may take different forms, and in the section that follows we describe some possible models.

Teaching and Training

The basic principle for diversity training is to have a structured framework. The components of the framework will be dictated by the resources available, curricula requirements, time allocated and the specific needs of students. Any approach that deals with diversity has to place diversity at the source and centre of the expected behaviours and past expectations. Group exercises will allow students to explore their own attitudes to diversity without feeling overawed. Throughout the process, skilled feedback is extremely important and the facilitators must be keenly aware of their own world view.

Learning about diversity can take place in a number of sessions, with identification of barriers in communication, building on existing knowledge, awareness of different types of messages and legal issues. Diversity profiles of the national and local populations can provide a useful introduction and information on setting up the right targets in teaching. Using role play and real scenarios can open up the possibility of exploring personal experiences. The trainees can identify changes in attitudes, behaviour and knowledge, built on discussions with additional written information. Web-based learning can contribute to the consolidation of attitudinal changes. A follow-up session a few months later can help in identifying changes in clinical practice, attitudes, skills and knowledge, and perceptions of the learning.

A number of models for the delivery of diversity training are suggested here, modified from Bhui and Bhugra.(35)

Developing specialists in the team

Training is team-based and each member of the group takes on the responsibility of liaising with one cultural or diverse group and becomes the educator for the team. The role of educators will depend on their skills and interests, and the focus for teaching may be (e.g.) policy, legal status or the development of services. As a result of this exercise, the individual becomes a cultural 'specialist' and his or her skills and knowledge can then be communicated to other team members. The major advantage in this approach is the ownership of change within the team, and the liaising person becomes the repository of information. A major disadvantage is that the individual may feel isolated and burdened if the rest of the team choose to not acquire necessary knowledge and skills.

Liaison with voluntary and independent providers

Here, voluntary and independent service providers act as liaison resources and brokers to provide delivery of training and supervision. The advantage of such a joint approach is mutual learning, support and respect. The service providers will also be seen as acceptable by users and carers. A key disadvantage is that the voluntary or independent sector may feel overwhelmed and compromised. Working with independent providers may be seen as unacceptable and unorthodox. These organisations may also appear to be less aware

of evidence-based practice in relation to diversity. It may also be difficult in practice to match up the two sets of values.

Using cultural brokers

A cultural broker is an individual from a specific culture who can provide a link between the services and the community. Such an individual educates both sides – one side on cultural norms and mores and the other side about the availability of services. Thus training and supervision can be two-way. The key advantage of such an approach is that the links with community are strengthened and learning is at the place of work. Its disadvantages include perceived situations where such an individual is seen as taking sides and may be wrongly aligned in the community's mind with the services.

Consulting expert panels

The use of expert advisory panels is another model(40) that has been successfully adopted in the assessment of health needs with North American Indian communities. This approach allows participation in identifying health needs by various diverse groups who can sanction appropriate treatments and provide directive guidance on taboos. This model can provide ongoing education for both qualified professionals and their trainees, and has the advantage of having committee liaison rather than a single individual being responsible. However, competing interests may create a multitude of problems and be cumbersome.

Supervision and Diversity

Cassimir and Morrison(41) suggest that the therapist must try and assume the internal frame of reference of the client and perceive the world as the client sees it, as well as seeing the client as they see themselves. Trainees and students can be viewed in the same light and trained in turn to see their patients in the same way. Even with adequate training and knowledge the health professional's skills and competencies need to be updated regularly with ongoing service-based training that reflects the demographic shifts. Initial training is therefore usefully supplemented by high-quality supervision for which various models have been described.(35) For students and trainees, such supervision may need to be based in their clinical settings when they are established as part of the team providing services.

In some situations supervision itself can raise complex diversity issues. For example, a student with a physical impairment may feel that his or her non-disabled supervisor is unable to understand issues to do with the barriers he or she faces. Similarly, if further aspects of identity are taken into account, there may be additional problems. For example, a visually impaired, female, Asian student may feel she is not being dealt with appropriately by a non-disabled, male, white supervisor.

In supervision settings the power relationship between teacher/trainer and student is unequal, and this may become further exaggerated by diversity matters. These unequal variables will include disability, ethnicity, gender and sexual orientation, as well as experiences and status differences. The supervisor/trainer should be able to set clear boundaries on the duration, type of supervision and the physical location of such an interaction. Supervision sessions will, and indeed must, involve discussion of feelings related to transference and counter-transference, which will include factors related to age, gender, ethnicity, sexual orientation and disability. Even though these are not specifically therapeutic sessions, sharing of experiences, some exploration of the feelings on both sides and discussions about future plans may all contribute to feelings of anger, frustration or contentment on either side. Students or trainees may hesitate in rebelling or transmitting their feelings in such a session. These interactions are rarely straightforward and can sometimes lead to sabotaging the session, miscommunication or subversion of the supervisor's task.

Conclusions

Although dealing with diversity may be daunting, the use of existing knowledge, classification of attributes and building on skills, can enable and empower teachers in dealing with students from diverse backgrounds with diverse needs. Identifying personal world views and using training methods at the individual and group levels will yield positive results. Students and trainees will have varying needs. Taking steps to understand and address those needs will help maximise learning outcomes and thus be positive for patient care. How organisational diversity impacts performance in the workplace and thus the quality of healthcare is not yet fully understood. It will also be subject to multiple stakeholder viewpoints, many of which will conflict. What is clear is that in an increasingly multicultural society with its expectations of social equality, a failure to engage with the broad range of issues that diversity raises is damaging to the credibility of both the organisation and the individual professional. Dealing with diversity is difficult, but diversity must be dealt with.

References

1 Brockner J, Chen Y-R, Mannix EA, Leung K and Skarlicki DP (2000) Culture and procedural fairness: when the effect of what you do depends on how you do it. *Administrative Science Quarterly*. **45**: 138–59.

2 Steiner DD and Gilliland SW (1996) Fairness reactions to personnel selection techniques in France and the United States. *Journal of Applied Psychology*. **81**: 134–41.

3 Jehn KA, Northcraft GB and Neale MA (1999) Why differences make a difference: a field study of diversity, conflict and performance in work groups. *Administrative Science Quarterly*. **44**: 741–63.

4 MacPherson W (1999) *The Stephen Lawrence Enquiry*. Report of an inquiry by Sir William MacPherson of Cluny. The Stationery Office, London (http://www.archive.official-documents.co.uk/document/cm42/4262/sli-00.htm).

5 Adams JS (1963) Toward an understanding of inequity. *Journal of Abnormal and Social Psychology*. **67**: 422–36.

6 Arvey RD and Sackett PR (1993) Fairness in selection: current developments and perspectives. In: Schmitt N and Borman WC (eds) *Personnel Selection in Organizations*. Jossey-Bass, San Francisco, CA.

7 Bagshaw M (2004) Is diversity divisive? A positive training approach. *Industrial and Commercial Training*. **36**: 153–7

8 Rajan A and Harris S (2003) The business impact of diversity. *Personnel Today*. **9**(February):18.

9 Cross TL, Barzon BJ, Dennis KW and Isaacs MR (1989) *Towards a Culturally Competent System of Care: a monograph on effective services for minority children who are severely emotionally disturbed*. CASSP Technical Assistance Center, Georgetown University Child Development Center, Washington, DC.

10 Secretary of State for Health (2002) *The NHS Plan. A Plan for Investment. A Plan for Reform* (CM 4818-I). Department of Health, London, p.109.

11 Babb P, Martin J and Haezewindt P (eds) (2004) *Focus on Social Inequalities*. London, HMSO.

12 Darzi A (2007) Healthcare for London: a framework for action. NHS, London (http://www.healthcareforlondon.nhs.uk/framework_for_action.asp).

13 Commission for Racial Equality (2002) *Framework for a Race Equality Policy – for higher education*. CRE, London (http://www.cre.gov.uk).

14 General Medical Council (2001) *Good Medical Practice*. GMC, London.

15 McKenzie KJ (1995) Racial discrimination in medicine (Editorial). *British Medical Journal*. **310**: 478–9.

16 Collier J and Broke A (1986) Racial and sexual discrimination in the selection of students for London medical schools. *Medical Education*. **20**: 86–90.

17 McManus IC, Richards P and Maitlis SL (1989) Prospective study of the disadvantage of people from ethnic minority groups applying to medical schools in the United Kingdom. *British Medical Journal*. **298**: 723–6.

18 McManus IC (1998) Factors affecting likelihood of applicants being offered a place in medical schools in the United Kingdom in 1996 and 1997: retrospective study. *British Medical Journal*. **317**: 1111–17.

19 McKeigue PM, Richards JDM and Richards P (1990) Effects of discrimination by sex and race on early careers of British medical graduates during 1981–7. *British Medical Journal*. **301**: 961–4.

20 Commission for Racial Equality (1996) *Appointing NHS Consultants and Senior Registrars: report of a formal investigation*. CRE, London.

21 Coker N (2001) *Racism in Medicine: an agenda for change*. King's Fund, London.

22 Royal College of Physicians (2001) Career Choices and Opportunities. A report of a working party of the Federation of Royal Colleges of Physicians. RCP, London (http://www.

rcplondon.ac.uk/pubs/wp/wp_womeninmed_summary.
htm).

23 Price EG, Gozu A, Kern DE *et al.* (2005) The role of cultural
diversity climate in recruitment, promotion and retention of
faculty in academic medicine. *Journal of General Internal
Medicine.* **20**: 565–71.

24 Kripalani S, Bussey-Jones J, Katz MG *et al.* (2006) A prescription for cultural competence in medical education. *Journal of
General Internal Medicine.* **21**: 1116–20.

25 Kilminster S, Downes J, Gough B *et al.* (2007) Women in medicine – is there a problem? A literature review of the changing
gender composition, structures and occupational cultures in
medicine. *Medical Education.* **41**: 39–49.

26 Melville C (2005) Discrimination and health inequalities experienced by disabled people. *Medical Education.* **39**: 122–6.

27 University Colleges and Admissions Services. Statistical
Services (http://www.ucas.co.uk/he_staff/stat_services1/
stats_online/data_tables/abusdis/).

28 Byron M, Cockshott Z, Brownett H *et al.* (2005) What does
disability mean for medical students? An exploration of the
words medical students associate with the term 'disability'.
Medical Education. **39**: 176–83.

29 Americano A (2006) Illness and disability. In: Hastie A (ed.)
Flexible Working and Training for Doctors and Dentists, pp. 173–
89. Radcliffe Publishing, Oxford.

30 *Collins English Dictionary* (2007). HarperCollins, London.

31 Bhui K, Warfa N, Edonya P, McKenzie K and Bhugra D (2007)
Cultural competence in mental health care: a review of model
evaluations. *BMC Health Services Research.* **7**: 15.

32 Barma L (1982) Stumbling blocks in intercultural communica-
tion: exercises, stories and syntheticultures. In: Samovar L and
Porter R (eds) *Intercultural Communication: a reader*, pp. 330–8.
Wadsworth, Belmont, CA.

33 Hofstede GJ, Pedersen PB and Hofstede G (2002) *Exploring
Culture: exercises, stories and syntheticultures.* Intercultural
Press, Yarmouth, ME.

34 Hampden-Turner C and Trompenaars F (2000) *Building Cross-
cultural Competence.* Yale University Press, New Haven, CT.

35 Bhui K and Bhugra D (1998) Training and supervision in effective cross-cultural mental health services. *Hospital Medicine.*
59: 861–5.

36 Bhugra D, Leff J, Mallet R, Der G *et al.* (1997) Incidence and
outcome of schizophrenia in whites, African-Caribbeans and
Asians in London. *Psychological Medicine.* **27**: 791–8.

37 Bhui K (1997) London's ethnic minorities and the provision of
mental health services. In: Johnson S, Ramsay R, Thornicroft
G and Brooks L (eds) *London's Mental Health Services*,
pp. 143–66. King's Fund Institute, London.

38 Bhugra D, Harding C and Lippett R (2004) Pathways into care
and satisfaction for black patients in south London. *Journal of
Mental Health.* **13**: 171–83.

39 Gray P (1998) Voluntary organisations. In: Bhugra D and Bahl
V (eds) *Ethnicity: an agenda for mental health*, pp. 202–10.
Gaskell, London.

40 Timpson J (1984) Indian mental health: changes in the delivery
of care in North Western Ontario. *Canadian Journal of Psychiatry.*
29: 234–41.

41 Cassimir G and Morrison BJ (1993) Re-thinking work with
multicultural population. *Community Mental Health Journal.* **29**:
547–9.

Further Reading

Americano A (2005) Educating doctors for diversity. In: Hastie A,
Hastie I, Jackson N *et al.* (eds) *Postgraduate Medical Education
and Training: a guide for primary and secondary care*, pp. 97–109.
Radcliffe Publishing, Oxford.

Americano A (2006) Illness and disability. In: Hastie A (ed.)
Flexible Working and Training for Doctors and Dentists, pp. 173–89.
Radcliffe Publishing, Oxford.

Bhugra D and Bhui K (2007) *Textbook of Cultural Psychiatry.*
Cambridge University Press, London.

Kandola R and Fullerton J (1998) *Diversity in Action: managing the
mosaic.* CIPD, London.

Tseng W-S and Streltzer D (eds) (2004) *Cultural Competence
in Clinical Psychiatry.* American Psychiatric Publishing,
Washington DC and London.

Web-based Resources

Advisory Conciliation and Arbitration Service (ACAS), http://
www.acas.org.uk. Helpline: +44 (0)845 747 4747

Chartered Institute of Personnel & Development, http://www.
cipd.co.uk

Commission for Equality and Human Rights, http://www.equal-
ityhumanrights.com

Department of Health (type in diversity or inequalities in the
search engine), http://www.dh.gov.uk

Department of Trade and Industry (discrimination in employment pages), http://www.dti.gov.uk/employment/discrimi-
nation/index.html

Equality and Diversity Forum, http://www.edf.org.uk

GLADD – site for lesbian, gay, bisexual and transgender doctors
and dentists, http://www.gladd.co.uk/index.htm

Developing medical educators: a journey, not a destination

Yvonne Steinert

KEY MESSAGES

- The notion of 'medical educator' encompasses a number of roles, including that of teacher, curriculum planner and evaluator, educational leader and administrator, researcher and scholar.

- There are many ways in which to develop as a medical educator. 'Formal' staff development activities are only one way to achieve this goal. Other approaches include 'learning on the job', belonging to a community of educators, mentorship and role modelling, and organisational support and development.

- The content of staff development activities should move beyond the enhancement of teaching effectiveness and target leadership abilities, the promotion of scholarship, and organisational change and development.

- Staff development activities should be guided by knowledge of core competencies for medical educators.

- Medical education is a social endeavour and the notion of community – and communities of practice – is fundamental to the development of medical educators.

Introduction

The root of the word 'doctor' is to teach. However, although the majority of doctors are expert in *what* they teach, most have had little or no training in *how* to teach.(1) They are also minimally prepared for the many roles that are subsumed under the term medical educator. As Jason and Westberg(2) state, 'the one task that is distinctively related to being a faculty member is teaching; all other tasks can be pursued in other settings; and yet, paradoxically, the central responsibility of faculty members is typically the one for which they are least prepared'.

In the past, it was assumed that intelligent people who have been students for many years have learnt – or can automatically learn – to be successful faculty members, and little or no support for staff development was provided.(3) This is no longer true. Increasing attention has been placed on the design and development of staff development programmes, in diverse contexts and settings.(4–7) Moreover, in recent years, a number of regulatory bodies have started to pay attention to the accreditation of teachers and teaching,(8,9) and they have highlighted the importance of staff development in the certification of educators.(10) In the UK, for example, the role of teacher is increas-

ingly recognised as a core professional activity for all doctors and one that cannot be left to chance, aptitude or inclination.(11)

The goal of this paper is to focus on the development of medical educators. To achieve this objective, we will try to define what is meant by a *medical educator*, describe the required core competencies and examine different ways of developing medical educators. Moreover, as staff development is one of the most common ways to achieve this objective, much of this paper will examine what is known about formal staff development programmes. However, we will also address the role and importance of work-based learning, communities of practice, mentorship and role modelling, and organisational support and development.

Who Is a Medical Educator?

The medical education literature tends to use the terms 'teacher' and 'medical educator' interchangeably, with no clear definitions. To inform this paper, we conducted a series of semi-structured interviews with 12 medical educators at McGill to ascertain their definitions and conceptions of being a medical educator.(12) Definitions included a broad range of conceptualisations, some of which are highlighted below:

> The medical educator is someone who critically reflects on the quality of the educational experience and tries to innovate and improve on what they have done.

Understanding Medical Education: Evidence, Theory and Practice. Edited by T Swanwick. © 2010 Association for the Study of Medical Education.

Medical educators have a passion, not just an interest, but a passion for bringing out the best, or finding ways to bring out the best, in students and learners that they work with to help develop the best physicians that we can …

A medical educator is someone who uses theories and principles of education in their activities. This includes teaching, scholarship, curricular design and evaluation, and research across the educational continuum …

What is striking in these definitions is the emphasis on reflection, passion, innovation and informed practice across a continuum of tasks and activities.

In this chapter, the term medical educator will encompass a broad spectrum of roles that include teaching, curriculum design and evaluation, educational leadership and innovation, and research and scholarship. Moreover, medical educators, whether in the clinical or classroom setting, will refer to individuals who actively *reflect* on what they do, using experience and available evidence to *inform* their educational practice and to *enhance* the teaching and learning of future healthcare professionals:

[We] continually ask ourselves how we can do this better: 'How can we get [our students] to be the best that they can be'… 'If my program is working, can I still make it better? If it is not working, why not and how can I improve it?'(12)

Either explicitly, or implicitly, we use what we have learned about education over the years to inform our teaching … (12)

What is Staff Development?

Staff development, or faculty development as it is often called, has become an increasingly important component of medical education. Staff development activities have been designed to improve teacher effectiveness at all levels of the educational continuum (e.g. undergraduate, postgraduate and continuing medical education), and diverse programmes have been offered to healthcare professionals in many settings.(13) In this paper, staff development will refer to that broad range of activities that institutions use to *renew* or *assist* faculty in their multiple roles.(14) That is, staff development is a planned programme designed to prepare institutions and faculty members for their various roles(15) and to improve an individual's knowledge and skills in the areas of teaching, research and administration.(16) The goal of staff development is to teach faculty members the skills relevant to their institutional and faculty position and to sustain their vitality, both now and in the future.

Staff development can provide medical educators with knowledge and skills about teaching and learning, curriculum design and delivery, student assessment and programme evaluation, and leadership and

administration, as well as research and scholarship. It can also reinforce or alter attitudes or beliefs about education and scholarly activity, provide a conceptual framework for what is often performed on an intuitive basis, and introduce clinicians and basic scientists to a community of medical educators interested in medical education and the enhancement of teaching and learning for students, patients and peers.

In addition, staff development can serve as a useful instrument in the promotion of organisational change.(5,17) That is, staff development can help build consensus, generate support and enthusiasm, and implement a change initiative; it can also help change the culture within the institution by altering the formal, informal and hidden curriculum(18,19) and by enhancing organisational capacities.(20) As Swanwick(21) states, staff development should be:

An institution-wide pursuit with the intent of professionalizing the educational activities of teachers, enhancing educational infrastructure, and building educational capacity for the future …

In many ways, staff development can play an important role at both the *individual* and the *organisational* level.(22) Moreover, although staff development activities predominantly focus on teaching and instructional effectiveness, there is a critical need for these activities to also address the other roles of medical educators, including that of curriculum designer, educational leader and administrator, and scholar.

A Curriculum for Staff Development?

Attributes and behaviours of effective clinical teachers have been identified in the literature. For example, Irby(23) reports that students value the following characteristics in their teachers:

* enthusiasm
* a positive attitude towards teaching
* rapport with students and patients
* availability and accessibility
* clinical competence
* subject matter expertise.

A number of core teaching skills have also been identified. These include:

* the establishment of a positive learning environment
* the setting of clear objectives and expectations
* the provision of timely and relevant information
* the effective use of questioning and other instructional methods
* appropriate role modelling
* the provision of constructive feedback and objective-based evaluations.(24)

It is interesting to note, however, that many staff development programmes have been developed independently of a curriculum for teachers and educators. As Purcell and Lloyd-Jones(11) state, 'in many countries there is a plethora of teacher training programmes for medical teachers. But what is good medical teaching? Unless we know what it is, how can we develop it?'

The literature provides us with some examples of developing core competencies for teachers. For example, Bland *et al.*(15) define an extensive set of essential skills, goals and objectives for successful medical faculty in five domains:

- education
- administration
- research
- written communication
- professional academic skills.

More recently, Harris *et al.*(3) presented a helpful overview of faculty members' roles, which include the following:

- *teacher/administrator*, which encompasses chair, residency director or clinic director
- *teacher/educator*, which includes director of education, pre-doctoral director or clerkship director
- *teacher/researcher*, which comprises director of research or research faculty
- *teacher/clinician*, which includes community preceptor or clinical faculty.

Harris *et al.*(3) also describe a series of competencies that incorporate leadership, administration, teaching and research.

Other researchers have compared student and faculty perceptions of effective clinical teaching. For example, Buchel and Edwards(25) asked residents and faculty members to rate the attributes of effective teachers. Both residents and faculty agreed that clinical competence is one of the most important attributes of an effective clinical teacher. They also agreed that better educators were those who demonstrated enthusiasm for their educational responsibilities. At the same time, residents commented that it was important for a quality educator to respect their autonomy and independence as clinicians, whereas faculty members reported that this was one of the least important traits of an effective teacher. In addition, faculty felt that serving as a role model worth emulating was essential, a factor stressed by previous authors.(26) Residents, however, did not believe that this was an important attribute and ranked it at the bottom of their list. Clearly, the perceptions of residents and faculty members are not always congruent, although an 'evidence-based' set of attitudes and behaviours should guide the development of staff development programmes.

It should also be noted that much less has been written about the roles of educational *leader* and *scholar*, roles that are often subsumed under the term 'medical educator'. In an interesting study, Bordage *et al.*(27) surveyed deans and associate deans to identify the educational and leadership skills required of 'programme directors with major educational and leadership responsibilities'. Their results indicate the importance of nine key skill areas:

- oral communication
- interpersonal abilities
- clinical competence
- educational goal definition
- educational design
- problem solving and decision making
- team building
- written communication
- budgeting and financial management.

Spencer and Jordan(28) also highlight the fact that educational change requires leadership and that we need to equip our colleagues to implement change. Clearly, the development of medical educators should address leadership competencies, as well as those that promote scholarship in its broadest sense.

Boyer(29) identifies four categories of scholarship:

- discovery
- integration
- application
- teaching.

Roughly considered, scholarship in education can involve the discovery of new knowledge (i.e. research), the integration or application of existing knowledge to new areas, and teaching.(30) Scholarship also provides a common ground for assessing the diverse roles and contributions of faculty members to the mission of the medical school and can take on many forms. For example, peer-reviewed publications and grants are products of the *scholarship of discovery*, which has been synonymous with research in the traditional sense. The scholarship of *integration* has been defined as making connections across the disciplines, illuminating data in a revealing way, whereas the scholarship of *application* has been likened to 'service' in one's own field of knowledge, to the application of theory into practice.

In medical education, fellowship programme development and web-based instructional materials are examples of the *scholarship of integration and application*. The *scholarship of teaching* involves the capacity to effectively communicate one's own knowledge, skills and beliefs. Moreover, teaching becomes scholarship when it is made public, is available for peer review and critique and can be reproduced and built on by other scholars.(31) The promotion of scholarship, and helping educators foster scholarly activities among their colleagues, is an important factor in the development of medical educators and yet one that is often neglected.

As this discussion suggests, the development of a curriculum for medical educators merits attention. At the same time, it would also be worth focusing on a better understanding of the teacher's experience. In an interesting study, Higgs and McAllister(32) studied the 'experience of being a clinical educator' and discovered that this experience consisted of six interactive and dynamic dimensions:

- a sense of self (or self-identity)
- a sense of relationship with others

- a sense of being a clinical educator
- a sense of agency, or purposeful action
- seeking dynamic self-congruence
- the experience of growth and change.

Based on this research, and our experience at McGill, it would be worthwhile to take a more careful look at the 'lived experience' of being an educator and to use this experience as a framework for training:

> My pride as a medical educator comes from watching the light go on in my students' eyes and knowing why the light goes off … (12)

> When I see junior colleagues work and demonstrate excellence in patient care, going the extra mile … I know that I have had an impact.(12)

In summary, medical teachers and educators need to be prepared for complex(33) and demanding roles that include teaching, leadership and administration, and scholarship in its broadest meaning.

How Can We Develop Medical Educators?

'Formal' approaches to developing medical educators

The most common staff development formats have included workshops and seminars, short courses, sabbaticals and fellowships.(34) Other methods include degree programmes, peer coaching, augmented feedback and online learning. A brief description of some of these formats follows.

Workshop, seminars and short courses

Workshops are popular because of their inherent flexibility and promotion of active learning. In particular, teachers value a variety of teaching methods within this format, including interactive lectures, small group discussions and exercises, role-plays and simulations, and experiential learning.(34) Workshops are commonly used to promote skill acquisition (e.g. lecturing or small group teaching skills),(35,36) prepare for new curricula (e.g. problem-based learning)(37,38) or help faculty adapt to new teaching environments (e.g. teaching in the ambulatory setting).(39,40) Workshops on leadership styles and skills(41) and/or curriculum design and innovation(42) can also help prepare educators for their leadership roles, whereas short courses on research methods(43) and writing for publication(44) can help prepare clinicians and basic scientists for their scholarly work.

To date, the majority of staff development programmes have focused on teaching improvement. That is, they aim to improve teachers' skills in clinical teaching, small group facilitation, feedback and evaluation.(34) A number of programmes also target specific core competencies (e.g. the teaching and evaluation of communication skills; professionalism) and the use of technology in teaching and learning. Less attention

has been paid to the personal development of healthcare professionals, educational leadership and scholarship, and organisational development and change. Although instructional effectiveness at the individual level is critically important, a more comprehensive approach is needed.(13) We clearly need to develop individuals who will be able to provide leadership to educational programmes, act as educational mentors, and design and deliver innovative educational programmes. As Cusimano and David(45) state, there is an enormous need for more healthcare professionals trained in methods of educating others so that medical education will continue to be responsive to driving forces of change. As previously stated, staff development also has an important role to play in promoting teaching as a scholarly activity and in creating an educational climate that encourages and rewards educational leadership, innovation and excellence.

Fellowships and other longitudinal programmes

Fellowships of varying length, format and emphasis have been utilised in many disciplines.(46–48) More recently, integrated, longitudinal programmes have been developed as an alternative to fellowship programmes or sabbaticals. These programmes, in which faculty commit 10–20% of their time over one to two years, allow healthcare professionals to maintain most of their clinical, research and administrative responsibilities while furthering their own professional development. Programme components typically consist of a variety of methods, including university courses, monthly seminars, independent research projects and participation in staff development activities. Integrated longitudinal programmes, such as a *Teaching Scholars Program*,(49–52) have particular appeal because teachers can continue to practise and teach while improving their educational knowledge and skills. Also, these programmes allow for the development of educational leadership and scholarly activity in medical education.

In summary, although fellowship and other longitudinal programmes vary in structure, duration and content, they all enable the acquisition of expertise and excellence in teaching, curricular design and evaluation, and educational leadership. Many of them also provide assistance in academic and career development(53,54) and help create a community of teachers and educators. In addition, they encourage the dissemination of new knowledge and understanding to further the field of medical education.

Degree programmes

Certificate or degree programmes are becoming increasingly popular in many settings. In part, this is due to what some authors have termed the 'professionalisation' of medical education.(10,11) Several authors have argued for the need to certify medical educators and thereby ensure global standards; others do not agree and worry about disenfranchising keen and committed educators (*see* Box 28.1).

Cohen *et al.*(57) provided an update on Master's degrees in medical education and reported on 21 different programmes in Holland (1), Canada (3), Australia (3), the US(6) and the UK (8). As these authors suggest, an advanced degree in medical edu-

---

BOX 28.1 Focus on: The professionalisation of medical educators

One of the Dutch terms for staff development is *Docentprofessionalisering,* which loosely translates to the professionalisation of teaching. This is of particular interest as we witness the professionalisation of medical education in a number of venues. For example, in the UK, the Dearing Report(55) makes a number of recommendations about faculty in higher education, including the following which is pertinent in this context:

> We recommend that institutions of higher education begin immediately to develop or seek access to programmes for teacher training of their staff, if they do not have them, and that all institutions seek national accreditation of such programmes from the Institute for Learning and Teaching in Higher Education.

The UK General Medical Council's *Good Medical Practice*(8) states that:

> Teaching, training, appraising and assessing doctors and students are important for the care of patients now and in the future. You should be willing to contribute to these activities … If you are involved in teaching you must develop the skills, attitudes and practices of a competent teacher.

In addition, the Postgraduate Medical Education and Training Board,(9) which is responsible for securing and maintaining standards and improving the quality of postgraduate medical education and training in the UK, has issued its own quality framework, which includes 'standards for trainers'. In particular, they state that 'trainers must be supported in their role by a postgraduate education team and have a suitable job plan with an appropriate workload and time to develop trainees'. They also assert that 'organizations providing postgraduate medical education must ensure that trainers have adequate support and resources to undertake their training role'.

Although the emphasis on accreditation for teaching and standards for teaching has not received the same attention in Canada or the US, there is clearly a movement towards increased accountability and accreditation of teaching, one of the roles of the medical educator.(56) Moreover, as Eitel *et al.*(10) suggest, staff development is one of the prerequisites for certification leading to professionalisation.

---

cation offers essential grounding in educational theory and practice and can provide the foundation for educational research and scholarship. Another review of Master's degrees in medical education was conducted by Pugsley *et al.*,(58) who commented on the variability in content and quality among these programmes and argued for increased standards and the need for quality assurance. Nonetheless, despite these concerns, most universities in the UK now require staff to undertake a university certificate in teaching and learning, and many medical schools, in partnership with the National Health Service (NHS) trusts, are providing opportunities for advanced educational training.(59) Degree programmes can be particularly helpful to individuals interested in educational leadership, administration or research.

Peer coaching

Peer coaching as a method of staff development has been described extensively in the education literature. Key elements of peer coaching include the identification of individual learning goals (e.g. improving specific teaching skills), focused observation of teaching by colleagues, and the provision of feedback, analysis and support.(60) This under-utilised approach, sometimes called *co-teaching* or *peer observation*, has particular appeal because it occurs in the teacher's own practice setting, enables individualised learning and fosters collaboration.(61) It also allows healthcare professionals to learn about each other as they teach together and, in this way, can nurture the development of medical educators.

'Informal' approaches to developing medical educators

Although staff development programmes are a popular way of developing medical educators, a number of alternative approaches should also be considered. Box 28.2 describes how medical educators at McGill University started the 'journey' of becoming a medical educator. For many, it started with their 'job responsibilities' and slowly evolved into a career path. The following section describes four of these important pathways.

Work-based learning

Work-based learning, often defined as learning *for* work, learning *at* work and learning *from* work,(21) is fundamental to the development of medical educators, for whom 'learning on the job' is often the first entry into teaching and education. In fact, it is in the everyday workplace – where educators conduct their clinical, research and teaching activities, and interact with faculty, colleagues and students – that learning most often takes place. It would therefore be extremely worthwhile to help medical educators see their everyday experiences as 'learning experiences' and encourage them to reflect with colleagues and students on

BOX 28.2 Ways of becoming a medical educator

Colleagues at the Centre for Medical Education at McGill University identified the following ways of 'becoming a medical educator':(12)

- **By the nature of my responsibilities** – *One of the nice things about medical education is that you can often have an administrative position that allows you to have a lab. I was undergraduate program director for quite a while ... by doing that it's given me a lab to try various innovations and evaluate them.*

- **By participating in staff development and other training opportunities** – *Participating in faculty development workshops introduced me to a community of educators and got me 'hooked' ... I haven't stopped learning since.*

- **By pursuing an advanced degree** – *My advanced degree allowed me to look at things with education glasses on. It also gave me the opportunity to immerse myself in a group with similar interests and needs.*

- **By wanting to** – *I had the interest and the desire. I have always wanted to be a teacher and I was good at teaching ... I followed my passion.*

- **By belonging to a community (of experts)** – *For me the most valuable part has been meeting regularly with a group of like-minded individuals committed to excellence and scholarship in medical education ... I have become immersed in the culture.*

- **By being mentored and through role modelling** – *I could not have done this alone. ...*

- **By *doing* medical education** – *I have learned by doing – and using, either explicitly, or implicitly, what I have learned over the years to inform my teaching.*

learning that has occurred in the clinical or classroom setting. It would also help bring staff development to the workplace.

It is interesting that staff development activities have traditionally been conducted away from the educator's workplace, requiring participants to take their 'lessons learnt' back to their own contexts. Perhaps it is time to reverse this tradition and think about how we can enhance the learning that takes place in the work environment.(62) By working together and participating in a larger community, clinicians and basic scientists can build new knowledge and understanding and develop approaches to problems faced in teaching and learning.(63)

Communities of practice

Closely related to 'learning at work' is the concept of situated learning and communities of practice. In my own setting, medical educators have commented on the role and value of a community of medical educa-

tors, brought together by a common interest in the enhancement of teaching and learning for students across the educational continuum and involvement in scholarly work in medical education, as a critical factor in their own development:

> For me it has been beneficial to be immersed in a group which is actually physically removed from where I do my clinical work ... where I come to regularly and am forced to engage in the discussions and try out new ideas.(12)

Barab *et al.*(64) define a community of practice as a 'persistent, sustaining, social network of individuals who share and develop an overlapping knowledge base, set of beliefs, values, history and experiences focused on a common practice and/or mutual enterprise'. Clearly, formal staff development programmes can play a pivotal role in developing communities of practice. At the same time, belonging to such a community can play a critical role in the development of medical educators.

Lave and Wenger(63) suggest that the success of a community of practice depends on five factors:

- the existence and sharing by the community of a common goal
- the existence and use of knowledge to achieve that goal
- the nature and importance of relationships formed among community members
- the relationships between the community and those outside it
- the relationship between the work of the community and the value of the activity.

In his later work, Wenger(65) also adds the notion that achieving the shared goals of the community requires a shared repertoire of common resources, including language, stories and practices (*see* Box 28.3).

In many ways, centres and/or departments of medical education, as well as the newer forms of academies,(67–69) can offer a setting for 'communities of practice' to develop. They can also help nurture and support both new and experienced teachers and educators. These centres and academies, which have been described in the literature and are increasing in number, can also help develop and sustain medical education as an academic discipline.(56) Critical to their success is a common purpose, open communication and opportunities for dialogue, guidance and institutional support.

Mentorship and role modelling

Mentoring is a common strategy to promote the development, socialisation and maturation of academic medical faculty.(15,70) However, although several formal mentorship programmes have been described,(71,72) this is an under-utilised approach for staff development, especially with regard to academic and career development. Daloz(73) describes a mentorship model that balances three key elements:

BOX 28.3 Focus on: Cultivating communities of practice

Wenger *et al.*(66) describe seven principles for cultivating communities of practice that have direct relevance for the development of medical educators. They include the following:

- *Design for evolution* – Communities should build on pre-existing personal networks and allow for natural growth and development. Design elements should be catalysts for the community's natural evolution.(66)

- *Open a dialogue between insider and outsider perspectives* – Good community design requires an insider's perspective to lead the discovery of what the community is about; however, an outside perspective is often needed to help members' see untapped possibilities.

- *Invite different levels of participation* – People participate in communities for different reasons (e.g. because the community provides value; for personal connections; to enhance skill development). Different levels of engagement (e.g. core, active, peripheral) are to be expected and encouraged. Successful communities often 'build benches' for those on the sidelines.(66)

- *Develop both public and private community spaces* – Most communities have public events where members gather to exchange ideas, solve problems or explore new concepts. However, communities are more than their 'calendar of events'.(66) The heart of the community is the one-on-one networking that occurs informally. All communities require both public and private interactions.

- *Focus on value* – Communities thrive because they deliver value to the organisation, to the teams on which community members serve and to the community members themselves. Articulation of its value helps a community to develop and grow.

- *Combine familiarity and excitement* – Successful communities offer the 'familiar comforts of a hometown' but also provide enough interest and variety to keep new ideas and new people cycling into the community.(66)

- *Create a rhythm for the community* – There are many rhythms in a community (e.g. the syncopation of familiar and exciting events, the frequency of private interactions, the ebb and flow of people from the sidelines into active participation and the pace of the community's overall evolution). The rhythm of a community is the strongest indicator of its being alive.

support, challenge and a vision of the individual's future career. This model can also serve as a helpful framework in staff development. Given the importance of mentoring for socialisation into the profession,

the development of meaningful academic activities, career satisfaction and the development of close collaborative relationships,(72) we must work to promote and recognise mentorship as a way of developing medical educators.

Role modelling, on the other hand, is instrumental in the development of all medical educators' roles, although it is not usually recognised as such. In our setting, educators have commented on the value of mentors and the importance of role modelling in their formation:

> Medical education involves risks. Without the support of my mentors and role models, I would not have had the courage to accomplish what I did.(12)

Learning from role models occurs through observation and reflection and is a complex mix of conscious and unconscious activities.(74) While we are all aware of the conscious observation of observed behaviours, understanding the power of the unconscious component is essential to effective role modelling. We should also remember that role models differ from mentors.(75) Role models inspire and teach by example – often while they are doing other things; mentors have an explicit relationship with a colleague over time.(76)

Organisational support and development

A recent survey of faculty members' needs for faculty development(77) highlights the necessity to look at staff development as 'development, orientation *and/or* support'. Interestingly, most programmes focus on the 'development' part. Much less has been written about faculty orientation and/or support.

Support for medical educators can take different forms, including managerial and organisational support, provision of information, recognition of teaching excellence and consideration of educational scholarship in promotion and tenure. As an example, support systems and materials are available in various areas of medical education(78) and range from textbooks tailored to the needs of those responsible for training doctors(79) to flexible and open learning materials and resources. Organisational support also includes:

- the development of institutional policies that support and reward excellence in teaching(10)
- a re-examination of the criteria for academic promotion and increased credit for educational initiatives(80)
- an increase in training and mentoring programmes
- enhanced resources for training teachers and junior faculty members.

In my own setting, the need for an orientation program for 'new' faculty members has been expressed as follows:

> You have to know how to navigate the system and there are certain expectations and if somebody doesn't make that explicit to you, it's very hard to figure out … (81)

As staff developers and medical educators, we often tend to focus on the individual teacher and overlook the importance of organisational support and development.(17)

What Is Known about Effectiveness?

Research on the impact of staff development activities has shown that overall satisfaction with programmes is high and that participants recommend these activities to their colleagues. Teachers also report a positive change in attitudes towards teaching as well as self-reported changes in knowledge about educational principles and specific teaching behaviours.(34) Other benefits include increased personal interest and enthusiasm, improved self-confidence, a greater sense of belonging to a community, and educational leadership and innovation. In our setting, participants in staff development activities have commented on the value of meeting like-minded colleagues and feeling a renewed sense of commitment and enthusiasm about teaching. As one participant reflected:

> I leave rejuvenated and ready to go out and teach a thousand students again!(49)

Others have identified the value of conceptual frameworks for what they do intuitively, as illustrated in the following quote:

> I was given new tools to teach. Not only were they described to me in words, but they were also used in front of me and I was part and parcel of the demonstration.(49)

In 2006, as part of the Best Evidence in Medical Education (BEME) collaboration, an international group of medical educators systematically reviewed the faculty development literature to ascertain the impact of faculty development initiatives on teaching effectiveness in medical education.(34) The results of this review indicate that the majority of the interventions targeted practising clinicians and included workshops, seminar series, short courses, longitudinal programmes and 'other' interventions, such as peer coaching, augmented feedback and site visits. The 53 reviewed articles included six randomised controlled trials and 47 quasi-experimental studies, of which 31 used a pre-test/post-test design. Box 28.4 summarises the findings of this review.

Despite numerous descriptions of staff development programmes, there has been a paucity of research demonstrating the effectiveness of most faculty development activities.(5,34) Few programmes have conducted comprehensive evaluations to ascertain what effect the programme is having on faculty, and data to support the efficacy of these initiatives have been lacking. Of the studies that have been conducted in this area, most have relied on the assessment of participant satisfaction; some have assessed the impact on cognitive learning or performance and several others have examined

---

BOX 28.4 Where's the evidence: Results of the BEME review(34)

The BEME review of faculty development initiatives designed to improve teaching effectiveness in medical education reported the following outcomes:

- *High satisfaction with staff development programmes* – Participants' overall satisfaction with staff development programmes was high. Moreover, they consistently found programmes to be acceptable, useful and relevant to their objectives. They also valued the methods used, especially those with a practical and skills-based focus.

- *Changes in attitudes towards teaching and staff development* – Participants reported positive changes in attitudes towards staff development and teaching as a result of their involvement in these activities. They cited a greater awareness of personal strengths and limitations, increased motivation and enthusiasm for teaching and learning, and a notable appreciation of the benefits of professional development.

- *Gains in knowledge and skills* – Participants reported increased knowledge of educational principles and strategies as well as gains in teaching skills. Where formal tests of knowledge were used, significant gains were shown.

- *Changes in teaching behaviour* – Self-perceived changes in teaching behaviours were consistently reported. While student evaluations did not always reflect participants' perceptions, observed changes in teaching performance were also detected.

- *Changes in organisational practice and student learning* – Although changes in organisational practice and student learning were not frequently investigated, changes did include greater educational involvement and establishment of collegial networks.

---

the long-term impact of these interventions. In addition, most of the research has relied on self-report rather than objective outcome measures or observations of change. More specifically, methods to evaluate staff development programmes have included:

- end-of-session evaluations
- follow-up survey questionnaires
- pre- and post-assessments of cognitive or attitudinal change
- direct observations of teaching behaviour
- student evaluations
- faculty self-ratings of post-training performance.

Common problems have included:

- lack of control or comparison groups
- heavy reliance on self-report measures of change
- small sample sizes.

There is clearly a need for more rigorous research designs and a greater use of qualitative and mixed methods to capture the complexity of faculty development interventions. The use of newer methods of performance-based assessment, incorporating diverse data sources, is also indicated, as is the value of process-oriented studies comparing different faculty development strategies and the maintenance of change over time.

What Theoretical Frameworks Can Guide the Development of Medical Educators?

MacDougall and Drummond(82) point out that there is no clear theoretical framework to describe how medical teachers and educators develop. In fact, despite an emphasis on educational 'know how' and practice, theory is noticeably absent from the staff development literature. In common with medical education itself, it would seem that a number of educational theories can be applied to faculty development and the development of medical educators. Many of these theoretical perspectives are covered in detail in other chapters; however, situated learning(83) appears to be one of the most useful overarching frameworks. Knowles' principles of adult learning(84,85) and Kolb's experiential learning cycle(86) are also pertinent, especially in the design and delivery of instructional programmes.

Situated learning

Situated learning is based on the notion that knowledge is *contextually situated* and fundamentally influenced by the *activity*, *context* and *culture* in which it is used.(83) This view of knowledge as *situated* in *authentic contexts* has important implications for our understanding of staff development and the design and delivery of instructional activities for faculty members.

Situated learning theory brings together the cognitive base and experiential learning that is needed to facilitate the acquisition of new behaviours. That is, it bridges the gap between the 'know what' and the 'know how' of teaching and learning by embedding learning in authentic activities. It also helps transform knowledge from the abstract and theoretical to the useable and useful.(87) The proponents of situated learning suggest that there should be a balance between the explicit teaching of a subject and the activities in which the knowledge learnt is used in an authentic context – both essential principles in staff development.

Some of the key components of situated learning include:

- cognitive apprenticeship
- collaborative learning
- reflection
- practice
- articulation of learning skills.(88)

Cognitive apprenticeship, a fundamental element of situated learning, has particular relevance to staff development. Apprenticeship is a familiar and pervasive method of learning in medicine.(89) Cognitive apprenticeship differs from a more traditional approach in that the process of carrying out the task that is to be learnt is not always observable; learning is not always situated in the workplace; and transfer of skills to new situations is required. Thus, to translate the model of traditional apprenticeship to cognitive apprenticeship, teachers need to:

- *identify the processes* of the task and make them visible, or explicit, to the student
- *situate* abstract tasks in authentic contexts, so that students understand the relevance of the work
- *vary* the diversity of learning situations
- *articulate* common aspects so that students can transfer their new knowledge and learning to new situations.(89)

Cognitive apprenticeship consists of four distinct phases: modelling, scaffolding, fading and coaching. (Further details about cognitive apprenticeship can be found in Box 5.1).

Collaborative learning is another important feature of situated learning and cognitive apprenticeship. Brown *et al.*(83) identify the following strategies to promote collaborative learning:

- collective problem solving
- displaying and identifying multiple roles
- confronting ineffective strategies and misconceptions
- developing collaborative work skills.

Small group work, peer teaching and group projects can also facilitate the acquisition of collaborative skills. As teamwork is a fundamental component of healthcare delivery, collaborative learning is essential in staff development.

Reflection, an essential ingredient of situated learning, has received increasing attention in the medical literature.(90) In practice, there are three kinds of reflective activity. Schön(90) describes a spontaneous reaction (i.e. 'thinking on your feet') as 'reflection *in* action'. This type of reflection, which is frequently described as a subliminal process of which the participant is only partially aware, most likely involves pattern recognition; as well, it is usually triggered by recognition that 'something doesn't seem right'.(90,91) Thinking of a situation after it has happened and initiating the ability to re-evaluate the situation is referred to as 'reflection *on* action'. This type of reflection, in which the participant is fully aware of what has occurred, allows the participant to mentally reconstruct the experience, paying particular attention to context. Reflection on action also forms a bridge between the re-lived situation and knowledge retrieved from internal memory or other external sources.(91)

While the development of the capacity to reflect 'in' and 'on' action has become an important feature of medical practice, 'reflection *for* action'(92) forms an additional avenue for professional training and improvement of practice, as it involves planning for the next step. As Lachman and Pawlina(92) have observed, 'The benefits of reflective practice, whilst meeting the objectives of new and revised curricula, extend beyond the construct of a medical curriculum. The process of reflection and its basis of critical thinking allows for the integration of theoretical concepts into practice, increased learning through experience, enhanced critical thinking and judgment in complex situations and the encouragement of student-centred learning.' Clearly, all of these benefits are of vital importance in the development of medical educators.

Practice is another central component of situated learning. Repeated practice serves to test, refine and extend skills into a web of increasing expertise in a social context of collaboration and reflection.(88) It also enables skills to become deeply rooted and 'automatically' mobilised as needed. The notion of experiential learning is closely tied to the concept of practice.

Articulation includes two aspects.(88) First, it refers to the concept of articulating or separating out different component skills in order to learn them more effectively. An example of this is effective communication with peers. Second, articulation refers to the goal of getting individuals to articulate their knowledge, reasoning or problem-solving processes in a specific domain. By articulating problem-solving processes, learners come to better understand their thinking processes, and they are better able to explain things to themselves and to others. Articulation also helps to make learning – and reflection – visible.

In summary, situated learning is based on the idea that knowledge is contextually situated and fundamentally influenced by the activity, context and culture in which it is used. In many ways, this model (and its key components of apprenticeship, collaboration, reflection, practice and articulation of skills) provides a useful framework by which to understand the development of medical educators.

Closely tied to the notion of situated learning is the concept of 'legitimate peripheral participation'.(63) This social practice, which combines 'learning by doing' (also known as experiential learning) and apprenticeship into a single theoretical perspective, is the process by which a novice becomes an expert. That is, from a situated learning perspective, learners build new knowledge and understanding through gradual participation in the community of which they are becoming a part. As learners, they begin at the edge – or periphery – of the community, where because of their status as learners, they have what is called 'legitimate peripheral participation'.(93)

In many ways, teachers go though a similar process. A key element of participation in the community is the opportunity to see and participate in the framing of problems and understand how knowledge is structured. According to Wenger,(65) social participation within the community is the key to informal learning.

It is also embedded in the practices and relationships of the workplace and helps create identity and meaning. In addition, it complements, and can substitute for, formal learning mechanisms. Informal learning is often not acknowledged as learning within organisations; rather, it is typically regarded as being 'part of the job'. However, learning at work is a key component of the development of medical educators, and there is value in rendering this learning as visible as possible so that it can be valued as an important component of staff development.

Principles of adult learning

Although some have argued that adult learning is not a theory(94) but merely a description of the adult learner, others believe that the principles of adult learning (also referred to as andragogy) form an important theoretical construct.(95) In either case, andragogy captures essential characteristics of adult learners and offers important guidelines for planning staff development programmes.

Knowles(84,85) coined the term andragogy, defining it as 'the art and science of helping adults learn'. Key principles include the following:

- Adults are independent.
- Adults come to learning situations with a variety of motivations and definite expectations about particular learning goals and teaching methods.
- Adults demonstrate different learning styles.
- Much of adult learning is 'relearning' rather than new learning.
- Adult learning often involves changes in attitudes as well as skills.
- Most adults prefer to learn through experience.
- Incentives for adult learning usually come from within the individual.
- Feedback is usually more important than tests and evaluations.

Clearly, the incorporation of these principles into the design of any educational programme will enhance receptivity, relevance and engagement. An understanding of these principles can also influence pacing, meaning and motivation.

The experiential learning cycle

Kolb and Fry(86) provide a description of the learning cycle that highlights the role of experience in the learning process. More specifically, they describe how experience is translated into concepts, which in turn guide the choice of new experiences.(96) In this model, which should be considered in the design of all instructional events, learning is viewed as a four-stage cycle (*see* Figure 2.2). Immediate concrete experience is the basis for observation and reflection; observations are then assimilated into a personal theory, from which new implications for action can be deduced, and all of these steps eventually lead to new experiences. According to Kolb and Fry,(86) learners need opportunities to experience each step of the learning cycle. That is, they need the ability to:

- experience diverse situations (in both the classroom and the clinical setting)
- observe and reflect on what they have learnt (often in a large group session)
- develop their own theory and understanding of the world
- experiment new ways of being in order for learning to occur.

Attention to the experiential learning cycle will facilitate teaching *and* learning and ensure that different learning styles are respected and nurtured in any staff development programme.

How Should We Design a Staff Development Programme?

As formal staff development programmes are one of the most common ways of developing medical educators, this section will highlight some general guidelines that have been previously described and can be of use to staff developers.(13)

Understand the organisational culture

Staff development programmes take place within the context of a specific institution or organisation. It is imperative to understand the culture of that institution and to be responsive to its needs. Staff development programmes should also capitalise on the organisation's strengths and work with the leadership to ensure success. In many ways, the cultural context can be used to promote or enhance staff development efforts. For example, as some authors have suggested, 'staff development during times of educational or curricular reform can take on added importance'.(97) It is also important to assess institutional support for staff development activities, ascertain available resources and lobby effectively. Clearly, staff development cannot occur in a vacuum.(13)

Determine appropriate goals and priorities

As with the design of any programme, it is imperative to define goals and priorities carefully. What are we trying to achieve – and why is it important to do so? It is equally important to determine programme objectives as they will influence our target audience, choice of programme, overall content and methodology. Determining priorities is not always easy, and it often involves consultations with key stakeholders. However, it is always essential to balance individual *and* organisational needs.

Conduct needs assessments to ensure relevant programming

As stated earlier, staff development programmes should base themselves on the needs of the individual as well as the institution. Student needs, patient needs and societal needs may also help direct relevant activities.(13) Assessing needs is necessary to refine goals, determine content, identify preferred learning formats and assure relevance. It is also a way of promoting early 'buy-in'. Common methods include:

- written questionnaires or surveys
- interviews or focus groups with key informants (e.g. participants, students, educational leaders)
- observations of teachers 'in action'
- literature reviews
- environmental scans of available programmes and resources.(98,99)

Whenever possible, we should try to gain information from multiple sources and distinguish between 'needs' and 'wants'. Clearly, an individual teacher's perceived needs may differ from those expressed by their students or peers. Needs assessments can also help further translate goals into objectives, which will serve as the basis for programme planning and evaluation of outcome.

Develop different programmes to accommodate diverse needs

Different staff development formats have been described in an earlier section. Clearly, we must design programmes that accommodate diverse goals and objectives, content areas, and the needs of the individual and the organisation. For example, if our goal is to improve our colleagues' lecturing skills, a half-day workshop on interactive lecturing might be the programme of choice. On the other hand, if we wish to promote educational leadership and scholarly activity among our peers, a teaching scholar programme or educational fellowship might be the preferred method.(13) In this context, it is also helpful to remember that staff *development* can include development, orientation, recognition and support, and different programmes are required to accommodate diverse objectives.

Incorporate principles of adult learning and instructional design

As previously mentioned, adults come to learning situations with a variety of motivations and expectations about teaching methods and goals. Incorporation of these principles into the design of a staff development programme is clearly needed, as physicians demonstrate a high degree of self-direction and possess numerous experiences that should serve as the basis for learning.(13)

Principles of instructional design should also be followed. For example, it is important to develop clear learning goals and objectives, identify key content areas, design appropriate teaching and learning strategies, and create appropriate methods of evaluation of both the students and the curriculum. It is equally important to integrate theory with practice(100) and to ensure that the learning is perceived as relevant to the work setting and to the profession. Learning should be interactive, participatory and experientially based, using the participants' previous learning and experience as a starting point. Detailed planning and organisation involving all stakeholders is critical, as is the creation of a positive learning environment. However, although theory should inform practice, staff development initiatives must remain relevant and practical (*see* Box 28.5).

Offer a diversity of educational methods

In line with principles of adult learning, staff development programmes should try to offer a variety of educational methods that promote experiential learning, reflection, feedback and immediacy of application. Common learning methods include interactive lectures, case presentations, small group discussions and individual exercises, role-plays and simulations, videotape reviews and live demonstrations. Practice with feedback is also key, as is the opportunity to reflect on personal values and attitudes. Computer-aided instruction, debates and reaction panels, journal clubs and self-directed readings are additional methods to consider. In line with our previous example, a workshop on interactive lecturing might include interactive plenary presentations, small group discussions and exercises, and opportunities for practice and feedback. A fellowship programme might include group semi-

nars, independent projects and structured readings. Whatever the method, the needs and learning preferences of the participants should be respected, and the method should match the objective. Healthcare professionals learn best 'by doing', and experiential learning should be promoted whenever possible.(13)

Promote buy-in and market effectively

The decision to participate in a staff development programme or activity is not as simple as it might at first appear. It involves the individual's reaction to a particular offering, motivation to develop or enhance a specific skill, being available at the time of the session and overcoming the psychological barrier of admitting need.(97) As faculty developers, it is our challenge to overcome reluctance and to market our 'product' in such a way that resistance becomes a resource to learning. In our context, we have seen the value of targeted mailings, professionally designed brochures and 'branding' of our product to promote interest. Continuing education credits, as well as free and flexible programming, can also help facilitate motivation and attendance. Buy-in involves agreement on importance, widespread support and dedication of time and resources at both the individual and the system level and must be considered in all programming initiatives.(101)

Work to overcome commonly encountered challenges

Common challenges faced by faculty developers include:
- lack of institutional support and resources for programme planning
- defining goals and priorities
- assessing needs and balancing individual and organisational needs
- motivating faculty to participate
- obtaining faculty buy-in
- promoting a 'culture change' that reflects renewed interest in teaching and learning.

Staff developers must inevitably work to overcome these problems through a variety of means that can include creative programming, skilled marketing and the delivery of high-quality activities. Flexible scheduling and collaborative programming, which address clearly identified needs, can also help ensure success at the system level.

Prepare staff developers

The recruitment and preparation of staff developers is rarely reported. However, it is important to recruit carefully, train effectively, partner creatively and build on previous experiences.(101) Medical educators can be involved in a number of ways: as co-facilitators, as programme planners or as consultants. In our own setting, we try to involve new faculty members in each staff development activity and conduct a preparatory

BOX 28.5 Where's the evidence: Key features of staff development(34)

The BEME review of faculty development initiatives designed to improve teaching effectiveness in medical education found that the following 'key features' contribute to the effectiveness of staff development activities:

The role of experiential learning – This includes the importance of applying what had been learned, practising skills and receiving feedback on these skills.

The provision of feedback – The role of feedback in promoting change is important, as is the use of feedback as a specific intervention strategy.

Effective peer and colleague relationships – This includes the value of peers as role models, the mutual exchange of information and ideas and the importance of collegial support to promote and retain change.

Well-designed interventions following principles of teaching and learning – Adherence to principles of instructional design and principles of adult learning promote effective learning and skill acquisition.

The use of multiple instructional methods to achieve intended objectives – This includes a diversity of educational methods within single interventions to accommodate learning styles and preferences.

meeting (or 'dry run') to review content and process, solicit feedback and promote 'ownership'. We also conclude each activity with a 'debriefing' session to discuss lessons learnt and plan for the future. Whenever possible, staff developers should be individuals who are well respected by their peers and have some educational expertise and experience in facilitating groups. It has been said that 'to teach is to learn twice'; this principle is clearly one of the main motivating factors for staff developers.

Evaluate – and demonstrate – effectiveness

The need to evaluate staff development programmes and activities is clear. In fact, we must remember that the evaluation of staff development is more than an academic exercise, and our findings must be used in the design, delivery and marketing of our programmes. It has also been stated earlier that staff development must strive to promote education as a scholarly activity; we must role model this approach in all that we do.(5)

In preparing to evaluate a staff development programme or activity, we should consider the goal of the evaluation (e.g. programme planning versus decision making, policy formation versus academic inquiry), available data sources (e.g. participants, peers, students or residents), common methods of evaluation (e.g. questionnaires, focus groups, objective tests, observations), resources to support assessment (e.g. institutional support, research grants) and models of programme evaluation (e.g. goal attainment, decision facilitation). Kirkpatrick's levels of evaluation(102) are also helpful in conceptualising and framing the assessment of outcome. They include the following:

- *reaction* – participants' views on the learning experience
- *learning* – change in participants' attitudes, knowledge or skills
- *behaviour* – change in participants' behaviour
- *results* – changes in the organisational system, the patient or the learner.

At a minimum, a practical and feasible evaluation should include an assessment of utility and relevance, content, teaching and learning methods, and intent to change. Moreover, as evaluation is an integral part of programme planning, it should be conceptualised at the beginning of any programme. It should also include qualitative and quantitative assessments of learning and behaviour change using a variety of methods and data sources.

Conclusion

As the demands for accountability in higher education gain momentum, pressures to change professional conduct in medical education will continue to grow.(10)

Moreover, as the emphasis on global standards in medical education increases,(103,104) so will the need for the professional development of medical educators. As Glicken and Merenstein(19) aptly state, faculty members often come to medical teaching with the 'wisdom and experience that dictates what their students need to know', although they have not been trained for the job at hand. Clearly, it is our responsibility to enable this training, either through formal or through informal approaches.

We also need to remember that medical education is a social endeavour. Faculty members at McGill University have identified core attributes (including reflection, passion, enthusiasm and pride) and skills (such as the ability to maintain multiple perspectives, situate learning, work with others and see the 'big picture') needed to become a medical educator.(12) They have also highlighted the benefit of a community of scholars in the formation of medical educators (as outlined in Box 28.2). In many ways, these suggestions can serve as a road map for developing medical educators, as each of us finds joy and satisfaction in this journey of discovery:

> To me a medical educator is someone who devotes part of their career and time and interests towards medical teaching and education. It is not the title that counts. It is more the effort and the amount of time and the process and the products that get produced that defines the level of medical educator we become.(12)

> You become a medical educator once you add the intangible – the passion and the commitment, the dedication and the creativity … (12)

Acknowledgements

I would like to thank Dr Peter McLeod, Dr Linda Snell and Dr Peter Cantillon for their helpful comments on this chapter. I would also like to gratefully acknowledge my colleagues at the Centre for Medical Education and the Faculty of Medicine at McGill University for their continued participation, insights and feedback on our faculty development programmes and activities. My own understanding of this complex process would not have been possible without this 'community of practice'.

Some of the material used in this chapter has been published previously in a contribution by the author to *A Practical Guide for Medical Teachers*(13) and to *Teaching Medical Professionalism*(105) and is reproduced here with permission.

References

1 Miller G (1980) *Educating Medical Teachers*. Harvard University Press, Cambridge, MA.
2 Jason H and Westberg J (1982) *Teachers and Teaching in US Medical Schools*. Appleton-Century-Crofts, New York.

3 Harris D, Krause K, Parish D and Smith M (2007) Academic competencies for medical faculty. *Family Medicine*. **39**(5): 343–50.

4 Skeff KM, Stratos GA, Bergen MR *et al.* (1999) Regional teaching improvement programs for community-based teachers. *American Journal of Medicine*. **106**: 76–80.

5 Steinert Y (2000). Faculty development in the new millennium: key challenges and future directions. *Medical Teacher*. **22**: 44–50.

6 Clark JM, Houston TK, Kolodner K *et al.* (2004) Teaching the teachers: national survey of faculty development in departments of medicine of US teaching hospitals. *Journal of General Internal Medicine*. **19**: 205–14.

7 McLean M, Cilliers F and Van Wyk J (2008) Faculty development: yesterday, today and tomorrow. *Medical Teacher*. **30**: 555–84.

8 General Medical Council (2006) Good medical practice (http://www.gmc-uk.org; accessed 15 October 2008).

9 Postgraduate Medical Education and Training Board (2008) Generic standards for training (http://www.pmetb.org.uk; accessed 15 October 2008).

10 Eitel F, Kanz KG and Tesche A (2000) Training and certification of teachers and trainers: the professionalization of medical education. *Medical Teacher*. **22**: 517–26.

11 Purcell N and Lloyd-Jones G (2003) Standards for medical educators. *Medical Education*. **37**: 149–54.

12 Steinert Y (2008) From teacher to medical educator: the spectrum of medical education. Unpublished report, Centre for Medical Education, Montreal.

13 Steinert Y (2005) Staff development. In: Dent J and Harden R (eds) *A Practical Guide for Medical Teachers*, pp. 390–9. Elsevier Churchill Livingstone, Edinburgh.

14 Centra J (1978) Types of faculty development programs. *Journal of Higher Education*. **49**: 151–62.

15 Bland C, Schmitz C, Stritter F, Henry R and Aluise J (1990) *Successful Faculty in Academic Medicine: essential skills and how to acquire them*. Springer Publishing Company, New York.

16 Sheets K and Schwenk T (1990) Faculty development for family medicine educators: an agenda for future activities. *Teaching and Learning in Medicine*. **2**(3): 141–8.

17 Steinert Y, Cruess R, Cruess S *et al.* (2007) Faculty development as an instrument of change: a case study on teaching professionalism. *Academic Medicine*. **82**: 1057–64.

18 Hafferty FW (1998) Beyond curriculum reform: confronting medicine's hidden curriculum. *Academic Medicine*. **73**: 403–7.

19 Glicken A and Merenstein G (2007) Addressing the hidden curriculum: understanding educator professionalism. *Medical Teacher*. **29**: 54–7.

20 Bligh J (2005) Faculty development. *Medical Education*. **39**: 120–1.

21 Swanwick T (2008) See one, do one, then what? Faculty development in postgraduate medical education. *Postgraduate Medical Journal*. **84**: 339–43.

22 Wilkerson L and Irby D (1998) Strategies for improving teaching practices: a comprehensive approach to faculty development. *Academic Medicine*. **73**: 387–96.

23 Irby D (1994) What clinical teachers in medicine need to know. *Academic Medicine*. **69**: 333–42.

24 Copeland H and Hewson M (2000) Developing and testing an instrument to measure the effectiveness of clinical teaching in an academic medical center. *Academic Medicine*. **75**: 161–6.

25 Buchel T and Edwards F (2005) Characteristics of effective clinical teachers. *Family Medicine*. **37**: 30–5.

26 Wright SM and Carrese JA (2002) Excellence in role modeling: insight and perspectives from the pros. *Canadian Medical Association Journal*. **167**: 638–43.

27 Bordage G, Foley R and Goldyn S (2000) Skills and attributes of directors of educational programmes. *Medical Education*. **34**: 206–10.

28 Spencer J and Jordan R (2001) Educational outcome and leadership to meet the needs of modern health care. *Quality in Health Care*. **10**: ii38–45.

29 Boyer E (1990) *Scholarship Reconsidered: priorities of the professoriate*. Princeton University Press, Princeton, NJ.

30 Simpson D and Fincher R (1999) Making a case for the teaching scholar. *Academic Medicine*. **74**: 1296–9.

31 Glassick CE (2000) Boyer's expanded definitions of scholarship, the standards for assessing scholarship and the elusiveness of the scholarship of teaching. *Academic Medicine*. **75**: 877–80.

32 Higgs J and McAllister L (2007) Educating clinical educators: using a model of the experience of being a clinical educator. *Medical Teacher*. **29**: e51–7.

33 Fraser SW and Greenhalgh T (2001) Coping with complexity: educating for capability. *British Medical Journal*. **323**: 799–803.

34 Steinert Y, Mann K, Centeno A *et al.* (2006) A systematic review of faculty development initiatives designed to improve teaching effectiveness in medical education: BEME guide No. 8. *Medical Teacher*. **28**: 497–526.

35 Nasmith L and Steinert Y (2001) The evaluation of a workshop to promote interactive lecturing. *Teaching and Learning in Medicine*. **13**: 43–8.

36 Nasmith L, Steinert Y, Saroyan A *et al.* (1997) Assessing the impact of a faculty development workshop: a methodological study. *Teaching and Learning in Medicine*. **9**: 209–14.

37 Nayer M (1995) Faculty development for problem-based learning programs. *Teaching and Learning in Medicine*. **7**: 138–48.

38 Olmesdahl PJ and Manning DM (1999) Impact of training on PBL facilitators. *Medical Education*. **33**: 753–5.

39 Quirk ME, DeWitt T, Lasser D *et al.* (1998) Evaluation of primary care futures: a faculty development program for community health center preceptors. *Academic Medicine*. **73**: 705–7.

40 Wilkerson L and Sarkin RT (1998) Arrows in the quiver: evaluation of a workshop on ambulatory teaching. *Academic Medicine*. **73**(s10): s67–9.

41 Steinert Y, Nasmith L and Daigle N (2003) Executive skills for medical faculty: a workshop description and evaluation. *Medical Teacher*. **25**: 666–8.

42 Steinert Y, Cruess S, Cruess R and Snell L (2005) Faculty development for teaching and evaluating professionalism: from programme design to curriculum change. *Medical Education*. **39**: 127–36.

43 Baldwin CD, Goldblum RM, Rason DK and Levine HG (1994) Facilitating faculty development and research through critical review of grant proposals and articles. *Academic Medicine*. **69**: 62–4.

44 Steinert Y, McLeod P, Liben S and Snell L (2008) Writing for publication in medical education: the benefits of a faculty development workshop and peer writing group. *Medical Teacher*. **30**: e280–5.

45 Cusimano M and David M (1998) A compendium of higher education opportunities in health professions education. *Academic Medicine*. **73**: 1255–9.

46 Hitchcock MA, Lamkin BD, Mygdal WK *et al.* (1986) Affective changes in faculty development fellows in family medicine. *Journal of Medical Education.* **61**: 394–403.

47 Searle N, Hatem C, Perkowski L and Wilkerson L (2006) Why invest in an educational fellowship program? *Academic Medicine.* **81**: 936–40.

48 Gruppen L, Simpson D, Searle N *et al.* (2006) Educational fellowship programs: common themes and overarching issues. *Academic Medicine.* **81**: 990–4.

49 Steinert Y, Nasmith L, McLeod P and Conochie L (2003) A teaching scholars program to develop leaders in medical education. *Academic Medicine.* **78**: 142–9.

50 Steinert Y and McLeod J (2006) From novice to informed educator: the teaching scholars program for educators in the health sciences. *Academic Medicine.* **81**: 969–74.

51 Rosenbaum ME, Lenoch S and Ferguson KJ (2005) Outcomes of a teaching scholars program to promote leadership in faculty development. *Teaching and Learning in Medicine.* **17**: 247–52.

52 Muller JH and Irby D (2006) Developing educational leaders: the teaching scholars program at the University of California, San Francisco, School of Medicine. *Academic Medicine.* **81**: 959–64.

53 Wilkerson L, Uijtdehaage S and Relan A (2006) Increasing the pool of educational leaders for UCLA. *Academic Medicine.* **81**: 954–8.

54 Hatem C, Lown B and Newman L (2006) The academic health centre coming of age: helping faculty become better teachers and agents of educational change. *Academic Medicine.* **81**: 941–4.

55 Dearing R (1997) *Higher Education in the Learning Society: report of the National Committee of Inquiry into Higher Education.* HMSO, London.

56 Walsh K (2007) Professionalism in medical education: could an academy play a role? *Medical Teacher.* **29**: 425–6.

57 Cohen R, Murnaghan L, Collins J and Pratt D (2005) An update on Master's degrees in medical education. *Medical Teacher.* **27**: 686–92.

58 Pugsley L, Brigley S, Allery L and Macdonald J (2008) Counting quality because quality counts: differing standards in Master's in medical education programmes. *Medical Teacher.* **30**: 80–5.

59 Hesketh E, Bagnall G, Buckley EG *et al.* (2001) A framework for developing excellence as a clinical educator. *Medical Education.* **35**: 555–64.

60 Flynn S, Bedinghaus J, Snyder C and Hekelman F (1994) Peer coaching in clinical teaching: a case report. *Family Medicine.* **26**: 569–70.

61 Orlander J, Gupta M, Fincke B *et al.* (2000) Co-teaching: a faculty development strategy. *Medical Education.* **34**: 257–65.

62 Boud D and Middleton H (2003) Learning from others at work: communities of practice and informal learning. *Journal of Workplace Learning.* **15**(5): 194–202.

63 Lave J and Wenger E (1991) *Situated Learning: legitimate peripheral participation.* Cambridge University Press, New York.

64 Barab SA, Barnett M and Squire K (2002) Developing an empirical account of a community of practice: characterizing the essential tensions. *The Journal of the Learning Sciences.* **11**: 489–542.

65 Wenger E (1998) *Communities of Practice: learning, meaning and identity.* Cambridge University Press, New York.

66 Wenger E, McDermott R and Snyder W (2002) *Cultivating Communities of Practice.* Harvard Business School Press, Boston, MA.

67 Bligh J and Brice J (2007) The Academy of Medical Educators: a professional home for medical educators in the UK. *Medical Education.* **41**: 625–7.

68 Cooke M, Irby D and Debas H (2003) The UCSF academy of medical educators. *Academic Medicine.* **78**: 666–72.

69 Irby D, Cooke M, Lowenstein D and Richards B (2004) The academy movement: a structural approach to reinvigorating the educational mission. *Academic Medicine.* **79**: 729–36.

70 Bligh J (1999) Mentoring: an invisible support network. *Medical Education.* **33**: 2–3.

71 Morzinski J, Diehr S, Bower D and Simpson D (1996) A descriptive, cross-sectional study of formal mentoring for faculty. *Family Medicine.* **28**: 434–8.

72 Pololi L, Knight S, Dennis K and Frankel R (2002) Helping medical school faculty realize their dreams: an innovative, collaborative mentoring program. *Academic Medicine.* **77**: 377–84.

73 Daloz L (1986) *Effective Teaching and Mentoring.* Jossey-Bass, San Francisco, CA.

74 Epstein RM, Cole DR, Gawinski BA *et al.* (1998) How students learn from community-based preceptors. *Archives of Family Medicine.* **7**: 149–54.

75 Ricer RE (1998) Defining preceptor, mentor, and role model. *Family Medicine.* **30**: 328.

76 Paice E, Heard S and Moss F (2002) How important are role models in making good doctors? *British Medical Journal.* **325**: 707–10.

77 Steinert Y and Walsh A (2006) *A Faculty Development Program for Teachers of International Medical Graduates.* Association of Faculties of Medicine of Canada, Ottawa.

78 Grant J (1998) Offering training and support to trainers. In: Paice E (ed.) *Delivering the New Doctor.* Association for the Study of Medical Education, Edinburgh.

79 Jolly B and Grant J (eds) (1997) *The Good Assessment Guide: a practical guide to assessment and appraisal for higher specialist training.* Joint Centre for Education in Medicine, London.

80 Azer S (2005) The qualities of a good teacher: how can they be acquired and sustained? *Journal of the Royal Society of Medicine.* **98**(2): 67–9.

81 Steinert Y, McLeod P, Boillat M *et al.* (2008) Faculty development: a field of dreams? *Medical Education.* **43**: 42–9.

82 MacDougall J and Drummond M (2005) The development of medical teachers: an enquiry into the learning histories of 10 experienced medical teachers. *Medical Education.* **39**: 1213–20.

83 Brown J, Collins A and Duguid P (1989) Situated cognition and the culture of learning. *Educational Researcher.* **18**: 32–42.

84 Knowles M (1985) *Andragogy in action.* Jossey-Bass, San Francisco, CA.

85 Knowles M (1980) *The Modern Practice of Adult Education: from pedagogy to androgogy.* Cambridge Books, New York.

86 Kolb D and Fry R (1975) Towards an applied theory of experiential learning. In: Cooper C (ed.) *Theories of Group Processes.* John Wiley, London.

87 Cruess R and Cruess S (2006) Teaching professionalism: general principles. *Medical Teacher.* **28**: 205–8.

88 McLellan H (1996) *Situated Learning Perspectives.* Educational Technology Publications, Englewood Cliffs, NJ.

89 Mann K (2006) Learning and teaching in professional character development. In: Kenney N (ed.) *Lost Virtue: professional character development in medical education.* Elsevier, New York.

90 Schön D (1983) *The Reflective Practitioner: how professionals think in action.* Basic Books, New York.

91 Hewson M (1991) Reflection in clinical teaching: an analysis of reflection-on-action and its implications for staffing residents. *Medical Teacher*. **13**: 227–31.

92 Lachman N and Pawlina W (2006) Integrating professionalism in early medical education: the theory and application of reflective practice in the anatomy curriculum. *Clinical Anatomy*. **19**: 456–60.

93 Robertson K (2005) Reflection in professional practice and education. *Australian Family Physician*. **34**: 781–3.

94 Norman G (1999) The adult learner: a mythical species. *Academic Medicine*. **74**: 886–9.

95 Merriam S (1996) Updating our knowledge of adult learning. *Journal of Continuing Education in the Health Professions*. **16**: 136–43.

96 Boud D, Keogh R and Walker D (1985) *Reflection: turning experience into learning*. Kogan Page, London.

97 Rubeck R and Witzke D (1998) Faculty development: a field of dreams. *Academic Medicine*. **73**(s9): S32–7.

98 Grant J (2002) Learning needs assessment: assessing the need. *British Medical Journal*. **324**: 156–9.

99 Lockyer J (1998) Needs assessment: lessons learned. *Journal of Continuing Education in the Health Professions*. **18**:190–2.

100 Kaufman D, Mann K and Jennett P (2000) *Teaching and Learning in Medical Education: how theory can inform practice*. Association for the Study of Medical Education, Edinburgh.

101 Steinert Y (2005) Staff development for clinical teachers. *The Clinical Teacher* **2**: 104–10.

102 Kirkpatrick D (1994) *Evaluating Training Programs: the four levels*. Berrett-Koehler Publishers, San Francisco, CA.

103 Karle H (2007) European specifications for global standards in medical education. *Medical Education*. **41**: 924–5.

104 World Federation for Medical Education (2007) Global standards programme (http://www.wfme.org; accessed 24 October 2008).

105 Steinert Y (2009) Educational theory and strategies for teaching and learning professionalism. In: Cruess R, Cruess S and Steinert Y (eds) *Teaching Medical Professionalism*, pp. 31–52. Cambridge University Press, New York.

Educational leadership

Judy McKimm and Tim Swanwick

KEY MESSAGES

- 'Leadership' is a social construct and a product of the preoccupations of the day.
- Leadership and strategic management are inextricably intertwined.
- The most effective leaders have well-developed self-awareness coupled with knowledge of and insight into the strengths and abilities of their 'followers'.
- Educational leadership in healthcare occurs within an environment of high complexity.

- Effective healthcare education leaders have to work across multiple boundaries: organisational, cultural, professional and sectoral.
- Leadership is about change: knowing your environment and horizon scanning are crucial.
- Leadership is about being and doing … leaders have to 'walk the walk'.

Introduction

Education leaders in the medical and allied professions carry a 'double burden'. They have to manage and lead universities and other educational institutions in a rapidly changing global environment while working in close collaboration with a range of healthcare delivery partners with their own financial and service-driven agendas. The complexity and pace of change in healthcare means that the need for effective leaders and leadership development has never been so important; however, in a sector that is continually focused on the achievement of targets and balancing budgets, training and development are not always given the highest priority.

In the UK, education is driven by a number of key governmental and European policy initiatives that set the context for educational leaders. These include aspirational policies, such as 'widening access' and the 'massification' of higher education, as well as an inexorable drive towards greater public accountability – a problematic area for leaders who work in universities traditionally run on collegial models of participative but autonomous decision making and consensus.

Bush(1) notes that it is vital for education leaders to maintain 'education' as their central concern. This is difficult to achieve in the healthcare sector, where there is an inbuilt tension between the purposes of *education* and the demands of *vocational training*, which has as its goal the production of a competent, safe future workforce. In the UK, this is further compli-

cated by the way that different government departments, across the four devolved countries, fund various parts of healthcare education and training, a situation that does not always lead to congruence on the ground.

In the UK, National Health Service (NHS) leadership development has been intrinsically linked to service redesign, improvements and delivery. The NHS Modernisation Agency, now the Institute for Innovation and Improvement, has been responsible for developing an *NHS Leadership Qualities Framework,*(2) a series of *Improvement Leaders' Guides* and more recently, a *Medical Leadership Competency Framework*.(3) Leadership in the NHS is firmly sited in service improvement, and the *NHS Leadership Framework* (see Figure 29.1) lays out an underpinning philosophy about leadership development – one that assumes that leadership skills can be learnt, aligns leadership qualities with management capabilities, locates leadership and leadership development at all levels within the organisation and aims to create an empowerment culture based on supporting people, the transformation of followers into leaders and the development and creation of a shared vision.

In higher education, which educates and trains the medical and healthcare workforce of the future at pre-registration level, public sector service improvement does not have the same priority, and, again, the policy agendas are different across the four UK countries. For example, the Higher Education Funding Council for England's strategic plan is focused around four core strategic aims:(4)
- enhancing excellence in learning and teaching
- widening participation and fair access
- enhancing excellence in research
- enhancing the contribution of higher education to the economy and society.

Understanding Medical Education: Evidence, Theory and Practice.
Edited by T Swanwick. © 2010 Association for the Study of Medical Education.

Figure 29.1 The NHS leadership framework.

Underpinning these aims are two cross-cutting aims:

- sustaining a high-quality higher education sector *and*
- enabling excellence.

There are then some inherent tensions and contradictions in leading change in today's public sector organisations. For healthcare education, this is exacerbated by differences between health service and education policies, values, systems and practices.

Another of the unique features that face healthcare educators is the challenge of leading education across professional boundaries. Leaders in healthcare education have to be aware of the needs and demands of multiple stakeholders in the current drive to produce competent healthcare practitioners, open to working in a flexible way. Working with academics, clinicians, healthcare managers and professionals with differing values and education systems means that leaders need to quickly establish credibility with different stakeholders, use and develop sound interpersonal skills and demonstrate effective management capabilities.

Training and development in leadership are often patchy and not easy to access for more junior staff. Higher education has traditionally been focused on developing the management skills of heads of departments and more senior management rather than forming part of succession planning and developing leadership capacity at all levels. Changes in skills mix and professional roles, changes in funding and commissioning arrangements and emerging organisational changes such as mergers, collaborations and partnerships will mean that tomorrow's healthcare education leaders will require higher-level leadership and management skills than ever before.

Leadership and Management

There are many definitions of leadership. Leadership theory looks not only at individuals but also at the relationship between leaders and followers and the context or situation in which they operate. In recent years, many theorists have found it useful to distinguish between *management* and *leadership*, and although there is considerable overlap and interdependency, differentiating between the two concepts will help us begin to explore what leadership is and some of the assumptions made about, and expectations of, people working in educational settings.

For Bennis and Nanus, 'managers are people who do things right and leaders are people who do the right thing'.(5) Managers are often described as performing *functions* in organisations, usually holding a particular formal title or fulfilling a particular role. Management is concerned with planning, organising, coordinating, commanding or controlling the activities of staff.(6) Leaders, by contrast, aim to influence and guide others into pursuing particular objectives or visions of the future and to motivate them into wanting to follow. Yukl suggests that 'leadership is the process of influencing others to understand and agree about what needs to be done and how it can be done effectively and the process of facilitating individual and collective efforts to accomplish the shared objectives'.(7)

Kotter(8) contrasts leadership and management and suggests that whereas leadership sets a direction and develops a vision for the future, that is, producing change and movement, management is more concerned with planning and with providing order and consistency in organisations rather than the process of producing change. Covey *et al.* put a slightly different slant on this, suggesting that managers work within an existing 'paradigm', solve problems and manage people, whereas leaders create new paradigms, challenge systems, seek new opportunities and lead people'.(9)

The differences between leadership and management identified by many authors over the years are succinctly summarised by Northouse(10) (*see* Box 29.1). However, contemporary leadership theory, for example, Blagg and Young,(11) Yukl(7) and Storey(12), suggests that in practice it is often the same person who operates in both capacities and that the most effective people in organisations are both managers and leaders.

Furthermore, in universities, administrators are often distinguished from academics, reflecting the way in which university systems have developed. The terms 'leaders' and 'managers' are not so widely used, although individuals clearly fulfil management and leadership functions. In practice, the barriers and constructs that often worked to place academics and administrators seemingly in opposition to one another

MANAGEMENT	LEADERSHIP
Produces order and consistency	*Produces change and movement*
Planning/Budgeting	Establishing direction
• Establish agendas	• Create a vision
• Set timetables	• Clarify big picture
• Allocate resources	• Set strategies
Organising/Staffing	Aligning people
• Provide structure	• Communicate goals
• Make job placements	• Seek commitment
• Establish rules and procedures	• Build teams and coalitions
Controlling/Problem solving	Motivating and inspiring
• Develop incentives	• Inspire and energise
• Generate creative solutions	• Empower subordinates
• Take corrective action	• Satisfy unmet needs

are breaking down, as educational organisations are becoming more aware of the need to operate efficiently and effectively in an increasingly competitive global market. Educational leaders can no longer rely wholly on formal positional authority but must seek to develop and display appropriate leadership characteristics and qualities, and it is increasingly recognised that people at all levels in an organisation have the potential to perform and display leadership.

A Brief History of Leadership

The next two sections look at leadership models and theories, charting their development and unpicking the contribution that these models and theories make to enhancing our understanding of what leaders do and what leadership is. It is important to remember that leadership itself is a social construct; therefore, the prevailing theories and models of leadership tend to be of their time and reflect the prevailing public 'mood' and the preoccupations of (largely) North American enterprise.

In the first half of the 20th century, leadership theory revolved around personal qualities, an approach based on the assumption that leaders are born rather than made. This gave rise to the pervasive idea of the 'great man' who will be a leader under any circumstances. The great man theories emphasised characteristics such as intelligence, energy and dominance, but several major reviews of the literature failed to consistently identify personality traits that differentiated leaders from non-leaders. Interestingly, trait theory

has made a comeback in recent years with the emotional intelligence theories of Goleman.(13)

From the 1950s onwards, attention shifted from personal characteristics of leaders to their behaviours, in particular, how their *style* and behaviours impacted on groups. Writers such as Blake and Mouton(14) consider the differences between 'task-focused' and 'people-focused' leaders and argue that high levels of concern for both is what is required.

While these models introduce the idea of leadership as a group of behaviours, they give little indication as to what sort of behaviours worked best in what circumstances. This was addressed through the work of, among others, Tannenbaum and Schmidt,(15) Fiedler(16) and Hersey and Blanchard.(17) The last two authors achieved widespread popularity through the *One Minute Manager* series with their explication of *situational* leadership. Hersey and Blanchard's argument is that leaders need to adapt their style to variations in the competence and commitment of followers. The four styles identified are directing, coaching, supporting and delegating. A situational approach to leadership is also adopted by Adair in his 'three circles model'.(18) Adair recommends that, depending on the circumstances, the focus of a leader's attention should be distributed flexibly between the *task*, the *team* and the *individual*.

It became apparent in the 1980s that none of the leadership theories to date offered advice on how to cope in environments of continuous change. Various authors highlighted that the models described so far were effectively managerial or transactional. Existing models helped plan, order and organise at times of stability but were inadequate at describing how people or organisations might be led through periods of significant change. A new paradigm emerged – that of *transformational* leadership(19), or leadership through the transformation of others to work towards the goal of some future desired state.

A fusion of the transformational notion of social influence and leadership trait theory led, in the 1980s and 1990s, to the emergence of *charismatic* leadership as a solution to organisational problems. Effective leaders were viewed as dominant personalities brimming with self-confidence and offering a clearly articulated ideology. They offered a strong role model and had high expectations of followers. However, it quickly became apparent that this culture of organisational 'heroes' was both unhealthy and unsustainable, and more recently there has been a shift towards thinking that emphasises the thoughtful, value-led leader, highlighting the needs of followers and bringing to the fore ideas of *distributed*, *collaborative* and *learning-oriented* leadership.(20–22)

However, as many authors, including Bryman(23) and Storey(12), have noted, these stages signal a change in emphasis – not a shift away – from previous models, and like the abominable snowman, a definitive model of leadership remains a tricky thing to track down.

Educational Management and Leadership

Writers and researchers who have focused on educational leadership and management, as opposed to general theories of leadership, tend to locate phenomena associated with educational leadership within various paradigms,(24) perspectives,(25) models(1) or metaphors.(26) All these terms tend to be applied in similar ways rather than reflect significant differences in meaning, and we will use them interchangeably here.

A significant chunk of current UK education policy emphasises the centrality of educational leadership and management. There is no shortage of leadership advice from government, consultants, academics and education authorities to leaders in schools, colleges and universities, but as Bush notes, 'many of these prescriptions are atheoretical in the sense that they are not underpinned by explicit values or concepts'.(27) Although leadership and management are practical activities, theories can help inform and influence practice by suggesting new ways and frameworks in which events, inter-relationships and situations can be seen. Pragmatic decisions might appear to be common sense, but 'common sense' is grounded in assumptions, limitations, a view about an organisation and a particular frame of reference. 'Theory-for-practice'(28) encourages us to look at organisations and relationships in a different light, helping us interpret and make sense of complexity and ambiguity and make relevant and informed management and leadership decisions.

Most of the theory and research on educational management and leadership relates to the context of schools and colleges, and very little has been done to consider leadership in the context of the education of health professionals. However, the broader research is useful in helping us look at the organisations and relationships involved in delivering medical education.

Bush and Glover(29) describe a typology of management models, building on previous work by Leithwood *et al.*(30) This framework, with its parallel grouping of leadership theories, is shown in Box 29.2. As discussed above, we believe that effective leadership is inextricably intertwined with strategic management, and for the remainder of this section shall consider general leadership theories alongside their analogous management paradigms. On the way, we will also consider the applicability of each model to the leadership and management of clinical education.

Formal management: managerial leadership

Formal management models view educational organisations as hierarchical, bounded bureaucratic systems with an official structure – represented by an organi-

---

BOX 29.2 Typology of management and leadership models

Management model	Leadership model
Formal	Managerial
Collegial	Participative
	Transformational
	Interpersonal
	Distributed
Political	Transactional
Subjective	Post-modern
Ambiguity	Contingency
Cultural	Moral

From Bush and Glover.(29)

---

sational chart – and relationships characterised by virtue of the legitimate authority vested in them. Managerial decisions are seen as objective, rational and goal oriented. Leaders have positional power over those beneath them but are accountable to internal and external bodies, such as the senate, councils or boards.

Theories drawn from structural or system sociology underpin these managerial models, most notably the concept of *bureaucracy*. Weber(31) describes a bureaucratic organisation as existing to achieve established purposes, with work best achieved through specialisation, division of labour, coordination and control, a description that sits well with contemporary education organisations.

In *managerial leadership*, leaders are responsible for:

- setting goals and ensuring the organisation reaches the goals
- maintaining the integrity of the educational structure and working within it using power and authority to the organisation's advantage
- 'bounding' the system in alignment with how the organisation sees the relationship with the external environment.

In these models, leaders are often seen, and revered, as holding much of the organisation's power and are expected to make decisions based on their own knowledge and expertise. In practice, most organisations invest power and authority across a senior management team rather than in a single leader, thus ensuring that the hierarchy stays in place and that the formal systems, structures and procedures are maintained. These 'Apollonian'(32) structures can provide a platform for the 'hero' leader; indeed, in education, such a figure may actively be sought out. Universities, for instance, often invest a huge amount of time, energy and resources in seeking out the best new vice-chancellor. Storey notes that in a managerial organisation, 'the need for leadership is often addressed in terms of the "reputational capital" that a celebrated leader can bring … this is very interesting and revealing because it highlights the importance of stakeholder perception'.(12)

In reality, modern educational organisations are complex and 'messy'; professional staff expect to be consulted and involved in decision making; goals are difficult to state and measure, as many of them are long term; and individuals do not necessarily behave in a prescribed way. In medical and healthcare education, there are additional areas of conflict because many individuals have authority and power in one arena – for instance, in their role as a consultant clinician – but may have little organisational power or authority in an academic setting. This, coupled with traditional power discrepancies between the professions in terms of authority, accountability, status and reward, means that there are additional tensions in healthcare education organisations that do not exist in schools, colleges or other university departments.

Therefore, whereas it is recognised that bureaucracy may be an appropriate organisational model for educational management,(33) there are inherent weaknesses – predominantly a tendency for the organisation to become preoccupied with the maintenance of its own structure and processes, thus forgetting its original educational purposes or relegating them to a position of subordinance.(34) Another general criticism is that bureaucracies are deprofessionalising, stripping away the autonomy of practitioners,(35) an issue explored in more detail by Mintzberg.(36)

Minztberg dissects organisations into five generic components and in doing so identifies a simple organisational taxonomy, namely, organisations as:

- a machine bureaucracy
- a professional organisation
- an entrepreneurial start-up
- an ad hocracy.

A *machine bureaucracy* can be conceptualised as a factory or production line, pumping out a standardised product under instructions from management. In the *entrepreneurial start-up*, the owner-manager takes the strategic decisions while remaining hands-on in the day-to-day business of the organisation. The *ad hocracy* is an ambiguous and organic form in which structural elements combine, disassociate and recombine to address complex problems. Healthcare education tends to be structured in *professional bureaucracies*, and this has profound implications for management and leadership.

In a professional organisation, Mintzberg(36) suggests that a small *strategic apex*, assisted by a supportive *technostructure* and *staff*, manages through a small *middle line* a large *operating core* of professionals. For the coordination of its work, a professional bureaucracy relies on the standardisation of skills through training and indoctrination, and although the operating professionals have considerable control, the standards to which they perform are set outside the structure of the organisation, usually by a self-governing association of fellow professional organisations. The pro-

fessional tends to resist rationalisation of their skills as this drives the structure towards that of a machine bureaucracy, thus destroying professional autonomy. Organisational strategy in the professional organisation is represented by the cumulative effect over time of multiple projects or initiatives undertaken by its members. As a consequence of these characteristics, the professional organisation tends to be rather inflexible, good at producing a standard unchanging product but ill suited to adaptation. Response to change is slow – evolution as opposed to revolution – and 'top-down' calls for reform are usually resisted.

In a professional organisation operating in a *collegial* management model, leaders and managers are seen to sit 'alongside' colleagues rather than manage from 'above'.(35) Collegiality assumes a common set of values, an authority of expertise and decisions reached through a process of discussion leading to consensus.(37) Collegiality has been shown in mainstream education to improve the quality of decision making, to bring about more effective implementation and, perhaps most importantly, to be the type of management teachers want.(37)

Unfortunately, as will be apparent, collegial management in the public sector is in conflict with the prevailing bureaucratic culture, a conflict heightened by governmental pressures for increased output and greater public accountability.

Collegial management: participative, transformational, interpersonal and distributed leadership

The collegial management model is normative; it is believed that members of the organisation share beliefs, values and norms and that decision making is made democratically. However, this belief is often illusory rather than grounded in reality, and leaders need to spend time ensuring that consultation and participation in decision making is real. They need to seek out and clearly define the beliefs and values that individuals and groups from different professional backgrounds share. Collegial decisions are founded on expert authority.

The collegial model is highly appropriate for small professional organisations. Larger units, such as universities, also retain many elements of collegiality in that they have extensive committee structures to facilitate representation and participation, and academic autonomy and freedom are valued at the 'bottom-up' approach. However, there has always been a separation between academic and non-academic staff and the right to participation in decision making that these roles enjoy. More recently, universities have been described as moving towards a more 'top-down', managerial model, partly in response to increased competition in a global marketplace. This shift also enables clear organisational goals that 'fit' all disciplines and professional groups within the educational organisation to be agreed. It has also led Hargreaves to describe the emergence of a phenomenon widespread in the pubic sector, that of 'contrived collegiality'(38) consultation without the possibility of control.

The management model of collegiality sits with participative, transformational, interpersonal and distributed leadership models, all of which rest on the notion of the leader as 'first among equals',(39) utilising the skills of influencing, negotiation, listening, facilitation and consensus building rather than acting in the role of a hero leader. Such leaders are aware of the complexity and interactivity of decision-making processes and are able to recognise and harness the expertise of the professionals whom they lead, as well as demonstrate sensitivity towards the 'informal codes of professional practice which govern expectations' between the leader and his or her staff.(40)

A number of what have come to be known as 'new paradigm' models of leadership(23) emerged in the 1980s. Transformational, charismatic and visionary leaders define organisational reality through the articulation of a clear vision and its supporting values. Thus new paradigm models depict leaders as managers of meaning rather than in terms of the way they influence processes. In the public sector, and notably in the NHS, transformational leadership has been seen as the key to addressing some of the limitations of a transactional approach, and the NHS leadership framework contains an interesting amalgam of the two paradigms where 'empowering others' can be found nestling alongside 'holding to account'.

> Leadership has experienced a major re-interpretation from representing an authority relationship (now referred to as management or transactional leadership which may or may not involve some form of pushing or coercion) to a process of influencing followers or staff for whom one is responsible, by inspiring them, or pulling them to a vision of some future state ... this new form of leadership is called transformational leadership because such individuals transform followers.(41)

Transformational leadership is characterised by the '4 Is' of Bass and Aviolo:(19)
- idealised influence
- inspirational motivation
- individualised consideration
- intellectual stimulation.

Transformational leadership and its near relative, *interpersonal leadership*,(1) are rooted in the philosophical belief that meaning is socially constructed. Grint describes the 'constitutive approach' as one in which leaders not only mould followers' interpretation of the environment but also present it as being the correct interpretation.(42) Here lies one of the critiques of transformational leadership, in that leaders may be tempted to manipulate meaning to suit their own ends. Writers such as Maccoby(43) highlight that there is a dark side to such charismatic leadership, that of a narcissistic leader, who can challenge change and disrupt the status quo but also can be arrogant and grandiose, thriving on risk and seeking power, glory and admiration. A wave of corporate scandals in the 1990s served to highlight the dangers of a narcissistic leader. Further on in this chapter, we shall see how the concept of 'value-led' leadership helps to compensate for some of the possibly negative aspects of the transformational approach.

Another post-charismatic model of leadership is described by Fullan,(44) a model based around embedded learning, devolved leadership in teams, and learning as a product of confrontation, mistakes and experimentation. Practice is made public in a collaborative culture. *Distributed leadership* or 'leadership at all levels' is currently receiving considerable attention in education and the NHS. The National College for School Leadership (NCSL) website,(45) for instance, notes:

> The NCSL is committed to helping schools to share leadership in a way that improves pupil outcomes. Distributed leadership is not a new idea. It has been around for a long time, either as delegated or as shared leadership. It is essentially about sharing out leadership across the organisation. ... schools need many leaders at all levels.

The case for distributed leadership is made on the basis of the following:
- a belief in leadership teams: a team being a more effective unit than an individual
- the fact that as schools become more complex places to manage and lead, there is a need for leadership at all levels, with 'coherence making'(22) as everyone's responsibility
- the development of pools of talent, from which tomorrow's leaders may be drawn.

All of these models value human capital, and for leaders and managers this has a clear message. An effective organisation will align the motivational goals of the individual employee with its own needs. The consequences of poor role/person fit are profound, and Argyris(46) found that over time, frustration intensified, leading to absenteeism, psychological withdrawal, restriction of output, feather bedding, sabotage and formation of power groups to redress the balance. The alternative strategy was to climb the hierarchy to, what was perceived to be a better job and perpetuate the whole sorry process.

To summarise a wealth of literature on the human side of organisations, successfully led organisations *empower* employees and *invest* in people (*see* Box 29.3).

Political management: transactional leadership

Power flows in educational organisations through three main conduits:
- bureaucratic processes (boards, committees, management hierarchies)
- collegiality (consensual decision making informed by expert knowledge)

BOX 29.3 Leading through people

Empower employees	Invest in people
redesign work	hire the right people
provide autonomy	reward them well
encourage participation	promote from within
focus on job enrichment	train and educate
emphasise teamwork	share the wealth
ensure upward influence	

- micro-politics(47) (negotiation, bargaining, conflict, subterfuge).

The potential sources of power in organisations have been analysed by a number of theorists.(48,49) Hoyle(28), for instance, has distinguished four main types:

- *structural* – power as the property of office
- *personality* – charisma and 'the aura of authority'
- *expertise* – which includes access to information as well as specialised knowledge
- *opportunity* – power through the occupancy of key administrative roles.

Sometimes, considerable power resides in the lowliest of roles, such as the hospital laundry lady or switchboard operator.

Politics then is ultimately about the deployment of such resources through the wielding and yielding of power, and the day-to-day interactions of people and their ideologies. Baldridge's work on universities in the US(39) highlights the role that interest and pressure groups have on influencing decision making and forcing change. His model of how policies emerge is iterative and dynamic: competition for scarce resources leading to formal and informal grouping jostling and positioning themselves for control, with power accruing to dominant coalitions. Personal and professional interests feed into the melee, the former in relation to status, working conditions and reward, and the latter to gain commitment to particular ways of working, curricular models, teaching and learning methods or student groupings.(28)

Hoyle describes how educational leaders can adopt political strategies to achieve their aims.(28) These include *dividing and ruling*, *co-optation*, *displacement*, *controlling information*, and *controlling meetings*, the last of these strategies achieved through the dubious strategies of rigging agendas, losing recommendations, nobbling members of the group, invoking outside bodies or massaging minutes (*see* Box 29.4).

The exercise of power is also a major preoccupation of *transactional leadership*, a leadership model based on four assumptions:

- people are motivated by reward and punishment
- social systems work best with a clear chain of command

BOX 29.4 Focus on: Power and authority

The relationship between power and authority is not straightforward. It is perfectly possible to have one without the other. Power, as has been described, is about the control and manipulation of scarce resources whether they be physical, economic, knowledge-based or to do with personal qualities.(5) Authority relates to the right, or perceived right, to exercise power.

According to the economist and sociologist Max Weber, all leaders are surrounded in a myth of superiority that derives from three forms of legitimate authority: charismatic, traditional and rational–legal domination.(50)

Charismatic domination derives from the personal qualities of the leader. Many religious leaders, and some political ones, derive their authority from this form of domination.

Traditional domination relates to positions that preserve long-established values and social relationships. In the UK, the Royal Family carry authority, not because of charisma but because an otherwise meritocrious society allows them to continue to adopt that social position derived purely from inheritance.

Rational or legal domination is the most advanced, and relates to authority as a function of delegated power within a bureaucraticy. Those in authority give orders (and expect to be obeyed) because their office gives them the right to give orders. However, there is a context-specific element to this, and orders are only to be obeyed if they are relevant to the situation in which they are given. The head of your department or school has rational–legal authority, and who knows, may also have charisma …

Power in educational institutions may go hand in hand with authority, such as those budgetary decisions made by the dean, head, principal or executive board. However, power in organisations is often wielded without authority through a process of 'influence' and micro-politics.

- authority resides within line management
- subordinates are there to do what their manager tells them.

Leadership of the transactional variety starts then to look very much like management, a similarity emphasised by Kotter,(51) who asserts that transformational leadership is about strategy and people, whereas transactional leadership revolves around systems and resources. Kotter *et al.*(52), though, are also clear that both leadership paradigms are needed in an effective organisation.

Leadership is different from management, but not for the reason people think. Leadership isn't mystical and mysterious. It has nothing to do with having charisma or other exotic personality traits. It's not the province of the chosen few. Nor is leadership necessarily better than management or a replacement for it: rather leadership and management are two distinctive and complementary activities. Both are necessary for success in an increasingly complex and volatile business environment.(8)

Subjective management: post-modern leadership

Bush(1) describes subjective management models as those which 'assume that organisations are the creations of people within them. Participants are thought to interpret situations in different ways, and these individuals' perceptions are derived from their background and values. Organisations have different meanings for each of their members and exist only in the experience of those members. Different writers vary in the emphasis they put on individuals rather than the organisation; some see the tension between the individual perspective and organisational collective as a 'chasm', whereas others see it more like a dialectic, with interdependence between individual and collective meanings.

Post-modern leadership is a relatively undefined concept; it has similarities to the interpersonal model in that it sees different actors as bringing multiple meanings and realities to any organisation or situation. 'Situations must be understood at local level with particular attention to diversity';(53) this emphasises the fluid and 'chaotic' nature of contemporary society in which power is *enacted* (ibid) through all members, thus leading to empowerment. Leaders need to rely on their skills as interpreters of meaning articulated in different ways by multiple stakeholders. The hero visionary does not fit in the post-modern world; leaders need to listen to, and focus on, people as individuals with their own world views.

Ambiguity management: situational leadership

Ambiguity models emphasise organisational change, uncertainty and unpredictability. Organisational goals and systems and processes are seen as unclear and not well understood, and participation in decision making is fluid as individuals opt in and out. Organisations are characterised by fragmentation and 'loose coupling',(54) particularly educational organisations in which members have a high degree of autonomy and discretion. The most famous of the models is the 'garbage can' model described by Cohen and March(55) in their research into colleges and universities, identifying that decisions are the result of fluid processes in which problems, solutions, participants and choice opportunities all interact to generate outcomes or decisions.

Gilbert(56) defines *situational* or *contingent leadership* as 'an approach based on the commonsensical idea that there will be interactions in most situations between the leader's attitude and attitudes, the tasks to be undertaken, the strengths and weaknesses of the team and the environment in which the leader and team have to operate'. The contingency leadership model sees leaders as having to adapt their stance and style to the particular situation rather than seeing one leadership approach as being the 'right' one. Peck *et al.*(57) note, for example, that 'transformational characteristics may be more appropriate in the earlier stages of a transition process, with the transactional characteristics required to stabilise transformational change'. It is not that one is superior or inferior to the other but rather that effective leaders appear to be able to utilise many styles and select those appropriate to the specific situation.

What are those styles? The Hay-McBer study of 3871 'randomly' selected executives identified six drivers of organisational climate or working atmosphere(13) (*see* Box 29.5). Effective leaders used all styles flexibly dependent on the situation, with the *authoritative* leadership style found to have the most positive effect of the six.

In the complex world of medical and healthcare education, effective leaders will be those who can respond to different situations in a measured way, selecting the appropriate leadership style to suit the situation. This point is particularly relevant for those who are coming from one leadership role (e.g. in clinical practice) into another (e.g. academia), as Gilbert(56) highlights: 'Success in one environment does not necessarily translate to another'.

Cultural models of management are very influential in mainstream education, and they emphasise the importance of informal modes of influence and of the centrality of values, beliefs and ideologies. Individuals are seen as actors who bring their ideas and values to their relationships with others. In turn, this influences the way in which an organisation develops norms and traditions – 'the way we do things around here'(58) – which are reinforced by symbols, ceremonies and rituals. Symbols are central to the construction of meaning, and in medical and healthcare education these abound as part of the undergraduate (pre-registration) socialisation process and continue throughout professional life. The importance of understanding the meaning ascribed to linguistic, behavioural and visual or physical symbols cannot be underestimated by leaders, particularly those who want to work interprofessionally or across organisations.

A strong organisational culture enables people to identify themselves and their aspirations with the purpose of the organisation and can heighten faith and confidence in an organisation in the midst of environmental turbulence and adversity. Organisational culture can be influenced in a myriad of small ways

BOX 29.5 Leadership that gets results(13): The leadership styles

	Coercive	Authoritative	Affiliatative	Democratic	Pace setting	Coaching
What the leader does?	Demands immediate compliance	Mobilises people towards a vision	Creates harmony and builds bonds	Forges consensus through participation	Sets high standards for performance	Develops people for the future
When it works best?	In a crisis	When a clear direction is needed	To heal rifts and motivate people in stressful circumstances	To get buy-in from valuable employees	To obtain quick results from a well-motivated team	To help an employee improve their performance
Overall effect on climate	–	++	+	+	–	+

through rituals, ceremonies, story telling, leading by example and even the books and magazines on display in the department. The academic trappings (gowns, maces, medals, crests, etc.) adopted by a number of Royal Colleges, some of them just a few decades old, are good examples of how cultural expression serves to define, or brand, an organisation. Small changes make big differences, and it is the leader's responsibility to pay attention to the detail as well as the big picture. Quite often, the solution to an underperforming organisation is not to undertake a massive restructuring exercise but to change the organisational culture, and cultural change again requires leadership at all levels.

Leaders also need to be aware of how changing demographics and widening participation impact on organisational and professional cultures; issues concerning gender, race, ethnicity and class can lead to a need to reframe cultural norms and values. Leaders may well have to deal with uncomfortable moments as once-dominant ideologies and positions are challenged and come under scrutiny. Leaders with a strong ethical and value-led approach, which acknowledges cultural shifts and responds appropriately, will be more effective than those who operate merely on exchange transactions.

Moral leadership is based on the notion of integrity, and although it is similar to transformational leadership in that it emphasises the commitment of followers, it emphasises values as well as vision. Leaders need to ensure that their central values accord with those in the educational organisation, or there will be dissonance and discomfort for all those involved. In times of financial hardship and competing agendas, maintaining integrity and an ethical stance can sometimes be very difficult, particularly so if we do not fully know ourselves.

Such self-knowledge features large in the writings of Goleman on emotional intelligence(7). Goleman(59) argues that in order to be successful in dealing with others, it is important to have effective awareness, control and management of your own emotions and a

deep understanding of your own goals, responses and behaviour patterns. This message is clearly incorporated into the *NHS Leadership Qualities Framework*, where 'personal qualities' lie at the framework's centre.

Personal values and concern for others are also at the heart of Greenleaf's(60) *servant leadership*, where, as Collins puts it, 'professional will is seen alongside personal self-effacement'.(61) The difference between the servant leader and other forms of leadership is that the servant leader 'is servant first ... It begins with the natural feeling that one wants to serve, to serve first. Then conscious choice brings one to aspire to lead'.(60) The primacy of serving a higher purpose has made Greenleaf's approach popular in the church and not-for-profit sectors.

Other leadership models: instructional and collaborative

Finally, we look at two other models that do not fit neatly into the framework above: instructional and collaborative leadership.

Bush(1) describes *instructional leadership* as 'focussing on the direction rather than the process of leadership ... with a firm emphasis on the purpose of education and the need to focus on teaching and learning as the prime purpose of educational institutions'. Although this model emerged out of school leadership, in professional education increasingly there is a renewed focus on teaching and learning, the behaviour of teachers and teachers' professional development. Examples of instructional leadership can be seen in the establishment of bodies such as the higher education academy and in the appointment of senior managers in the NHS and in universities with named responsibilities for 'teaching and learning' or education and the recent establishment of a national Faculty of Medical Educators(62) in the UK.

Collaborative leadership, which focuses on a commitment to partnership working for the good of the service users, draws on many of the approaches outlined above. However, it also demands a specific set of qualities and behaviours, such as being able to

- assess the environment
- demonstrate clarity of values
- see commonalities and common interests and make connections
- share vision and build and mobilise people and resources
- build, promote and sustain trust
- share power and influence
- develop people and reflect on oneself.

Collaborative leadership shares the burden but also the power and resources. This requires that 'collaborative leaders are personally mature. They have a solid enough sense of self that they do not fear loss of control'.(63)

Above all, collaborative leaders must listen, and be seen to do so. As van Zwanenberg(64) notes: 'the person in a position of leadership who is not open to actively listening, questioning and reflecting in a very conscious way will be judged as a hypocrite if they continue to talk the language of partnership …

Leading Teams

Recent thinking then has shifted the leadership focus back from whole organisations to distributed leadership involving small groups and teams.(45,65) *Team building* has long been a part of organisational and professional development activities. Manz and Sims suggest that a new management style will be needed for team-based organisations – *super-leadership* – with the locus of control shifting from the leader to the team.(66)

Teachers use team-leading and team-building concepts all the time when they are managing groups of students and trainees, and the majority of teacher training programmes include small-group teaching, looking at the role of the teacher as facilitator in helping a group achieve its outcomes in terms of both task and process. In educational leadership, aspiring or existing leaders can draw on their educational expertise and use their skills in a transferable way with the teams they are leading.

Recent research by the UK government's Performance and Innovation Unit(67) suggests that the climate within a given team can account for up to 30% of its performance and that the leader of the team has a primary role in creating the appropriate climate. The climate of a team is difficult to break down into its component parts but includes elements such as levels of personal autonomy, adequate reward and recognition, and clarity of roles and boundaries. An effective leader then will need an understanding of the nature of teams and the necessary conditions for them to function well. Adair(18) proposes that a team leader should strive to maintain a balance between three key

areas of need in order to achieve team and organisational objectives in a sustainable way. It would be difficult to imagine any situation where a perfect balance between the three needs is always achieved, but the task of the leader is to attempt to maintain balance and also to manage the situation when one of the three (usually task) takes precedence over the others.

Team leaders need to have certain behaviours that facilitate teamworking. Kozlowski *et al.*(68) identify the following helpful behaviours:

- developing shared knowledge among team members
- acting as a mentor
- instructing others
- facilitating group processes
- providing information
- monitoring performance
- promoting open communication
- providing goals
- allocating resources efficiently.

Other skills include the ability to lead participative meetings, listening skills, the ability to handle conflict, group-centred decision-making skills, team-building skills, and coaching and developing skills.

Teams are dynamic units that are constantly evolving, and this evolution involves a number of identifiable stages famously identified by Tuckman.(69) The stage at which a team finds itself – forming, storming, norming or performing – is directly related to the quality and quantity of its output. A team leader needs to know which stage his or her team is at and support the team through its various transitions.

For a team to achieve its potential, it is also essential that the operational roles of its members are matched as closely as possible to their individual working and social style. People function within teams in different ways, but these can be identified and roles can be allocated accordingly to ensure that the team reaches its full potential. Belbin famously classifies individual behaviours in teams into nine distinct 'roles' – observable tendencies of individuals to relate with their colleagues and contribute to the team (*see* Box 29.6).

A number of tools are available to help analyse the membership of the team. However, the ability of the leader to identify preferred roles using a degree of intuition should not be underestimated. It must also be borne in mind that team roles are tendencies, not fixed patterns, and most team members will have at least one secondary tendency. Not every team will have all roles at its disposal, but Belbin's research found that teams that did, tended to perform more effectively. If there are elements missing, it falls on the leader to find ways to address the shortfall.

Perhaps the most important caveats that should accompany such an approach, particularly in the context of higher education, are that no single team role is more important than another and that the

BOX 29.6 Belbin team roles(70)

Plant: an 'ideas person'. Thoughtful, creative, brilliant, radical. Better at thinking than communicating. Not interested in details.

Coordinator: the 'chairperson'. A good team captain. Involves all team members and plays a mediator role in discussions. Coordinates work rather than does it.

Monitor evaluator: the 'critic'. Evaluates everything carefully, seeing both sides of every argument. Cold and objective. Can be perceived as negative and/or unenthusiastic.

Implementer: a 'doer'. A reliable worker who puts ideas into action and gets on with it. May not be very imaginative or flexible.

Completer finisher: the conscientious details person. Pays attention to detail and completes the job. Can be a worrier.

Resource investigator: the 'networker'. The group's ambassador and detective, making friends and tracking down information and resources. Initial enthusiasm can fade before the project is completed.

Shaper: the 'driver'. Pushes through ideas and keeps projects moving, enjoying the cut and thrust of the action. Can upset others as they do this.

Teamworker: the 'peacemaker'. Lubricates the team with diplomacy and helps keep the team working effectively. Everybody's friend. Can be indecisive.

Specialist: the 'expert'. Provides technical or other specialist knowledge to the team. Input is usually restricted to their own specialism.

potential weaknesses of each role should be seen as allowable. Successful teams thrive on their diversity and allow members to play on their strengths. Attempting to change behaviours may be counterproductive and stifle individuality. The task of the leader is to exploit the strengths, allow for the weaknesses and exploit the natural motivation that an understanding of the needs and capacities of everyone in the team engenders.

Leading Change

Like leadership, change is an elusive concept, and literature on change and change management is vast.(71–73) As a working definition, change can be considered as the transformation of an individual or a system from one state to another, a process that may be initiated by internal factors or external forces or both. An understanding of the nature of change and change management is essential for any educational leader, none more so than those who work in the health sector, and in considering recent developments in healthcare education, we wish to emphasise a shift in the concep-

tualisation of change and change management that has occurred in recent years.

Mintzberg(74) summarises this shift in thinking in arguing that change can be thought of as either a pre-planned and predictable event or alternatively as an open-ended, ongoing and unpredictable process aimed at aligning and realigning in response to a changing environment. Early attempts at delineating change, such as that of Lewin,(75) focused on defining phases or stages of the process that might be managed before moving on to the next. Lewin's model describes unfreezing the present situation, moving to a new situation and refreezing. Bullock and Batten(76) similarly define a four-stage model of exploration–planning–action–integration. Implicit in both, and indeed in many other models, is the constancy of both the existing and the new state and the assumption that, given the appropriate skills and resources, the movement to the new state can be brought about in a controlled manner. Yet more models of change emphasise the problem-solving approach of problem identification, solution generation, choice of solution, implementation and evaluation,(77,78) again stressing a rational, linear progression through the change process.

More recently, there has been twofold acceptance that a rational approach to change will only get you so far and that it is change, not stability, that is the steady state.

House(25) notably outlines a trilogy of perspectives on educational change: *technological, cultural* and *political*. Not only does this provide a useful model for the analysis of change events but it acknowledges the importance of issues other than the innovation itself, particularly how innovations are interpreted and integrated into their destination social fabric (the cultural perspective) and how power, authority and competing interests are played against each other (the political perspective). That is not to say that a techno-rational approach to change is wrong, but as we have discussed, having multiple perspectives or frames through which to examine problems enables a richer repertoire of management strategies to be deployed.

The second emerging theme is the acceptance that change is here to stay. Furthermore, as Fullan points out, 'it is a mug's game to hope for the speed of change to slow down'.(79) Change and reform in education, and indeed the health service, have become a way of life. In recent years, seemingly disconnected and often conflicting policies have rained down on health and education professionals with increasing rapidity as politicians attempt to make their mark in a rapidly revolving political cycle. However, this is not a new phenomenon, and Baker has concluded after a lifetime of study of educational reform that: 'Planned change for (educators) is not the cumulative development of a comprehensive strategy. Rather, it is "one dammed thing after another" '.(80)

Multiple perspectives on change and the 'acceleration of just about everything'(81) are then acknowledged features of our social era, a period that has been labelled variously as postmodernity,(82) late capitalism(83), and the informational society.(84) These key features have led naturally to an interest in complex systems by social scientists. Indeed, Hargreaves(85) adds a fourth 'post-modern' perspective to House's original typology acknowledging *complexity* – alongside two other characteristic elements of late capitalism, consumerism and diversity – as a key feature of 21st-century educational change. New paradigms of change management are developing, borne out of the language of chaos and complexity theory, a relatively new area of scientific enquiry, a little more than 15 years old, which offers insights into the behaviour of large-scale physical, biological and social systems. Complexity theory arises from the observation that order will often spontaneously emerge out of what appears to be chaos. Complexity deals with the nature of emergence, innovation, learning and adaptation.(86)

Human systems have a tendency to avoid the onset of chaos if at all possible. Sometimes, this occurs to such a great extent in organisations that stability and equilibrium set in, leading to stereotypical patterns of behaviour and poor change responsiveness. However, the environment is sufficiently chaotic and elements within in it sufficiently inter-related not to allow the state to persist for long, and an oscillation sets in between the twin pulls of the urge to maintain integrity (autopoeisis) and the impulse to explore and adapt to the changing environment.

In social systems, stasis occurs where there is a high level of agreement and an equally high level of certainty. Chaos ensues when there is neither agreement nor certainty. Between these two extremes lies an area of variable agreement and variable certainty, and this is the zone of complexity where anything is possible, the 'swampy lowlands'(87) wherein lie the really important problems worth grappling with.

Businesses,(88) schools (38) and healthcare organisations(89) have all been viewed as 'complex adaptive systems'. In complex situations, as described, 'order is not totally predetermined and fixed, but the universe (however defined) is creative, emergent (through iteration, learning and recursion), evolutionary and changing, transformative and turbulent'.(71) Despite this constant disequilibrium, the complex adaptive system strives to create order out of chaos, constantly reorganising in response to the changing environment. Complex adaptive systems display 'perpetual novelty'(90) and a propensity for problem solving. Fraser and Greenhalgh(91) summarise a number of complexity concepts applicable to education and training.

- Neither the system nor its external environment is, or ever will be, constant.
- Individuals within a system are independent and creative decision makers.
- Uncertainty and paradox are inherent within the system.
- Problems that cannot be solved can nevertheless be 'moved forward'.
- Effective solutions can emerge from minimum specification.
- Small changes can have big effects.
- Behaviour exhibits patterns (that can be termed 'attractors').
- Change is more easily adopted when it taps into attractor patterns.

What does complexity mean for educational leadership? Mintzberg *et al.*(92) suggest a non-directive approach to change management:

> The best way to manage change is to allow for it to happen, to be pulled by the concerns out there rather than being pushed by the concepts in here.

Pascale *et al.*(93) similarly advocate perturbing the system and standing back to observe the results. Fullan(22) too countenances 'never a check list – always complexity' but does set out a series of observations on complex change (*see* Box 29.7), which provide useful guidance for the instigators of educational reform. Importantly though, in addition to recognising the self-determination of complex systems,

---

BOX 29.7 Complex change lessons(22)

- Give up the idea that the pace of change will slow down

  Change is always piecemeal, incoherent and fragmented

- Coherence making is a never-ending proposition and is everyone's responsibility

  Policy alignment at the top is only the start

- Changing context is the focus

  Even small changes in the social context will yield big results

- Premature clarity is a dangerous thing

  Sustainability relies on internalisation of change by individuals – which takes time

- The public's thirst for transparency is irreversible (and on balance this is a good thing)

  Develop open, interactive and quality information systems

- You can't get large-scale reform through bottom-up strategies alone

  System change may require top-down intervention

- Mobilise the social attractors – moral purpose, quality relationships and knowledge

  People will organise themselves around the powerful social attractors

- Charismatic leadership is negatively associated with sustainability

  Develop leadership at all levels

Fullan also emphasises the importance of leadership to the change process.

Both Fraser and Greenhalgh and Fullan acknowledge the confused and complex nature of educational change and that self-organisation of an educational system can occur given minimal direction. Both also acknowledge the importance of *attractors* or traits within systems that set the direction for this self-organisation. Values, principles, goals, theories and leadership can all act as attractors, pulling together ideas, information, people and energy in generating new and emergent patterns.

Strategic Planning

As we identified earlier, one of the key features of leadership, as opposed to management, is the setting of direction through the articulation of a vision and the development of a strategy.

Strategy, though, is a word that has multiple meanings concisely summarised by Mintzberg *et al.*,(92) namely:

- *a plan* – a guide to take one along a path from a current state to some future state
- *a pattern* – a consistent pattern of behaviour
- *a position* – the location of a particular product in a market
- *a perspective* – a way of interacting
- *a ploy* – a tactic designed to outwit a competitor.

Also, one, some or all of these constructions may be employed in the process of strategic planning.

Strategic planning has a number of functions. It sets direction, focuses effort, defines the organisation and provides a consistency of approach and behaviour. However, there are downsides, as a strategic plan, beautifully written and long in gestation, may encourage 'groupthink', blinding the leadership of an organisation to new opportunities. Consistency, too, is not always desirable, as it may serve to overlook the rich diversity within any organisation. A strategic plan needs therefore to be flexible enough to take into account changes in the environment or new ideas and ways of doing things that emerge during the plan's lifetime.

The classic model of strategic planning traces a journey from a vision (often expressed as 'purpose' or a 'mission'), through aims, objectives and action plans, to monitoring arrangements (*see* Figure 29.2). It is a pathway underpinned by the expressed and (one hopes) lived values of the organisation.

To be successful, strategic planning needs to take account of the views of all stakeholders. For a medical school department, these might include the university, students, teachers and tutors, the hospital, the local postgraduate deanery, other medical schools, patient groups, royal colleges and the General Medical Council. Taking people with you is key, and to settle on a stra-

Figure 29.2 Strategic planning.

tegic direction too early in the process is fraught with danger. In Claxton's words, 'slow knowing' is the key.

> One needs to be able to soak up experience of complex domains – such as human relationships – through one's pores, and to extract subtle, contingent patterns that are latent within it. And to do that one needs to be able to attend to a whole range of situations patiently without comprehension; to resist the temptation to foreclose on what that experience may have to teach.(94)

Strategic planning should therefore have at its heart a reiterative process of evaluative analysis, a gauging and regauging of the operating environment of the organisation, canvassing the views of stakeholders, understanding trends and developing an awareness of the shaping forces at work. Through this process, leaders may also act to 'seize the future'(2) as they work outside their own organisation to shape the key uncertainties that lie ahead. A number of approaches may be used to gather information to inform a strategic plan, and some of these are illustrated in Box 29.8.

Having articulated a vision and, through an iterative process, agreed on a number of strategic aims or broad statements of intent, organisational objectives can be defined. To be effective, objectives should be SMART: specific, measurable, achievable, realistic, time bounded. Tactics and action plans can then be developed to meet the stated objectives and plans put in place for monitoring and evaluation.

Throughout the process, the leader needs to ensure that at all levels, the strategic plan is concordant with the organisation's agreed values. Without a strong backbone of values, a strategic plan becomes meaningless, and commitment will be lacking. In order to keep organisational values fresh and meaningful, they themselves should be reviewed and rearticulated on a regular basis.

BOX 29.8 How to: Develop a strategic plan

A number of tools may assist the process of strategic planning.

SWOT analysis

SWOT enables the organisation to identify its specific competencies, and alongside consideration of its values ensures that there is good alignment between the external environment and internal situation. The mnemonic stands for: the organisation's internal **S**trengths; the organisation's **W**eaknesses; the **O**pportunities presented by the external environment; and **T**hreats in the external environment.

Gap analysis

Gap analysis is done to map the gap that exists between implied and specified future requirements and the existing situation. Gap analysis highlights services and/or functions that have been accidentally left out, deliberately eliminated or are yet to be developed or procured. The underlying method is simple and revolves around two simple questions: Where are we now, i.e. where will we be if we don't change anything? Where do we want to be, i.e. what does the environment demand of us?

PEST analysis

PEST provides a means of identifying possible futures facing an organisation and is useful for broadening perspectives on future strategy. The four PEST headings are: **P**olitical, **E**conomic, **S**ocial and **T**echnological.

Porter's 'Five Forces'

Another model developed by Michael Porter of the Harvard Business School is designed to aid an analysis of the organisation's environment and the attractiveness of the industry. The five forces are the:

- risk of new competitors
- threat of substitute products
- bargaining power of buyers
- bargaining power of providers
- degree of competitive rivalry between existing institutions.

Through choosing an appropriate strategy, the organisation can alter the impact of these forces to its advantage, e.g. by collaborating rather than competing with rivals.

Stakeholder analysis

Stakeholder analysis provides a tool to explore how the views of others might affect the implementation of your strategy. All individuals or groups that might have an interest in your plan are listed and defined as 'opposed', 'neutral' or 'supportive'. How far would you have to move an individual or group for the plan to succeed? It may be enough just to shift some stakeholders to neutral, but essential to obtain the active support of others. How might the plan be presented differently to meet the needs of each group (think politically here) and/or what changes might you have to make in order to make it acceptable or desirable.

Scenario planning

Traditional forecasting methods often fail to predict significant changes, particularly when the environment is turbulent and unpredictable. Scenario planning enables us not to predict the future, but to devise a number of possible futures for the organisation concerned. A strategy can then be devised that would best equip the organisation to survive in those possible worlds. Scenario planning is best carried out by a group that includes representation from all walks of the organisation as the idea is to devise scenarios that take into account as many different perspectives as possible.

Leading Improvement and Getting Results

Donald Berwick, one of the great contemporary thinkers on healthcare improvement, defined what he called the 'central law of improvement',(95) namely, that *every system is perfectly designed to achieve the results it achieves.* From this, he developed the idea that real improvement can only occur from changing systems, not changing within systems. Effective leaders of improvement then, rather than exhorting or cajoling people to work harder within a system, challenge the very system itself and provide a vision of a superior alternative.

A simple model for achieving change that results in improvement – and change and improvement are not necessarily the same thing – asks three basic questions:(96)

- What are we trying to achieve?
- How will we know if a change leads to an improvement?
- What changes could we make that we think will result in improvement?

There are several leadership elements to these questions. Clarity about what is to be achieved is an absolute obligation on the leader, to set the aims and mission of the organisation and to communicate these clearly. The more clearly aims are articulated, the greater the chance of them being realised.

The second of the questions relates to the measurement of outcomes, not as a way of instituting punishment or reward (e.g. star ratings and league tables) but as a means to learn. If we introduce this new assessment system, how will we know that it makes a difference? How will we know whether a problem-based learning curriculum will lead to better doctors?

Also, in an educational field full of self-determining professionals, a third key leadership task is to provide an environment that encourages innovation and experimentation. Constant small improvements that involve everyone in the organisation expand the available 'gene pool' of ideas and potential solutions. The 'never-ending proposition' of 'coherence making'(79) then becomes everyone's responsibility.

Change-adept organisations empower their members and build capacity through personal professional development. In a change-responsive organisation, blame is eliminated, innovation is encouraged, and there is an open environment of continuous improvement. In schools, promoting the professional development of colleagues has been found to be central in helping teachers cope with and instigate change.(97) In addition, Lomax(98) suggests that a research perspective is needed, encouraging all staff to think critically about their work. In this way, a professional learning community can be developed.

In developing a climate of continuous learning and improvement, we are in effect building a *learning organisation*. Learning organisations concern themselves with learning at all levels and place a high value on both individual and organisational development. As such, they are said to be quicker to adapt to change.(99)

Improvement as described becomes predominantly a developmental issue and one of getting the organisational culture right. What if things go wrong? As discussed in the section on human resources above, rewarding people well, both materially and through positive feedback, is important in terms of motivation. However, there is a flip side to this. The leader who does not intervene when performance is slipping or praises contributions that are substandard, as well as those that are excellent, cheapens their positive regard and will lose the respect of their followers. Without clear and consistent standards to which followers are held accountable, praise and reward will have no value.

Challenges for Healthcare Education Leaders

Leading in medical and healthcare education, especially at senior level, can lead to particular issues and challenges not encountered by those working in other educational disciplines or contexts. One of the main reasons is that medical education is developed and delivered across professional, subject discipline and organisational boundaries. The organisations involved are bound by their own structures, systems, funding mechanisms, cultures, norms and values, and it is often difficult to straddle the clinical–academic 'divide'.

McKimm(100) carried out interviews with a small number of established leaders in medical and healthcare education in the UK and identified a set of issues and challenges consistently noted by the interviewees.

Personal issues

- Maintaining an appropriate work–life balance is difficult, especially for those with domestic commitments.
- The culture of senior management practice in both clinical and academic life has impact on career progression for those with domestic responsibilities.
- Some women noted the existence of the 'glass ceiling' and impact of taking career breaks.
- Leaders who had trained as clinicians had to make decisions on how to manage both clinical and academic careers and when/if to leave clinical practice.
- Leaving clinical practice is tied in with maintaining credibility as a leader.
- Aspiring leaders with non-traditional career backgrounds feel that they will be overlooked in consideration for senior management positions, especially at medical schools.

Organisational and cultural issues

- There are many organisational barriers to leadership; leaders need to understand the culture and anthropology of their own organisation to succeed.
- Some leaders felt that their profession, discipline or clinical specialty is perceived in a stereotyped or 'less serious' way by others, and this has impeded progress into a leadership role in medical education.
- Clinicians from some specialties may be better able to cope with the dual demands of clinical and academic life than those from other specialties.

Balancing competing agendas

- An overwhelming issue identified is working within a rapidly changing and complex NHS.
- Dual demands of working in higher education (which is highly accountable) and the NHS (which is subject to rapid change) put a strain on healthcare education leaders not found in other sectors of higher education.
- Tensions between management styles, cultures, values and demands of higher education and the NHS – 'crowded stage' with multiple task masters.

The wider agenda

- Healthcare education leaders need to be aware of their influential role in changing and improving healthcare systems.

- There is a need for an accessible forum for discussion of advanced medical education and change by senior medical education leaders.
- Leaders need to be aware of the wider educational and healthcare agendas and help drive issues such as inter-professional learning and collaboration, promoting diversity and innovation in educational management and leadership.

The issues and challenges raised by the leaders in the study highlight that most leaders in medical and healthcare education will at some point have to make decisions about their leadership direction and whether that lies predominantly in higher education, a clinical setting, undergraduate or postgraduate education. There are many opportunities for leading at various levels and in different contexts in medical education. Becoming aware of the opportunities available and matching this to experience and capabilities are a part of the leadership journey, often revisited many times during a career.

Leadership Development

As Storey points out: 'the public sector has ... addressed the leadership development agenda in a particularly high profile and emphatic way'.(12) In parallel with the shifting perspectives on leadership itself from trait and style, through task versus people and transformational and other 'new paradigm' approaches, to the current position that explores what McDermott(101) calls 'leadership from within' (emphasising reflection, emotions, values and openness to experience), traditional approaches to learning leadership from 'experts' have given way to experiential and learner-centred approaches. Learning capability is now seen as a key strategic resource, and leadership is seen as central to the development of 'learning organisations'.(102,103)

In addition to the management and leadership programmes offered by universities and the NHS, different professional groups have taken different approaches to leadership development, and there is a range of leadership development programmes on offer to healthcare educators. Some of these emphasise the value of leadership development in an inter-professional context (learning from and with other professionals), but most are focused either on clinical leadership or strategic management and leadership development in higher education. There are very few programmes that are discipline based or that specifically aim to cross the NHS and higher education divide.

Aspiring or current educational leaders can access a range of programmes to support their ongoing professional development. The most effective of these provide a mixture of strategic management, organisational and leadership theory coupled with practical exercises geared to the context in which the leader is or will be working. Many programmes use tools and exercises designed to deepen self-awareness and reflection and encourage support for individuals in the form of action learning sets, coaching or mentoring. However, effective programmes need also to be longitudinal and oriented around individuals and the organisations in which they work. For this to happen, management and leadership development must be embedded in the culture of every educational organisation.

Summary

Leadership is one of those concepts that seems very easy to define, until you try to do so. This chapter offers an overview of the way in which leadership theory has developed over the past 50 or so years, illuminating some of the most influential concepts and indicating how these might apply to the healthcare education leaders of today and tomorrow. We have not had room to do justice to all the ideas surrounding leadership nor have we explored some of the pressing issues facing leaders of diverse organisations, such as those concerned with gender or race. In some sections, we have focused on developments in the UK and the close relationship between higher education and the NHS, but the theoretical concepts are applicable to a wider international audience.

We hope that this guide to leadership highlights what healthcare education might require of its leaders of the future: what kind of leader and what attributes, skills and qualities those leaders might need to demonstrate. If we are to develop a healthcare workforce capable of delivering high-quality services, then we will need to develop excellence in healthcare education, and this in turn will require educational leaders at all levels who can manage as well as lead and who can work effectively and collaboratively across boundaries.

References

1 Bush T (2003) *Theories of Educational Management and Leadership*. Sage, London.
2 NHS Leadership Centre (2003) *NHS Leadership Qualities Framework*. NHS Leadership Centre, London.
3 Academy of Medical Royal Colleges and NHS Institute for Innovation and Improvement (2008) *Medical Leadership Competency Framework*. AoMRC, London.
4 HEFCE (Higher Education Funding Council for England) Strategic Plan 2006–11 (http://www.hefce.ac.uk/pubs/hefce/2006/06_13/06_13.pdf; accessed 16 September 2006).
5 Bennis W and Nanus N (1985) *Leaders: the strategies for taking charge*. Harper & Row, New York.
6 Fayol H (1949) *General and Industrial Management*. Pitman Publishing, London.
7 Yukl G (2002) *Leadership in Organisations (5e)*. Prentice Hall, Upper Saddle River, NJ.

8 Kotter JP (1990) What leaders really do. *Harvard Business Review.* **May/Jun**: 103–11.

9 Covey S, Merrill AR and Merrill RR (1994) *First Things First.* Simon & Schuster, New York.

10 Northouse P (2004) *Leadership: theory and practice* (3e). Sage, London.

11 Blagg D and Young S (2001) What makes a good leader? *Harvard Business School Bulletin.* **April** (http://hbswk.hbs.edu/item/2141.html).

12 Storey J (ed.) (2004) *Leadership in Organisations: current issues and key trends.* Routledge, London.

13 Goleman D (2000) Leadership that gets results. *Harvard Business Review.* **Mar/Apr**: 78–90.

14 Blake R and Mouton J (1964) *The Managerial Grid.* Gulf, Houston, TX.

15 Tannenbaum R and Schmidt W (1958) How to choose a leadership pattern: should a leader be democratic or autocratic or something in between? *Harvard Business Review.* **36**: 95–101.

16 Fiedler F (1964) A contingency model of leadership effectiveness. In: Berkowitz L (ed.) *Advances in Experimental Social Psychology*, pp. 149–90. Academic Press, New York.

17 Hersey P and Blanchard K (1988) *Management of Organizational Behaviour.* Prentice Hall, Englewood Cliffs, NJ.

18 Adair J (1973) *Action-centred Leadership.* McGraw-Hill, New York.

19 Bass B and Avolio B (1994) *Improving Organizational Effectiveness Through Transformational Leadership.* Sage, Thousand Oaks, CA.

20 Vanderslice V (1988) Separating leadership from leaders: an assessment of the effect of leader and follower roles. *Human Relations.* **41**: 677–96.

21 Alimo-Metcalfe B (2002) *Leadership and Gender: a masculine past; a feminine future.* University of Leeds, Leeds.

22 Fullan M (2001) *Leading in a Culture of Change.* Jossey-Bass, San Francisco, CA.

23 Bryman A (1996) Leadership in organisations. In: Clegg SR, Harvey C and Nord WR (eds) *Handbook of Organisational Studies*, pp. 276–292. Sage, London.

24 Boyd W (1992) The power of paradigms: reconceptualising educational policy and management. *Educational Administration Quarterly.* **28**(4): 504–28.

25 House E (1981) Three perspectives on innovation: technological, political and cultural. In: Lehming R and Kane M (eds) *Improving Schools: using what we know*, pp. 42–114. Sage, Beverley Hills, CA.

26 Morgan G (1998) *Images of Organization: the executive edition.* Berrett-Kochler Publications, San Francisco, CA and Sage, Thousand Oaks, CA.

27 Bush T (1999) Crisis or crossroads? The discipline of educational management in the late 1990s. *Educational Management and Administration.* **27**(3): 239–52.

28 Hoyle E (1986) *The Politics of School Management.* Hodder & Stoughton, London.

29 Bush T and Glover D (2002) *School Leadership: concepts and evidence.* National College for School Leadership, Nottingham.

30 Leithwood K, Jantzi D and Steinbach R (1999) *Changing Leadership for Changing Times.* Open University Press, Buckingham.

31 Weber M (1947) *The Theory of Social and Economic Organization.* Free Press, New York.

32 Handy C (1995) *Gods of Management: the changing work of organizations.* Doubleday, New York.

33 Lungu G (1985) In defense of bureaucratic organization in education. *Education Management and Administration.* **13**: 172–8.

34 Osborne A (1990) The nature of educational management. In: West-Burnham J (ed.) *Education Management for the 1990s*, pp. 9–10. Longman, Harlow.

35 Bush T (1995) *Theories of Educational Management* (2e). Paul Chapman, London.

36 Mintzberg H (1992) *Structure in Fives: designing effective organisations.* Prentice Hall, Harlow.

37 Bush T (2002) Educational management: theory and practice. In: Bush T and Bell L (eds) *The Principles and Practice of Education Management*, pp. 15–31. Paul Chapman, London.

38 Hargreaves A (1994) *Changing Teachers, Changing Times: teachers' work and culture in a postmodern age.* Cassell, London.

39 Baldridge JV, Curtis DV, Ecker G and Riley GL (1978) *Policy Making and Effective Leadership.* Jossey-Bass, San Francisco, CA.

40 Coulson A (1986) *The Managerial Work of Headteachers.* Sheffield City Polytechnic, Sheffield.

41 Alimo-Metcalfe B (1998) *Effective Leadership.* Local Government Management Board, London.

42 Grint K (1995) *Management: a sociological introduction.* Polity Press, Oxford.

43 Maccoby M (2000) Narcissistic leaders: the incredible pros, the inevitable cons. *Harvard Business Review.* **Jan/Feb**: 69–77.

44 Fullan M (2001) *The New Meaning of Educational Change* (3e). Routledge Falmer, London.

45 National College for School Leadership (2003) *Distributed Leadership Review Summary* (http://www.ncsl.org.uk/media/3C4/95/distributed-leadershipliterature-review-summary.pdf; accessed 10 September 2006).

46 Argyris C (1964) *Integrating the Individual and the Organization.* Wiley, New York.

47 Ball S (1987) *The Micropolitics of the School: towards a theory of school organisation.* Methuen, London.

48 Hales C (1997) Power, authority and influence. In: Harris A, Preedy M and Bennett N (eds) *Organizational Effectiveness and Improvement in Education*, pp. 22–30. Open University Press, Buckingham.

49 Handy C (1993) *Understanding Organisations* (4e). Penguin Books, London.

50 Weber M (1998) The types of legitimate domination. In: Roth G and Wittich C (eds) *Economy and Society*, pp. 215–54. University of California Press, Berkeley, CA.

51 Kotter J (1996) *Leading Change.* Harvard Business School Press, Boston, MA.

52 Westley F and Minztberg H (1989) Visionary leadership and strategic management. *Strategic Management Journal.* **10**: 17–37.

53 Keough T and Tobin B (2001) Postmodern leadership and the policy lexicon: from theory, proxy to practice. Paper presented at the Pan-Canadian Education Research Agenda Symposium, Quebec.

54 Weick K (1976) Educational organizations as loosely coupled systems. *Administrative Science Quarterly.* **21**(1): 1–19.

55 Cohen MD and March JG (1976) *Leadership and Ambiguity: the American college president.* Harvard Business School Press, Boston, MA.

56 Gilbert P (2005) *Leadership: being effective and remaining human.* Russell House Publishing, Lyme Regis.

57 Peck E, Dickinson H and Smith J (2006) Transforming or transacting? The role of leaders in organisational transition. *British Journal of Leadership in Public Services.* **2**(3): 4–14.

58 Deal TE (1985) The symbolism of effective schools. *Elementary School Journal.* **85**(5): 601–20.

59 Goleman D (1996) *Emotional Intelligence*. Bloomsbury, London.

60 Greenleaf RK (1977) *Servant Leadership: a journey into the nature of legitimate power and greatness*. Paulist Press, Mahwah, NJ.

61 Collins J (2001) *Good to Great*. Random House, London.

62 FAQ sheet for the proposed academy of medical educators (2006) (http://www.asme.org.uk/academy/academy_faq.htm).

63 Turning Point Leadership Development National Excellence Collaborative (2003) Academics and practitioners on collaborative leadership (http://www.collaborativeleadershiporg/pages/pdfs/LDC_panels_lowres_pdf; accessed 4 September 2006).

64 Van Zwanenberg Z (2003) *Modern Leadership for Modern Services*. Scottish Leadership Foundation, Alloa.

65 Alimo-Metcalfe B and Alban-Metcalfe J (2004) Leadership in public sector organisations. In: Storey J (ed.) *Leadership in Organisations: current issues and key trends*, pp. 173–202. Routledge, London.

66 Manz CC and Sims HP (1991) Super-leadership: beyond the myth of heroic leadership. *Organisational Dynamics*. **19**: 18–35.

67 Performance and Innovation Unit (2000) Strengthening leadership in the public sector (http://www.cabinet-office.gov.uk/innovation; accessed 11 September 2006).

68 Kozlowski SWJ, Gully SM, Salas E and Cannon-Bowers JA (1995) Team leadership and development: theory, principles, and guidelines for training leaders and teams. Third Symposium on Work Teams, University of North Texas, Dallas, TX.

69 Tuckman B (1965) Developmental sequence in small groups. *Psychological Bulletin*. **63**: 384–9.

70 Belbin RM (1991) *Management Teams: why they succeed or fail*. Heinemann, London.

71 Morrison K (1998) *Management Theories for Educational Change*. Paul Chapman, London.

72 Handy C (1989) *The Age of Unreason*. Business Books, London.

73 Iles V and Sutherland K (2001) *Organisational Change: a review for healthcare managers, researchers and professionals*. National Coordinating Centre for NHS Service Delivery and Organisation, London.

74 Mintzberg H (1987) Crafting strategy. *Harvard Business Review*. **Mar/Apr** (2): 66–75.

75 Lewin K (1958) Group decisions and social change. In: Swanson G, Newcomb T and Hartley L (eds) *Readings in Social Psychology*, pp. 459–73. Rinehart & Winston, New York.

76 Bullock R and Batten D (1985) It's just a phase we're going through: a review and synthesis of OD phase analysis. *Group and Organisation Studies*. **10**: 383–412.

77 Buchanan D and Boddy D (1992) *The Expertise of the Change Agent*. Prentice Hall, Hemel Hempstead.

78 Bank J (1992) *The Essence of Total Quality Management*. Prentice Hall, London.

79 Fullan M (2003) *Change Forces with a Vengeance*. Routledge Falmer, London.

80 Baker P, Curtis D and Beneson W (1991) Structures and processes of planned change. *The School Community Journal*. **Fall/Winter**(1): 11–19.

81 Gleick J (1999) *Faster: the acceleration of just about everything*. Pantheon, New York.

82 Harvey D (1989) *The Condition of Postmodernity*. Polity Press, Cambridge, MA.

83 Jameson F (1991) *Postmodernism, Or, The Cultural Logic of Late Capitalism*. Verso, London.

84 Castells M (1996) *The Rise of the Network Society*. Blackwell, Oxford.

85 Hargreaves A, Earl L and Schmidt M (2002) Perspectives on alternative assessment reform. *American Educational Research Journal*. **39**(1): 69–95.

86 Battram A (1998) *Navigating Complexity*. The Industrial Society, London.

87 Schön D (1983) *The Reflective Practitioner: how professionals think in action*. Basic Books, New York.

88 Lewin R and Regine B (2000) *The Soul at Work*. Simon & Schuster, New York.

89 Plesk P and Greenhalgh T (2001) The challenge of complexity in health care. *British Medical Journal*. **323**: 625–8.

90 Waldrop M (1992) *Complexity: the emerging science at the edge of order and chaos*. Penguin, Harmondsworth.

91 Fraser S and Greenhalgh T (2001) Coping with complexity: educating for capability. *British Medical Journal*. **323**: 799–803.

92 Mintzberg H, Ahlstrand B and Lampel J (1998) *Strategy Safari: a guided tour through the wilds of strategic management*. Free Press, New York.

93 Pascale R, Milleman M and Gioja L (2000) *Surfing the Edge of Chaos*. Crown Business Publishing, New York.

94 Claxton G (1997) *Hare Brained and Tortoise Mind*. Fourth Estate, London.

95 Berwick D (1996) A primer on the improvement of systems. *British Medical Journal*. **312**: 619–22.

96 Langley GJ, Nolan KM and Nolan TW (1992) *The Foundation of Improvement*. API Publishing, Silver Spring, MD.

97 Moyles J, Suchuitsky W and Chapman L (1998) *Teaching Fledglings to Fly: report on mentoring in primary schools*. Association of Teachers and Lecturers, London.

98 Lomax P (1990) *Managing Staff Development in Schools: an action research approach*, BERA Dialogues 3. Multilingual Matters, Clevedon.

99 Senge P (1990) *The Fifth Discipline: the art and practice of the learning organization*. Doubleday, New York.

100 McKimm J (2004) *Case Studies in Leadership in Medical and Health Care Education: special report 5*. Higher Education Academy Subject Centre for Medicine, Dentistry and Veterinary Medicine, Newcastle-upon-Tyne.

101 McDermott GR (1994) Partnering with God: Ignatian spirituality and leadership in groups. In: Conger JA (ed.) *Spirituality at Work: discovering the spirituality in leadership*, pp. 132–61. Jossey-Bass, San Francisco, CA.

102 Shewhart WA (1931) *Economic Control of Manufacturing Product*. Van Nostrand, New York.

103 Drath WH and Palus CJ (1994) *Making Common Sense: leadership as meaning making in a community of practice*. Center for Creative Leadership, Greensboro, NC.

Further Reading

Adair J (2002) *Effective Strategic Leadership*. Macmillan, London.

Belbin R (1999) *Management Teams: why they succeed or fail*. Butterworth Heinneman, Oxford.

Bolden R (2004) *What is Leadership?* University of Exeter Leadership South West Research Report (available from http://www.leadershipsouthwest.com; accessed 20 April 2006).

Bush T and Bell L (eds) (2002) *The Principles and Practice of Education Management*. Paul Chapman, London.

Fullan M (2005) *Leadership and Sustainability: systems thinkers in action*. Corwin Press (Sage), Thousand Oaks, CA.

Hoyle E and Wallace M (2005) *Educational Leadership: ambiguity, professionals and managerialism*. Sage, London.

Iles V and Sutherland K (1997) *The Literature on Change Management*. National Co-ordinating Centre for NHS Service Delivery and Organisation, London. Review for healthcare managers, researchers and professionals.

Kotter J (1990) *A Force for Change: how leadership differs from management*. Free Press, New York.

Kydd L, Anderson A and Newton W (eds) (2003) *Leading People and Teams in Education*. Sage, London.

Lewin R (1993) *Complexity: life on the edge of chaos*. Phoenix, London.

McKimm J (2004) *Developing Tomorrow's Leaders in Health and Social Care Education: special report 5*. Higher Education Academy, Newcastle.

Mullins LJ (1999) *Management and Organisational Behaviour* (5e). Financial Times Pitman Publishing, London.

Open University (2005) *Systems Thinking and Practice – a primer*. Open University, Milton Keynes.

Rost JC (1991) *Leadership for the 21st Century*. Praeger, New York.

Sweeney K and Griffiths F (eds) (2002) *Complexity and Healthcare: an introduction*. Radcliffe Publishing, Oxford.

Index